Fitness for Life Canada

PREPARING TEENS FOR HEALTHY, ACTIVE LIFESTYLES

Guy C. Le Masurier
Vancouver Island University

Charles B. Corbin
Arizona State University

Kellie Baker
Memorial University of Newfoundland

John Byl

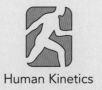

Human Kinetics

Library of Congress Cataloging-in-Publication Data

Names: Le Masurier, Guy C., author. | Corbin, Charles B., author. | Baker,
  Kellie, author. | Byl, John., author.
Title: Fitness for life Canada : preparing teens for healthy, active
  lifestyles / Guy C. Le Masurier, Charles B. Corbin, Kellie Baker, John Byl.
Description: Champaign, IL : Human Kinetics, [2017] | Includes webography and
  index.
Identifiers: LCCN 2016023424 (print) | LCCN 2016039475 (ebook) | ISBN
  9781492511731 (print) | ISBN 9781492546054 (ebook)
Subjects: LCSH: Physical fitness for youth--Study and teaching
  (Secondary)--Canada--Textbooks.
Classification: LCC GV225.A1 L46 2017 (print) | LCC GV225.A1 (ebook) | DDC
  613.7083--dc23
LC record available at https://lccn.loc.gov/2016023424

ISBN: 978-1-4925-1173-1 (print)

The web addresses cited in this text were current as of September 2016, unless otherwise noted.

Acquisitions Editor: Diana Vincer; **Senior Developmental Editor:** Melissa Feld; **Managing Editor:** Derek Campbell; **Copyeditor:** Joyce Sexton; **Indexer:** Nancy Ball; **Permissions Manager:** Dalene Reeder; **Graphic Designers:** Nancy Rasmus and Dawn Sills; **Cover Designer:** Keith Blomberg; **Photographs (cover):** © Human Kinetics, unless otherwise noted; first two photos in top row © Fotolia; fourth photo in bottom row © Getty Images; **Photographs (interior):** © Human Kinetics, unless otherwise noted; **Photo Asset Manager:** Laura Fitch; **Photo Production Manager:** Jason Allen; **Senior Art Manager:** Kelly Hendren; **Illustrations:** © Human Kinetics, unless otherwise noted; **Printer:** Walsworth

The video contents of this product are licensed for educational public performance for viewing by a traditional (live) audience, via closed circuit television, or via computerized local area networks within a single building or geographically unified campus. To request a license to broadcast these contents to a wider audience—for example, throughout a school district or state, or on a television station—please contact your sales representative (**www.HumanKinetics.com/SalesRepresentatives**).

Printed in the United States of America   10   9   8   7   6   5   4   3   2   1

The paper in this book was manufactured using responsible forestry methods.

Human Kinetics
Website: www.HumanKinetics.com

United States: Human Kinetics
P.O. Box 5076
Champaign, IL 61825-5076
800-747-4457
e-mail: info@hkusa.com

Canada: Human Kinetics
475 Devonshire Road Unit 100
Windsor, ON N8Y 2L5
800-465-7301 (in Canada only)
e-mail: info@hkcanada.com

Europe: Human Kinetics
107 Bradford Road
Stanningley
Leeds LS28 6AT, United Kingdom
+44 (0) 113 255 5665
e-mail: hk@hkeurope.com

Australia: Human Kinetics
57A Price Avenue
Lower Mitcham, South Australia 5062
08 8372 0999
e-mail: info@hkaustralia.com

New Zealand: Human Kinetics
P.O. Box 80
Mitcham Shopping Centre, South Australia 5062
0800 222 062
e-mail: info@hknewzealand.com

E6580

Contents

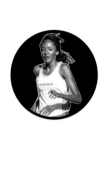
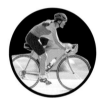
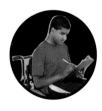

UNIT II   Preparing for Lifelong Activity and Health

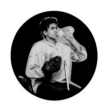

UNIT III   Being Active and Building Fitness

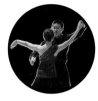

UNIT IV Building Muscle Fitness and Flexibility

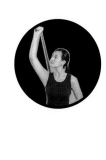
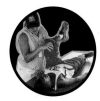

UNIT V Making Healthy Food and Fitness Choices

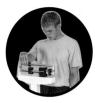

UNIT VI Creating Positive and Healthy Experiences

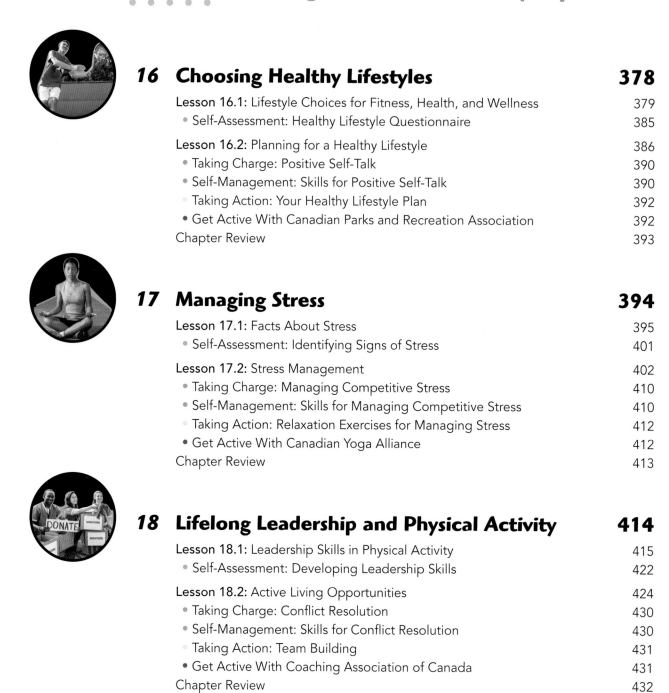

UNIT VII   Making Lifestyle Choices

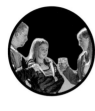

19 Alcohol, Drugs, and Tobacco   **434**

Lesson 19.1: Alcohol Use and Abuse   435
• Self-Assessment: My Alcohol Knowledge   444

Lesson 19.2: Drugs and Tobacco   445
• Taking Charge: Building Strong Refusal Skills   456
• Self-Management: Skills for Strong Refusal   456
  Taking Action: Raising Your Awareness About Alcohol, Drug,
  and Tobacco Abuse   458
• Get Active With MADD Canada   458
Chapter Review   459

20 Reproductive and Sexual Wellness   **460**

Lesson 20.1: Sexuality and Sexual Orientation   461
• Self-Assessment: Sexuality Survey   467

Lesson 20.2: Birth Control, Pregnancy, and Sexually Transmitted Infections   469
• Taking Charge: Improving Social Self-Perception   480
• Self-Management: Skills for Improving Self-Perception   480
  Taking Action: Sexual Well-Being   482
• Get Active With SexandU   482
Chapter Review   483

21 Healthy Relationships   **484**

Lesson 21.1: Family Life and Family Structure   485
• Self-Assessment: Rate Your Relationships   490

Lesson 21.2: Building and Supporting Healthy Relationships   491
• Taking Charge: Dating Coercion and Violence   501
• Self-Management: Skills for Reducing Your Risk of Experiencing
  Dating Coercion and Violence   501
  Taking Action: Taking Dating Violence Seriously   503
• Get Active With WAVAW Rape Crisis Centre   503
Chapter Review   504

Glossary   505
Index   517

Touring *Fitness for Life Canada*

Do you want to be healthy and fit? Do you want to look your best and feel good?

Fitness for Life Canada is based on the proven HELP philosophy: **H**ealth for **E**veryone for a **Life**time in a very **P**ersonal way.

H = Health

E = Everyone

L = Lifetime

P = Personal

The HELP philosophy allows you to take personal control of your future fitness, health, and wellness.

Fitness for Life Canada helps you become a physically literate person so that you can

- understand and apply important concepts and principles of fitness, health, and wellness;
- understand and use self-management skills that promote healthy lifestyles for a lifetime;
- be an informed consumer and critical user of fitness, health, and wellness information; and
- adopt healthy lifestyles now and later in life.

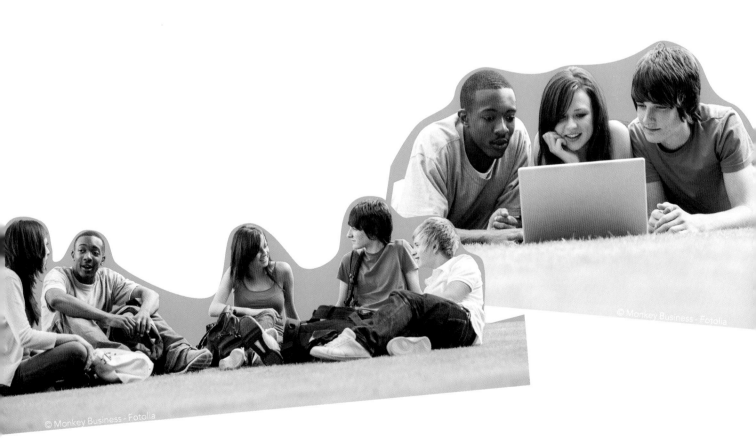

Fitness for Life Canada will help you meet your fitness and physical activity goals. Take this guided tour to learn about all of the features of this textbook. Two lessons are included in each chapter to help you learn key concepts relating to fitness, health, and wellness.

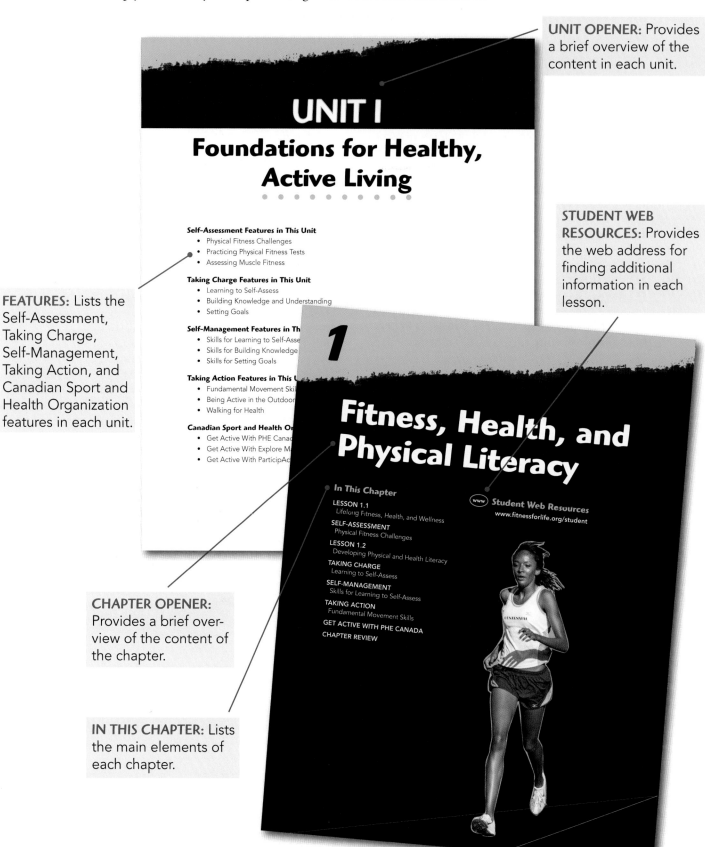

UNIT OPENER: Provides a brief overview of the content in each unit.

STUDENT WEB RESOURCES: Provides the web address for finding additional information in each lesson.

FEATURES: Lists the Self-Assessment, Taking Charge, Self-Management, Taking Action, and Canadian Sport and Health Organization features in each unit.

CHAPTER OPENER: Provides a brief overview of the content of the chapter.

IN THIS CHAPTER: Lists the main elements of each chapter.

UNIT I

Foundations for Healthy, Active Living

Self-Assessment Features in This Unit
- Physical Fitness Challenges
- Practicing Physical Fitness Tests
- Assessing Muscle Fitness

Taking Charge Features in This Unit
- Learning to Self-Assess
- Building Knowledge and Understanding
- Setting Goals

Self-Management Features in Th...
- Skills for Learning to Self-Asse...
- Skills for Building Knowledge...
- Skills for Setting Goals

Taking Action Features in This U...
- Fundamental Movement Skill...
- Being Active in the Outdoor...
- Walking for Health

Canadian Sport and Health Or...
- Get Active With PHE Canad...
- Get Active With Explore M...
- Get Active With ParticipAc...

1

Fitness, Health, and Physical Literacy

In This Chapter

LESSON 1.1
Lifelong Fitness, Health, and Wellness

SELF-ASSESSMENT
Physical Fitness Challenges

LESSON 1.2
Developing Physical and Health Literacy

TAKING CHARGE
Learning to Self-Assess

SELF-MANAGEMENT
Skills for Learning to Self-Assess

TAKING ACTION
Fundamental Movement Skills

GET ACTIVE WITH PHE CANADA

CHAPTER REVIEW

(www) **Student Web Resources**
www.fitnessforlife.org/student

LESSON OBJECTIVES: Describes what you will learn in each lesson.

LESSON VOCABULARY: Lists key terms in each lesson, which are defined in the glossary and on the student website.

FITNESS QUOTES: Provide quotes from famous people about fitness, health, and wellness.

Lesson 2.1
Adopting Healthy Lifestyles

Lesson Objectives

After participating in this lesson, you should be able to
1. name and describe the five types of determinants of fitness, health, and wellness;
2. name and describe the five benefits of a healthy lifestyle; and
3. explain the Stairway to Lifetime Fitness, Health, and Wellness and how it can be used.

Lesson Vocabulary

determinant, priority healthy lifestyle choice, self-management skill, state of being

Do you consider yourself healthy? Do you think you have good fitness? How would you rate your overall wellness? Let's take a moment to consider the nature of fitness, health, and wellness. Each is a **state of being** that an individual person can possess to his or her benefit and that of those around them. If you possess fitness, you can more easily complete daily tasks and meet the challenges of life in a positive way. If you possess health and wellness, you are free from disease and can enjoy a good quality of life. These states are interrelated, so if you do something to change one, you affect the others. Your fitness, health, and wellness are also affected by many other factors. Medical and scientific experts refer to these factors as **determinants**.

> " I guess that one of the most important things I've learned is that nothing is ever completely bad. Even cancer. It has made me a better person. It has given me courage and a sense of purpose I never had before. But you don't have to do like I did . . . wait until you lose a leg or get some awful disease, before you take the time to find out what kind of stuff you're really made of. You can start now. Anybody can. "
>
> —Terry Fox, Canadian athlete, humanitarian, and cancer research activist

Determinants of Fitness, Health, and Wellness

As shown in figure 2.1, your fitness, health, and wellness are affected by five types of determinants: (1) personal, (2) environmental, (3) health care, (4) social and individual, and (5) healthy lifestyle choices. Some are more within your control than others. The figure shows the determinant types in varying shades of orange—the lighter the colour, the less control you have; the darker the colour, the more control.

Personal Determinants

You have relatively little control, or none at all, over personal determinants, such as heredity, age, sex, and disability; thus they are shaded in light orange in the figure. Nonetheless, these factors can greatly affect your fitness, health, and wellness. For example, a person might inherit genes that put him or her at risk for certain diseases, and disease risk also increases with age. Sex is also a factor. For example, males, especially after the teen years, tend to have more muscle than females do. As for age, up to a certain point in life, muscles grow, and some parts of fitness improve just because of normal changes in the body. We also know that women have a longer life expectancy than men. Another potential factor is disability, which can affect a person's capacity to perform certain tasks but does not necessarily affect her or his health or quality of life.

You'll learn more about personal determinants and their effects on fitness, health, and wellness in other chapters of this book. Although you cannot

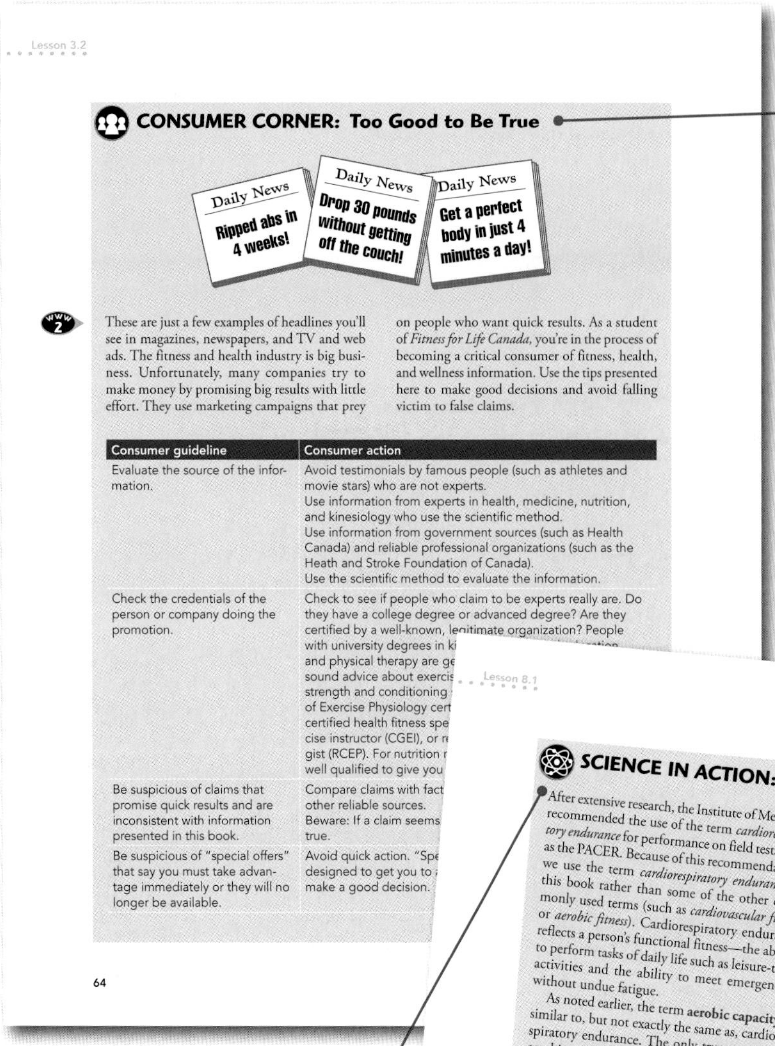

Lesson 3.2

CONSUMER CORNER: Too Good to Be True

Daily News
Ripped abs in 4 weeks!
Daily News
Drop 30 pounds without getting off the couch!
Daily News
Get a perfect body in just 4 minutes a day!

These are just a few examples of headlines you'll see in magazines, newspapers, and TV and web ads. The fitness and health industry is big business. Unfortunately, many companies try to make money by promising big results with little effort. They use marketing campaigns that prey on people who want quick results. As a student of *Fitness for Life Canada*, you're in the process of becoming a critical consumer of fitness, health, and wellness information. Use the tips presented here to make good decisions and avoid falling victim to false claims.

Consumer guideline	Consumer action
Evaluate the source of the information.	Avoid testimonials by famous people (such as athletes and movie stars) who are not experts. Use information from experts in health, medicine, nutrition, and kinesiology who use the scientific method. Use information from government sources (such as Health Canada) and reliable professional organizations (such as the Heath and Stroke Foundation of Canada). Use the scientific method to evaluate the information.
Check the credentials of the person or company doing the promotion.	Check to see if people who claim to be experts really are. Do they have a college degree or advanced degree? Are they certified by a well-known, legitimate organization? People with university degrees in ki… and physical therapy are ge… sound advice about exercis… strength and conditioning … of Exercise Physiology cert… certified health fitness spe… cise instructor (CGEI), or r… gist (RCEP). For nutrition … well qualified to give you…
Be suspicious of claims that promise quick results and are inconsistent with information presented in this book.	Compare claims with fact… other reliable sources. Beware: If a claim seems… true.
Be suspicious of "special offers" that say you must take advantage immediately or they will no longer be available.	Avoid quick action. "Spe… designed to get you to … make a good decision.

64

CONSUMER CORNER: Provides information to help you become a good consumer and avoid quackery.

STUDENT ACTIVITY: Engages you with the concept.

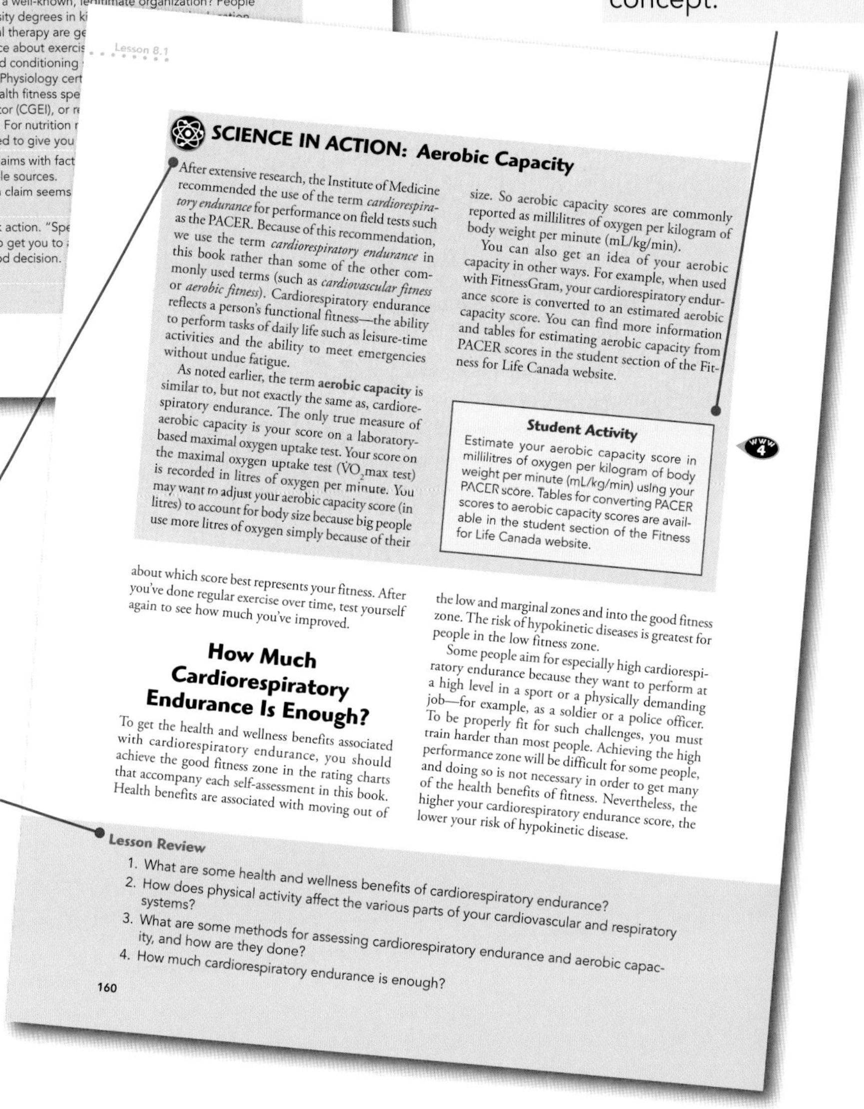

Lesson 8.1

SCIENCE IN ACTION: Aerobic Capacity

After extensive research, the Institute of Medicine recommended the use of the term *cardiorespiratory endurance* for performance on field tests such as the PACER. Because of this recommendation, we use the term *cardiorespiratory endurance* in this book rather than some of the other commonly used terms (such as *cardiovascular fitness* or *aerobic fitness*). Cardiorespiratory endurance reflects a person's functional fitness—the ability to perform tasks of daily life such as leisure-time activities and the ability to meet emergencies without undue fatigue.

As noted earlier, the term **aerobic capacity** is similar to, but not exactly the same as, cardiorespiratory endurance. The only true measure of aerobic capacity is your score on a laboratory-based maximal oxygen uptake test. Your score on the maximal oxygen uptake test (VO_2max test) is recorded in litres of oxygen per minute. You may want to adjust your aerobic capacity score (in litres) to account for body size because big people use more litres of oxygen simply because of their size. So aerobic capacity scores are commonly reported as millilitres of oxygen per kilogram of body weight per minute (mL/kg/min).

You can also get an idea of your aerobic capacity in other ways. For example, when used with FitnessGram, your cardiorespiratory endurance score is converted to an estimated aerobic capacity score. You can find more information and tables for estimating aerobic capacity from PACER scores in the student section of the Fitness for Life Canada website.

Student Activity

Estimate your aerobic capacity score in millilitres of oxygen per kilogram of body weight per minute (mL/kg/min) using your PACER score. Tables for converting PACER scores to aerobic capacity scores are available in the student section of the Fitness for Life Canada website.

about which score best represents your fitness. After you've done regular exercise over time, test yourself again to see how much you've improved.

How Much Cardiorespiratory Endurance Is Enough?

To get the health and wellness benefits associated with cardiorespiratory endurance, you should achieve the good fitness zone in the rating charts that accompany each self-assessment in this book. Health benefits are associated with moving out of the low and marginal zones and into the good fitness zone. The risk of hypokinetic diseases is greatest for people in the low fitness zone.

Some people aim for especially high cardiorespiratory endurance because they want to perform at a high level in a sport or a physically demanding job—for example, as a soldier or a police officer. To be properly fit for such challenges, you must train harder than most people. Achieving the high performance zone will be difficult for some people, and doing so is not necessary in order to get many of the health benefits of fitness. Nevertheless, the higher your cardiorespiratory endurance score, the lower your risk of hypokinetic disease.

Lesson Review

1. What are some health and wellness benefits of cardiorespiratory endurance?
2. How does physical activity affect the various parts of your cardiovascular and respiratory systems?
3. What are some methods for assessing cardiorespiratory endurance and aerobic capacity, and how are they done?
4. How much cardiorespiratory endurance is enough?

160

SCIENCE IN ACTION: Helps you understand how new information is generated using the scientific method.

LESSON REVIEW: Helps you review and remember the information you learned in the lesson.

FITNESS TECHNOLOGY: Helps you become aware of new technological information related to fitness, health, and wellness and helps you try out and use new technology.

FITNESS TECHNOLOGY: Pedometers and Accelerometers

A **pedometer** is a small, battery-powered device that can be worn on your belt. It counts each step you take and displays the running count on a meter. You simply open the face of the pedometer or push a button to see how many steps you've taken. Some pedometers also contain a small computer that allows you to enter the length of your step (your stride length) and your body weight so that the computer can estimate the distance you walk and the number of calories you expend. More expensive pedometers can also track the total time you spend in activity during the day and the number of bouts of activity that you perform lasting 10 minutes or longer. Less expensive pedometers must be reset at the end of the day, but some more expensive ones can store steps for several days. There are also numerous free or inexpensive apps for Apple and Android devices.

Accelerometers are similar to pedometers but measure physical activity in more detail. Specifically, accelerometers can record the *intensity* of your movements (for more about intensity, see the discussion of METs and recall the "I" in the FITT formula), as well as the amount of *time* (the first "T" in the FITT formula) you spend at different intensities. Like a pedometer, an accelerometer is worn on your belt and contains a small computer and a device (the accelerometer itself) that measures the intensity of your movements. Most accelerometers can count your steps taken per day and estimate the calories you expend in activity. There are also numerous free or inexpensive apps for Apple and Android devices. Be sure to check the customer reviews when searching for apps.

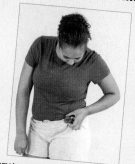

A pedometer counts steps and is a good way to self-monitor moderate activity.

Using Technology

Estimate the number of steps you take on a typical weekday and a typical weekend day. Then wear a pedometer to see how many steps you actually take (weekday and weekend day). See if you're as active as you think you are!

WEB ICONS: Indicate that additional information is available on the student website.

www 5

FIT FACT

The average person in Canada accumulates 3,500 to 5,000 steps per day. This is considerably less than the averages in some other countries—for example, 9,000 or more in Australia and Switzerland and 7,000 or more in Japan—where obesity rates are much lower.

such as an accelerometer (see the Fitness Technology feature). Heart rate monitors can also be used, and as with the accelerometer, there are heart rate monitor apps. An accelerometer both counts your steps and gives you a better idea of your exercise intensity than a pedometer can. You can determine the distance you've walked by finding out the length of your step (your stride length), then multiplying it by the number of steps you take.

FIT FACT: Offers interesting information about key topics.

EXERCISES: Provide instructions and pictures to teach you correct technique for exercises.

CORE MUSCLE FITNESS EXERCISES

CURL-UP

The curl-up is considered to be among the best abdominal exercises because it isn't risky like some other abdominal exercises. The curl-up is sometimes referred to as the crunch, and it's a good substitute for the straight-leg sit-up and hands-behind-the-head sit-up.

1. Lie on your back with your knees bent at 90 degrees and your arms extended.
2. Curl up by rolling your head, shoulders, and upper back off the floor. Roll up only until your shoulder blades leave the floor.
3. With a controlled motion, slowly return to the starting position and repeat.

Caution: Do not hold your feet while doing a trunk curl. Do not clench your hands behind the head or neck.

Variations
- **Arms across chest or hands by face (more difficult):** Fold your hands across your chest rather than keeping them

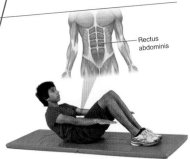
Rectus abdominis

This exercise uses your abdominal muscles.

straight, or place your hands on your face by your cheeks (not behind your head or neck).
- **Twist curl (builds oblique muscles):** Fold your arms across your chest, turn your trunk to the left, and touch your right elbow to your left hip. Repeat to the opposite side.

TRUNK LIFT (BENCH)

1. Lie facedown on a padded bench (or a bleacher with a towel on it) that is 41 to 46 centimetres (16 to 18 inches) high. Your upper body (from your waist up) should extend off the bench.
2. Have your partner hold your calves just below the knees.
3. Place one hand over the other on your forehead with your palms facing away and your elbows held to the side at the level of your ears.
4. Start with your upper body lowered. Lift slowly until your upper body is even with the bench (in line with your legs). Caution: Do not lift the trunk higher than horizontal.
5. With a controlled movement, lower to the beginning position and repeat.

Safety tip: As you do these exercises, lift slowly, move only as far as the directions specify, and use slow, controlled movements to return to the starting position. This exercise is appropri-

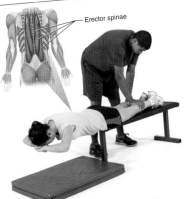
Erector spinae

This exercise uses your back extensor muscles.

ate when performed properly; but as noted earlier, using the trunk muscles for lifting or carrying is not recommended.

SELF-ASSESSMENT: Body Composition and Flexibility

In this self-assessment, you'll perform two tests: the body mass index (BMI) test and the back-saver sit and reach. Body mass index is an indicator of your body composition. The back-saver sit and reach measures the flexibility of your lower back and your hamstrings (the muscles on the back of your thighs). If you have not done so already, practice this test before performing it for a score. You will have an opportunity later to do other self-assessments of body composition and flexibility. For these two tests, record your scores and fitness ratings as directed by your teacher. These tests give you information that you can use to develop your personal needs profile (step 1) for your personal physical activity plan. If you're working with a partner, remember that self-assessment information is personal and considered confidential. It shouldn't be shared with others without the permission of the person being tested.

SELF-ASSESSMENT: Helps you learn more about your fitness and behaviours that affect your health and wellness and helps you prepare a personal plan for improvement.

Body Mass Index

1. Measure your height in metres (or inches) without shoes.
2. Measure your weight in kilograms (or pounds) without shoes. If you're wearing street clothes (as opposed to lightweight gym clothing), subtract 0.9 kilograms (2 pounds) from your weight.
3. Calculate your BMI using the chart or either of the following formulas.

$$\frac{\text{weight (lb)}}{\text{height (in.)} \times \text{height (in.)}} \times 703 = \text{BMI}$$

$$\frac{\text{weight (kg)}}{\text{height (m)} \times \text{height (m)}} = \text{BMI}$$

Use table 4.2 to find your BMI rating, and record your BMI score and rating.

Height

ft/in	cm																								
6' 4"	192.5	12	13	13	14	15	16	17	18	19	20	21	22	22	23	24	24	26	26	27	28	29	29	30	31	32	33	34
6' 3"	190	12	13	14	15	16	16	17	18	19	20	20	21	22	23	24	24	25	26	27	28	29	29	30	31	32	33	34	34
6' 2"	187.5	13	13	14	15	16	17	18	18	19	20	21	22	23	24	24	25	26	27	28	29	29	30	31	32	33	34	34	36
6' 1"	185	13	14	15	15	16	17	18	19	20	21	22	22	23	24	25	26	27	28	28	29	30	31	32	33	34	34	36	37
6' 0"	182.5	13	14	14	15	16	17	18	18	19	20	20	21	22	23	24	24	26	27	28	28	29	30	31	32	33	34	34	36	37	38
5' 11"	180	14	15	16	17	18	19	20	21	22	23	24	24	26	27	27	28	29	30	31	32	33	34	34	36	37	38	39
5' 10"	177.5	14	15	16	17	18	19	20	21	22	23	24	24	25	26	27	28	2						37	38	39	40
5' 9"	175	14	15	16	17	18	19	20	21	22	23	24	25	26	27	28	29	3		
5' 8"	172.5	15	15	16	17	18	19	20	21	22	23	24	24	26	27	28	29	29
5' 7"	170	15	16	17	18	19	20	21	22	24	24	26	27	28	29	29	31
5' 6"	167.5	16	17	18	19	20	21	22	23	24	25	26	27	28	29	30	32	33
5' 5"	165	16	17	18	19	21	22	23	24	24	26	27	28	29	30	32	33
5' 4"	162.5	17	18	19	20	21	22	23	24	26	27	28	29	30	31	33	34
5' 3"	160	17	18	20	21	22	23	24	26	27	28	29	30	31	33	34	36
5' 2"	157.5	18	19	20	21	23	24	24	26	27	29	29	31	32	33	34	36
5' 1"	155	18	20	21	22	23	24	26	27	28	29	31	32	33	34	36	37
5' 0"	152.5	19	20	21	23	24	25	27	28	29	31	32	33	34	36	37	38
4' 11"	150	20	21	22	24	24	26	28	29	30	32	33	34	36	37	38	40
4' 10"	147.5	20	22	23	24	26	27	28	29	31	33	34	35	37	38	40	41
4' 9"	145	21	22	24	25	27	28	29	31	32	34	35	37	38	39	41	4
4' 8"	142.5	22	23	24	26	27	28	29	31	33	34	36	38	39	41	42	4
Weight (kg)		44	47	50	53	56	59	62	65	68	71	74	77	80	83	86	
Weight (lbs)		97	103	110	117	123	130	136	143	150	156	163	169	176	183	189	1

Body mass index calculation chart. Locate your height in the left c box where the selected row and column intersect is your BMI sco

TABLE 4.2 Rating Chart: Body Mass Index

	13 years old		14 years old		15 years old		16 years old		17 years old		18 years old	
	Male	Female	Male	Female	Male	Female	Male	Female	Male	Female	Male	Female
Very lean	≤15.4	≤15.3	≤16.0	≤15.8	≤16.5	≤16.3	≤17.1	≤16.8	≤17.7	≤17.2	≤18.2	≤17.5
Good fitness	15.5–21.3	15.4–22.0	16.1–22.1	15.9–22.8	16.6–22.9	16.4–23.5	17.2–23.7	16.9–24.1	17.8–24.4	17.3–24.6	18.3–25.1	17.6–25.1
Marginal fitness	21.4–23.5	22.1–23.7	22.2–24.4	22.9–24.5	23.0–25.2	23.6–25.3	23.8–25.9	24.2–26.0	24.5–26.6	24.7–27.6	25.2–27.4	25.2–27.1
Low fitness	≥23.6	≥23.8	≥24.5	≥24.6	≥25.3	≥25.4	≥26.0	≥26.1	≥26.7	≥27.7	≥27.5	≥27.2

Data based on *FitnessGram*.

Back-Saver Sit and Reach

1. Place a measuring stick, such as a metre stick or yardstick, on top of a box that is 30 centimetres (12 inches) high with the stick extending 23 centimetres (9 inches) over the box and the lower numbers toward you. You may use a flexibility testing box if one is available.
2. To measure the flexibility of your right leg, fully extend it and place your right foot flat against the box. Bend your left leg, with the knee turned out and your left foot 5 to 8 centimetres (2 to 3 inches) to the side of your straight right leg.
3. Extend your arms forward over the measuring stick. Place your hands on the stick, one on top of the other, with your palms facing down. Your middle fingers should be together with the tip of one finger exactly on top of the other.
4. Lean forward slowly; do not bounce. Reach forward with your arms and fingers, then slowly return to the starting position. Repeat four times. On the fourth reach, hold the position for three seconds and observe the measurement on the stick below your fingertips.
5. Repeat the test with your left leg straight.
6. Record your score to the nearest centimetre (2.54 centimetres equals 1 inch). Consult table 4.3 to determine your fitness rating for each side of your body.

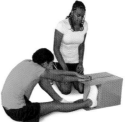

The back-saver sit and reach assesses flexibility.

TABLE 4.3 Rating Chart: Back-Saver Sit and Reach (Centimetres)

	13 or 14 years old		15 years or older	
	Male	Female	Male	Female
High performance	≥25	≥30	≥25	≥35.5
Good fitness	20–23	25–28	20–23	30–33
Marginal fitness	15–18	20–23	15–18	25–28
Low fitness	≤13	≤18	≤13	≤23

To convert centimetres to inches, multiply centimetres by 0.39. Alternatively, you can use the Internet to find a calculator that converts centimetres to inches.

Data based on *FitnessGram*.

TAKING CHARGE AND SELF-MANAGEMENT: Provide guidelines for learning self-management skills that help you adopt healthy behaviours.

TAKING CHARGE: Finding Social Support

Social support involves your family members, friends, teachers, and community members encouraging your physical activities or participating with you. You're more likely to begin or continue an activity if the people you associate with also do it.

Shannon's family has always enjoyed bike riding. As a toddler, she would ride in the child's seat behind her mother. Every evening, the family would ride through the neighbourhood. By the time she was in school, Shannon had her own two-wheeler. Now a teenager, Shannon still loves to ride, but school activities sometimes prevent her from riding with her family. She wants to continue riding but doesn't want to do it alone.

Aleem's family has never been very active. Most of his friends tend to watch television, play video games, or just hang out rather than doing anything active. Sometimes Aleem watches while a group of his classmates plays a quick game of volleyball after school. They often invite

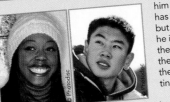

him to join the game. He has been tempted to join but has hesitated because he is not friends with any of the players. He has enjoyed the activities he has tried in the past but has never continued them for very long.

Both Shannon and Aleem need social support. Shannon needs it to continue an activity she already enjoys. Aleem needs it to encourage him to begin an activity and then reinforce his participation.

For Discussion

Who might Shannon ask to go riding with her? What could Aleem do to become involved in physical activity? What other suggestions can you offer for finding social support? What groups might Shannon and Aleem identify with to get social support? Consider the guidelines presented in the Self-Management feature when you answer the discussion questions.

FOR DISCUSSION: Helps you take charge by making good decisions.

SELF-MANAGEMENT: Skills for Finding Social Support

Experts indicate that people who experience support from others are more likely to participate in regular physical activity, especially over the course of a lifetime. Social support is also helpful to people in reaching and maintaining a healthy body weight, building muscle fitness, and improving eating habits. Consider the following guidelines to help you gain others' support for your physical activity.

- **Do a self-assessment of your current level of social support.** Ask your teacher about the social support worksheet that can help you do this assessment. Use the self-assessment to determine areas in which you can improve your social support.
- **Birds of a feather flock together.** Find friends who are interested in the activities that interest you, or encourage your current friends to support you or join you in your participation.

- **Join a club or team.** If no club or team exists for your chosen activity, talk to a teacher, family member, or community recreation leader about starting one.
- **Contact local organizations.** Organizations such as the R.E.A.L. (Recreation Experiences and Leisure) program financially support children and teens to join clubs and teams, and they also provide equipment when possible.
- **Discuss your interests with family and teachers.** Ask them for their support. Ask them to help you learn the activity.
- **If possible, take lessons.** In addition to formal lessons, you can also ask teachers and others to support you by helping you learn to perform an activity properly.
- **Family matters.** Encourage your family members to try the activity.
- **Get proper equipment.** Ask for equipment for your birthday or other special occasion.

TAKING ACTION: Lets you try out teacher-directed activities that can help you become fit and active for a lifetime.

GET ACTIVE: Spotlights Canadian sport and health organizations, describing who they are, what they do, and how you can get active with them.

TAKING ACTION: Fundamental Movement Skills

One key component of physical literacy is learning movement skills. In fact, before you can perform complex and sport-specific movement skills (e.g., kicking a soccer ball, performing a trick on a skateboard, hitting a tennis forehand, catching a lacrosse ball), you need to learn the fundamental movement skills. Fundamental movement skills include kicking, striking (objects), throwing, catching, jumping, and running. When you are confident and competent with these fundamental movement skills, you can develop sport-specific and complex movement skills that allow you to enjoy sport and physical activity. Most importantly, having a firm grasp of the fundamental movement skills will help you enjoy a long life of physical activity. You will take action here by performing a circuit of fundamental movement skills with your teacher. After you have tried the different stations, you can reflect on your performance and identify the fundamental movement skills that you need to work on and those that you have mastered.

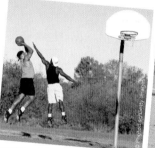
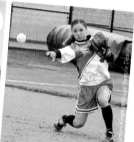

Jumping and throwing are fundamental movement skills used in many different activities.

GET ACTIVE WITH PHE CANADA

©Physical and Health Education Canada

Who We Are

Physical and Health Education Canada (PHE Canada) is a national not-for-profit organization supporting the healthy development of children and youth by advocating for, increasing access to, and developing programs and resources to support the delivery of high-quality health education, physical education, and sport programming. Established in 1933, PHE Canada strives to have all children and youth live physically active and healthy lives now and in their future.

What We Do

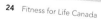

PHE Canada works with your teachers, coaches, and recreation leaders and develops fun and educational programs, resources, and activities to help you achieve your personal goals and be your best self. PHE Canada wants you to be happy and healthy. That means helping you develop the skills to participate in sports or any physical activities you have an interest in, understand the importance of proper nutrition, and establish positive self-esteem and mental resiliency.

Our experienced staff and expert advisors ensure that our programs, resources and activities are appropriate for your age level yet challenging to help you improve; meet the highest standards of educational content to ensure optimal understanding and knowledge transfer; and, perhaps most important, are fun and engaging so you are excited and have a positive experience toward living a healthy, active lifestyle.

Get Involved

PHE Canada has a variety of programs, resources, and activities for children of all ages. We invite you, your parents, your teachers, your coaches, and your recreation leaders to learn more about us. Visit PHECanada on the web at www.phecanada.ca, Facebook at www.facebook.com/PHECanada, and Twitter at @PHECanada.

Reprinted, by permission, from Jordan Burwash. ©Physical and Health Education Canada.

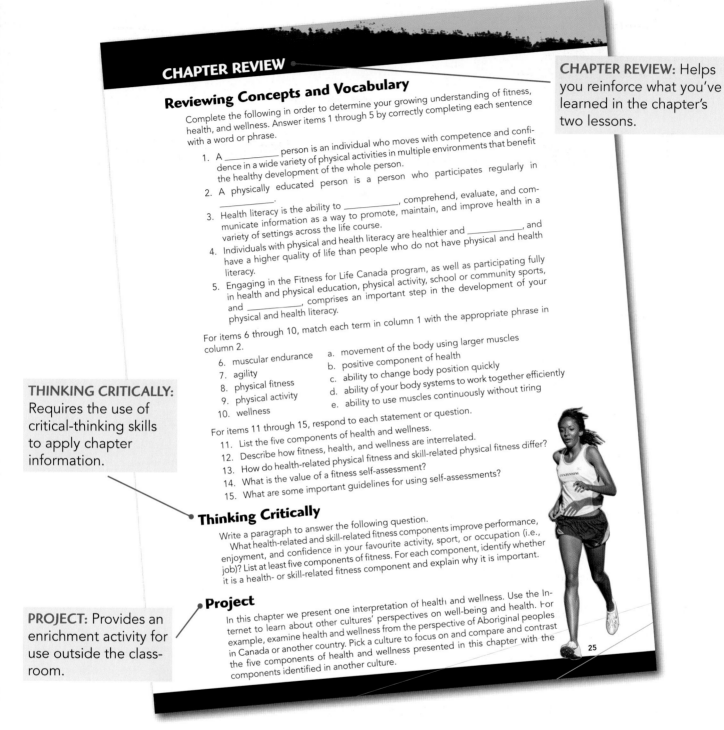

CHAPTER REVIEW

Reviewing Concepts and Vocabulary

Complete the following in order to determine your growing understanding of fitness, health, and wellness. Answer items 1 through 5 by correctly completing each sentence with a word or phrase.

1. A _____ person is an individual who moves with competence and confidence in a wide variety of physical activities in multiple environments that benefit the healthy development of the whole person.

2. A physically educated person is a person who participates regularly in _____.

3. Health literacy is the ability to _____, comprehend, evaluate, and communicate information as a way to promote, maintain, and improve health in a variety of settings across the life course.

4. Individuals with physical and health literacy are healthier and _____, and have a higher quality of life than people who do not have physical and health literacy.

5. Engaging in the Fitness for Life Canada program, as well as participating fully in health and physical education, physical activity, school or community sports, and _____, comprises an important step in the development of your physical and health literacy.

For items 6 through 10, match each term in column 1 with the appropriate phrase in column 2.

6. muscular endurance
7. agility
8. physical fitness
9. physical activity
10. wellness

a. movement of the body using larger muscles
b. positive component of health
c. ability to change body position quickly
d. ability of your body systems to work together efficiently
e. ability to use muscles continuously without tiring

For items 11 through 15, respond to each statement or question.

11. List the five components of health and wellness.
12. Describe how fitness, health, and wellness are interrelated.
13. How do health-related physical fitness and skill-related physical fitness differ?
14. What is the value of a fitness self-assessment?
15. What are some important guidelines for using self-assessments?

Thinking Critically

Write a paragraph to answer the following question.
What health-related and skill-related fitness components improve performance, enjoyment, and confidence in your favourite activity, sport, or occupation (i.e., job)? List at least five components of fitness. For each component, identify whether it is a health- or skill-related fitness component and explain why it is important.

Project

In this chapter we present one interpretation of health and wellness. Use the Internet to learn about other cultures' perspectives on well-being and health. For example, examine health and wellness from the perspective of Aboriginal peoples in Canada or another country. Pick a culture to focus on and compare and contrast the five components of health and wellness presented in this chapter with the components identified in another culture.

25

CHAPTER REVIEW: Helps you reinforce what you've learned in the chapter's two lessons.

THINKING CRITICALLY: Requires the use of critical-thinking skills to apply chapter information.

PROJECT: Provides an enrichment activity for use outside the classroom.

In addition to all the textbook features, the Fitness for Life Canada program includes several other components:

- **Student Web Resource:** You have access to a wide variety of resources at www.fitnessforlife.org/student. These resources will aid your understanding of the textbook content and include video clips that demonstrate how to do the self-assessment exercises in each chapter, worksheets, interactive review questions, and expanded discussions of topics that are marked by web icons throughout this book.

- **Teacher Web Resource:** Your teacher has access to a special web resource with lessons and activities that you can do to better learn and understand the information in this textbook.

Now read on, and enjoy *Fitness for Life Canada*!

UNIT I

Foundations for Healthy, Active Living

● ● ● ● ● ● ● ● ● ●

Self-Assessment Features in This Unit
- Physical Fitness Challenges
- Practicing Physical Fitness Tests
- Assessing Muscle Fitness

Taking Charge Features in This Unit
- Learning to Self-Assess
- Building Knowledge and Understanding
- Setting Goals

Self-Management Features in This Unit
- Skills for Learning to Self-Assess
- Skills for Building Knowledge and Understanding
- Skills for Setting Goals

Taking Action Features in This Unit
- Fundamental Movement Skills
- Being Active in the Outdoors
- Walking for Health

Canadian Sport and Health Organization Features in This Unit
- Get Active With PHE Canada
- Get Active With Explore Magazine
- Get Active With ParticipAction

1

Fitness, Health, and Physical Literacy

In This Chapter

 Student Web Resources
www.fitnessforlife.org/student

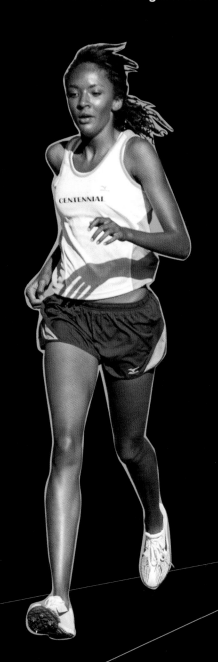

Lesson 1.1
Lifelong Fitness, Health, and Wellness

Lesson Objectives

After participating in this lesson, you should be able to

1. define *physical fitness*, *health*, and *wellness* and describe how they are interrelated;
2. describe the five components of health and wellness; and
3. identify the six parts of health-related physical fitness and the five parts of skill-related physical fitness.

Lesson Vocabulary

agility, balance, body composition, body fat level, cardiorespiratory endurance, coordination, flexibility, functional fitness, health, health-related physical fitness, hypokinetic condition, muscular endurance, physical activity, physical fitness, power, public health scientist, reaction time, skill-related physical fitness, speed, strength, wellness

If you could have one wish come true, what would it be? Some people would wish for material things, such as the latest video game console, the newest phone, a new car, a new house, or money. But if you think about it a little more and consider what it would be like to live with sickness or injury, you might wish for good fitness, health, and wellness for yourself and your family. If you possess fitness, health, and wellness, you can enjoy life to its fullest. Without them, no amount of money will allow you to do all of the things you would like to do. More than 90 percent of all people, including teens, agree that good health is important because it helps you feel good, look good, and enjoy life with the people you care about most.

As you read this book, you'll learn more about healthy lifestyle choices that can help you be fit, healthy, and well. You'll learn how to prepare a personal fitness plan and a healthy personal lifestyle plan, and how to use self-management skills to stick with your plan. The goal of this book is to help you become an informed consumer of information who makes effective decisions about your lifelong fitness, health, and wellness. The book content and the daily lesson activities will help you develop specific knowledge, skills, and attitudes that will help you develop physical literacy and accomplish this goal.

> " The first wealth is health. "
>
> —Ralph Waldo Emerson, poet

Before you can start developing a plan, you need some basic information. In this lesson, you'll learn definitions for some key words used throughout this course. You'll better understand the meaning of the words "fitness," "health," and "wellness," and you'll learn about their components.

What Is Health? What Is Wellness?

Early definitions of **health** focused on illness. The first medical doctors concentrated on helping sick people overcome their health problems; in other words, their main job was treating people who were ill.

But in 1947, the World Health Organization (WHO), which now includes representatives from 194 countries, issued a statement indicating that health meant more than freedom from disease or illness. This recognition led people to develop a more comprehensive definition of health, which now includes **wellness**. According to the WHO statement, the sheer fact of not being sick doesn't mean you are well. Wellness is the positive component of health that includes having a good quality of life and a good sense of well-being exhibited by a positive outlook on life.

Figure 1.1 shows that a healthy person both is not ill (the blue half) and has a strong wellness component (the green half). Illness is the negative component of health that we want to treat or

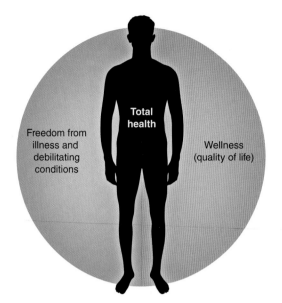

FIGURE 1.1 Being healthy means having wellness in addition to not being ill.

prevent, whereas wellness is the positive component of health that we want to promote.

Health and wellness have many components, and a chain is often used to show how the components are linked (figure 1.2). For a chain to be strong, each link must be strong. Likewise, to have good health and wellness, you must have all of the health and wellness components, not just one or two. The goal is to promote the positive while avoiding the negative in each component, as shown in figure 1.2. If you're happy, informed, involved, fit, and fulfilled, then you have incorporated the positive aspects of the health components into your life. You possess wellness, and your risk of illness is reduced. The bottom line is this: Health is freedom from disease and debilitating conditions as well as optimal wellness in all five components (physical, emotional-mental, social, intellectual, and spiritual).

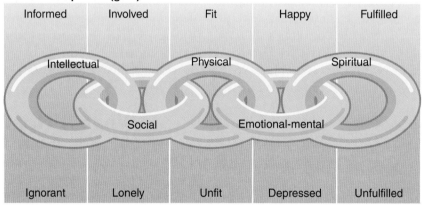

FIGURE 1.2 The total health and wellness chain.

Based on Corbin et al. 2011.

❤ FITNESS TECHNOLOGY: World Wide Web

The World Wide Web has given many people immediate access to all kinds of health and fitness information. As you'll learn elsewhere in this book, some of the information available on the web is good. However, there is a lot of inaccurate information, especially health information. In each chapter of this book, you'll find a web address that leads you to sound information about fitness, health, and wellness. Look for special web symbols included throughout the book; just type in the address from the first page of the chapter, and you'll find good, reliable information. These

web pages will also give you links to other reliable sources of fitness and health information.

Using Technology

Access the web address provided at the beginning of each chapter in this book. You will find additional information related to topics in each lesson. Explore the topics to learn more. Explore some of the websites provided to find good fitness and health information.

Personal Health and Community Health

One major goal of this book is to help each reader achieve good personal health and wellness. Another important goal is to promote community health, which refers to the health of a group rather than an individual—from small groups such as families and networks of friends, to larger groups such as towns and cities, and on to very large groups such as states and countries. Just as each person sets health goals, communities do so as well. Your school is a community, and many schools have an established comprehensive school health (CSH) program. A CSH program aims to improve student learning and health by creating a healthy school environment. Comprehensive school health programs affect the whole school environment by taking actions that address four distinct but interrelated pillars that provide a strong foundation for comprehensive school health: social and physical environment, teaching and learning, healthy school policy, and partnerships and services.

An example of a large-scale program designed to promote health in a large community is the Active Canada 2020 project, in which over 1,000 organizations throughout Canada work together to increase the physical activity level of every person in Canada by the year 2020. **Public health scientists** working with physical activity, recreation, education, and health promotion professionals from across Canada developed the goals.

What Is Physical Fitness?

Physical fitness refers to the ability of your body systems to work together efficiently to allow you to be healthy and perform activities of daily living. Being efficient means doing daily activities with little wasted effort. A fit person is able to perform schoolwork, meet home responsibilities, and still have enough energy to enjoy sport and other leisure

FIT FACT

In order to apply for work as a lifeguard, a firefighter, a police officer, an airplane pilot, or military personnel, you will have to pass a number of different fitness tests.

SCIENCE IN ACTION: Kinesiology (Exercise Science)

The past two centuries have sometimes been called the golden age of medicine because they have seen many of the most significant advances in health and medical science. Toward the end of the 20th century, a relatively new science called kinesiology emerged as more and more evidence accumulated showing the health and wellness benefits of physical activity and exercise. The Natural Sciences and Engineering Research Council of Canada recognizes kinesiology as a major area of science.

Put simply, kinesiology is the study of human movement. There are, of course, many types of human movement. Some involve small-muscle movements, such as the movement of your eyes when reading, the movement of your fingers when typing, and the movement of your hands when playing a musical instrument. Kinesiology is the study of all human movement, but it focuses on large-muscle physical activity; in fact,

the phrase "**physical activity**" is a very general term for large-muscle movement. There are many types of physical activity, including moderate-intensity activities such as walking, vigorous-intensity activities such as aerobics, sport and recreational activities, and exercise for muscle fitness and flexibility. These activity types are included in the Physical Activity Pyramid, which is described in more detail throughout this book.

Student Activity

Take a closer look at the Physical Activity Pyramid introduced in chapter 6 (and on the back of your textbook) and identify what step your favourite activities are on. Talk to your friends and family and determine what steps their favourite activities are on.

activities. A fit person can respond effectively to normal life situations, such as raking leaves at home, stocking shelves at a part-time job, and marching in the band at school. A fit person can also respond to emergency situations—for example, by running to get help or aiding a friend in distress.

The Parts of Physical Fitness

Physical fitness is made up of 11 parts—6 of them health related and 5 skill related. All of the parts are important to good performance in physical activity, including sports. But the six are referred to as contributing to **health-related physical fitness** because scientists in kinesiology have shown that they can reduce your risk of chronic disease and promote good health and wellness. These parts of fitness are **body composition**, **cardiorespiratory endurance**, **flexibility**, **muscular endurance**, **power**, and **strength**. They also help you function effectively in daily activities.

As the name implies, **skill-related physical fitness** components help you perform well in sports and other activities that require motor skills. For example, **speed** helps you in sports such as track and field. These five parts of physical fitness are also linked to health but less so than the health-related components. For example, among older adults,

balance, **agility**, and **coordination** are very important for preventing falls (a major health concern), and **reaction time** relates to risk for automobile accidents. Each part of physical fitness is described in more detail in the two following features: The Six Parts of Health-Related Fitness and The Five Parts of Skill-Related Fitness.

Health-Related Physical Fitness

Think about a runner. She can probably run a long distance without tiring; thus she has good fitness in at least one area of health-related physical fitness. But does she have good fitness in all six parts? Run-

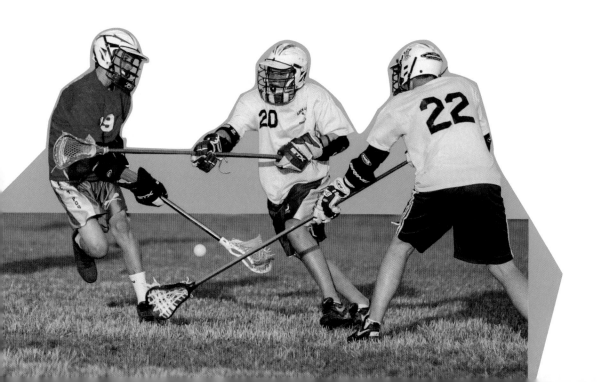

FIT FACT

Power, formerly classified as a skill-related part of fitness, is now classified as a health-related part of fitness. A report by the independent Institute of Medicine provides evidence of the link between physical power and health. The report indicates that power is associated with wellness, higher quality of life, reduced risk of chronic disease and early death, and better bone health. Power, and activities that improve power, have also been found to be important for healthy bones in children and teens.

ning is an excellent form of physical activity, but being a runner doesn't guarantee fitness in all parts of health-related physical fitness. Like the runner, you may be more fit in some parts of fitness than in others. The feature named The Six Parts of Health-Related Fitness describes each part and shows an example. As you read about each part, ask yourself how fit you think you are in that area.

How do you think you rate in each of the six health-related parts of fitness? To be healthy, you should be fit in relation to each of the six parts. Totally fit people are less likely to develop a **hypo-kinetic condition**—a health problem caused partly by lack of physical activity—such as heart disease,

The Six Parts of Health-Related Fitness

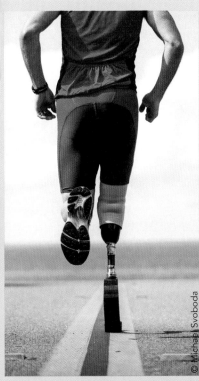

© Michael Svoboda

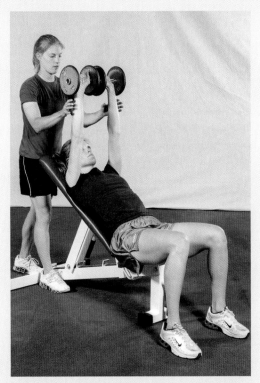

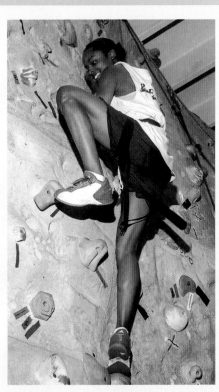

Cardiorespiratory endurance is the ability to exercise your entire body for a long time without stopping. It requires a strong heart, healthy lungs, and clear blood vessels to supply your large muscles with oxygen. Examples of activities that require good cardiorespiratory endurance are distance running, swimming, snowshoeing, and cross-country skiing.

Strength is the amount of force your muscles can produce. It is often measured by how much weight you can lift or how much resistance you can overcome. Examples of activities that require good strength are lifting a heavy weight and pushing a heavy box.

Muscular endurance is the ability to use your muscles many times without tiring—for example, doing many push-ups or curl-ups (crunches) or climbing a rock wall.

> continued

The Six Parts of Health-Related Fitness

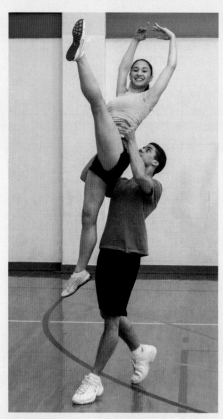

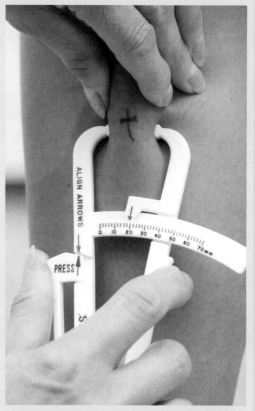

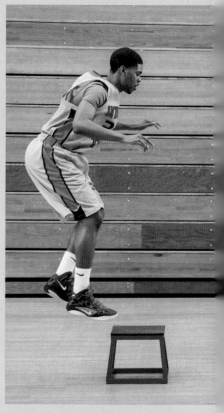

Flexibility is the ability to use your joints fully through a wide range of motion without injury. You are flexible when your muscles are long enough and your joints are free enough to allow adequate movement. Examples of people with good flexibility include dancers, gymnasts, surfers, and skateboarders.

Body composition refers to the different types of tissues that make up your body, including fat, muscle, bone, and organ. Your level of body fat is often used to assess the component of body composition related to health. Body composition measures commonly used in schools include body mass index (based on height and weight), skinfold measures (which estimate body fatness), and body measurements such as waist and hip circumferences.

Power is the ability to use strength quickly; thus it involves both strength and speed. It is sometimes referred to as explosive strength. People with good power can, for example, jump far or high, take a fast slap shot, throw a fast ball, and swim fast.

high blood pressure, diabetes, osteoporosis, colon cancer, or a high **body fat level**. You'll learn more about hypokinetic conditions in other chapters of this book. People who are physically fit also enjoy better wellness. They feel better, look better, and have more energy. You don't have to be a great athlete in order to enjoy good health and wellness and be physically fit. Regular physical activity can improve anyone's health-related physical fitness.

Skill-Related Physical Fitness

Just as the runner in our example may not achieve a high rating in all parts of health-related physical fitness, she also may not rate the same in all parts of skill-related physical fitness. Though most sports require several parts of skill-related fitness, different sports can require different parts. For example, a skater might have good agility but lack good reaction time. Some people have more natural ability in some areas than in others. No matter how you score on the skill-related parts of physical fitness, you can enjoy some type of physical activity.

Remember, too, that good health doesn't come from being good in skill-related physical fitness. It comes from doing activities designed to improve your health-related physical fitness and eating a nutritious diet, and it can be enjoyed both by great

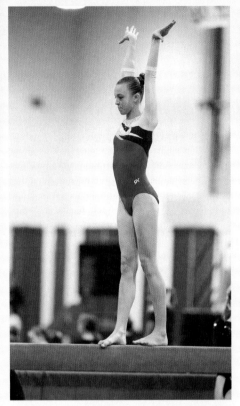

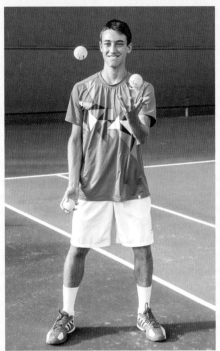

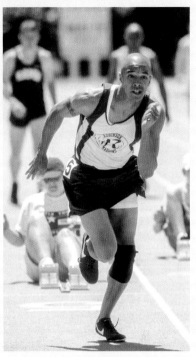

Balance is the ability to keep an upright posture while standing still or moving. People with good balance are likely to be good, for example, at gymnastics, snowboarding, archery, and ice skating.

Coordination is the ability to use your senses together with your body parts or to use two or more body parts together. People with good eye–hand or eye–foot coordination are good at juggling and at hitting and kicking games, such as soccer, baseball, volleyball, badminton, tennis, and golf.

Speed is the ability to perform a movement or cover a distance in a short time. For example, people with good leg speed can run fast, and people with good arm speed can throw fast or hit a ball that is thrown fast.

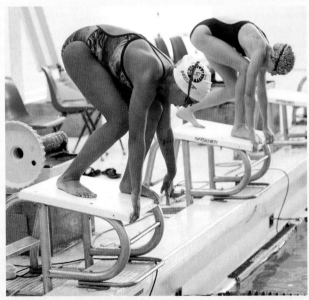

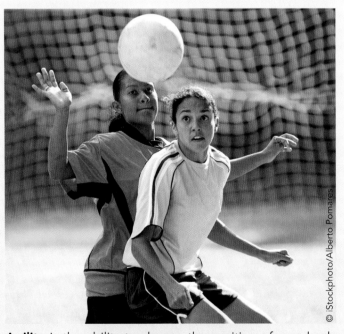

Reaction time is the amount of time it takes you to move once you recognize the need to act. People with good reaction time can make fast starts in track and swimming and can dodge fast attacks in fencing and karate. Goalies in sports like lacrosse, ringette, and handball need good reaction time.

Agility is the ability to change the position of your body quickly and control your body's movements. People with good agility are likely to be good, for example, at wrestling, diving, soccer, Ultimate, and ice skating.

athletes and by people who consider themselves nonathletic.

As noted earlier, health-related fitness offers a double benefit. It not only helps you stay healthy but also helps you perform well in sport and other physical activities. For example, cardiorespiratory endurance helps you resist heart disease and helps you perform well in sports such as swimming and cross-country skiing. Similarly, strength helps you perform well in sports such as rugby and wrestling; muscular endurance is important in soccer and tennis; flexibility helps in sports such as gymnastics and rock climbing; power helps in track activities such as the discus throw and the long jump; and having a healthy amount of body fat makes your body more efficient in many activities.

Functional Fitness

Functional fitness refers to the ability to function effectively when performing normal daily tasks. You have functional fitness if you can do your school-work, get to and from school, participate in leisure activities without fatigue, respond to emergency situations, and perform other daily tasks safely and without fatigue (e.g., riding a bike, driving a car, or doing housework and yard work). From this point of view, health-related fitness not only helps you stay healthy but also helps you function; for example, it helps you avoid fatigue when working or playing. Similarly, skill-related fitness not only helps you perform well in sports but also can help you function

> **"** I associate beauty with health, physically and mentally. Health and beauty go together. **"**
>
> —Sophie Grégoire Trudeau, women's health advocate and former television host

in life, such as when you need to stop quickly while driving a car or sledding down a hill. As you work your way through this book, you'll learn how each part of health- and skill-related fitness contributes to your functional fitness.

Fitness, Health, and Wellness Are Interrelated

Fitness, health, and wellness are all states of being, and you can maximize all three by living a healthy lifestyle. The interrelationship of fitness, health, and wellness is shown in figure 1.3. For example, if you're active on a regular basis, your fitness improves. That reduces your risk of disease, which improves your health. Your wellness and quality of life are also improved because you feel better and can better enjoy the activities of daily life.

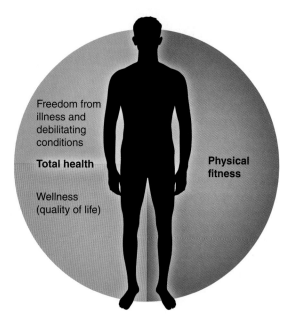

FIGURE 1.3 Interrelationship of fitness, health, and wellness.

Lesson Review

1. How are physical fitness, health, and wellness interrelated?
2. What are the five components of health and wellness?
3. List the six parts of health-related physical fitness and the five parts of skill-related physical fitness.

Each chapter of this book includes a feature titled Self-Assessment. In most chapters, the self-assessment is designed to help you determine your personal fitness level. You'll record and analyze your assessment results. In this chapter's self-assessment, you'll try 11 challenges. They're called challenges rather than tests because they are not meant to be tests of fitness, nor are they meant to be exercises that you do to get fit. Instead, trying these challenges is a fun and active way to better understand the differences between the various parts of physical fitness. Please do not draw conclusions about your fitness based on your performance in these challenges. As you work your way through this book, you'll learn many self-assessments to help you determine your true fitness level.

The cardiorespiratory endurance and flexibility challenges will help you warm up before performing the other challenges. You may also want to consider additional warm-up exercises recommended by your instructor.

Part 1: Health-Related Physical Fitness Challenges

Running in Place (Cardiorespiratory Endurance)

1. Determine your resting heart rate for one minute. To do this, use your index and middle fingers to feel your pulse at your wrist (on the side of the thumb) or neck (start with your two fingers at the side of your nose and move your fingers straight downward to your neck), then count your pulse (heartbeats) for one minute.
2. Run 120 steps in place for one minute. Count one step every time a foot hits the floor.
3. Rest for 30 seconds, then count your pulse (heart rate) for one minute.

People with good cardiorespiratory endurance recover quickly after exercise. Is your heart rate after this exercise within 15 beats per minute of your resting heart rate before running in place?

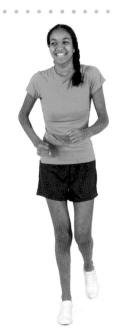

This challenge focuses on cardiorespiratory endurance.

Two-Hand Ankle Grip (Flexibility)

1. Squat with your heels together. Lean the upper body forward and reach with your hands between your legs and behind your ankles.
2. Clasp your hands in front of your ankles.
3. Interlock your hands for the full length of your fingers. Keep your feet still. Hold the position for five seconds.

Good flexibility benefits people at work (e.g., plumbers, electricians, painters) and at play (e.g., dancers, gymnasts, surfers).

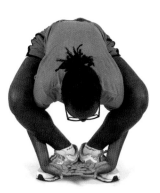

This challenge focuses on flexibility.

Single-Leg Raise (Muscular Endurance)

1. Bend forward at your waist so that your upper body rests on a table and your feet are on the floor.
2. Raise one leg so that it is extended straight out behind you. Complete several such raises with each leg. Performing multiple repetitions (8 or more) requires muscular endurance. Stop if you reach 25 with each leg.

Good muscular endurance allows you to participate in activities that you might do for a long time (e.g., hiking, shopping, dancing).

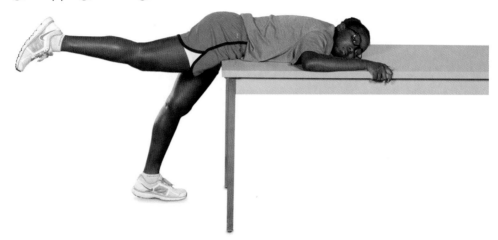

This challenge focuses on muscular endurance.

Arm Skinfold (Body Fat Level)

1. Let your right arm hang relaxed at your side. Have a partner gently pinch the skin and the fat under the skin on the back of your arm halfway between your elbow and shoulder. Together the skin and fat under the skin is called a skinfold.
2. Several skinfolds in different body locations can be used to determine the total amount of fat in the body. At this point there is no need to measure the skinfold. The skinfold on the arm is used only to illustrate the concept of body composition.

Body composition affects both health and performance.

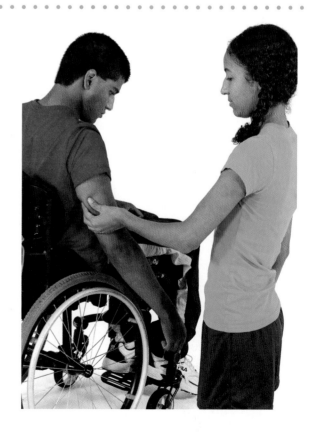

This challenge focuses on body composition.

90-Degree Push-Up (Strength)

1. Lie facedown on a mat or carpet with your hands under your shoulders, your fingers spread, and your legs straight. Your legs should be slightly apart and your toes should be tucked under, or flexed, so that the pads of your toes are in contact with the floor.

2. Push up until your arms are straight. Keep your legs and back straight—your body should form a straight line.

3. Lower your body by bending your elbows until your upper arms are parallel to the floor (elbows at a 90-degree angle—not to the point that your body touches the floor again), then push up until your arms are fully extended. Do one push-up every three seconds. You may want to have a partner say "up-down" every three seconds to help you. Performing up to five push-ups requires muscular strength.

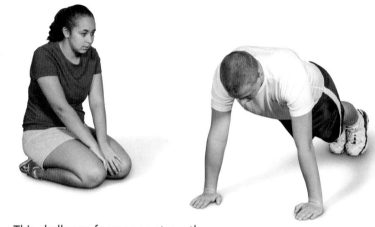

This challenge focuses on strength.

Strength is important for everyday activities (e.g., opening jars, lifting objects), certain types of work (e.g., carpentry, firefighting), and most sports.

Kneel Jump (Power)

1. Kneel so that your shins and knees are on a mat. Hold your arms back. Point your toes straight backward so that the instep of both feet (i.e., laces of your sneakers) are in contact with the floor.

2. Without curling your toes under you or rocking your body backward, swing your arms upward and spring to your feet.

3. Hold your position for three seconds after you land.

Power is important for sprinters, jumpers, and throwers.

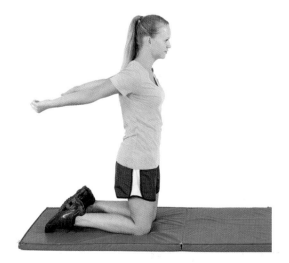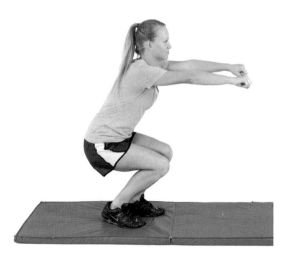

This challenge focuses on power.

Part 2: Skill-Related Physical Fitness Challenges

Line Jump (Agility)

1. Balance on your right foot on a line on the floor.
2. Leap onto your left foot so that it lands to the right of the line.
3. Leap across the line onto your right foot; land to the left of the line.
4. Leap onto your left foot, landing on the line.

Agility is important for cross-country runners, figure skaters, and most team sport athletes.

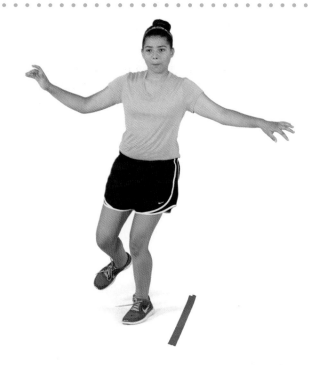

This challenge focuses on agility.

Double Heel Click (Speed)

1. Jump into the air and click your heels together twice before you land. If you need to, start by clicking your heels once, working your way up to clicking twice.
2. Your feet should be at least eight centimetres (three inches) apart when you land.

Speed in the legs benefits people who like to run. Speed in the arms benefits people who throw and strike objects.

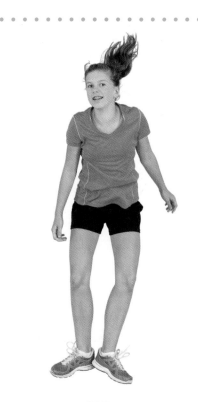

This challenge focuses on speed.

Backward Hop (Balance)

1. With your eyes closed, hop backward on one foot five times.
2. After the last hop, hold your balance for three seconds.

Balance is important for performance in activities such as skateboarding, ice skating, and surfing. Balance is also important for preventing injuries from falls.

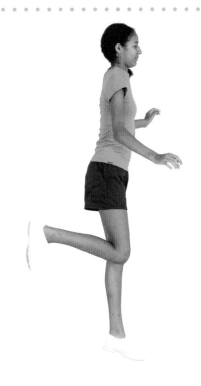

This challenge focuses on balance.

Double-Ball Bounce (Coordination)

1. In each of your hands, hold a volleyball or basketball. Make sure you are holding the same size and type of ball in each hand for this activity. Beginning at the same time with each hand, bounce both balls at the same time, at least knee high.
2. Bounce both balls three times in a row without losing control of them.

Eye–hand coordination helps in activities like table tennis and lacrosse. Eye–foot coordination is important for soccer and rugby.

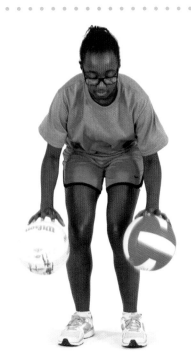

This challenge focuses on coordination.

Coin Catch (Reaction Time)

1. Point your right elbow outward in front of you. Your right hand, palm up, should be beside your right ear. If you're left-handed, do this activity with your left hand.
2. Balance a coin as close to the end of your elbow as possible.
3. Quickly lower your elbow and grab the coin in the air with the hand of the same arm.

Reaction time helps people avoid obstacles when riding bikes or driving cars. Sprinters, baseball batters, and drag racers need very good reaction time to be successful.

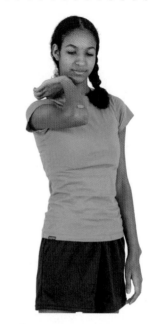

This challenge focuses on reaction time.

Lesson 1.2

Developing Physical and Health Literacy

Lesson Objectives

After participating in this lesson, you should be able to

1. define health and physical literacy,
2. explain why physical and health literacy are important, and
3. list the characteristics of a physically educated person.

Lesson Vocabulary

health education, health literacy, physical education, physical literacy

Imagine that you have graduated from high school and you are living the life that you have dreamed about. What are you doing? Who are you with? How does this vision make you feel?

Now imagine that it's Friday morning and you receive a text that says a bunch of your friends are going camping at the lake for the weekend. You quickly text back "I'm in!" You pack up your swimsuit, towel, warm clothes for sitting by the fire, some food and drinks, sunglasses, sunscreen, sleeping bag, and tent. Is there anything else you need? Maybe you need to charge your phone and bring your portable speakers? What about a good book or magazine? What about a deck of cards or a volleyball? After you pack, you drive over to a friend's place, load more gear into your car, and drive to the meeting spot. When you arrive, your group of friends is all there. Now you need to hike into the camping area; it's a secret spot that you have been going to for years. After the hike in, you start to set up camp. The fire pit is still there and you begin to collect wood, chop kindling, get the tents set up, and make your camping spot comfortable. It's only 5 p.m., so you all decide to head to the lake for a swim. Some people jump right in, others wade in slowly, and a few stay on shore to read magazines and play volleyball. After some beach time, you all head back to the camp and get the fire started, cook food, play some cards, and talk and laugh. After a great day and a late night you put your head on your pillow inside your warm tent and think about how lucky you are. You still have another day or two at the lake with your friends, so there's a lot to look forward to.

Maybe your vision of a great weekend happens in the city. Maybe you look forward to different experiences. Whatever visions you hold for the future, it is important to realize that you will have those experiences in your body. Human bodies are amazing and you will need to use yours for the rest of your life. Consider all of the physical activities you engaged in on the camping trip just described; texting, driving, hiking, constructing a tent, gathering and splitting firewood, swimming, volleyball, cooking, eating, and playing cards. Having a healthy body is an important part of participating fully in life whether on a camping trip with friends, going to school, or going to work. You probably know what it feels like to be injured, sick, and unable to participate fully in life. An active and healthy lifestyle gives you the best chance to participate fully in life. People who develop the skills, knowledge, and attitudes to more easily live active and healthy lifestyles are considered to have **physical literacy** and **health literacy**.

What Is Physical Literacy?

Literacy refers to being educated or "cultured." Early definitions of literacy referred only to the ability to read and write. The definitions of literacy have been expanded to include other skills, such as quantitative (i.e., math literacy), computer and technical (i.e., computer literacy), health and hygiene (i.e., health literacy), and physical (i.e., physical literacy). The types of literacy apply to all subject matter areas, including the sciences, the humanities, the arts, math, **health education**, and physical education. **Physical education** is the one subject in school that is primarily dedicated to helping you develop physical literacy.

Canada has a definition of physical literacy that was approved by a number of different Canadian organizations. All of the organizations encourage regular physical activity, including involvement in physical education and sports. The Canadian definition was adopted from the International Physical Literacy Association (IPLA) and states, "physical literacy can be described as the motivation, confidence, physical competence, knowledge and understanding to value and take responsibility for engagement in physical activities for life." This definition focuses on lifelong physical activity.

Physical and Health Education Canada, an organization of physical and health educators, has endorsed the Canadian consensus definition of physical literacy but also has an alternate definition: "Individuals who are physically literate move with competence and confidence in a wide variety of physical activities in multiple environments that benefit the healthy development of the whole person." Table 1.1 provides some examples of the characteristics of a physically literate individual. Fitness for Life Canada is designed to help each individual achieve all characteristics of a physically literate person.

It is important to recognize that the characteristics of a physically literate person are interdependent.

That is, they affect one another. For example, as you increase your knowledge about the health benefits of physical activity, you are more likely to have a positive attitude toward physical activity. If you have a positive attitude toward physical activity, you will probably go out and participate more often and develop your skills. As you participate more often and develop your skills, you are likely to become more knowledgeable about that activity, more physically fit, and more motivated to continue with participation.

> " Individuals who are physically literate move with competence and confidence in a wide variety of physical activities in multiple environments that benefit the healthy development of the whole person. "
>
> —Mandigo, Francis, Lodewyk, & Lopez, 2009, *Physical Literacy for Educators* (Physical and Health Education Canada)

TABLE 1.1 Characteristics of a Physically Literate Individual and Examples of Each Characteristic

Characteristic	Examples for an adolescent
Demonstrates physical competence	• Has the basic skills to participate in a variety of individual sports, team sports, and recreational activities and can create a practice plan to improve performance for self-selected skills • Has the ability to participate in activities on land, on snow or ice, in the air, and in the water • Has a healthful level of physical fitness
Demonstrates knowledge and understanding of, and the ability to apply, concepts, principles, strategies, and tactics related to movement and performance	• Understands the health and psychological benefits of physical activity • Understands concepts and principles of movement that enhance motor skill performance • Understands strategies and tactics that enable successful participation in sports and other physical activities • Understands the risk of having marginal health-related fitness levels and living a sedentary life • Has learned a variety of self-management skills that enable effective personal physical activity program planning and that contribute to maintaining a lifelong active healthy life (e.g., self-assessment, goal setting, self-planning, self-monitoring, time management)
Values and takes responsibility for engagement in physical activity for life	• Appreciates the value of physical activity for living a healthy, engaged life • Demonstrates the ability to make informed personal decisions relating to physical activity and to take personal responsibility for healthy behaviours
Is confident in physical activity and in personal decisions that relate to active healthy living	• Exhibits confidence in a variety of physical activities • Exhibits confidence in personal decisions that relate to active healthy living
Is motivated to participate in lifelong physical activity	• Is motivated to learn basic skills, to become physically fit, to improve knowledge and understanding, and to value and take responsibility for engaging in physical activity

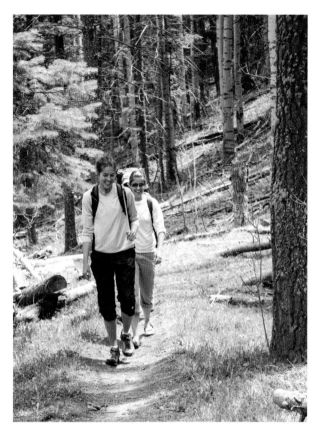

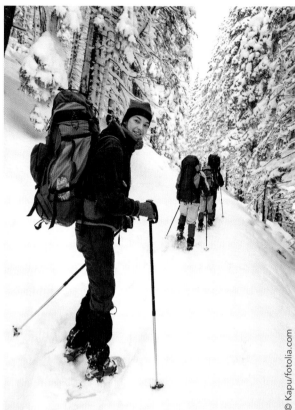

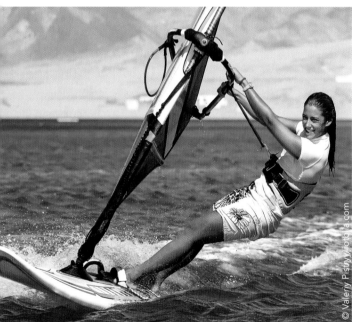

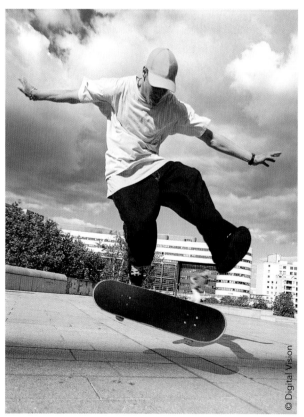

Being able to move confidently and competently on land, on snow or ice, in water, and in the air is an important part of physical literacy.

What Is Health Literacy?

The Public Health Agency of Canada defines health literacy as the ability to access, comprehend, evaluate, and communicate information as a way to promote, maintain, and improve health in a variety of settings across the life course. The Fitness for Life Canada program will help you develop both physical and health literacy. For example, in the first lesson of this chapter you learned about the definitions of health and wellness. You also learned about the five components of health and wellness. In upcoming chapters you will read about and engage in learning experiences about health topics such as nutrition, managing stress, substance use and abuse, and sexual reproduction. Many experts believe that adolescence is a critical stage for developing health literacy because of the rapid physical, social, and psychological changes that occur during the teenage years.

Why Are Physical and Health Literacy Important?

It is important to recognize that everyone is on his or her own path to developing physical and health literacy and will acquire and be able to apply their skills, knowledge, and attitudes at different times. Individuals with physical and health literacy lead active and healthy lifestyles and are happier, are healthier, and have a higher quality of life than people who do not have physical and health literacy. You might be thinking that you are as healthy and happy as you want to be. That's great! You might also think that you have a lot of the skills necessary to be considered physically and health literate. That's great too. However, scientific research clearly shows that as teenagers move into adulthood they become less physically active, begin to lose physical fitness, and gain weight. Low activity and fitness levels

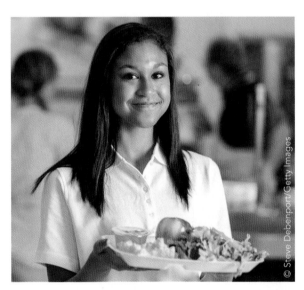

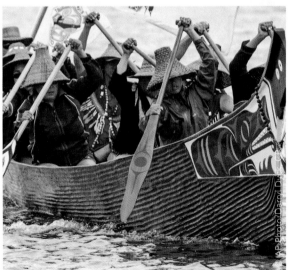

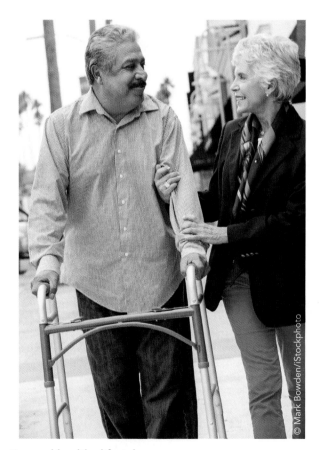

Health and physical literacy skills will help you lead an active and healthy lifestyle.

combined with weight gain are a leading cause of disease and death among adults. In a few short years you will graduate from high school and take the next step in your life's journey. No one will be telling you what to eat, what to wear, how to act, or who to hang out with. You get to make those decisions, and it will be helpful to have some tools to live a healthy and fulfilling life. One way to prepare yourself for living an active and healthy adult life is to make an effort to develop your physical and health literacy in health and physical education classes in school.

How Can I Develop Physical and Health Literacy?

You are lucky that you have a health and physical education teacher who has chosen to use the Fitness for Life Canada program. This program was designed to help you acquire and apply the knowledge, skills, and attitudes to develop your own personal healthy lifestyle plan whether you like to bike, climb, dance, grow vegetables, participate in gymnastics, hunt, play hockey, play lacrosse, run, skateboard, snowboard, swim, play soccer, walk, or participate in Zumba. Learning specific kinds of knowledge, skills, and attitudes contributes toward your physical and health literacy and helps you as

you plan your personal program. For example, the Fitness for Life Canada program helps you develop essential decision-making skills that will help you move from dependence on others for fitness, health, and wellness toward independence. The Stairway to Lifetime Fitness (see figure 1.4) illustrates how learning self-management skills such as self-assessing fitness, physical activity, and healthy eating; finding social support; and goal setting can help you move from having others make decisions for you to making good decisions on your own. Fitness for Life Canada was also designed to help you learn about making healthy choices related to nutrition, stress management, and substance abuse. Engaging in the Fitness for Life Canada program, as well as participating fully in health and physical education, physical activity, school or community sports, and healthy eating, represents an important step in the development of your physical and health literacy. Whatever you like to do, wherever you live, and whatever job you end up working in, the Fitness for Life Canada program will help you make good decisions and plans for active and healthy living. Developing physical and health literacy does not stop after you complete your school health and physical education classes. Developing physical and health literacy is a lifetime pursuit. We all change as we grow older, so you will need to develop new knowledge, skills, and attitudes to remain an active and healthy adult.

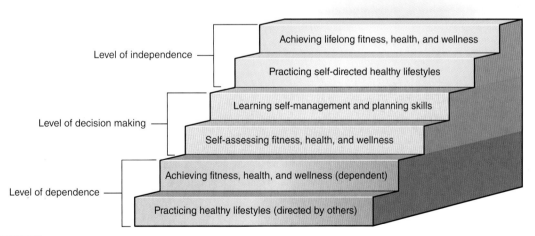

FIGURE 1.4 The Stairway to Lifetime Fitness, Health, and Wellness.

Lesson Review
1. What is the definition of physical literacy? What is the definition of health literacy?
2. What are some benefits of developing physical and health literacy?
3. What are the five characteristics of a physically educated person?

TAKING CHARGE: Learning to Self-Assess

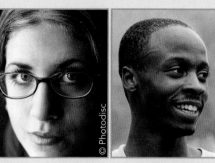

Self-management skills help you adopt a healthy lifestyle both now and throughout life. Self-assessment is a type of self-management skill that enables you to test yourself to see what you can do. You can perform many kinds of self-assessment. For example, you can assess your physical fitness, eating patterns, stress level, health risks, knowledge, and ability to perform in a sport or a recreational activity. This book includes many self-assessments focused on physical fitness, as well as some that address health, wellness, and healthy lifestyle choices. The following example focuses on health-related physical fitness.

Julia and Trey were friends who wanted to know more about their health-related physical fitness. They had taken fitness tests in school but had learned little about why they were doing the tests or how to test themselves. They wanted to learn how to assess their own fitness.

Julia remembered some of the tests she had taken in elementary school, such as running a 40-metre dash and performing something called a "shuttle run." Trey had not taken a fitness test in physical education, but he had been tested for his baseball team to see how far he could throw a ball and how fast he could run to first base.

Julia and Trey thought about doing a self-assessment that included all of the tests Julia had been given in school and all of the tests Trey had done for his baseball team. But they weren't sure how to do the tests in the correct way, and they weren't sure that these were the best tests. What they really wanted to learn was how to do a self-assessment for health-related physical fitness.

For Discussion

Do you think the tests Julia performed in elementary school assessed health-related physical fitness? Why or why not? Do you think the tests Trey performed for his baseball team measured health-related physical fitness? Why or why not? What do you think the tests they performed really measured? Discuss a plan of self-assessment that Julia and Trey could follow to determine their health-related physical fitness.

The guidelines in the following Self-Management feature will help you as you answer the discussion questions and will be useful as you try the various self-assessments included in this book.

SELF-MANAGEMENT: Skills for Learning to Self-Assess

Before you go on a road trip, you probably use a map provided by Google maps or a global positioning system (GPS) to make plans. The map helps you decide where you want to go. Assessing your own fitness is much like using a map. You can assess your current fitness and physical activity in order to help you learn where you need to improve and make your plans for doing so. You can also use the assessment information to develop strategies and tactics to commit to your plan. Use the following guidelines as you learn to do personal fitness and activity self-assessments.

- **Try a wide variety of tests.** Fitness and physical activity include many parts, and performing a variety of self-assessments

enables you to get a total picture of your fitness and activity needs. You will learn various self-assessment techniques in this class.

- **Choose self-assessments that work best for you.** You'll try all the self-assessments you learn in this book, but ultimately you won't need to use them all. You should choose at least one assessment for each type of health-related physical fitness and one assessment to determine your current activity level. After you've tried many self-assessments, you'll be prepared to select the ones that meet your current needs.

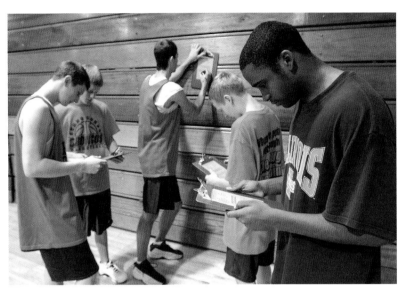
Learning to assess your own fitness is an important life skill.

- **Practice.** When you first started texting, it wasn't easy, but your skill improved with practice. Similarly, the first time you do self-assessments, you'll make mistakes, but the more you practice, the better you'll get. So, once you decide which assessments to use on a regular basis, practice using them!

- **Use self-assessments for personal improvement.** Once you've learned to use self-assessments, repeat them from time to time to monitor your progress. Avoid making assessments too often, but check yourself periodically to see how you're doing. It takes several weeks to see improvement in health-related physical fitness after starting a new activity program. Avoid daily or even weekly self-assessments in favour of self-assessing after several weeks when improvement is more likely.

- **Use health standards rather than comparing yourself with others.** Sometimes people are discouraged when they get test results, often because they had unrealistic expectations. Rather than comparing yourself with others, evaluate yourself in relation to health standards and to your own previous performances. This type of comparison helps you stay realistic. The standards used in this book are based on the level of fitness needed for good health and wellness—not on comparisons of one person with another.

- **Information from self-assessments is personal.** Self-assessments are done to gain information that will help you build an accurate personal profile and plan for healthy active living. In many assessments you will work with a partner. Partners must agree to keep test results confidential. Information may be submitted to an instructor, parent, or guardian—again with the expectation that information is kept private. Information should not be shared with others without the permission of the person being tested. Think of doing a self-assessment as like hiring a personal trainer. A certified personal trainer would have you do a series of tests to determine your strengths and weaknesses and then work with you to come up with a plan to meet your goals. The personal trainer should keep your information totally confidential.

One key component of physical literacy is learning movement skills. In fact, before you can perform complex and sport-specific movement skills (e.g., kicking a soccer ball, performing a trick on a skateboard, hitting a tennis forehand, catching a lacrosse ball), you need to learn the fundamental movement skills. Fundamental movement skills include kicking, striking (objects), throwing, catching, jumping, and running. When you are confident and competent with these fundamental movement skills, you can develop sport-specific and complex movement skills that allow you to enjoy sport and physical activity. Most importantly, having a firm grasp of the fundamental movement skills will help you enjoy a long life of physical activity. You will take action here by performing a circuit of fundamental movement skills with your teacher. After you have tried the different stations, you can reflect on your performance and identify the fundamental movement skills that you need to work on and those that you have mastered.

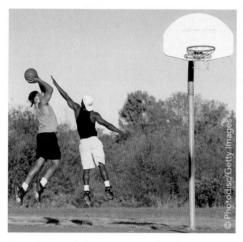 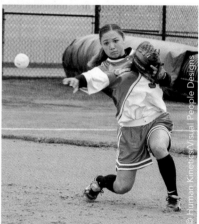

Jumping and throwing are fundamental movement skills used in many different activities.

GET ACTIVE WITH PHE CANADA

©Physical and Health Education Canada

Who We Are

Physical and Health Education Canada (PHE Canada) is a national not-for-profit organization supporting the healthy development of children and youth by advocating for, increasing access to, and developing programs and resources to support the delivery of high-quality health education, physical education, and sport programming. Established in 1933, PHE Canada strives to have all children and youth live physically active and healthy lives now and in their future.

What We Do

PHE Canada works with your teachers, coaches, and recreation leaders and develops fun and educational programs, resources, and activities to help you achieve your personal goals and be your best self. PHE Canada wants you to be happy and healthy. That means helping you develop the skills to participate in sports or any physical activities you have an interest in, understand the importance of proper nutrition, and establish positive self-esteem and mental resiliency.

Our experienced staff and expert advisors ensure that our programs, resources and activities are appropriate for your age level yet challenging to help you improve; meet the highest standards of educational content to ensure optimal understanding and knowledge transfer; and, perhaps most important, are fun and engaging so you are excited and have a positive experience toward living a healthy, active lifestyle.

Get Involved

PHE Canada has a variety of programs, resources, and activities for children of all ages. We invite you, your parents, your teachers, your coaches, and your recreation leaders to learn more about us. Visit PHECanada on the web at www.phecanada.ca, Facebook at www.facebook.com/PHECanada, and Twitter at @PHECanada.

Reprinted, by permission, from Jordan Burwash. ©Physical and Health Education Canada.

Reviewing Concepts and Vocabulary

Complete the following in order to determine your growing understanding of fitness, health, and wellness. Answer items 1 through 5 by correctly completing each sentence with a word or phrase.

1. A _____ person is an individual who moves with competence and confidence in a wide variety of physical activities in multiple environments that benefit the healthy development of the whole person.

2. A physically educated person is a person who participates regularly in _____.

3. Health literacy is the ability to _____, comprehend, evaluate, and communicate information as a way to promote, maintain, and improve health in a variety of settings across the life course.

4. Individuals with physical and health literacy are healthier and _____, and have a higher quality of life than people who do not have physical and health literacy.

5. Engaging in the Fitness for Life Canada program, as well as participating fully in health and physical education, physical activity, school or community sports, and _____, comprises an important step in the development of your physical and health literacy.

For items 6 through 10, match each term in column 1 with the appropriate phrase in column 2.

6. muscular endurance   a. movement of the body using larger muscles
7. agility   b. positive component of health
8. physical fitness   c. ability to change body position quickly
9. physical activity   d. ability of your body systems to work together efficiently
10. wellness   e. ability to use muscles continuously without tiring

For items 11 through 15, respond to each statement or question.
11. List the five components of health and wellness.
12. Describe how fitness, health, and wellness are interrelated.
13. How do health-related physical fitness and skill-related physical fitness differ?
14. What is the value of a fitness self-assessment?
15. What are some important guidelines for using self-assessments?

Thinking Critically

Write a paragraph to answer the following question.

What health-related and skill-related fitness components improve performance, enjoyment, and confidence in your favourite activity, sport, or occupation (i.e., job)? List at least five components of fitness. For each component, identify whether it is a health- or skill-related fitness component and explain why it is important.

Project

In this chapter we present one interpretation of health and wellness. Use the Internet to learn about other cultures' perspectives on well-being and health. For example, examine health and wellness from the perspective of Aboriginal peoples in Canada or another country. Pick a culture to focus on and compare and contrast the five components of health and wellness presented in this chapter with the components identified in another culture.

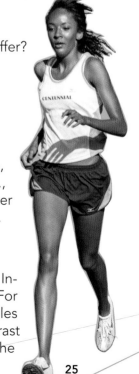

2

Adopting Healthy Lifestyles and Self-Management Skills

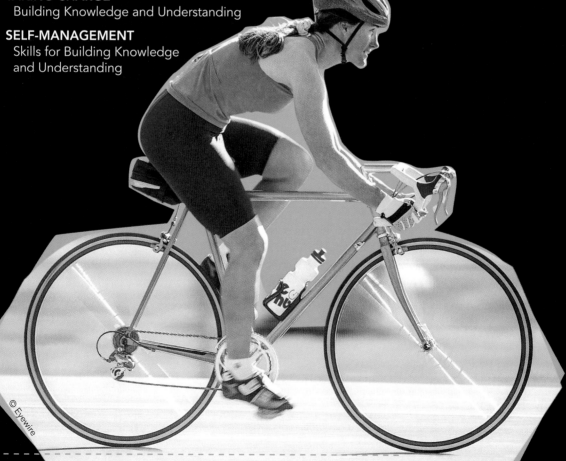

© Eyewire

Lesson 2.1
Adopting Healthy Lifestyles

Lesson Objectives

After participating in this lesson, you should be able to

1. name and describe the five types of determinants of fitness, health, and wellness;
2. name and describe the five benefits of a healthy lifestyle; and
3. explain the Stairway to Lifetime Fitness, Health, and Wellness and how it can be used.

Lesson Vocabulary

determinant, priority healthy lifestyle choice, self-management skill, state of being

Do you consider yourself healthy? Do you think you have good fitness? How would you rate your overall wellness? Let's take a moment to consider the nature of fitness, health, and wellness. Each is a **state of being** that an individual person can possess to his or her benefit and that of those around them. If you possess fitness, you can more easily complete daily tasks and meet the challenges of life in a positive way. If you possess health and wellness, you are free from disease and can enjoy a good quality of life. These states are interrelated, so if you do something to change one, you affect the others. Your fitness, health, and wellness are also affected by many other factors. Medical and scientific experts refer to these factors as **determinants**.

> " I guess that one of the most important things I've learned is that nothing is ever completely bad. Even cancer. It has made me a better person. It has given me courage and a sense of purpose I never had before. But you don't have to do like I did . . . wait until you lose a leg or get some awful disease, before you take the time to find out what kind of stuff you're really made of. You can start now. Anybody can. "

—Terry Fox, Canadian athlete, humanitarian, and cancer research activist

Determinants of Fitness, Health, and Wellness

As shown in figure 2.1, your fitness, health, and wellness are affected by five types of determinants: (1) personal, (2) environmental, (3) health care, (4) social and individual, and (5) healthy lifestyle choices. Some are more within your control than others. The figure shows the determinant types in varying shades of orange—the lighter the colour, the less control you have; the darker the colour, the more control.

Personal Determinants

You have relatively little control, or none at all, over personal determinants, such as heredity, age, sex, and disability; thus they are shaded in light orange in the figure. Nonetheless, these factors can greatly affect your fitness, health, and wellness. For example, a person might inherit genes that put him or her at risk for certain diseases, and disease risk also increases with age. Sex is also a factor. For example, males, especially after the teen years, tend to have more muscle than females do. As for age, up to a certain point in life, muscles grow, and some parts of fitness improve just because of normal changes in the body. We also know that women have a longer life expectancy than men. Another potential factor is disability, which can affect a person's capacity to perform certain tasks but does not necessarily affect her or his health or quality of life.

You'll learn more about personal determinants and their effects on fitness, health, and wellness in other chapters of this book. Although you cannot

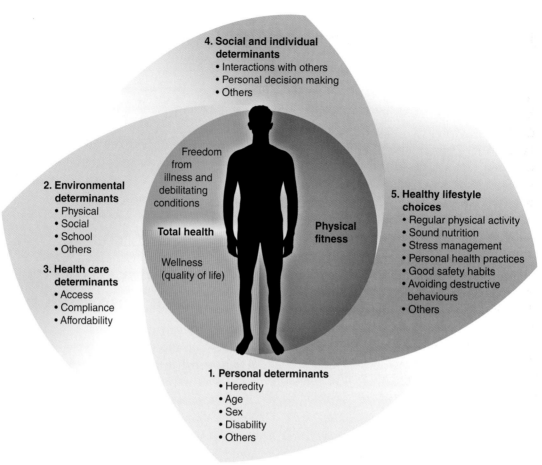

4. Social and individual determinants
• Interactions with others
• Personal decision making
• Others

Freedom from illness and debilitating conditions

Total health

Wellness (quality of life)

2. Environmental determinants
• Physical
• Social
• School
• Others

3. Health care determinants
• Access
• Compliance
• Affordability

Physical fitness

5. Healthy lifestyle choices
• Regular physical activity
• Sound nutrition
• Stress management
• Personal health practices
• Good safety habits
• Avoiding destructive behaviours
• Others

1. Personal determinants
• Heredity
• Age
• Sex
• Disability
• Others

FIGURE 2.1 The five determinants of fitness, health, and wellness.

Based on C. Corbin et al., 2013, *Concepts of fitness and wellness: A comprehensive lifestyle approach*, 10th ed. (St. Louis, MO: McGraw-Hill).

FIT FACT

A disability is an objective condition (i.e., physical or mental impairment). Adapted physical educators and health professionals adapt activities, equipment, and environments to ensure that people with disabilities can pursue physical activity. For example, a person with a hearing impairment (i.e., disability) can play ice hockey, and a person with one leg (i.e., disability) can still go snow skiing. We are all physically different, and various personal determinants affect what you can and cannot do. Understanding your own strengths and limitations helps you be the best you can be and allows you to help others be the best they can be.

control personal determinants, you can be aware of them. Being aware can help you decide to alter other determinants over which you do have control, such as healthy lifestyle choices.

Environmental and Health Care Determinants

Fitness, health, and wellness are also affected by environmental and health care determinants. In figure 2.1, they are coloured in a darker shade of orange than the personal determinants because you have more control over them. For example, as an adult, you can choose to live or work in a healthy environment; you can also recycle in order to help protect the environment. There are other ways you can take action to improve the environment but, of course, there are limits on your control. For example, you cannot directly control the quality of the air in your neighbourhood. Environmental determinants are discussed throughout this book.

SCIENCE IN ACTION: Heredity and Fitness, Health, and Wellness

Exercise physiologists have studied human genes to determine whether heredity plays a role in fitness, health, and wellness. Their studies show that the genes we inherit from our parents do make a difference. For example, some people inherit genes that make them more likely to have a specific disease; other genes make it more likely that a person will be able to build muscle mass. And of course genes make a difference in how tall you are and how much you weigh. Recently, scientists have also discovered that, because of genetics, people respond differently to exercise. They learned this by studying groups of people who all did the same exercise. Despite performing the same exercise program, some people benefited more than others. This is how researchers identified the role of heredity in fitness (a personal determinant).

Even though heredity surely makes a difference in your fitness, health, and wellness, scientists also emphasize that making healthy lifestyle choices can help counteract heredity. Early in life, heredity plays a major role in your health, fitness, and wellness. However, people who practice a healthy lifestyle throughout life are among the healthiest people regardless of their heredity. What you inherit matters, but over the long haul what you do can be even more important to being healthy, fit, and well.

Student Activity

In the preceding chapter on fitness, health, and physical literacy we learned about health-related fitness. Choose one part of health-related fitness and describe how your own heredity influences it.

Health care refers to being able to see a doctor or other health care professional as needed and having access to health care facilities and medicine. Health care also includes opportunities to learn about prevention of illness and promotion of wellness. People who receive good health care live longer and have higher-quality lives compared to those who don't. This factor is shown in a darker shade of orange because you have some control over it. Having access to good health care, seeking health care when it's needed, and complying with health care recommendations are all important to your health and wellness.

Social and Individual Determinants

As an individual in a free society, you have the freedom to make choices and decisions that affect your fitness, health, and wellness. For example, you choose your friends and make decisions about how you interact with them, and these social choices make a difference. Teens who choose friends who avoid destructive habits and practice healthy ones are more likely to be fit, healthy, and well themselves. Individual determinants are also important. Being a good consumer—for example, by using

good information to choose healthy foods—is a way each individual can contribute to good fitness, health, and wellness. In figure 2.1, social and individual determinants are coloured in a relatively dark shade of orange because you can exercise a lot of control over the choices you make, both as an individual and with your friends and other people. Personal decision making and peer interactions are discussed in the special features titled Taking Charge throughout this book.

Healthy Lifestyle Choices

By far the most important determinants of your fitness, health, and wellness are your lifestyle choices. A healthy lifestyle is made up of behaviours that you adopt to improve your fitness, health, and wellness. Because you generally have a lot of control over these determinants, they are coloured in dark orange in figure 2.1. With good information and good **self-management skills**, you can adopt each of the healthy lifestyle behaviours illustrated in the figure. Self-management skills help you become more active and eat better; they also help you adapt well in stressful situations. You'll learn more about self-management skills in lesson 2.

Adopting a healthy lifestyle gives you many benefits. First, it reduces your risk of disease and early death. In fact, about three of every five early deaths result from unhealthy lifestyle choices. Healthy choices, on the other hand, can help you prevent and treat various illnesses. For example, eating well and being active can help prevent heart disease and manage diabetes. You might assume that because illness and disease are more common in later life, you don't have to worry about them now. You might even share an attitude that is common among teenagers: "I'm young and healthy; it can't happen to me." But evidence indicates that the disease process begins early in life. Therefore, choosing and adopting a healthy lifestyle early in your life can do a lot to prevent disease and illness later on.

FIT FACT

Smokers lose, on average, 13 to 14 years of life because of smoking.

Benefits of a Healthy Lifestyle for Teens

Living a healthy lifestyle helps you not only later in life—you can also enjoy many benefits now. Examples include looking your best and feeling good, learning better, enjoying daily life, and effectively handling emergencies.

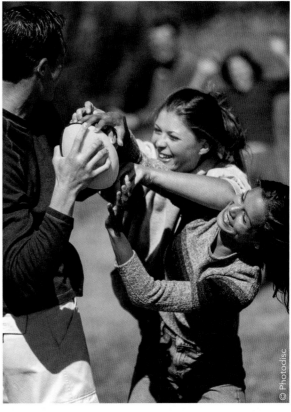

Regular physical activity can help you feel good on the inside and outside.

Feeling Good (Inside and Out)

People who do regular physical activity feel better on the inside. If you're active and therefore physically fit, you can resist fatigue, you're less likely to be injured, and you're capable of working more efficiently. National surveys indicate that active people sleep better, do better in school, and experience less depression than people who are less active. Research indicates that regular activity can increase brain chemicals called endorphins that give you a sensation of feeling great after exercise such as running. You can also help yourself feel your best by eating well and managing stress wisely (for diet and stress management strategies, see the separate chapters on nutrition and stress). Experts also agree that regular physical activity is one healthy lifestyle

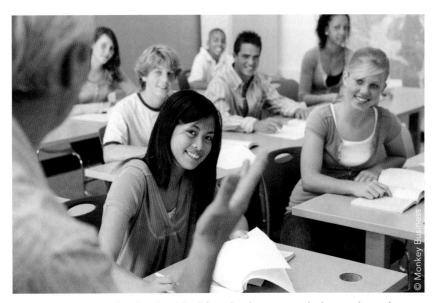

Physical activity and other healthy lifestyle choices can help you learn better.

choice that can help you feel good about yourself on the outside by looking your best. Other ways to feel good inside and out are proper nutrition, good posture, and good body mechanics.

Learning Better

Did you know that in recent years scientists have proven that you learn better if you are active, eat well, get enough sleep, and manage stress effectively? More specifically, studies show that teens who are active and fit score better on tests and are less likely to be absent from school. In addition, teens who are active and eat regular healthy meals, especially breakfast, are more alert at school and less likely to be tired in the classroom. And recent studies show that regular exercise and good fitness are associated with high function in the parts of the brain that promote learning. So being fit applies to your brain as well.

Enjoying Life

Everyone wants to enjoy life. But what if you're too tired on most days to participate in the activities

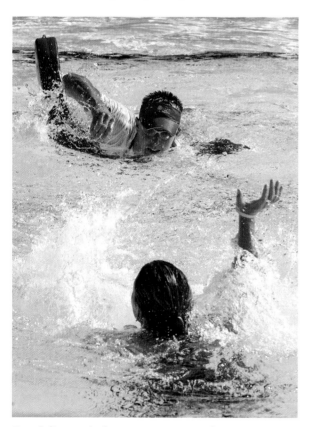

Good fitness helps you to respond in emergency situations.

you really like? Regular physical activity increases your physical fitness, which is the key to being able to do more of the things you want to do. People who are fit, healthy, and well are able to enjoy life to the fullest.

Meeting Emergencies

Sometimes challenging situations arise suddenly in life. You can prepare yourself to meet emergencies, as well as day-to-day demanding situations, by engaging in regular physical activity and making other healthy lifestyle choices. For example, if you're physically fit and active, you'll be able to run for help, change a flat tire, and offer various kinds of assistance to others as needed.

Program Overview

Throughout this book, you'll learn how determinants influence your fitness, health, and wellness. We focus especially on three **priority healthy lifestyle choices** that are very important in helping you prevent disease, get and remain fit, and enjoy a good quality of life. These three choices are regular physical activity, sound nutrition, and effective stress management. The fact that these are choices means, of course, that they are largely in your control.

Stairway to Lifetime Fitness, Health, and Wellness

Do you live a healthy lifestyle? Do you eat well? If you eat meals at home, you are more likely to eat well, but will you continue doing so when you're on your own? Are you physically active? Many teens are. But will you remain active as you grow older? Will you do the same kinds of activity you do now? If you answered no to any of these questions, you need to begin developing a lifetime plan for practicing a healthy lifestyle. One way to accomplish this goal is to climb what is called the Stairway to Lifetime Fitness, Health, and Wellness. As you can see in figure 2.2, when you climb this stairway, you move from a level of dependence to a level of independence. You move from having others make decisions for you to making positive decisions on your own.

Step 1: Making Healthy Lifestyle Choices—Directed by Others

Think about the way you eat, the various physical activities you're involved in, and your other lifestyle practices—even simple things such as brushing your teeth. When you were a kid, other people made most decisions about your lifestyle at home, at school, and in the community. As you've grown older, you've started making more decisions for yourself. Ultimately, you'll be almost totally responsible for making your own decisions. In the not so distant future, school programs will no longer serve as your incentive to exercise, and other opportunities for physical activity will probably decrease. You'll also choose your own food. Living out the healthy lifestyle choices made for you (or facilitated) by other people is a good first step, but it's up to you to keep climbing the stairway.

Step 2: Achieving Fitness, Health, and Wellness—Dependent

The first step is about taking action based on what others expect. If you stick with the healthy living practices described in step 1, you will improve your fitness, health, and wellness (step 2). The resulting fitness, health, and wellness that you enjoy are dependent on others. In other words, you are not primarily responsible; others are. For example, if you get fit because of exercise prescribed by coaches and physical education teachers, you are dependent on them for the benefit you gain from the exercise.

You may also eat well because of choices made by a parent who buys the food and prepares most or all of your meals. It's good that others help you to be active and adopt healthy lifestyles (step 1). It's also good when these lifestyles lead to fitness, health, and wellness (step 2). But it's not until you move to the third step on the stairway that you begin to make your own decisions.

Step 3: Self-Assessment

Self-assessments help you set appropriate goals, make positive decisions, and become more independent. A self-assessment is an evaluation that you make of yourself. You can evaluate (self-assess) your fitness, health, and wellness, as well as the lifestyle choices that produce them. In each chapter of this book, you'll try many kinds of self-assessments. Once you learn to self-assess, you'll have reached the third step on the stairway. You can use the skill of self-assessment throughout your life to help you develop and implement your lifetime plan.

Step 4: Self-Management Skills and Self-Planning

Self-management skills help you implement healthy lifestyle choices that lead to good fitness, health, and wellness. One self-management skill was discussed in the previous step—self-assessment—and many others are discussed throughout this book (one per chapter). A brief introduction to these self-management skills is provided in the next lesson of

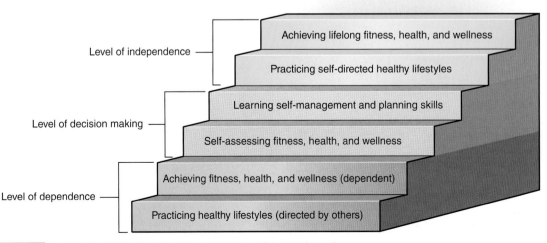

FIGURE 2.2 The Stairway to Lifetime Fitness, Health, and Wellness.

FITNESS TECHNOLOGY: Surf the Net for Self-Assessments

The Internet contains numerous sites that provide instructions for health- and skill-related fitness assessments. You can also find self-assessments for physical activity, healthy eating, sleep, and almost any other health behaviour you can imagine. YouTube is a great place to find videos of different self-assessments that require you to perform activity. The online student web resource also provides some videos of health-related fitness assessments. If you want to self-assess your physical activity level, a lot of free web-based applications are available. Within this textbook are instructions for several fitness, nutrition, and health self-assessments. By the end of the Fitness

for Life Canada program, you should be able to create a personalized self-assessment of your fitness and health that reflects your unique interests.

> ## Using Technology
>
> Surf online for the terms "free fitness assessments" or "fitness test battery" and look at some of the resources that are available. Compare some of the fitness assessments to the fitness assessments throughout this book. Look for similarities and differences. In many cases you will find calculators that will compute your fitness score after you have performed a test.

this chapter. After you've learned a variety of self-management skills, you'll be equipped to move on to the next step of the stairway.

Step 5: Practicing a Self-Directed Healthy Lifestyle

With this step, you will move to the level of decision making and problem solving. You'll have learned why fitness, health, and wellness are important, what your personal needs are, and how to plan for a lifetime. Because no two people have identical needs, no two people will have exactly the same program. But you will now have the necessary tools (self-management skills) to succeed in independent planning. You'll be able to develop your own personal fitness, health, and wellness programs by implementing the healthy choices discussed in this book. In a way, then, this step is much like the first step in the stairway, but now you're making your own decisions instead of having other people make decisions for you.

Step 6: Achieving Lifelong Fitness, Health, and Wellness

When you reach the top step of the stairway, you will have taken responsibility for your own lifetime fitness, health, and wellness. You'll have moved from depending on others to making independent decisions, and you'll now implement the programs you developed in the previous step. You'll continue to use self-assessment and other self-management skills (such as self-monitoring) to modify your plans as your needs and interests change. You'll also use other self-management skills to overcome barriers that might prevent you from sticking to your plan.

Making Healthy Lifestyle Choices

This book and this class are designed to help you make healthy lifestyle choices that enable you to achieve lifetime fitness, health, and wellness. In the remaining chapters, you'll learn how to climb the stairway and reach the highest step.

Lesson Review

1. What are the five types of determinants of fitness, health, and wellness, and which are most within your personal control?
2. What are the major benefits of healthy lifestyle choices such as regular physical activity and good nutrition?
3. What is the Stairway to Lifetime Fitness, Health, and Wellness, and how can it be used?

In this book, you'll read about many physical fitness tests. The overall goal is to be able to select appropriate tests (self-assessments) to use both now and throughout your life. Several groups have developed physical fitness assessments specifically for young people. One of these, called FitnessGram, is the most widely used test battery in many countries. A test battery is a group of items designed to test several parts of fitness, and the FitnessGram test battery assesses various parts of health-related physical fitness.

 There are other test batteries in addition to FitnessGram. The Canadian Society for Exercise Physiology (CSEP) developed a health-related fitness test battery as part of their Physical Activity Training for Health (PATH) program. The CSEP-PATH test battery was developed for Canadians aged 15 to 69 years. CSEP-PATH contains some of the same tests as FitnessGram but also some different ones. For example, CSEP-PATH includes the modified Canadian Aerobic Fitness Test (mCAFT) and the vertical jump test. The Alpha-Fit test battery is another example of a fitness test battery for youth and adults that assesses health-related fitness. Alpha-Fit was developed in Europe and, like FitnessGram, is used throughout the world. Alpha-Fit contains some of the same items as FitnessGram but

also some different ones. For example, Alpha-Fit includes the long jump and grip strength tests. These same two test items are included in the Institute of Medicine (IOM) Fitness Test Battery developed for youth fitness surveys in the United States. Recent research has shown a relationship between grip strength and long jump tests and good health.

Before using a physical fitness test, learn about the test and what it measures, then practice each test item that you plan to use. Practice helps you get better at taking the test properly so that you're truly measuring fitness rather than just learning test-taking skills. For best results, give your best effort when doing the self-assessment. For now, the goal is not to determine a score or rating on the test items but to practice the tests so that you know how to perform them properly. Because body composition assessments are not performance tests, they don't require practice and thus are not described here, but you'll learn more about them later.

If you're working with a partner, remember that self-assessment information is personal and confidential. It should not be shared with others without the permission of the person being tested. Record your results as directed by your teacher.

Test of Cardiorespiratory Endurance

PACER
(Progressive Aerobic Cardiovascular Endurance Run, or 20-Metre Shuttle Run)

This test is included in FitnessGram, Alpha-Fit, and the IOM Fitness Test Battery.

1. The test objective is to run back and forth across a 20-metre distance as many times as you can at a predetermined pace (pacing is based on signals from a special audio recording provided by your instructor).

2. Start at a line located 20 metres from a second line. When you hear the beep from the audio track, run across the 20-metre area to the second line, arriving just before the audio track beeps again, and touch the line with your foot. Turn around and get ready to run back.

3. At the sound of the next beep, run back to the line where you began. Touch the line with your foot. Make sure to wait for the beep before running back.

4. Continue to run back and forth from one line to the other, touching the line each time. The beeps will come faster and faster, causing you to run faster and faster. The test is finished when you twice fail to reach the opposite side before the beep.

Practice Tips

1. Practice running at the correct pace so that you arrive just before the beep that signals you to change directions.

2. Practice adjusting your pace as the beeps come faster and faster.

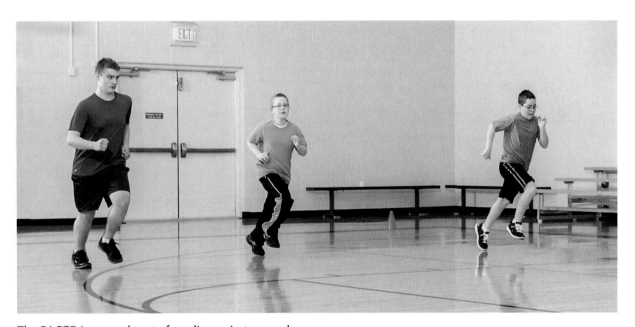

The PACER is a good test of cardiorespiratory endurance.

Tests of Muscle Fitness

Curl-Up (Abdominal Muscle Strength and Muscular Endurance)

This test is included in FitnessGram.

1. Lie on your back on a mat or carpet. Bend your knees approximately 140 degrees. Your feet should be slightly apart and as far as possible from your buttocks while still allowing your feet to be flat on the floor. (The closer your feet are to your buttocks, the more difficult the movement is.) Your arms should be straight and parallel to your trunk with your palms resting on the mat.

2. Place your head on a piece of paper. The paper will help your partner judge whether your head touches down on each repetition. Place a strip of cardboard (or rubber, plastic, or tape) 11.5 centimetres wide and 1 metre long under your knees so that the fingers of both hands just touch the near edge of the strip. You can tape the strip down or have a partner stand on it to keep it stationary.

3. Keeping your heels on the floor, curl your shoulders up slowly and slide your arms forward so that your fingers move across the cardboard strip. Curl up until your fingertips reach the far side of the strip.

4. Slowly lower your back until your head rests on the piece of paper.

5. Repeat this procedure so that you do one curl-up every three seconds. A partner can help you by saying "up, down" every three seconds.

Practice Tips

1. Practice keeping your buttocks and heels in the same location (that is, not moving them) as you do repetitions.

2. Practice doing one repetition (up, down) every three seconds.

3. Practice reaching to the end of the strip for each repetition.

4. Practice lowering your head to the mat on each repetition.

5. Next, practice as many repetitions as you can (up to 15). Have a partner check your form to make sure you are performing each curl-up correctly.

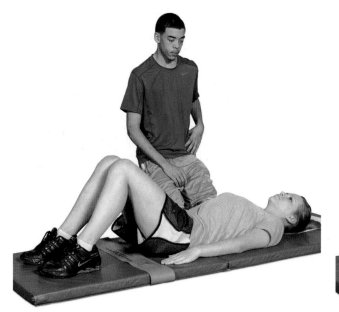 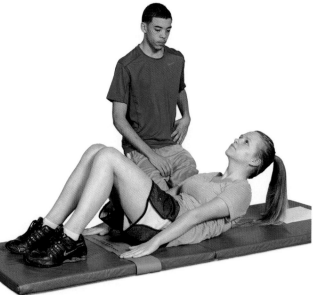

When properly performed, the curl-up is a good measure of muscle fitness of the abdominal muscles.

Push-Up (Upper Body Strength and Muscular Endurance)

This test is included in the CSEP-PATH test battery and FitnessGram.

1. Lie facedown on a mat or carpet with your hands (palm down) under your shoulders, your fingers spread, and your legs straight. Your legs should be slightly apart and your toes tucked under.

2. Push up until your arms are straight. Keep your legs and back straight. Your body should form a straight line from your head to your heels.

3. Lower your body by bending your elbows until your upper arms are parallel to the floor (elbows at a 90-degree angle), then push up until your arms are fully extended. Do one push-up every three seconds. You may want to have a partner say "up, down" every three seconds to help you.

Practice Tips

1. Practice lowering until your elbows are bent at 90 degrees. You may want to have a partner hold a yardstick parallel to the floor (at the elbow) to help you determine when your elbows are properly bent.

2. Practice pushing up all the way so that your arms are at full extension at the top of each push-up.

3. Practice doing one repetition (up, down) every three seconds.

4. Next, practice as many repetitions as you can (up to 15). Have a partner check your form to make sure you are performing each push-up correctly.

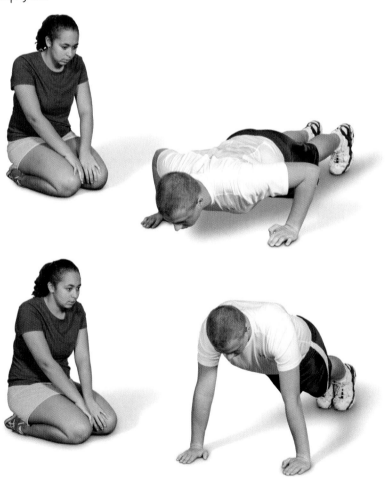

The 90-degree push-up is a measure of muscle fitness of the upper body.

Handgrip Strength (Isometric Hand and Arm Strength)

This test is included in the CSEP-PATH test battery, Alpha-Fit, and the IOM Fitness Test Battery.

1. Use a dynamometer to measure isometric strength. Adjust the dynamometer to fit your hand size.
2. Squeeze as hard as possible for two to five seconds. Your arm should be extended with your elbow nearly straight. Do not touch your body with your arm or hand.
3. Repeat with each hand. Alternate hands to allow a rest between each attempt.
4. Results are most often reported in kilograms.

Practice Tips

1. Try the grip at different settings to see which enables you to perform the best.
2. Try bending your knees a bit as you squeeze to help maintain good balance, which may help your score.

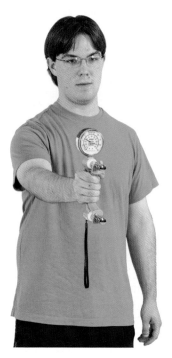

The handgrip strength test measures muscle fitness, and scores are related to total body strength.

Standing Long Jump (Leg Power, or Explosive Strength)

This test is included in Alpha-Fit and the IOM Fitness Test Battery.

1. Use masking tape or another material to make the necessary line on the floor.
2. Stand with your feet shoulder-width apart behind the line on the floor. Bend your knees and hold your arms straight in front of your body at shoulder height.
3. Swing your arms downward and backward, then vigorously forward as you jump forward as far as possible, extending your legs.
4. Land on both feet and try to maintain your balance on landing. Do not run or hop before jumping.

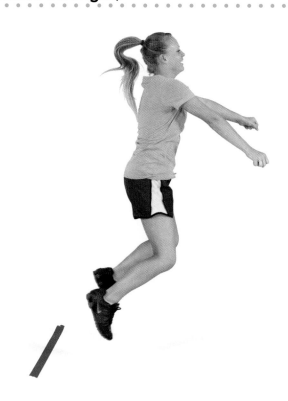

The standing long jump is a test of power (explosive strength).

Practice Tips

1. For best performance, lean forward just before you jump. Practice to get the best timing of the lean followed by the forward arm swing just before you jump.
2. Try the test several times so that you can land without losing your balance. To help you avoid falling when you land, keep your arms extended in front of you. Also bend your knees when you land to help you absorb the shock of landing and to help you maintain your balance.
3. Try bending your knees more or less before different jumps to see which amount of knee bend gives you the best jump.

Test of Muscle Fitness and Flexibility

Trunk Lift (Back Muscle Fitness and Back and Trunk Muscle Flexibility)

This test is included in FitnessGram.

1. Lie facedown with your arms at your sides and your hands under or just beside your thighs.
2. Lift the upper part of your body very slowly so that your chin, chest, and shoulders come off the floor. Lift your trunk as high as possible, to a maximum of 30 centimetres. Hold this position for three seconds while a partner measures how far your chin is from the floor. Your partner should hold the ruler at least 2.5 centimetres in front of your chin. Look straight ahead so that your chin is not tipped abnormally upward.

Caution: The ruler should not be placed directly under your chin, in case you have to lower your trunk unexpectedly.

Practice Tips

1. Practice lifting your trunk 30 centimetres off the floor. Hold the trunk off the floor at 30 centimetres (do not lift higher) for three seconds.
2. Practice three to five times to see if you are able to hold the lift for the required three seconds.
3. Practice looking straight ahead so that your chin is not tipped up.

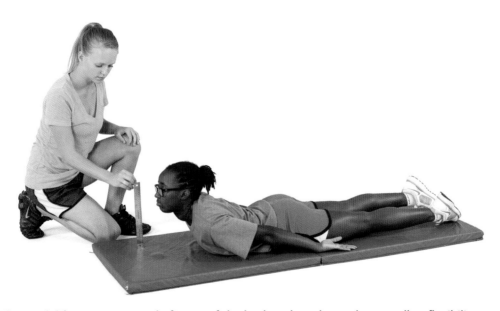

The trunk lift measures muscle fitness of the back and trunk muscles as well as flexibility.

Test of Flexibility

Back-Saver Sit and Reach (Range of Motion, or Flexibility, of the Hip)

This test is included in the CSEP-PATH test battery and FitnessGram.

1. Place a measuring stick, such as a yardstick or metre stick, on top of a box that is 30 centimetres high with the stick extending 23 centimetres over the box and the lower numbers toward you. You may use a flexibility testing box if one is available.

2. To measure the flexibility of your right leg, fully extend it and place your right foot flat against the box. Bend your left leg, with the knee turned out and your left foot 5 to 8 centimetres to the side of your straight right leg.

3. Extend your arms forward over the measuring stick. Place your hands on the stick, one on top of the other, with your palms facing down. Your middle fingers should be together with the tip of one finger exactly on top of the other.

4. Lean forward slowly; do not bounce. Reach forward with your arms and fingers, then slowly return to the starting position. Repeat four times. On the fourth reach, hold the position for three seconds and observe the measurement on the stick below your fingertips.

5. Repeat with your left leg.

Practice Tips

1. Do the PACER practice or another general warm-up before practicing this test.

2. Practice keeping your extended leg straight (a very slight bend is okay).

3. Practice keeping your other leg bent and the foot of that leg about 5 to 8 centimetres from your straight leg.

4. Practice keeping one middle finger on top of the other.

5. Practice holding your stretch for three seconds.

6. Practice three to five times with each leg.

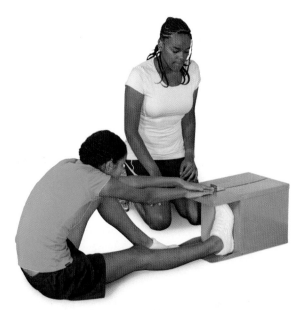

The back-saver sit and reach measures flexibility (range of motion) of the hip.

Lesson 2.2
Stages of Change and Learning Self-Management Skills

Lesson Objectives

After participating in this lesson, you should be able to

1. describe the stages of change in adopting a healthy lifestyle,
2. describe several self-management skills, and
3. explain how to use self-management skills for living a healthy life.

Lesson Vocabulary

exercise, motor skill, physical activity, sedentary, skill

In the first lesson of this chapter, you learned about what it means to live a healthy lifestyle. You also learned about many determinants of health, fitness, and wellness. In this lesson, you'll learn about making lifestyle changes to enhance your fitness, health, and wellness. First, you'll learn about the stages of change. People do not change overnight; change takes time, and people who are making a change typically progress through five stages. These stages were identified by psychologists working to help people stop smoking. They found that most smokers do not quit all at once but go through stages instead. Later, exercise psychologists and nutrition scientists found that these five stages of change apply to other lifestyle choices, such as physical activity and nutrition. Understanding these stages can help you make positive changes in your lifestyle.

FIT FACT

Physical activity refers to movement that uses your large muscles. Thus it includes a wide range of pursuits, such as sport, dance, recreational activities, and activities of daily living. Exercise is a form of physical activity specifically designed to improve your fitness.

Stages of Change for a Healthy Lifestyle

Healthy lifestyle behaviours—such as being active, eating well, and managing stress—are within your control. With effort, almost anyone can make healthy lifestyle changes in these areas. There are five stages of change for modifying behaviours to improve fitness, health, and wellness: precontemplation (not thinking of change), contemplation, planning for change, taking action to change, and maintenance. Figure 2.3 shows the five stages of change for physical activity.

- **Precontemplation:** A person at stage 1 chooses not to be active. Another term for being inactive is **sedentary**, and more than one-third of all adults are sedentary and thus are included in this stage. You might think there are no sedentary teens, but there are. It's true that this category includes fewer teens than adults, but nearly one in four teens can also be included here. In an ideal world, all people would be active exercisers, but sometimes people move slowly from one stage to the next.

- **Contemplation:** A sedentary person might read about the importance of physical activity and even start to think about being active—but take no action. This person has moved from being sedentary to being an inactive thinker (stage 2). An inactive thinker does little physical activity but is thinking about becoming active.

- **Planning:** At stage 3, a person starts planning to be active. For example, he or she might visit an exercise facility or buy a new tennis racket. The person has now become a planner, even though he or she is not yet active.

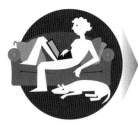 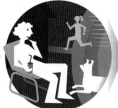 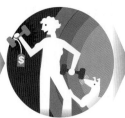 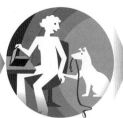 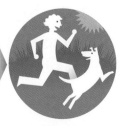

Sedentary
I'm inactive, and I plan to stay that way.

Inactive thinker
I'm inactive, but I'm thinking about becoming active.

Planner
I'm taking steps to start to be active.

Activator
I'm active, but not yet as active as I should be.

Active exerciser
I'm regularly active and have been for some time!

FIGURE 2.3 The five stages of change for physical activity.

- **Taking action:** Stage 4 involves actually becoming active. The person, now an activator, goes to the exercise facility to work out, for example, or plays tennis with a friend.

- **Maintenance:** Stage 5 involves maintaining regular activity. The ultimate goal is to help all people progress to the stage of the active exerciser (stage 5). When this stage is reached, a person is active on a regular basis for a long time (at least several months).

The same five stages of change apply to other healthy lifestyle choices. For example, figure 2.4 shows the stages as they might relate to eating well. Only about one in every four teens eats the recommended number of fruits and vegetables each day, and about one in 10 has avoided eating meals for as long as 24 hours. Teens who do not eat well are at stage 1, whereas those who do eat well on a regular basis are at stage 5. For any healthy lifestyle choice, the goal is to move to stage 5.

Living a healthy lifestyle means making good choices in various areas of your life. You can be at one level of change in one area and at another level in a different area. For example, perhaps you're not active on a regular basis but are thinking about becoming more active; therefore, you're at stage 2 for physical activity. At the same time, you might regularly eat well and therefore be at stage 5 for healthy eating.

FIT FACT

Changes in behaviour don't always occur from stage 1 to 5 without interruption. Sometimes people move forward a few stages, then fall back a stage, and then move forward again. With effort, progress is made gradually from one stage to another.

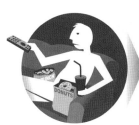 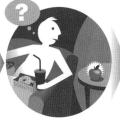 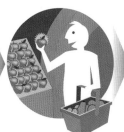 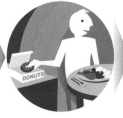 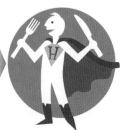

Unhealthy eater
I don't eat well, and I don't plan to.

Thinker
I don't eat well, but I'm thinking about eating healthier.

Planner
I'm taking steps to eat healthier.

Improved eater
I eat well some of the time, but I need to do better.

Healthy eater
I regularly eat healthy meals and avoid empty calories.

FIGURE 2.4 The five stages of change for eating well.

Self-Management Skills: Adopting a Healthy Lifestyle

How do you change your lifestyle? How do you move from stage 1 to stage 5 for being active or eating well?

The best way is to learn self-management skills for change. A **skill** is an ability that allows you to perform a specific task effectively. You improve your skills through practice. For example, writing and typing are skills that help you communicate; if you practice them, you get better at doing them. Similarly, **motor skills**—such as throwing, kicking, and catching—help you perform better in sports and games. They also improve with practice.

Self-management skills are abilities that help you change your lifestyle. There are three kinds: those that help you begin to change, those that help you make change, and those that help you maintain change (see figure 2.5).

> " Happiness lies, first of all, in health. "
>
> —George William Curtis, author and social reformer

Skills That Help You Think About Change

Table 2.1 lists the names and descriptions of 21 self-management skills. Some of these are especially helpful to people who need to make changes but have not begun a plan of action (people in stages 1 and 2). Self-assessment skills, for example, help you see that you need to make changes and determine what changes to make. Building knowledge and understanding helps you see why it is important to change. Knowing the benefits of healthy lifestyle choices—such as being active and eating right—can also motivate you to make positive changes. More specifically, identifying risk factors for disease helps you see the need to adopt a healthy lifestyle not only for now but also for your future.

Two other self-management skills that help you begin to change are positive attitude and self-confidence. If you think you can make a change and you feel good about the change, then you're more likely to be motivated to actually do it! You'll learn more about the self-management skills that help you start making changes as you progress through this book.

Skills That Help You Make Changes

Once you have reached stage 3 of the change process, you're ready to take action, but you must

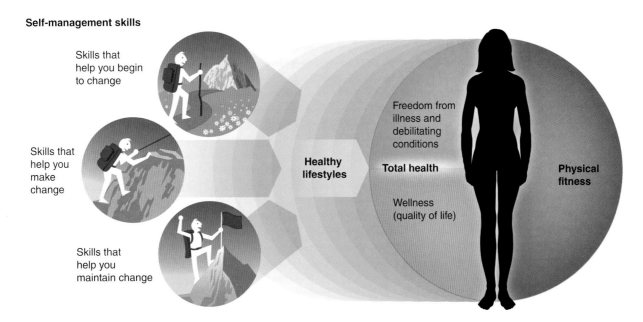

Self-management skills

- Skills that help you begin to change
- Skills that help you make change
- Skills that help you maintain change

Healthy lifestyles

Total health
- Freedom from illness and debilitating conditions
- Wellness (quality of life)

Physical fitness

FIGURE 2.5 Self-management skills help you change your lifestyle to improve your fitness, health, and wellness.

TABLE 2.1 Self-Management Skills for Fitness, Health, and Wellness

Skill	Description
Skills that help you think about change	
Self-assessment	This skill helps you see where you are and what to change in order to get where you want to be.
Building knowledge and understanding	Being able to gather fitness, health, and wellness information from reliable sources is a skill that can help you learn about the benefits of a healthy lifestyle and make healthy changes in your life.
Identifying risk factors	Identifying your health risks enables you to assess and then reduce them.
Positive attitude	This skill helps position you to succeed in adopting healthy lifestyles.
Self-confidence	This skill helps you build the feeling that you're capable of making healthy changes in your lifestyle.
Skills that help you make changes	
Goal setting and self-planning	These skills create a foundation for developing your personal plan by setting goals that are SMART (specific, measurable, attainable, realistic, and timely) and preparing a written schedule.
Time management	This skill helps you be efficient so that you have time for the important things in your life.
Choosing good activities	This skill involves selecting the activities that are best for you personally so that you will enjoy and benefit from doing them.
Learning performance skills	This skill helps you to perform well and with confidence. For example, learning motor skills helps you become active; learning stress management skills helps you avoid or reduce stress; and learning nutrition skills helps you eat well.
Improving self-perception	This skill helps you think positively about yourself so that you're more likely to make healthy lifestyle choices and feel that they will make a difference in your life.
Stress management	This skill involves preventing or coping with the stresses of daily life.
Skills that help you maintain changes	
Self-monitoring	This skill involves keeping records (logs) to see whether you are in fact doing what you think you're doing.
Overcoming barriers	This skill helps you find ways to stay active despite barriers, such as lack of time, temporary injury, lack of safe places to be active, inclement weather, and difficulty in selecting healthy foods.
Finding social support	This skill enables you to get help and support from others (such as your friends and family) as you adopt healthy behaviours and work to stick with them.
Saying no	This skill helps keep you from doing things you don't want to do, especially when you're under pressure from friends or other people.
Preventing relapse	This skill helps you stick with healthy behaviours even when you have problems getting motivated.
Thinking critically	This skill enables you to find and interpret information that helps you make positive decisions and solve problems in living a healthy lifestyle.
Resolving conflicts	This skill helps you solve problems and avoid stress.
Positive self-talk	This skill helps you perform your best and make healthy lifestyle choices such as being active by thinking positive thoughts rather than negative ones that detract from success.
Developing good strategy and tactics	This skill helps you focus on a specific plan of action and successfully execute the plan.
Finding success	Finding success is not technically a skill, but it comes from using a variety of self-management skills to change behaviour. If you use the self-management skills described here and believe that they will help you succeed, you are much more likely to achieve success.

know how to take the right action. Six of the self-management skills help you begin to actually make the lifestyle changes that are right for you (see table 2.1). Goal setting and self-planning skills help you design a plan for change. Time management skills help you make time for carrying out your personal plan. Goal setting, self-planning, and time management skills apply to all types of lifestyle change.

Other self-management skills that help you become more active are choosing good activities and learning performance skills. As you do so, the skill of improving self-perception helps you think positively about yourself. Also, people who think positively and know how to manage stress are more likely to make changes because they believe that change is possible and aren't worried about confronting change.

Skills That Help You Maintain Changes

The remaining self-management skills presented in table 2.1 help you stick with your healthy lifestyle changes. Once you've made a lifestyle change (that is, achieved stage 4 or 5 in that area of your life), these skills help you stay there. Self-monitoring helps you track your progress. You can also learn to overcome barriers, find support from others, and say no to those who might deter you. And you can learn specific skills that help keep you from quitting your healthy lifestyle (preventing relapse).

Several other skills can also help you stay on the right track. Learning to think critically helps you make positive decisions and avoid mistakes that can hurt your health. Learning to resolve conflicts helps you avoid stress. Using positive self-talk and good strategy and tactics helps you find success so that you are much more likely to stick with your lifestyle plan.

This book is intended to help you live an active, healthy life. To accomplish this goal, you must learn about and practice the self-management skills listed in table 2.1.

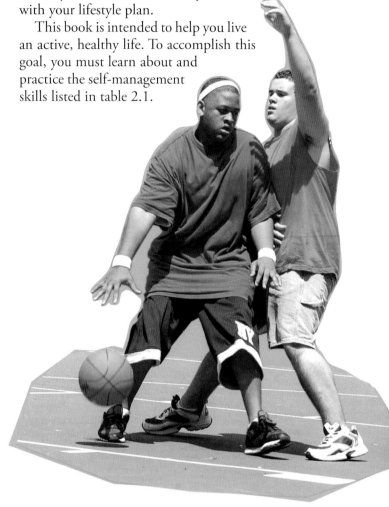

Lesson Review

1. What are the five stages of change, and how are they useful to you?
2. What are some examples of self-management skills for each of the different stages of change?
3. How can you use self-management skills for living a healthy life?

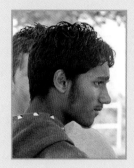

Anish's mother, Mrs. Bhalla, made a New Year's resolution to be more active. She did not know a lot about how to exercise, so she searched the web for information about fitness programs. She found a website with the following claim: "Get fit in five minutes a day without getting sweaty!" Anish was concerned because he had learned in class that it takes weeks of regular exercise to improve fitness.

Anish told his mom, "I think you need to learn more about fitness and physical activity before you get started because you're always telling me 'if it's too good to be true, it probably is.'" But his mother decided to try the plan anyway. Several months later, her fitness had not improved, and she felt discouraged.

At this point, she talked with Anish about the fitness and activity strategies he was learning at school. They both decided that it was important for her to gain good knowledge about fitness before trying a new program. Anish had also learned the value of understanding the

"why" of exercise if a person wants to get best results: Why should I exercise (what are the benefits)? Why is this plan best for me (what are my personal needs)?

Anish and his mother agreed that she would learn along with him as he studied fitness and physical activity at school so that she could do things right the next time she tried.

For Discussion

Mrs. Bhalla made one positive decision and one bad decision. How can someone who wants to make a healthy New Year's resolution avoid making a bad decision about fitness and physical activity? Why do you think people choose programs such as the one Mrs. Bhalla tried? What would you tell someone who said to you "it's possible to get fit in five minutes a day"? How might Anish help his mother in the future? Consider the guidelines presented in the following Self-Management feature as you answer these discussion questions.

SELF-MANAGEMENT: Skills for Building Knowledge and Understanding

Knowledge based on thorough information can help you make positive decisions. But knowledge alone does not always lead to positive decisions. You must understand the information you take in. A person with knowledge knows facts, but a person with understanding comprehends the significance of the facts and can use that understanding to make positive decisions.

In this book, you gain knowledge about fitness, health, and wellness. You also build higher-level understanding that helps you apply the information you've learned. The following guidelines will help you use this book to build both your knowledge and your understanding.

- **Learn the facts first.** Learning the facts is a necessary first step toward building higher-level understanding.

- **Use the scientific method.** Investigate (collect information) to gain as many facts as possible. The facts help you analyze and test hypotheses. For example, you might have a hypothesis that you can get fit in five minutes a day. After acquiring the facts and analyzing them, you would learn that the hypothesis is false. The scientific method helps you understand the information you learn and make sound decisions.

- **Ask why.** When studying healthy lifestyle choices, ask yourself "why" questions: Why do I need this? Why should I believe this information? Why will this information be beneficial?

- **Consult reliable sources.** Whether you're consulting a website, magazine article, or book, check with trusted people to help you find good sources. Your knowledge and understanding are only as good as the sources you use. The chapter titled Making Good Consumer Choices provides more information about how to find reliable source material.

- **Try to apply.** When learning new information, ask, "How can I apply this?" Applying new information to real situations helps you understand it, which in turn helps you apply it more effectively. For example, regarding the dangers of fat in your diet, ask yourself questions like these: What else do I need to know? How much fat is too much? What changes can I make in my diet to reduce my fat intake?

- **Put it all together.** When you learn about something new, you often find many pieces of information. Taking time to fit the pieces together will help you make sense of what you've learned. Another word for putting all the facts together is "synthesizing." For example, if you know you feel stressed out, and you know that there are several reasons for the stress, how do you use all of the information together—synthesize it—to make a positive decision?

TAKING ACTION: Being Active in the Outdoors

Fresh air, nature, and fitness? Yes, please! Canadians are known for being rugged, outdoor people. Canadians are fortunate to have so many beautiful outdoor places with clean air and water to experience. Most communities have natural spaces where you can walk, jog, run, or bike. Some communities have also created "fitness trails"—pathways through parks or woodlands designed especially for walking, jogging, running, and sometimes bicycling. Some fitness trails include human-made or natural structures intended for particular exercises. These structures allow walkers, joggers, and runners to mix their movement activity with muscle fitness and flexibility exercises. Fitness trails are sometimes considered "outdoor gyms," and there's probably one near you!

Take action by learning about, visiting, or even helping create a fitness trail near you. Many fitness trails are already well established by city parks and recreation departments or federal agencies such as Parks Canada. Although they may differ from remote trails, urban areas can have fitness trails.

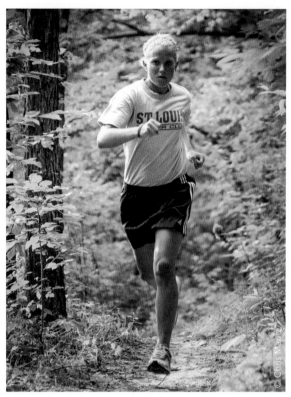

Being outdoors dramatically increases the amount of activity that people perform.

explore GET ACTIVE WITH EXPLORE MAGAZINE

Who We Are

Explore is the award-winning national lifestyle magazine that delivers the information and inspiration that active outdoor-loving Canadians want or, more accurately, can't do without. For starters, we reveal the destinations that crank up our readers' heart rates long before they can actually lace up their trail runners, pick up paddles, or jump on their bikes. We also provide high-quality consumer tips and highlight events from coast to coast to coast that will keep readers interested all year long. Since 2001, Explore has been nominated for 190 magazine awards.

What We Do

Our experienced writers and photographers are a savvy group who care deeply about exploring the outdoors and share the most relevant information to help our passionate audience achieve their exploration goals and dreams. This group takes you with them on the most exciting adventures from the most remote corners of Canada and beyond.

Some of the themes we feature include adventure travel, bucket-list journeys, practical tips and gear reviews, and articles on outdoor sport such as hiking, biking, climbing, backcountry skiing, paddling, adventure racing, and camping.

Get Involved

Get outside and explore. Whether it's an ambitious trip to a remote corner of Canada, an exotic kayak getaway in Central America, or a fun camping excursion with friends, find the adventure that calls to you and do it again and again. One day your stories could inspire others. If writing or photography on these topics is a goal, enthusiasts can submit well-written, researched, and original ideas to explore@explore-mag.com for consideration.

Reviewing Concepts and Vocabulary

Complete the following in order for you to determine your growing understanding of fitness, health, and wellness. Answer items 1 through 5 by correctly completing each sentence with a word or phrase.

1. Factors that affect my fitness, health, and wellness are called _____.
2. Determinants that I have little control over are called _____ determinants.
3. Determinants that I have the most control over are called _____ determinants.
4. The steps that lead me from dependence to independence in my personal fitness, health, and wellness are referred to together as the _____.
5. _____ is a skill that helps you see where you are and what to change in order to get where you want to be.

For items 6 through 10, match each term in column 1 with the appropriate phrase in column 2.

6. sedentary   a. I'm active, but not as active as I should be.
7. activator   b. I'm regularly active and have been for some time.
8. inactive thinker   c. I'm inactive and I plan to stay that way.
9. planner   d. I'm inactive, but I am thinking about becoming active.
10. active exerciser   e. I'm taking steps to start being active.

For items 11 through 15, respond to each statement or question.

11. Explain what a self-management skill is and why it can be useful.
12. Describe why healthy lifestyle choices are the most important determinants of fitness, health, and wellness.
13. What are some of the fitness test items used in major fitness test batteries such as FitnessGram, and what do they measure?
14. What are fitness trails, and how can they be useful in staying active?
15. What are some guidelines for building knowledge and understanding?

Thinking Critically

Write a paragraph to answer the following question.

Of all the self-management skills described in Stages of Change and Learning Self-Management Skills, which one would most help you be more active or eat better? Give three or more reasons for your answer.

Project

Assume that you are the head of a marketing company assigned to create an ad campaign promoting healthier eating and more active living. Prepare a script for a television commercial for the promotion. If resources are available, create a video of the commercial. If you are musically inclined, create a jingle. If you are creative with words, develop a slogan. If you like to draw, create a comic strip or a single cartoon that makes a strong statement about active living or healthy eating.

3

Setting Goals and Planning Personal Programs

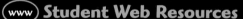 **Student Web Resources**
www.fitnessforlife.org/student

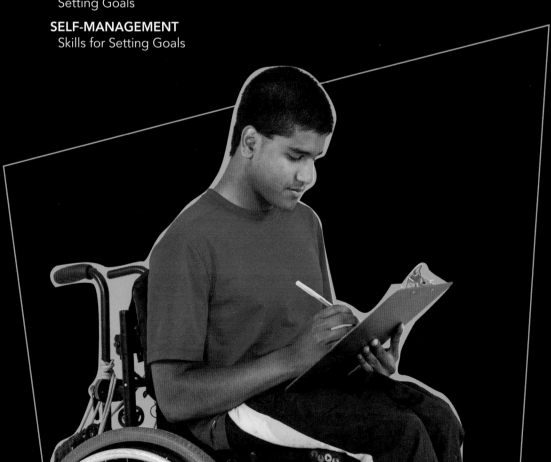

Lesson 3.1
Goal Setting

Lesson Objectives

After participating in this lesson, you should be able to

1. explain the SMART formula for setting goals,
2. explain how long-term and short-term goals differ, and
3. describe process and product goals and explain how they differ.

 ### Lesson Vocabulary

acronym, goal setting, long-term goal, mnemonic, process goal, product goal, short-term goal, SMART goal

How do you turn your dreams into realities? **Goal setting** is one strategy used by many successful people as part of their overall planning to achieve success; they decide ahead of time what they plan to accomplish, then they go about doing it. You can use goals to plan a personal fitness program, a program of good eating, or any other type of program. In this lesson, you'll learn to use long-term and short-term goals. You'll also learn about other goals that can help you make good lifestyle choices, such as being physically active and eating well.

> " The goal you set must be challenging. At the same time, it should be realistic and attainable, not impossible to reach. It should be challenging enough to make you stretch, but not so far that you break. "
>
> —Rick Hansen, Canadian Paralympian, activist, and philanthropist for people with disabilities

SMART Goals

 You may have already learned about **SMART goals**. Here's a quick review to help you remember the five rules for setting goals as you work your way through this book and set your own goals.

S = specific. Your goal should include details of what you want to accomplish.

M = measurable. You should be able to measure (evaluate and assess) your progress in order to accurately determine whether you've accomplished your goal.

A = attainable. Your goals should challenge you. They should not be too easy or too hard.

R = realistic. You should be able to reach your goal if you put in the time and effort and have the necessary resources.

T = timely. Your goal should be useful to you at this time in your life and one that can be met in the time allotted.

FIT FACT

A **mnemonic** (pronounced ni-mon'-ik) is a trick for remembering something. The mnemonic SMART helps us remember five guidelines for creating goals. Specifically, SMART is an **acronym**, which means that each letter in the word is the first letter of a key word related to goal setting.

SMART Long-Term Goals

Long-term goals take you months or even years to accomplish, whereas you can reach **short-term goals** in a short time, such as a few days or weeks. One example of a long-term goal is completing a marathon after one year of training. If you plan to train safely, you could make your long-term goal of completing a marathon a reality.

In order to complete a marathon (i.e., 42 kilometres [26 miles]), you will have to make time for training. Building up the cardiorespiratory fitness and muscular endurance to run a marathon takes time. If you were able to set aside three to five days per week to train, it would take you several months to develop the necessary fitness to run a marathon. Now let's see whether this would be a SMART goal.

Specific. Completing a marathon is a very specific long-term goal.

Measurable. Completing a marathon is measurable. You can know exactly if you have completed the 42-kilometre distance on a single day. At different times during your training you can measure how much distance you can cover. This will give you an idea of how close you are getting to your goal.

Attainable. Completing a marathon is possible for people who walk, run, use a wheelchair, or need support to make their way on the race course (e.g., people who have vision impairments). The goal is probably unattainable for a person without arms or legs.

Realistic. If you put aside the time to train and allow yourself several months to build up your cardiorespiratory fitness and muscular endurance, completing a marathon is realistic. Of course, you must also consider other commitments, such as homework, activities, and family responsibilities.

Timely. The goal of completing a marathon after a year of training has a specific and workable time line.

SMART Short-Term Goals

Short-term goals can usually be reached in a few days or weeks. Thus you might set a series of short-term

© Galina Barskaya

goals to help you accomplish a long-term goal. For example, to meet your long-term goal of completing a marathon, you might set a short-term goal of walking, running, or rolling (i.e., wheelchair) three times a week for 30 minutes over the next two weeks. Doing so would be a manageable way to start working toward meeting your long-term goal. After completing this short-term goal, you could establish a new one.

Let's now consider whether this short-term goal would be a SMART one.

Specific. You've made the goal specific by listing the number of times you will train over the next two weeks (i.e., six times), and the specific amount of time you will train for each time.

Measurable. You can measure your progress toward the goal by tracking each training session. You can add up the number of training sessions and time yourself each session to make sure you trained for 30 minutes.

Attainable. Your short-term goal is attainable because it depends only on your making the effort to fit 30 minutes of training into six of the next 14 days. You could have set a goal of training more days per week, but that is not recommended if you are a beginner; and it might not be attainable because if you train too hard too soon, you might injure yourself (look up "principle of progression" in the glossary).

Realistic. Setting a realistic number of training days and a realistic amount of training time depends on other factors, such as homework, activities, and family responsibilities. However,

FIT FACT

Each year, millions of Canadians make New Year's resolutions to eat better and exercise more. And each year, many of them fail to stick with their resolutions. Scientists have discovered that one of the main reasons for this failure is that people choose long-term goals that cannot be accomplished in the time allotted. In other words, they fail to set SMART goals. This pattern illustrates why scientists urge people to focus short-term goals on lifestyle change rather than on results such as fitness or weight loss.

you have the time to train 90 minutes a week (three sessions of 30 minutes per week) and still meet other responsibilities, so this is a realistic goal.

Timely. Training for 30 minutes three times per week over the next two weeks is a timely goal because you've specified the time frame for completing the goal and it fits your current schedule.

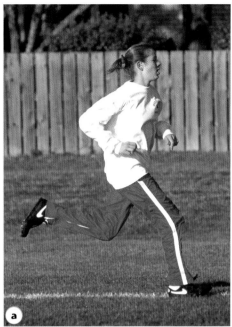
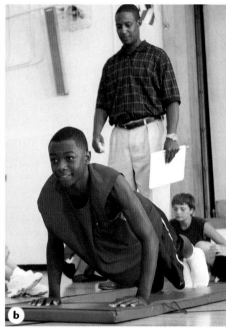

Product and Process Goals

FIGURE 3.1 Product and process goals: *(a)* Running a mile in eight minutes is a product goal, and *(b)* doing five push-ups a day for three weeks is a process goal.

The long-term goal of completing a marathon is a **product goal**. A product is something tangible that results from work or effort. It's not what you do, but what you get as a result of what you do. Examples of product goals for fitness, health, and wellness include being able to perform 25 push-ups, being able to run a mile in eight minutes, and losing 5 pounds (figure 3.1*a*). In each case, the goal is a product or outcome of work and effort. Product

goals make appropriate long-term goals because it may take you a fair amount of work and time to reach them.

Process goals involve performing behaviours, such as replacing all of your soda intake with water. Process refers to what you do rather than to the product resulting from what you do. Examples for fitness, health, and wellness include exercising 60 minutes, eating five fruits and vegetables every day,

♥ FITNESS TECHNOLOGY: Apps

Smartphones, iPods, tablets, and other portable electronic devices use software, or applications (more commonly known as apps), to perform a wide variety of functions. Some companies have developed apps that can help you plan and monitor your physical activity and healthy eating. For example, you can record your self-assessment results and your program schedule and track your exercise and food intake.

Using Technology

Create an idea for a fitness or health app. Describe the app and how it would be used.

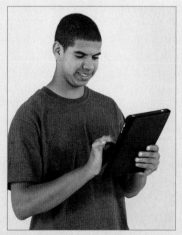

Smartphones, iPods, and tablets have apps that help you meet healthy lifestyle goals.

⚛ SCIENCE IN ACTION: Optimal Challenge

Scientists in many fields have collaborated to find ways to help people stay active, eat well, and stick with other healthy lifestyle behaviours. They have discovered that in order to be successful, you must set goals that provide "optimal challenge." The key is giving effort (trying hard). If a challenge is too easy, there's no need to try hard—it's not really a challenge. On the other hand, if a goal is too hard, we fail, which may lead us to give up or quit because our effort seems hopeless (see figure 3.2).

An optimal challenge requires reasonable effort. Meeting an optimal challenge provides us with success and makes us want to try again. In fact, providing optimal challenge is one reason that video games are so popular. They challenge you by making the task more difficult as you improve, and this optimal challenge makes you want to play again and again. You can use optimal challenge when setting your own goals to help yourself succeed.

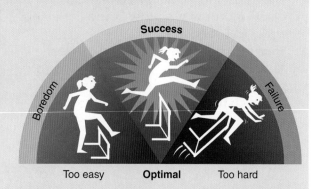

Figure 3.2   Some challenges can lead to boredom or failure, but optimal challenges can lead to success.

Student Activity

Imagine that you want to help a friend learn a skill—for example, hitting a tennis ball, learning to swim, or doing a forward tuck on a trampoline. How could you use optimal challenge to help your friend learn the skill?

and doing five push-ups a day for three weeks (figure 3.1*b*). Process goals make good short-term goals because you can easily monitor your progress and, with effort, succeed. In contrast, product goals do not make especially good short-term goals because they can be discouraging, especially for a person who is just beginning to change. For example, if you chose a product goal of performing, say, 25 push-ups, it might (depending on your current fitness level) take you so long to meet the goal that you would give up. But a short-term process goal—such as performing 5 to 10 push-ups each day for two weeks—would be possible for you to achieve with effort. Thus, as you meet a series of short-term process goals, you work toward meeting long-term product goals.

The Taking Charge and Self-Management features in this chapter focus on setting goals for physical activity and building physical fitness. Elsewhere in the book, you'll get the chance to set long-term goals for fitness, health, and wellness (product goals) and for making healthy lifestyle changes (process goals) that lead to good fitness, health, and wellness. You'll also get the chance to set short-term goals that help you move toward achieving your long-term goals.

> " If you want to live a happy life, tie it to a goal, not to people or things. "
>
> —Albert Einstein, Nobel Prize–winning physicist

Lesson Review

1. Describe how you can use the SMART formula to help you set goals.
2. Describe how you can use long-term and short-term goals to plan your program. In your answer, use fitness and physical activity examples.
3. What is the difference between a process goal and a product goal? In your answer, use fitness and physical activity examples.

SELF-ASSESSMENT: Assessing Muscle Fitness

Throughout this book you are introduced to national and international fitness test batteries and get a chance to practice test items to make sure you know how to do them properly. In this self-assessment, you'll perform four tests that measure your muscle fitness: curl-up, push-up, handgrip strength, and long jump (but remember, there are other tests that would be appropriate to use as well that you'll learn about throughout the text). For each item,

you'll learn how to rate your performance. For the tests included in this chapter, you'll record your scores and ratings as directed by your teacher so that you can use the information when you plan your personal fitness program. If you're working with a partner, remember that self-assessment information is personal and considered confidential. It shouldn't be shared with others without the permission of the person being tested.

Curl-Up
(Abdominal Muscle Strength and Muscular Endurance)

1. Lie on your back on a mat or carpet. Bend your knees approximately 140 degrees. Your feet should be slightly apart and as far as possible from your buttocks while still allowing your feet to be flat on the floor. Your arms should be straight and parallel to your trunk with your palms resting on the mat.

2. Place your head on a piece of paper. Place a strip of cardboard (or rubber, plastic, or tape) 11.5 centimetres (4.5 inches) wide and 1 metre (3 feet) long under your knees so that the fingers of both hands just touch the near edge of the strip.

3. Keeping your heels on the floor, curl your shoulders up slowly and slide your arms

forward so that your fingers move across the cardboard strip. Curl up until your fingertips reach the far side of the strip.

4. Slowly lower your back until your head rests on the piece of paper.

5. Repeat the curl-up procedure so that you do one curl-up every three seconds. A partner could help you by saying "up, down" every three seconds. You are finished when you can't do another curl-up or when you fail to keep up with the three-second count.

6. Record the number of curl-ups you completed, then find your rating in table 3.1 and record it.

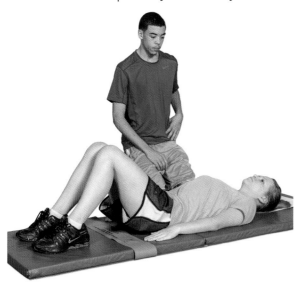
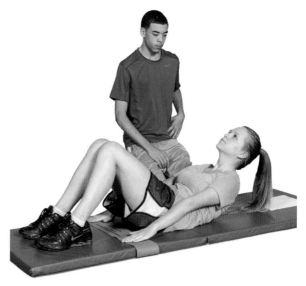

The curl-up assesses muscle fitness of the abdominal muscles.

TABLE 3.1   Rating Chart: Curl-Up (Number of Repetitions)

	13 years old		14 years old		15 years or older	
	Male	Female	Male	Female	Male	Female
High performance	≥41	≥33	≥46	≥33	≥48	≥36
Good fitness	21–40	18–32	24–45	18–32	24–47	18–35
Marginal fitness	18–20	15–17	20–23	15–17	20–23	15–17
Low fitness	≤17	≤14	≤19	≤14	≤19	≤14

Data based on *FitnessGram*.

Push-Up
(Upper Body Strength and Muscular Endurance)

1. Lie facedown on a mat or carpet with your hands (palm down) under your shoulders, your fingers spread, and your legs straight. Your legs should be slightly apart and your toes tucked under.

2. Push up until your arms are straight. Keep your legs and back straight. Your body should form a straight line from your head to your heels.

3. Lower your body by bending your elbows until your upper arms are parallel to the floor (elbows at a 90-degree angle), then push up until your arms are fully extended.

4. Do one push-up every three seconds. You may want to have a partner say "up, down" every three seconds to help you. You are finished when you are unable to complete a push-up with proper form for the second time or are unable to keep the pace for a second time.

5. Record the number of push-ups you performed, then find your rating in table 3.2 and record it.

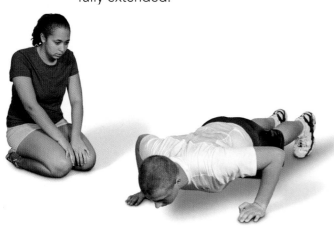
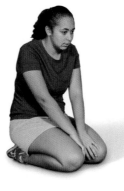
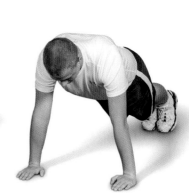

The push-up assesses muscle fitness of the upper body.

TABLE 3.2   Rating Chart: Push-Up (Number of Repetitions)

	13 years old		14 years old		15 years old		16 years or older	
	Male	Female	Male	Female	Male	Female	Male	Female
High performance	≥26	≥16	≥31	≥16	≥36	≥16	≥36	≥16
Good fitness	12–25	7–15	14–30	7–15	16–35	7–15	18–35	7–15
Marginal fitness	10–11	6	12–13	6	14–15	6	16–17	6
Low fitness	≤9	≤5	≤11	≤5	≤13	≤5	≤15	≤5

Data based on *FitnessGram*.

Handgrip Strength (Isometric Hand and Arm Strength)

1. Use a dynamometer to measure isometric strength. Adjust the dynamometer to fit your hand size.
2. Squeeze as hard as possible for two to five seconds. Your arm should be extended with your elbow nearly straight. Do not touch your body with your arm or hand.
3. Do two tests with each hand. Record your best score for each hand. Add your best right-hand score to your best left-hand score, then divide the total by 2 to get your average score.
4. Record your average score, then find your rating in table 3.3 and record it.

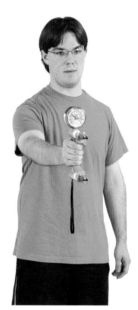

The handgrip strength test assesses isometric hand and arm strength.

TABLE 3.3   Rating Chart: Handgrip Strength in Kilograms

	13 years old		14 years old		15 years old		16 years old		17 years or older	
	Male	Female	Male	Female	Male	Female	Male	Female	Male	Female
High performance	≥29	≥26	≥36	≥28	≥41	≥28	≥49	≥28	≥51	≥32
Good fitness	26–28	24–25	32–35	27	37–40	27	45–48	27	48–50	29–31
Marginal fitness	24–25	23	29–31	25–26	34–36	25–26	42–44	26	44–47	27–28
Low fitness	≤23	≤22	≤28	≤24	≤33	≤25	≤41	≤25	≤43	≤26

Ratings are based on the average of the best right-hand and left-hand scores. Values are rounded off to the nearest whole number. To convert kilograms to pounds, multiply kilograms by 2.2. Alternatively, you can use the Internet to find a calculator that converts kilograms to pounds.

Standing Long Jump (Leg Power, or Explosive Strength)

1. Use masking tape or another material to make the necessary line on the floor.
2. Stand with your feet shoulder-width apart behind the line on the floor. Bend your knees and hold your arms straight in front of your body at shoulder height.
3. Swing your arms downward and backward, then vigorously forward as you jump forward as far as possible, extending your legs.
4. Land on both feet and try to maintain your balance on landing. Do not run or hop before jumping.
5. Perform the test two times. Measure the distance from the line to where your heels landed. Record the better of your two scores, then find your rating in table 3.4 and record it.

The standing long jump assesses leg power.

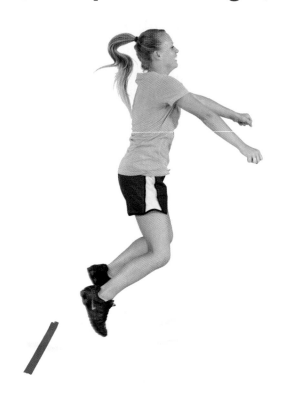

TABLE 3.4   Rating Chart: Standing Long Jump in Centimetres

	13 years old		14 years old		15 years old		16 years old		17 years or older	
	Male	Female	Male	Female	Male	Female	Male	Female	Male	Female
High performance	≥185	≥150	≥203	≥152	≥216	≥155	≥224	≥157	≥231	≥173
Good fitness	170–184	145–149	185–202	147–151	198–215	150–154	208–223	152–156	218–230	160–172
Marginal fitness	155–169	136–144	170–184	140–146	185–197	142–149	196–207	145–151	203–217	147–159
Low fitness	≤154	≤135	≤169	≤139	≤184	≤141	≤195	≤144	≤202	≤146

To convert centimetres to inches, multiply centimetres by 0.39. Alternatively, you can use the Internet to find a calculator that converts centimetres to inches.

Lesson 3.2
Personal Program Planning

Lesson Objectives

After participating in this lesson, you should be able to

1. describe the five steps in program planning,
2. describe and explain the purpose of a personal needs profile, and
3. describe what you would include in a written program plan.

Lesson Vocabulary

personal lifestyle plan, personal needs profile, personal program

Have you ever prepared a written plan to change to a healthy lifestyle? If not, would you know how to prepare a good plan? You can use self-management skills to help you adopt healthy lifestyles. You've already learned about the self-management skill of goal setting. In this lesson, you'll learn about another self-management skill—self-planning—in which you prepare personal plans for various aspects of a healthy lifestyle, such as being active, eating well, and managing stress. Eventually, you'll put all of these plans together to prepare a comprehensive **personal lifestyle plan**.

The Five Steps of Program Planning

The steps used in program planning are described in detail in the sections that follow. Figure 3.3 provides a visual representation of the program planning steps. Can you see how the process is a cycle?

Step 1: Determine Your Personal Needs

The first step toward preparing a good **personal program** plan is to collect information about your personal needs. Throughout this book, you'll do many self-assessments of personal fitness, physical activity patterns, foods you eat, and other health-related areas. You'll use the information you gather to build a personal fitness, physical activity, or nutrition profile. This personal profile will help you focus on your own personal needs as you plan your program. If you don't know your needs, it will be

difficult to perform the next steps in personal program planning such as considering program options (step 2) or setting goals (step 3). For example, before planning a fitness and activity program, you assess your fitness level and physical activity patterns. Before planning a nutrition program, you assess your eating habits. In fact, before you plan to change any aspect of your lifestyle, you should perform a self-assessment in that particular area.

FIT FACT

According to Statistics Canada, about 50 percent of teens aged 12 to 17 years report consuming less than the *minimum* recommended five servings of fruit and vegetables per day.

Once you complete your self-assessment in a specific lifestyle area, you summarize your scores and ratings in a chart called a **personal needs profile**. You'll build a personal needs profile for each healthy lifestyle plan you develop as you work your way through this book. The following example addresses muscle fitness and muscle fitness exercises. It will help you see what a profile looks like.

Procrastination is one of the most common and deadliest of diseases and its toll on success and happiness is heavy.

—Wayne Gretzky, Hall of Fame hockey player

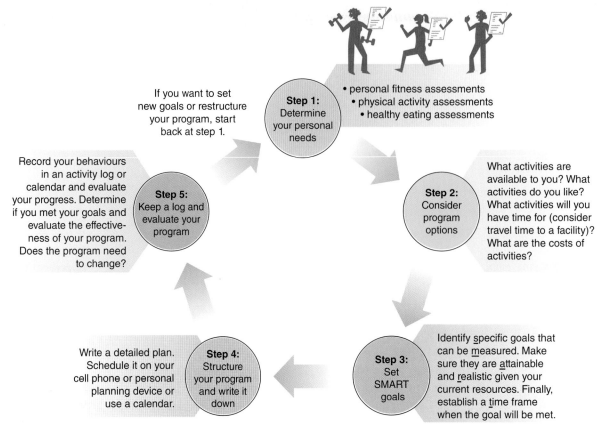

FIGURE 3.3 Program planning process.

Jordan is a freshman in high school. She has always wanted to play on the lacrosse team and felt that improving her muscle fitness would help her be a better player. She also felt that building muscle fitness would help her look better, which for her meant having more lean muscle. To evaluate her current overall body muscle fitness, Jordan performed three self-assessments: the curl-up, the push-up, and the long jump. She felt that these tests would give her a good indication of her overall body muscle fitness because they assess both upper and lower body muscles and also body areas that are most relevant to improving performance in her sport. She also answered some questions about her current muscle fitness activities. She summarized her results in a personal needs profile (see figure 3.4).

Step 2: Consider Your Program Options

After determining your personal needs, the next step is to consider your program options. For physical

Activity self-assessment	Yes	No	Comment
Do you do muscle fitness exercises 2 or 3 days per week?		✓	Stretch every day for 10 min.
Fitness self-assessments	Score	Rating	
Push-up	6	Marginal	
Curl-up	19	Good fitness	
Standing long jump	145 cm	Marginal	

FIGURE 3.4 Jordan's personal needs profile.

Elastic band exercises		Calisthenics	Free weights	Resistance machine exercises	Isometric exercises	
✓	Arm curl	✓ Prone arm lift	Bench press	Bench press	✓	Biceps curl
✓	Arm press	✓ Push-up	Biceps curl	Biceps curl	✓	Bow exercise
✓	Upright row	✓ Bridging	Dumbbell row	Lat pull-down	✓	Hand push
✓	Leg curl	✓ Curl-up	Seated French curl	Seated row	✓	Back flattener
✓	Two-leg press	✓ Trunk lift	Seated press	Triceps press	✓	Knee extender
✓	Toe push	✓ High-knee jog	Half squat	Hamstring curl	✓	Leg curl
		✓ Side leg raise	Hamstring curl	Heel raise	✓	Toe push
		✓ Stride jump	Heel raise	Knee extension	✓	Wall push
			Knee extension			

FIGURE 3.5 Jordan's exercise options for muscle fitness.

activity, you determine what types of activity are available to you. Since Jordan was interested in muscle fitness, she used a checklist of the muscle fitness activities available to her. As you can see from the chart (figure 3.5), there are many types of muscle fitness exercise. Jordan checked elastic band exercises, calisthenics, and isometric exercises because she could do them at home and had the necessary equipment. She decided to hold off on considering other types of exercise until she learned more about them.

Step 3: Set Goals

The next step in self-planning is to set SMART goals. Jordan reviewed the example of writing SMART goals to train for a marathon (presented in the Goal Setting lesson), then used the SMART formula to write down her own long-term and short-term goals (see figure 3.6). She chose exercise (process) goals for her short-term goals. For her long-term goals, she listed fitness (product) goals.

S = specific. Jordan set her goals for muscle fitness and physical activity by choosing specific exercises and a specific number of exercise days per week. She grounded these decisions in the information recorded in her personal needs profile.

M = measurable. Jordan made her goals measurable by deciding on the number of weeks, the number of exercise days per week, and, for her long-term fitness goals, the number of repetitions or distance for each outcome.

Short-term goals	Long-term goals
1. Perform the push-up and elastic band biceps curl exercises 3 days a week.	1. Perform 10 push-ups.
2. Perform the long jump, the elastic band leg curl, and the elastic band toe push exercises 3 days a week.	2. Long jump 1.5 m.
3. Perform the curl-up exercise for the abdominal muscles 3 days a week.	3. Perform 25 curl-ups.

FIGURE 3.6 Jordan's goals for fitness and physical activity included both short-term and long-term goals.

A = attainable. To keep her goals attainable, Jordan's short-term goals addressed only activity (not fitness). She chose fitness goals for her long-term goals. She took this approach because muscle fitness takes time to build, which means that short-term fitness goals are often not attainable. In addition, for her long-term fitness goals, she chose scores that are higher than she can currently achieve—but not too high. For her activity goals, Jordan chose two weeks of exercise as her short-term goal. In this way, she will first focus on her short-term goal as a step toward achieving her long-term goal. Jordan also sought out help from her physical education teacher in selecting her exercises and setting attainable goals.

R = realistic. Because Jordan has various commitments—such as homework, family activities, and school activities—she limited the number of her goals (both short- and long-term) so that she has a realistic chance to meet them all.

T = timely. Jordan also set a specific amount of time for reaching both her long-term and her short-term goals. Since she needs more muscle fitness to make the lacrosse team, she needs to improve her fitness in time for tryouts.

> " You are never too old to set another goal or to dream a new dream. "
>
> —C.S. Lewis, author

Step 4: Structure Your Program and Write It Down

In the fourth step, you use information gained during steps 1, 2, and 3 to structure your program. Once you establish your goals, you prepare a detailed written plan. As you work through this book, you'll create written plans for several programs; they will all be similar to Jordan's planning.

Jordan used a chart to prepare her exercise plan for muscle fitness. Since muscle fitness exercises should not be done every day, Jordan's teacher helped her decide which days to do each exercise

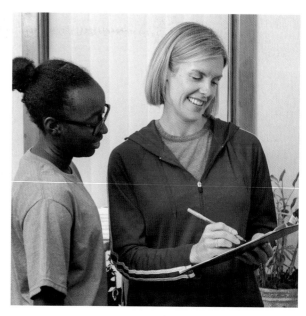

Experts can provide assistance in choosing exercises and determining how often to perform them.

and how many to do. Her teacher also helped her select the right elastic band to use in her exercises. Jordan decided on the best time of day based on her free time and the times when she most enjoyed exercising. She also considered times when she was not likely to be interrupted. A sample of Jordan's written plan is shown in figure 3.7. The last column allowed Jordan to checkmark each day on which she did her exercises.

Step 5: Keep a Log and Evaluate Your Program

After you've tried your program for some time (the exact amount of time depends on your goals), evaluate it. Did you meet your goals? Was your program plan a good one? After your evaluation, make a new plan using the program planning steps.

Jordan tried her plan for two weeks. She placed checkmarks beside the days on which she completed the exercises in her plan. As you can see in figure 3.7, she missed her planned exercises on only one day during the two-week period. Given this success, she decided to keep doing the same plan for another two weeks on her way to meeting her long-term goals. She hoped to reach her long-term goal in eight weeks.

Day	Activity (exercise)	Time	Repetitions	Completed Week 1	Week 2
Mon.	Warm-up (jog)	4 p.m.	5 min	✓	✓
	Biceps curl (exercise band)		3 sets of 10	✓	✓
	Toe push (exercise band)		3 sets of 10	✓	✓
	Curl-up		2 sets of 15	✓	✓
	Long jump		3 sets of 10	✓	✓
Tues.	Warm-up (walk)	4 p.m.	5 min	✓	✓
	Push-up		2 sets of 5	✓	✓
	Leg curl		3 sets of 10	✓	✓
Wed.	Warm-up (jog)	4 p.m.	5 min	✓	✓
	Biceps curl (exercise band)		3 sets of 10	✓	✓
	Toe push (exercise band)		3 sets of 10	✓	✓
	Curl-up		2 sets of 15	✓	✓
	Long jump		3 sets of 10	✓	✓
Thurs.	Warm-up (walk)	4 p.m.	5 min	✓	
	Push-up		2 sets of 5	✓	
	Leg curl		3 sets of 10	✓	
Fri.	Warm-up (jog)	4 p.m.	5 min	✓	✓
	Biceps curl (exercise band)		3 sets of 10	✓	✓
	Toe push (exercise band)		3 sets of 10	✓	✓
	Curl-up		2 sets of 15	✓	✓
	Long jump		3 sets of 10	✓	✓
Sat.	Warm-up (walk)	4 p.m.	5 min	✓	✓
	Push-up		2 sets of 5	✓	✓
	Leg curl		3 sets of 10	✓	✓
Sun.	No exercise				

FIGURE 3.7 Jordan's two-week written program plan.

CONSUMER CORNER: Too Good to Be True

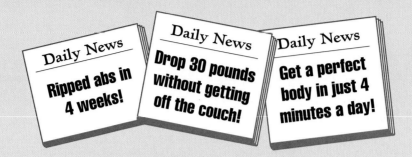

These are just a few examples of headlines you'll see in magazines, newspapers, and TV and web ads. The fitness and health industry is big business. Unfortunately, many companies try to make money by promising big results with little effort. They use marketing campaigns that prey on people who want quick results. As a student of *Fitness for Life Canada*, you're in the process of becoming a critical consumer of fitness, health, and wellness information. Use the tips presented here to make good decisions and avoid falling victim to false claims.

Consumer guideline	Consumer action
Evaluate the source of the information.	Avoid testimonials by famous people (such as athletes and movie stars) who are not experts. Use information from experts in health, medicine, nutrition, and kinesiology who use the scientific method. Use information from government sources (such as Health Canada) and reliable professional organizations (such as the Heath and Stroke Foundation of Canada). Use the scientific method to evaluate the information.
Check the credentials of the person or company doing the promotion.	Check to see if people who claim to be experts really are. Do they have a college degree or advanced degree? Are they certified by a well-known, legitimate organization? People with university degrees in kinesiology, physical education, and physical therapy are generally well equipped to give you sound advice about exercise. The same is true for a certified strength and conditioning specialist (CSCS), Canadian Society of Exercise Physiology certified personal trainer (CSEP-CPT), certified health fitness specialist (CHFS), certified group exercise instructor (CGEI), or registered clinical exercise physiologist (RCEP). For nutrition needs, a registered dietician (RD) is well qualified to give you information.
Be suspicious of claims that promise quick results and are inconsistent with information presented in this book.	Compare claims with facts you've learned from this book and other reliable sources. Beware: If a claim seems too good to be true, it probably isn't true.
Be suspicious of "special offers" that say you must take advantage immediately or they will no longer be available.	Avoid quick action. "Special offers" that quickly expire are designed to get you to act fast without taking the time to make a good decision.

Using Self-Planning Skills

You can use the five steps of program planning presented in this lesson to help you do your self-planning—that is, to plan your own program. Once you've developed a personal program plan, you're on your way to becoming independent rather than dependent on others.

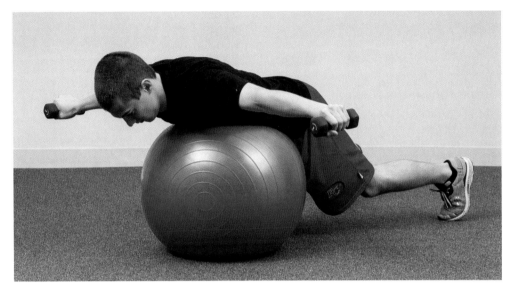

Keeping a log or journal of the activities you perform can help you determine if you have met your goals.

Lesson Review

1. What are the five steps in program planning? Describe each step.
2. What information do you need when preparing your personal needs profile? Why are these pieces of information important?
3. What are some things you should write down when doing your personal program plan? How will these help you?

TAKING CHARGE: Setting Goals

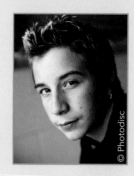

You probably know people who are sedentary or who eat a lot of unhealthy food. They may be in stage 1 of the process of change for physical activity or nutrition. They may have tried to make lifestyle changes but been ineffective because they failed to set good goals. This feature highlights SMART goals for nutrition.

Ms. Booker, a physical education teacher, noticed that Kevin seemed a bit listless in class. She stopped by his desk and asked, "Are you all right, Kevin? You seem a bit tired."

Kevin said, "I'm okay. I was in a hurry this morning so I missed breakfast."

Later, as she passed through the cafeteria, Ms. Booker couldn't help noticing that Kevin was eating food from a vending machine for lunch. He was sitting by himself at an isolated table.

Ms. Booker walked over, sat down, and asked, "Are you feeling better now?"

Kevin replied, "Yes, but I know I need to eat better."

Ms. Booker said, "Maybe you need to make a plan to eat better. Do you remember the SMART formula we learned in class? Maybe you could use the formula to set some goals." Kevin agreed that this was a good idea.

For Discussion

How could Kevin use the SMART formula to set good nutrition goals? What might be some good long-term goals for him? What might be some good short-term goals? What kinds of advice do you think Ms. Booker gave Kevin about goal setting? What advice would you have for Kevin? Consider the guidelines presented in the following Self-Management feature as you answer these discussion questions.

SELF-MANAGEMENT: Skills for Setting Goals

Now that you know more about different types of goal setting, you can begin developing some goals of your own. Use the following guidelines to help you as you identify and develop your personal goals.

- **Know your reasons for setting your goals.** People who set goals for reasons other than their own personal improvement often fail. Ask yourself, *Why is this goal important for me?* Make sure you're setting goals for yourself based on your own needs and interests.

- **Choose a few goals at a time.** As you work your way through this book, you'll establish goals for fitness, physical activity, food choices, weight management, stress management, and other healthy lifestyle behaviours. But rather than focusing on all of these goals at once, you'll choose a few goals at a time. Trying to do too much often leads to

failure. Choosing a few goals at a time can help you be successful.

- **Use the SMART formula.** The SMART formula helps you set goals that are specific, measurable, attainable, realistic, and timely.

- **Set long-term and short-term goals.** The SMART formula helps you establish both long-term and short-term goals. When setting short-term goals, focus not on results but on making good lifestyle changes (that is, focus on process goals).

- **Put your goals in writing.** Writing down a goal represents a personal commitment and increases your chances of meeting that goal. You'll get the opportunity to write down your goals as you do the activities in this book.

- **Self-assess periodically and keep logs.** Doing self-assessments helps you set your goals and determine whether you've met them. Focus on improvement by working toward goals that are slightly higher than your current self-assessment results.

- **Reward yourself.** Achieving a personal goal is rewarding. Allow yourself to feel good. Congratulate yourself for your accomplishment.
- **Revise if necessary.** If you find that a goal is too difficult to accomplish, don't be afraid to revise it. It's better to revise your goal than to quit because you didn't reach an unrealistic goal.
- **Consider maintenance goals.** Improvement is not always necessary. Once you reach the highest level of change, setting a goal of maintenance can be a good idea. For example, an active, fit person cannot continue to improve in fitness forever. At some point, enough is enough, and following a regular workout schedule to maintain good fitness is a reasonable goal. Likewise, once you achieve the goal of eating well, maintaining your healthy eating pattern is a worthwhile goal.

Walking can be done by most people, in most places, and with little or no equipment. Research shows that 30 minutes or more of daily walking can

- help you maintain a healthy weight,
- reduce your risk of hypokinetic disease,
- improve your wellness and mental health,
- strengthen your bones and muscles, and
- increase your chances of living longer.

Because walking is a moderate-intensity activity, it can typically be done while talking with others. As a result, you can use it as a way of not only relaxing and helping your body but also of building healthy relationships as you walk and talk with friends and family members. If you have not been active up until now, walking is also a great way to slowly build your fitness before you start an exercise program. In fact, some people have begun with a walking program and ended up running a marathon. If you want to start looking and feeling your best but don't know where to start, take action and try walking!

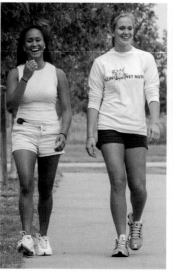 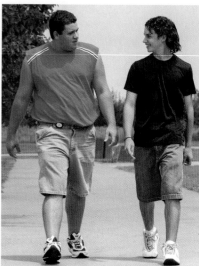

Taking action by walking can improve health and promote social relationships.

GET ACTIVE WITH PARTICIPACTION

©ParticipACTION

Who We Are

ParticipAction is a national nonprofit organization that helps Canadians sit less and move more. Originally established in 1971, ParticipAction works with its partners, which include sport, physical activity, and recreation organizations and government and corporate sponsors, to make physical activity a vital part of everyday life.

What We Do

ParticipAction is a pioneering social marketing organization best known for its mass-media campaigns that promote awareness of the importance of physical activity for Canadians of all ages. These days, ParticipAction focuses on two major things: initiatives that enable behaviour change and thought leadership. That means we provide opportunities for people to get more active through a variety of programs, and we work with other researchers and experts to educate people about the latest and greatest physical activity research. Did you know that sitting for long periods is bad for you, even if you're an otherwise active person?

Get Involved

ParticipAction is a go-to source for tips, opportunities, information, and inspiration about all things physical activity. Check out www.participaction.com to find out about programs like the ParticipAction Teen Challenge, which provides microgrants to help 13- to 19-year-olds work with local organizations to overcome barriers to being active, or Sports Day in Canada, a national celebration of the power of sport to build community and get Canadians moving with more than 2,000 local events in every province and territory in Canada. Plus, find tips and inspiration on the blog Pep Talk at blog.participaction.com, or find more on Twitter (@ParticipAction), Facebook (ParticipAction) or Instagram (@ParticipAction). ParticipAction promises to move you to move more!

Reprinted, by permission, from ParticipACTION.

Reviewing Concepts and Vocabulary

Complete the following in order for you to determine your growing understanding of fitness, health, and wellness. Answer items 1 through 5 by correctly completing each sentence with a word or phrase.

1. The acronym used to remember the characteristics of effective goals is _____.

2. Performing several exercises three days a week for two weeks is an example of a _____-term goal.

3. Deciding to walk 30 minutes a day for the next two months is an example of a _____-term goal.

4. Being able to run a kilometre in four minutes is an example of a _____ goal.

5. Deciding to do flexibility exercises three days a week is an example of a _____ goal.

For items 6 through 10, match each step of the program planning process in column 1 with the appropriate phrase in column 2.

6. step 1   a. setting goals
7. step 2   b. considering program options
8. step 3   c. structuring your program
9. step 4   d. determining your personal needs
10. step 5   e. evaluating your program

For items 11 through 15, respond to each statement or question.

11. Describe the five rules for setting SMART goals.
12. Describe the five steps in program planning.
13. What are some tests you can use to assess and rate your muscle fitness? Why did you choose these?
14. Describe how process goals are different than product goals and explain why this difference is important.
15. What are some guidelines for using the self-management skill of goal setting?

Thinking Critically

Write a paragraph to answer the following question.

Why is it important to understand the concept of optimal challenge when setting goals? Provide an example to help you make your point.

Project

Imagine that in December you are hired as health consultant to help other teens make New Year's resolutions for eating better and being more active. Prepare a brief blog posting that contains advice for making effective New Year's resolutions.

UNIT II

Preparing for Lifelong Activity and Health

● ● ● ● ● ● ● ● ● ● ● ● ● ● ● ● ● ●

Self-Assessment Features in This Unit
- Body Composition and Flexibility
- Assessing Social Support
- PACER and Trunk Lift

Taking Charge Features in This Unit
- Reducing Risk Factors
- Finding Social Support
- Learning to Self-Monitor

Self-Management Features in This Unit
- Skills for Reducing Risk Factors
- Skills for Finding Social Support
- Skills for Learning to Self-Monitor

Taking Action Features in This Unit
- The Warm-Up
- Accessing Social Support
- Physical Activity Pyramid Circuit

Canadian Sport and Health Organization Features in This Unit
- Get Active With CSEP
- Get Active With Right To Play
- Get Active With Sport for Life Society

4

Engaging in Safe and Smart Physical Activity

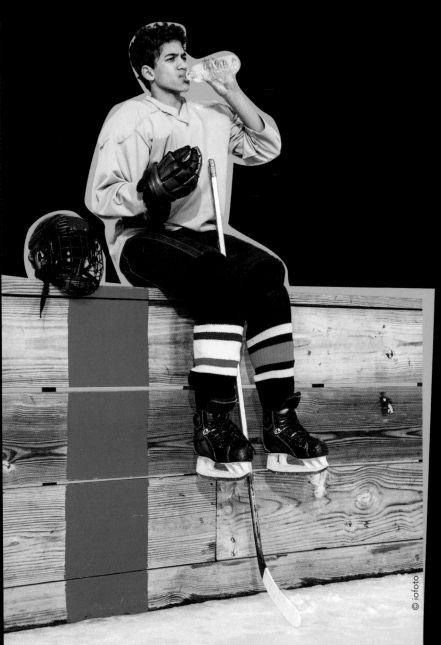
© iofoto

In This Chapter

LESSON 4.1
Safe and Smart Physical Activity

SELF-ASSESSMENT
Body Composition and Flexibility

LESSON 4.2
Health and Wellness Benefits

TAKING CHARGE
Reducing Risk Factors

SELF-MANAGEMENT
Skills for Reducing Risk Factors

TAKING ACTION
The Warm-Up

GET ACTIVE WITH CSEP

CHAPTER REVIEW

 Student Web Resources
www.fitnessforlife.org/student

Lesson 4.1
Safe and Smart Physical Activity

Lesson Objectives

After participating in this lesson, you should be able to

1. describe medical readiness and explain how to assess it,
2. explain how the environment affects physical activity, and
3. describe some steps in dressing appropriately for physical activity in normal environmental conditions.

Lesson Vocabulary

air quality index, dynamic warm-up, graded exercise test, heat index, humidity, hyperthermia, hypothermia, Physical Activity Readiness Questionnaire (PAR-Q), windchill factor

Are you prepared to be active? Whether you are a beginner, are a competitive athlete, or have been physically active for some time, you need to know how to exercise safely in all conditions. If you're a beginner, the first step is to be physically and medically ready. Answering some simple questions about yourself is the first step to exercising safely. You should also be ready for a variety of environmental conditions—such as heat, cold, pollution, and high altitude—that could necessitate a change in your exercise habits. In this lesson, you'll learn how to prepare yourself for physical activity.

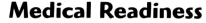

> " An ounce of prevention is worth a pound of cure. "
>
> —Benjamin Franklin, statesman and scientist

Medical Readiness

Have you ever been injured during physical activity? Do you know how to prepare yourself for exercise so as to avoid injury and participate safely? Before you begin a regular physical activity program for health and wellness, you should assess your medical and physical readiness. For this purpose, Canadian experts have developed a seven-item questionnaire called the **Physical Activity Readiness Questionnaire (PAR-Q)**. If you answer yes to any of the seven questions, you are advised to seek medical consultation before beginning or continuing an exercise program. You can get a copy of the questionnaire

from your teacher. You may also want to show the PAR-Q to your parents or other adults who are important to you. Of course you should consider any current health problems as you prepare for exercise. For example, some people have short-term illnesses such as a cold or the flu that will alter their plans for exercise. Others, with chronic conditions such as asthma, have to alter their exercise according to their doctor's instructions. Older people are also more likely to be at risk when doing exercise. You may want to encourage older adults who are important to you to answer the PAR-Q questions before they begin an exercise program.

As for yourself, you may even be required to have a medical examination if you're going to participate in an interscholastic sport or other program of similar intensity, such as a community sport or other rigorous physical challenge. Medical exams help ensure that you are free from disease and can also help you prevent health problems in the future. You should also answer the questions included in the sport readiness questionnaire available from your teacher.

Later in life, you may need to do a **graded exercise test**, which is administered by a health professional and is sometimes called an exercise stress test. The test is done on a treadmill and can help identify people at high risk for health problems such as heart attack (figure 4.1). It is an expensive test and is not necessary for everyone, and a health professional can use screening to determine whether it is appropriate for you. Even seemingly fit athletes can be at risk, although risk is very low among young athletes.

SCIENCE IN ACTION: Guidelines for Warming Up and Cooling Down

The time you spend doing physical activity each day is your physical activity session. The activity session has three phases: warm-up, workout, and cool-down. The warm-up is the activity you perform before your workout in order to get ready for it. The workout is the main part of your activity session. It can involve exercise to build fitness, participation in a competitive event, or activity done just for fun. The cool-down is the activity you perform after your workout to help you recover. You can use the information presented here about warming up and cooling down to prepare yourself for the various workouts described in this book.

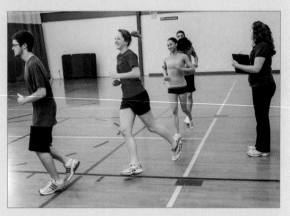

The general warm-up helps your heart and other body systems get ready for more vigorous physical activity.

The Warm-Up

Experts have studied the warm-up for nearly 100 years. For many years, exercise physiologists thought that a stretching warm-up was the preferred method of getting ready for a workout. For this reason, the most common type of warm-up includes static stretching (slowly stretching a muscle beyond its normal length and holding the stretch for several seconds). The Canadian Society of Exercise Physiology (CSEP) and the American College of Sports Medicine (ACSM) note that a warm-up improves range of motion and may reduce the risk of injury. But some recent research has raised questions about whether the traditional stretching warm-up really prevents injury. Additionally, questions have been raised about the effects of a stretching warm-up on certain types of performance. The best evidence now suggests that your warm-up can vary depending on the workout you plan to perform. Here are some warm-up guidelines:

You don't need to perform a warm-up before a workout of low to moderate intensity (such as walking or slow jogging). Low to moderate physical activity is used as a general warm-up, so a workout consisting of low- to moderate-intensity exercise doesn't require a special warm-up.

CSEP recommends 10 minutes of general warm-up involving low- to moderate-intensity physical activity before a vigorous workout or competition. The goal is to increase your body and muscle temperature. This general warm-up helps your heart and other body systems get ready for more vigorous exercise. The general warm-up can include walking, jogging, and calisthenics, such as the activities included in a **dynamic warm-up** (see the Taking Action feature near the end of the chapter).

The National Strength and Conditioning Association (NSCA) recommends a series of dynamic exercises before a workout or competition that requires strength, speed, and power. Examples of dynamic exercises include jogging, skipping, hopping, jumping, and calisthenics using your arms, legs, shoulders, and hips (see this chapter's Taking Action feature). You can also perform sport-related movements that use your body parts similarly to how you'll use them in sport competition. Examples include jumping and shooting drills for basketball and swinging a club or bat with gradually increasing intensity. Dynamic warm-up exercises are good for increasing your body temperature and for getting your muscles ready for more vigorous exercise. They can serve as all or part of the general warm-up recommended by ACSM.

A stretching warm-up may be performed before a workout or competition, including activities that require strength, speed, and power, if the stretch is not held too long. The NSCA recommends dynamic movement exercises as the preferred warm-up before activities requiring strength, speed, and power. For this reason, some may choose not to perform a stretching warm-up before these activities. However, for those who enjoy a stretching warm-up, stretching exercises can be included as long as each stretch is not held for more than 60 seconds, even before a strength, speed, and power workout. Recent research indicates that as long as the stretches don't exceed 60 seconds, they don't inhibit performance. Research also indicates that abruptly stopping a stretching warm-up after regularly performing one increases risk of injury. If you choose a stretching warm-up, you should use a variety of stretching exercises to address all of your major muscle groups and joints (see this chapter's Taking Action feature). Stretches should be held for 15 to 30 seconds. Stretching is more effective when your muscles are warm, so you should stretch only after performing a general warm-up.

Stretching exercises used to build flexibility, rather than for warming up, are best performed as a separate part of your workout. The stretching warm-up and the stretching workout are not the same thing. A stretching warm-up is used to prepare you for physical activity. The stretching workout includes exercises to build flexibility, a health-related component of physical fitness. The ACSM recommends that stretching for flexibility be done after the general warm-up as part of the workout or as a separate workout session after the cool-down. The flexibility workout is typically much more comprehensive than a warm-up. You will have the opportunity to study flexibility and the flexibility workout later in this book.

The Cool-Down

After a workout, your body needs to recover from the demands of physical activity; to aid this process, ACSM recommends a cool-down of 5 to 10 minutes after a vigorous workout. The cool-down usually consists of slow to moderate activity, such as walking or slow jogging, that allows your heart and muscles to gradually recover. The cool-down helps prevent dizziness and fainting. Hard exercise increases the flow of blood to your muscles; for example, running causes more blood to be pumped to your arms and legs than to your head. If you suddenly stop running, the blood can pool in your legs. This leaves your heart with less blood to pump to your brain, which may cause you to feel dizzy or faint. But if you continue moving after a hard run, your muscles will squeeze the veins of your legs. This helps return the blood to your heart, which can then pump more blood to your brain, making you less likely to feel dizzy or faint. The following list provides some more cool-down guidelines.

- Do not lie down or sit down immediately after vigorous activity.
- Gradually reduce the intensity of activity during the cool-down (for example, if you were running, slow to a jog, then a walk, and then consider gentle stretching).
- Walk or do other moderate total body movements.
- You may choose to do some of the stretching exercises presented in chapter 12 after your general cool-down while your muscles are still warm.

Student Activity

How does the information in this feature change the way you would warm up before, and cool down after, a workout? Apply the best warm-up and cool-down approaches to your workouts or precompetition routine.

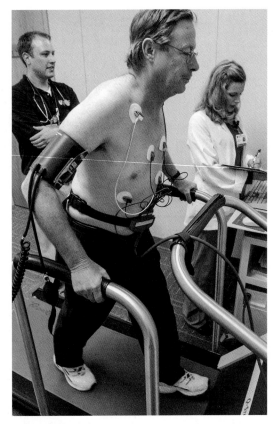

FIGURE 4.1 The graded exercise test can be used to screen adults with risk factors for health problems.

Readiness for Extreme Environmental Conditions

Environmental conditions play an important role in determining when and how strenuously you should exercise. Whether you are just beginning a physical activity program or have been exercising for a while, you must understand how environmental conditions can affect your body during exercise. Your body can adapt to environmental factors such as heat, cold, altitude, and air quality. That adaptability is why people who have been exposed to an environment for a long time can function better in it than those who have just become exposed. This lesson presents guidelines to help you adapt to weather and other environmental factors in order to prevent injury and health problems. All people should follow these guidelines, but they are especially important for people who are new to exercise or new to a particular environment.

Hot, Humid Weather

Be careful when performing physical activity in high heat and **humidity**, which can cause your body temperature to rise too high—a situation referred to as **hyperthermia** or overheating. When exercise causes your body temperature to rise, you start to perspire (sweat). As your sweat evaporates, your body is cooled. But when the humidity is high, evaporation is less effective in cooling your body, and hyperthermia is more likely to occur. Hyperthermia causes three main conditions, which are described in table 4.1.

FIT FACT

Hyper means too much or excessive, and *thermia* refers to heat, so *hyperthermia* means too much heat. *Hypo* means too little or less than normal, so *hypothermia* means too little heat.

TABLE 4.1 Heat-Related Conditions

Condition	Definition
Heat cramps	Muscle cramps caused by excessive heat exposure and low water consumption.
Heat exhaustion	Condition caused by excessive heat exposure and characterized by paleness, clammy skin, profuse sweating, weakness, tiredness, nausea, dizziness, muscle cramps, and possibly vomiting or fainting. Body temperature may be normal or slightly above normal.
Heatstroke	Condition caused by excessive heat exposure and characterized by high body temperature up to 41 °C (106 °F); hot, dry, flushed skin; rapid pulse; lack of sweating; dizziness; and possibly unconsciousness. This serious condition can result in death and requires prompt medical attention.

Use the following guidelines to prevent and cope with heat-related conditions.

- **Begin gradually.** As your body becomes accustomed to physical activity in hot weather, it becomes more resistant to heat-related injury. Start with short periods of activity and gradually increase the duration.

- **Drink water.** In hot weather, your body perspires more than usual to cool itself. In order to replace the water your body loses through perspiration, you need to drink plenty of water before and after activity. If you are exercising in the heat or for many hours in a row, you should try to drink some water during exercise if you can.

- **Wear proper clothing.** Wear porous clothing that allows air to pass through to cool your body. Also wear light-coloured clothing—lighter colours reflect the sun's heat, whereas darker colours absorb it. Clothing made of fibres that wick away moisture and keep you cool (for example, Coolmax and Drymax) are now available.

- **Rest frequently.** Physical activity creates body heat. Periodically stop to rest in a shady area to help your body lower its temperature.

- **Avoid extreme heat and humidity.** You can use the **heat index** chart shown in figure 4.2 to determine whether the environment is too hot and humid for activity. If the heat

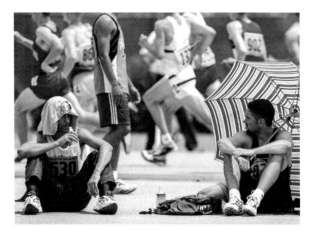

When you exercise in hot weather, wear light-coloured clothing and drink plenty of water to help cool your body.

index is too high, you should postpone or cancel your activity. You should do physical activity in the caution zones only if you are well adapted to hot environments and should follow all of the basic guidelines. The amount of time it takes to adapt to these conditions varies from person to person.

- **If heat-related injury occurs, get out of the heat and cool your body.** Find shade; apply cool, wet towels to your body; spray your body with water; drink water; and seek medical help if you feel you are exhibiting signs of possible heatstroke. If you see heatstroke symptoms in another person, take the same actions and seek medical attention for them.

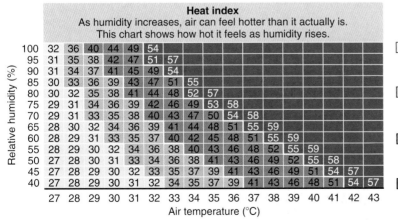

Heat index
As humidity increases, air can feel hotter than it actually is. This chart shows how hot it feels as humidity rises.

Relative humidity (%)	27	28	29	30	31	32	33	34	35	36	37	38	39	40	41	42	43
100	32	36	40	44	49	54											
95	31	35	38	42	47	51	57										
90	31	34	37	41	45	49	54										
85	30	33	36	39	43	47	51	55									
80	30	32	35	38	41	44	48	52	57								
75	29	31	34	36	39	42	46	49	53	58							
70	29	31	33	35	38	40	43	47	50	54	58						
65	28	30	32	34	36	39	41	44	48	51	55	59					
60	28	29	31	33	35	37	40	42	45	48	51	55	59				
55	28	29	30	32	34	36	38	40	43	46	48	52	55	59			
50	27	28	30	31	33	34	36	38	41	43	46	49	52	55	58		
45	27	28	29	30	32	33	35	37	39	41	43	46	49	51	54	57	
40	27	28	29	30	31	32	34	35	37	39	41	43	46	48	51	54	57

Air temperature (°C)

☐ Caution: Fatigue is possible with prolonged exposure and activity. Continuing activity could result in heat cramps.

☐ Extreme caution: Heat cramps and heat exhaustion are possible. Continuing activity could result in heatstroke.

☐ Danger: Heat cramps and heat exhaustion are likely; heatstroke is probable with continued activity.

☐ Extreme danger: Heatstroke is imminent.

FIGURE 4.2 Heat index chart.

Cold, Windy, and Wet Weather

It can also be dangerous to exercise in cold, windy, and wet weather. Extreme cold can result in **hypothermia**, or excessively low body temperature. Hypothermia is accompanied by shivering, numbness, drowsiness, muscular weakness, and confusion or disorientation. Extreme cold can also cause a condition called frostbite, in which a body part becomes frozen. A person with frostbite often feels no pain, which makes the condition even more dangerous. Use the following guidelines when exercising in cold, windy, and wet weather.

• **Avoid extreme cold and wind.** Before dressing for physical activity, use the chart in figure 4.3 to determine the **windchill factor**. Exercising when the temperature is cold and the wind is blowing is especially dangerous because the air feels colder and the body cools down faster due to evaporative cooling (when the wind blows on the sweat produced by the body). The windchill chart shows how long it takes to get frostbite when your skin is exposed to various windchill levels. Experts agree that if the time to frostbite is 30 minutes or less, you should postpone activity. If you're active when the windchill factor is excessive, be sure to dress properly and be aware of the symptoms of frostbite:

○ Skin becomes white or greyish-yellow and looks glossy.

○ Pain may be felt early and then subside, though often feeling is lost and no pain is felt.

○ Blisters may appear later.

○ The affected area feels intensely cold and numb.

• **Dress appropriately.** Wear several layers of lightweight clothing rather than a heavy jacket or coat. The clothing closest to your body (base layer) helps wick away body moisture to keep you warm and dry. Silk and special wicking materials made of synthetic fibres such as Polartec and Primaloft are good for this layer. Cotton is not recommended for the base layer because it tends to get wet and stay wet. The second layer is often called the insulating layer. This layer helps retain body heat but should also wick away moisture. Polyester fleece and wool are good for this layer. The outer layer is designed to protect you against wind and moisture (rain, snow) but should also allow heat and moisture to be released. For this reason jackets made of plastic, rubber, or other materials that do not "breathe" are not recommended. Jackets made of synthetic fibres (for example, GORE-TEX, eVent) that breathe are recommended. Wearing a jacket with a zipper allows you to regulate heat retained and released by the body. Wear a high collar on one of the inner layers. If needed, wear a knit cap, ski mask, or mittens (which keep hands warmer than gloves do).

• **Avoid exercising in weather that is icy or cold and wet.** These conditions can cause special problems. Your shoes, socks, and pant legs can get wet, which increases your risk of foot injuries and falls.

FIT FACT

Health scientists recently discovered an inaccuracy in the windchill factor system that had been used for years. Specifically, the importance of wind had been overemphasized. Now, Canadian experts aided by U.S. scientists have developed a new formula, which is used in the windchill chart shown in figure 4.3.

Pollution and Altitude

The effectiveness and safety of your exercise can also be affected by conditions other than weather, such as air pollution and altitude. Air pollution can affect your ability to breathe, and experts have identified levels of pollution (ozone and particulate matter) that are unhealthful. Pollution levels are rated by means of an **air quality index** that ranges from good to very unhealthful. When the air pollution level is high, you can find warnings on radio, television, and reliable websites. During such times, avoid exercising outdoors. A table showing air quality levels is

Frostbite occurs in 30 minutes or less

Wind speed (kph)	5	0	−5	−10	−15	−20	−25	−30	−35	−40	−45	−50
60	−2	−9	−16	−23	−30	−36	−43	−50	−57	−64	−71	−78
55	−2	−8	−15	−22	−29	−36	−43	−50	−57	−63	−70	−77
50	−1	−8	−15	−22	−29	−35	−42	−49	−56	−63	−69	−76
45	−1	−8	−15	−21	−28	−35	−42	−48	−55	−62	−69	−75
40	−1	−7	−14	−21	−27	−34	−41	−48	−54	−61	−68	−74
35	0	−7	−14	−20	−27	−33	−40	−47	−53	−60	−66	−73
30	0	−6	−13	−20	−26	−33	−39	−46	−52	−59	−65	−72
25	1	−6	−12	−19	−25	−32	−38	−44	−51	−57	−64	−70
20	1	−5	−12	−18	−24	−30	−37	−43	−49	−56	−62	−68
15	2	−4	−11	−17	−23	−29	−35	−41	−48	−54	−60	−66
10	3	−3	−9	−15	−21	−27	−33	−39	−45	−51	−57	−63
5	4	−2	−7	−13	−19	−24	−30	−36	−41	−47	−53	−58

Temperature (°C)

FIGURE 4.3 Windchill chart.

available in the student section of the Fitness for Life Canada website.

People who live at high altitude are able to exercise there with little trouble, but people who live at lower altitude may have trouble adjusting to being active at higher altitude. It takes time for the body to adjust, even for very fit people. For this reason, if you exercise at a higher altitude than you are used to (for example, if you go skiing), lower the intensity of your physical activity until your body adapts. It usually takes two to three weeks for your heart, lungs, muscles, and blood to adapt to a change in altitude.

General Readiness: Dressing for Physical Activity

As you've seen, special environmental circumstances—such as intense heat and cold—require special dress for physical activity. But even under normal circumstances, the way you dress has a lot to do with your comfort and enjoyment. Consider the following guidelines when dressing for physical activity.

- **Wear comfortable and appropriate clothing for the environmental conditions.** Guidelines for dressing for cold and hot weather were presented earlier. In addition to following these guidelines, wearing comfortable clothing will make your workout more enjoyable.

- **Use sun screen and wear clothing that protects you from the sun.** These will help protect your skin from harmful ultraviolet rays.

- **Wash exercise clothing regularly.** Clean clothing is more comfortable than soiled clothing, and it reduces the chance of fungal growth and infection, which also cause odour.

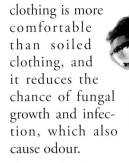

- **Dress in layers when exercising outdoors.** You can remove layers of clothing as you become warmer while exercising and put them back on when you cool down.

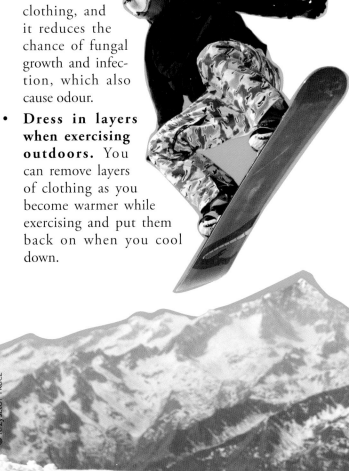

• **Wear proper socks.** Moisture-wicking fabrics are now used in making socks and other apparel (see the Fitness Technology feature). Socks made with these fabrics reduce foot moisture and can help prevent blisters. Thick socks made of cotton or another traditional fabric can help cushion your feet but are not as effective at keeping them dry.

• **Wear proper shoes.** Most people can use a good pair of multipurpose exercise or sport shoes. However, if you plan to do special activities, you might prefer shoes designed just for those. Try shoes on before buying them. When you try them on, wear the kind of socks you normally wear and walk around to see how the shoes feel. They should not feel too heavy, because extra weight makes exercise more tiring. Avoid vinyl or plastic shoes that do not let air pass through to help cool your feet. As an alternative to cloth and leather shoes (which do allow some air passage), new shoes made from fabrics that wick away excess moisture have proven effective in keeping feet dry. Before buying shoes, consider the features shown in figure 4.4.

• **Consider lace-up ankle braces.** Ankle braces can help prevent ankle injuries, especially for activities that involve quick changes in direction, such as basketball and racquetball. Studies show that lace-up ankle braces reduce the number of ankle injuries among those who have a history of them. Some people prefer high-top shoes for sports with high rates of ankle injury.

Other General Preparation Guidelines

In this chapter, you've learned about medical readiness, environmental factors that affect your activity, and dressing appropriately for activity. Here are some additional steps you can take to make your activity sessions safe and effective.

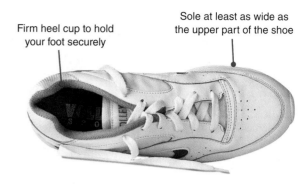

Firm heel cup to hold your foot securely

Sole at least as wide as the upper part of the shoe

Wedge sole at least 1.25 centimetres higher at the heel than the toe

Good arch support

FIGURE 4.4 Characteristics of proper shoes.

• **Start slow and gradually improve.** When you begin a new program, start gradually so you don't hurt yourself. As your fitness improves, you can do more. Safe exercise depends on good health-related fitness of all kinds.

• **Warm up before your workout.** Scientists have recently discovered that different types of warm-up are necessary for different kinds of activity. As you continue to study *Fitness for Life Canada,* you'll try a variety of warm-up activities depending on the workout you plan to do.

• **Cool down after your workout.** The cool-down helps you recover after your workout by bringing your heart rate down and returning blood circulation back to normal levels. The immediate stoppage of vigorous activity without a cool-down can cause dizziness and, in some cases, cause a person to pass out.

FITNESS TECHNOLOGY: High-Tech Exercise Clothing

Modern technology has produced clothing that is especially good for exercising in both hot and cold weather. As noted in the guidelines for exercising in hot or cold environments, clothing made of special synthetic fibres are available that wick moisture away from the body to help it stay cool (for example, Coolmax and Drymax) or warm (for example, Polartec and Primaloft). Clothing made of wicking fibres can aid your performance in the heat and cold. Jackets made of a synthetic material such as Gore-Tex or eVent block the wind but allow your body heat to be released. This type of garment also works well as an outer layer in cold weather. These synthetic fibres are engineered to function in different ways.

Using Technology

Research one type of synthetic fibre used in making exercise clothing in hot or cold environments. What are the special characteristics of the fibre you selected? How does this work to protect you when being active in a variety of conditions?

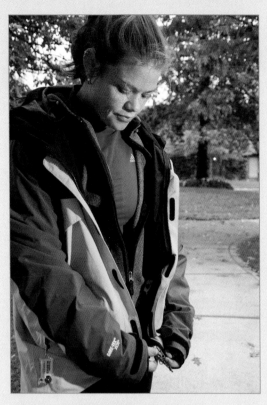
Wearing specially engineered clothing can help you when you exercise in the heat or cold.

Lesson Review

1. What are some steps you can take to make sure you're medically ready to participate in physical activity and sport? Why is this important?
2. What are some environmental factors that can make activity unhealthy or unsafe?
3. What are some guidelines for dressing properly for physical activity in normal environmental conditions?

✓ SELF-ASSESSMENT: Body Composition and Flexibility

In this self-assessment, you'll perform two tests: the body mass index (BMI) test and the back-saver sit and reach. Body mass index is an indicator of your body composition. The back-saver sit and reach measures the flexibility of your lower back and your hamstrings (the muscles on the back of your thighs). If you have not done so already, practice this test before performing it for a score. You will have an opportunity later to do other self-assessments of body composition and flexibility. For these two tests, record your scores and fitness ratings as directed by your teacher. These tests give you information that you can use to develop your personal needs profile (step 1) for your personal physical activity plan. If you're working with a partner, remember that self-assessment information is personal and considered confidential. It shouldn't be shared with others without the permission of the person being tested.

Body Mass Index

1. Measure your height in metres (or inches) without shoes.
2. Measure your weight in kilograms (or pounds) without shoes. If you're wearing street clothes (as opposed to lightweight gym clothing), subtract 0.9 kilograms (2 pounds) from your weight.
3. Calculate your BMI using the chart or either of the following formulas.

$$\frac{\text{weight (lb)}}{\text{height (in.)} \times \text{height (in.)}} \times 703 = \text{BMI}$$

$$\frac{\text{weight (kg)}}{\text{height (m)} \times \text{height (m)}} = \text{BMI}$$

Use table 4.2 to find your BMI rating, and record your BMI score and rating.

Height ft/in	cm																												
6' 4"	192.5	12	13	13	14	15	16	17	18	18	19	20	21	22	22	23	24	24	26	26	27	28	29	29	30	31	32	33	34
6' 3"	190	12	13	14	15	16	16	17	18	19	20	20	21	22	23	24	24	25	26	27	28	29	29	30	31	32	33	34	34
6' 2"	187.5	13	13	14	15	16	17	18	18	19	20	21	22	23	24	24	25	26	27	28	29	29	30	31	32	33	34	34	36
6' 1"	185	13	14	15	15	16	17	18	19	20	21	22	22	23	24	25	26	27	28	29	29	30	31	32	33	34	34	36	37
6' 0"	182.5	13	14	15	16	17	18	19	20	20	21	22	23	24	24	26	27	28	29	29	30	31	32	33	34	34	36	37	38
5' 11"	180	14	15	15	16	17	18	19	20	21	22	23	24	24	26	27	27	28	29	30	31	32	33	34	34	36	37	38	39
5' 10"	177.5	14	15	16	17	18	19	20	21	22	23	23	24	25	26	27	28	29	30	31	32	33	34	34	36	37	38	39	40
5' 9"	175	14	15	16	17	18	19	20	21	22	23	24	25	26	27	28	29	30	31	32	33	34	34	36	37	38	39	40	41
5' 8"	172.5	15	16	17	18	19	20	21	22	23	24	24	26	27	28	29	29	31	32	33	34	34	36	37	38	39	40	41	42
5' 7"	170	15	16	17	18	19	20	21	22	24	24	26	27	28	29	29	31	32	33	34	34	36	37	38	39	40	41	42	43
5' 6"	167.5	16	17	18	19	20	21	22	23	24	25	26	27	29	29	31	32	33	34	34	36	37	38	39	40	41	42	43	45
5' 5"	165	16	17	18	19	21	22	23	24	24	26	27	28	29	30	32	33	34	34	36	37	38	39	40	42	43	44	45	46
5' 4"	162.5	17	18	19	20	21	22	23	24	26	27	28	29	30	31	33	34	34	36	37	38	39	41	42	43	44	45	46	47
5' 3"	160	17	18	20	21	22	23	24	25	27	28	29	30	31	32	34	34	36	37	38	39	41	42	43	44	45	46	48	49
5' 2"	157.5	18	19	20	21	23	24	24	26	27	29	29	31	32	33	34	36	37	38	40	41	42	43	44	46	47	48	49	50
5' 1"	155	18	20	21	22	23	24	26	27	28	29	31	32	33	34	36	37	38	40	41	42	43	45	46	47	48	50	51	52
5' 0"	152.5	19	20	21	23	24	25	27	28	29	31	32	33	34	36	37	38	40	41	42	43	45	46	47	49	50	51	52	54
4' 11"	150	20	21	22	24	24	26	28	29	30	32	33	34	36	37	38	40	41	42	44	45	46	48	49	50	52	53	54	56
4' 10"	147.5	20	22	23	24	26	27	28	29	31	33	34	35	37	38	40	41	42	44	45	46	48	49	51	52	53	55	56	57
4' 9"	145	21	22	24	25	27	28	29	31	32	34	35	37	38	39	41	42	44	45	47	48	49	51	52	54	55	57	58	59
4' 8"	142.5	22	23	24	26	28	29	31	32	33	34	36	38	39	41	42	44	45	47	48	50	51	53	54	56	57	59	60	62
Weight (kg)		44	47	50	53	56	59	62	65	68	71	74	77	80	83	86	89	92	95	98	101	104	107	110	113	116	119	122	125
Weight (lbs)		97	103	110	117	123	130	136	143	150	156	163	169	176	183	189	196	202	209	216	222	229	235	242	249	255	262	268	275

Body mass index calculation chart. Locate your height in the left column and your weight in the bottom row. The box where the selected row and column intersect is your BMI score.

TABLE 4.2 Rating Chart: Body Mass Index

	13 years old		14 years old		15 years old		16 years old		17 years old		18 years old	
	Male	Female	Male	Female	Male	Female	Male	Female	Male	Female	Male	Female
Very lean	≤15.4	≤15.3	≤16.0	≤15.8	≤16.5	≤16.3	≤17.1	≤16.8	≤17.7	≤17.2	≤18.2	≤17.5
Good fitness	15.5–21.3	15.4–22.0	16.1–22.1	15.9–22.8	16.6–22.9	16.4–23.5	17.2–23.7	16.9–24.1	17.8–24.4	17.3–24.6	18.3–25.1	17.6–25.1
Marginal fitness	21.4–23.5	22.1–23.7	22.2–24.4	22.9–24.5	23.0–25.2	23.6–25.3	23.8–25.9	24.2–26.0	24.5–26.6	24.7–27.6	25.2–27.4	25.2–27.1
Low fitness	≥23.6	≥23.8	≥24.5	≥24.6	≥25.3	≥25.4	≥26.0	≥26.1	≥26.7	≥27.7	≥27.5	≥27.2

Data based on *FitnessGram*.

Back-Saver Sit and Reach

1. Place a measuring stick, such as a metre stick or yardstick, on top of a box that is 30 centimetres (12 inches) high with the stick extending 23 centimetres (9 inches) over the box and the lower numbers toward you. You may use a flexibility testing box if one is available.

2. To measure the flexibility of your right leg, fully extend it and place your right foot flat against the box. Bend your left leg, with the knee turned out and your left foot 5 to 8 centimetres (2 to 3 inches) to the side of your straight right leg.

3. Extend your arms forward over the measuring stick. Place your hands on the stick, one on top of the other, with your palms facing down. Your middle fingers should be together with the tip of one finger exactly on top of the other.

4. Lean forward slowly; do not bounce. Reach forward with your arms and fingers, then slowly return to the starting position. Repeat four times. On the fourth reach, hold the position for three seconds and observe the measurement on the stick below your fingertips.

5. Repeat the test with your left leg straight.

6. Record your score to the nearest centimetre (2.54 centimetres equals 1 inch). Consult table 4.3 to determine your fitness rating for each side of your body.

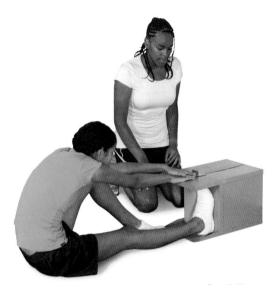

The back-saver sit and reach assesses flexibility.

TABLE 4.3 Rating Chart: Back-Saver Sit and Reach (Centimetres)

	13 or 14 years old		15 years or older	
	Male	Female	Male	Female
High performance	≥25	≥30	≥25	≥35.5
Good fitness	20–23	25–28	20–23	30–33
Marginal fitness	15–18	20–23	15–18	25–28
Low fitness	≤13	≤18	≤13	≤23

To convert centimetres to inches, multiply centimetres by 0.39. Alternatively, you can use the Internet to find a calculator that converts centimetres to inches.

Data based on *FitnessGram*.

Lesson 4.2
Health and Wellness Benefits

Lesson Objectives

After participating in this lesson, you should be able to

1. explain, using examples, how physical activity is related to hypokinetic conditions;
2. list some benefits of physical activity that contribute to health and wellness; and
3. explain, using examples, how physical activity is related to hyperkinetic conditions.

Lesson Vocabulary

activity neurosis, atherosclerosis, blood pressure, cardiovascular disease (CVD), coronary artery disease (CAD), diabetes, diastolic blood pressure, eating disorder, heart attack, hyperkinetic condition, hypertension, hypokinetic disease, metabolic syndrome, osteoporosis, peak bone mass, risk factor, stroke, systolic blood pressure

Have you ever wondered why many people now live twice as long as most people did a few hundred years ago? Do you know the leading causes of death today? Do you understand the roles played by physical activity and nutrition in living a long, high-quality life?

Before 1900, the leading cause of death in Canada and other developed countries was pneumonia, and infections from other bacteria and viruses accounted for many of the other common causes of death. Science has found cures or vaccinations for many of these conditions, and today they are no longer the leading health problems for people with access to modern health care. Instead, the leading health threats today are conditions that are hypokinetic—caused in part by sedentary living—such as heart disease, cancer, and stroke (in that order). In this lesson, you'll learn more about how physical activity reduces your risk of hypokinetic conditions and increases your personal wellness; similar benefits are provided by good nutrition.

Hypokinetic Diseases and Conditions

Hypokinetic diseases are health problems caused by doing too little physical activity. Health Canada and the U.S. Centers for Disease Control and Prevention indicate that regular physical activity is one of the most important things you can do for your health. Canada could save $2.6 billion by 2030 if just 10 percent of the population became

" This may be the first generation of children not to live as long as their parents. "

—Dr. David Butler-Jones, Chief Public Health Officer, 2004-2013

more active. Increases in physical activity would also mean a reduction in premature death. The ACSM lists 27 different health benefits of regular exercise. Sometimes teenagers feel that these statistics are not relevant to them; they think illness happens only to old people. As you'll see next, however, many hypokinetic diseases are now prevalent among teens, and many teens are not active enough to resist these conditions.

Cardiovascular Disease

Did you know that **cardiovascular disease (CVD)** is the second leading cause of death in Canada? In 2011, about one in every three Canadians lost her or his life to at least one form of CVD.

Cardiovascular disease encompasses various conditions, for example **coronary artery disease (CAD)**. *Coronary* means related to the heart, and an *artery* is a kind of blood vessel. Your heart is a muscle that acts as a pump to push blood, and your arteries are the pipelines that carry your blood from your heart to various parts of your body. Coronary artery disease exists when the arteries become clogged—a condition called **atherosclerosis**, which occurs when substances including fats, such as cholesterol, build up on the inside walls of the arteries. This buildup narrows the openings through the arteries. As a result, the heart must work harder to pump blood. See figure 4.5 for the difference between a clear artery and one that is partially blocked. Atherosclerosis typically develops with age but can begin early in life.

A **heart attack** occurs when the blood supply within the heart is severely reduced or cut off; as a result, an area of the heart muscle can die. The main reasons for heart attacks are arteries blocked by atherosclerosis, blood clots in narrowed arteries, spasms in the muscle of the artery, or a combination of these causes. During a heart attack, the heart may beat abnormally or even stop beating. Treatments often include medicines that stabilize the heartbeat and cardiopulmonary resuscitation (CPR) to restore circulation of oxygen.

Another form of CVD is **stroke**, which is the third leading cause of early death in Canada and other developed countries. It occurs when the oxygen supply to the brain is severely reduced or cut off. A stroke can be caused when an artery that supplies blood to the brain bursts or is blocked by a blood clot or atherosclerosis. Because a stroke damages the brain, it can affect a person's ability to move, think, and speak. Some strokes are severe enough to cause death.

A primary risk factor for CVD is **hypertension**, or, as it is commonly called, high blood pressure. Each time your heart beats, it forces blood through your arteries, causing blood to push against your

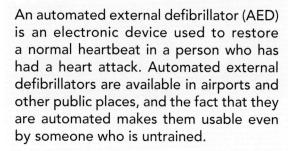

FIT FACT

An automated external defibrillator (AED) is an electronic device used to restore a normal heartbeat in a person who has had a heart attack. Automated external defibrillators are available in airports and other public places, and the fact that they are automated makes them usable even by someone who is untrained.

artery walls. The force of this pushing is called **blood pressure**. When the doctor checks your blood pressure, he or she looks for two readings. The pressure in your arteries immediately after your heart beats is called **systolic blood pressure**. It is the higher of the two readings. The lower of the two numbers, your **diastolic blood pressure**, is the pressure in your artery just before the next beat of your heart.

You can see what counts as normal blood pressure in table 4.4. The table also shows the range for prehypertension, a new category indicating blood pressure that is higher than normal but not high enough to be considered hypertension. People with prehypertension should take precautions to prevent developing even higher blood pressure. There are three stages of high blood pressure. Stage 1 is the least severe and stage 3 the most. When you have your blood pressure checked, you should be rested and relaxed. Blood pressure will be higher if you exercise immediately before having a reading. Also, your blood pressure is often elevated when you're excited or anxious. The incidence of high blood pressure has decreased in recent years because of improved medicines and early screening. Because high blood pressure is a hypokinetic condition, regular physical activity can help decrease it. A healthy low-sodium diet is also helpful in reducing high blood pressure.

An active person's coronary arteries are more likely to be free from atherosclerosis and generally

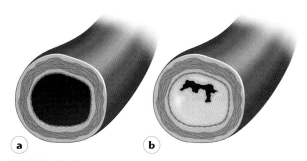

FIGURE 4.5 (a) A healthy heart has open arteries. (b) An unhealthy heart has clogged arteries that can cause a heart attack.

TABLE 4.4 Blood Pressure Readings

	Normal	Prehypertension	Stage 1	Stage 2	Stage 3
Systolic	≤119	120–139	140–159	160–179	≥180
Diastolic	≤79	80–89	90–99	100–109	≥110

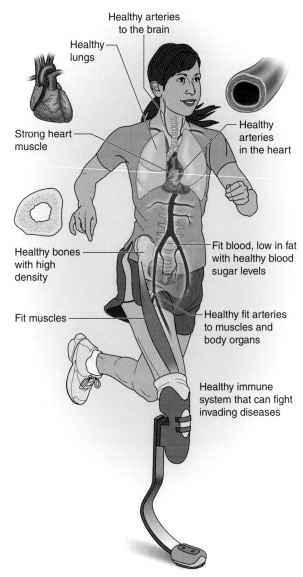

Healthy arteries
to the brain

Healthy
lungs

Strong heart
muscle

Healthy
arteries
in the heart

Healthy bones
with high
density

Fit blood, low in fat
with healthy blood
sugar levels

Fit muscles

Healthy fit arteries
to muscles and
body organs

Healthy immune
system that can fight
invading diseases

FIGURE 4.6 Physical activity benefits associated with reduced risk of hypokinetic conditions and cardiovascular disease.

healthy. An active person also has healthy arteries in his or her brain, muscles, and organs; has a strong heart muscle capable of pumping adequate blood to the body; has fit blood that is low in fat, such as cholesterol; and has blood pressure in the healthy range. Regular physical activity not only reduces your risk of heart attack and stroke but also is often prescribed by doctors to help people recovering from these conditions. Figure 4.6 illustrates some ways in which regular physical activity reduces the risk of hypokinetic conditions, including CVD.

People get CVD for many reasons, each of which is called a **risk factor**. The more risk factors you have, the more chance you have of getting a disease.

Two kinds of risk factor exist: primary (more important) and secondary (less important). Because one primary risk factor is sedentary (inactive) living, CVD is considered a hypokinetic condition. Other primary risk factors for heart disease include smoking, high blood pressure, high fat levels in the blood, too much body fat, and diabetes. Secondary risk factors include stressful living and excessive alcohol use. More information is available in the Taking Charge feature near the end of this chapter.

As you get older, your doctor will likely test your cholesterol, blood pressure, blood sugar, and other potential CVD risk factors. Your doctor will also provide you a rating or standard for each of these tests that indicates how those levels might affect your health. Research shows that your activity and nutrition influence conditions like high cholesterol, high blood pressure, and other risk factors.

Cancer

According to the Canadian Cancer Society, cancer includes more than 50 types, all characterized by the uncontrollable growth of abnormal cells. Cancer's uncontrolled cells invade normal cells, steal their nutrition, and interfere with the cells' normal functioning.

Cancer is the leading cause of death in Canada, accounting for 30 percent of all deaths. When diagnosed early, many forms of cancer can be treated and even cured through surgery, chemical or radiation therapy, or medication. Many of the risk factors for cancer are the same as those for heart disease. We know that the death rate from all forms of cancer is lower in active people than in inactive people. Certain forms of cancer (breast, colon, prostate, and rectal) are considered hypokinetic conditions because people who are physically active are less likely to get them than people who are inactive. It is not clear why physical activity helps reduce the risk of cancer, but, as shown in figure 4.6, one of the health benefits of physical activity is an immune system that is more capable of fighting diseases that invade the body. Another good way to help prevent or minimize cancer is to get regular physical exams.

Diabetes

When a person's body cannot regulate its sugar level, the person has a disease called **diabetes**. A person with diabetes has excessively high blood sugar unless she or he gets medical assistance. People with diabetes may also have trouble using insulin effectively because the cells may become resistant to it. Insulin is a hormone made in the pancreas that helps control blood sugar level. Over time, diabetes can damage the blood vessels, heart, kidneys, and eyes. A very high level of sugar in the blood can cause coma and death. Fortunately, several effective medical treatments can help people with diabetes regulate their blood sugar and lead a normal life.

There are two types of diabetes. Type 1, which accounts for about 10 percent of cases, is not a hypokinetic condition and is often hereditary. People with type 1 diabetes take insulin. In people without diabetes, the body automatically produces insulin to keep blood sugar in a normal range. At one time, it was thought that people with type 1 diabetes should avoid physical activity. Now we know that physical activity can help people manage diabetes. Most people with type 1 diabetes take a blood sample one or more times a day in order to test their blood sugar. If the level is high, they take insulin to lower their blood sugar. In the past, it was necessary to puncture the skin to take a blood sample, but new technology allows some people with diabetes to wear a computerized watch that automatically tests blood sugar without having to draw blood.

The most common kind of diabetes—type 2—is a hypokinetic condition because people who are physically active are less likely to have it. As shown in figure 4.6, active people are more likely to have a healthy level of blood sugar. Diabetes has many of the same risk factors as heart disease, including sedentary living. Exercise helps reduce your risk of type 2 diabetes by lowering your blood sugar level, helping your body tissues use insulin more efficiently, and helping control body fat. Having too much body fat is a major risk factor for type 2 diabetes. In fact, so many obese people have diabetes that one expert coined the term *diabesity*—a combination of the words "diabetes" and "obesity."

FIT FACT

Type 2 diabetes used to be called adult-onset diabetes because adults got it, not teens and children. This name is no longer used because in recent years the disease has become common among youth.

Obesity

Obesity, in which a person has a high percentage of body fat, often results from inactivity, though many other factors can contribute. The Canadian Medical Association views obesity as a chronic condition affected by many factors. The American Medical Association now classifies obesity as a disease. Having too much body fat contributes to conditions such as heart disease and diabetes. From 1978 to 2007, the incidence of overweight and obesity among children in Canada almost doubled, rising from 15 to 29 percent, and a similar upward trend is found in other developed nations.

Osteoporosis

Osteoporosis exists when bone structure deteriorates (see figure 4.7) and bones become weak. It is most common among older people but has its beginnings in youth. You develop your greatest bone mass—also called your **peak bone mass**—when you're young. People who exercise regularly develop stronger bones than those who are sedentary. Choose physical activities that cause you to bear weight and thus stress your bones in a healthy way. Examples of weight-bearing activities are walking, running, jumping, and resistance training. If you do the right kind of activity when you're young, you'll build a higher peak bone mass. As a result, even if you lose bone mass as you get older, you'll have stronger bones than if you hadn't exercised while young.

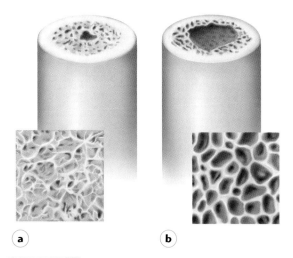

a   **b**

FIGURE 4.7 Osteoporosis involves a decrease in bone density: *(a)* healthy bone in an active person; *(b)* unhealthy bone (osteoporosis) more common among sedentary people.

One contributor to osteoporosis is a lack of sufficient calcium in the diet, especially when a person is young. Women are more likely to have osteoporosis than men because the hormonal changes they experience later in life cause their body to absorb calcium less efficiently. Whether you are female or male, you can maximize your bone health throughout life by getting good nutrition, regular activity, and proper medical attention.

Other Hypokinetic Conditions

Evidence suggests that regular physical activity can also reduce the risk or relieve the symptoms of the following diseases and conditions.

- **Mental health conditions.** One-third of all adults report that they often feel depressed, and one in eight adolescents suffers from depression. People who participate regularly in physical activity are less likely to be depressed. Being active can also help reduce feelings of anxiety and improve brain function in older people.

- **Back problems.** More than 80 percent of all adults experience back pain at some point, but exercise can help reduce the incidence of back problems by strengthening core muscles and hamstring muscles and by lengthening lower back and hamstring muscles.

- **Metabolic health conditions.** "Metabolism" is a word that refers to the many chemical reactions that allow the body, and the cells of the body, to live and function effectively. You are metabolically healthy when the chemical reactions work normally, allowing the cells to function well. When this does not happen, metabolic problems occur. People with metabolic problems such as high blood fat (high cholesterol), high blood pressure, a large waistline, and high blood sugar have a condition called **metabolic syndrome**. This syndrome is associated with heart disease, diabetes, and other hypokinetic diseases. Regular exercise can improve metabolic health and reduce the symptoms of metabolic syndrome.

- **Immune system conditions.** Regular physical activity has been shown to enhance the function of the immune system, thus helping the body resist infections such as the common cold and the flu.

- **Arthritis.** Moderate activity has been shown to help reduce symptoms of some forms of arthritis.

- **Alzheimer's disease and dementia.** Research shows that doing regular exercise and challenging mental tasks can improve brain health and reduce the risk of memory loss disorders.

Physical Activity and Wellness

As you can see, physical activity plays an important role in preventing hypokinetic diseases and conditions and thus is a key to good health. But remember—health is more than freedom from disease; it also includes positive health, or wellness. Some of the benefits of physical activity that contribute to wellness are illustrated in figure 4.8.

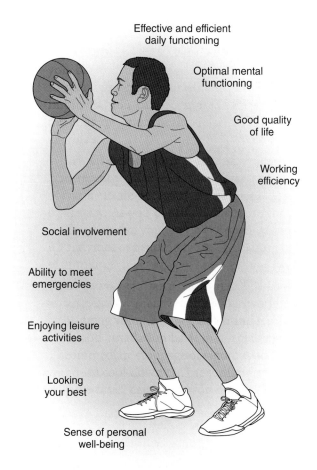

Effective and efficient
daily functioning

Optimal mental
functioning

Good quality
of life

Working
efficiency

Social involvement

Ability to meet
emergencies

Enjoying leisure
activities

Looking
your best

Sense of personal
well-being

FIGURE 4.8 The wellness benefits of regular physical activity.

FIT FACT

Studies conducted by experts in exercise physiology, exercise psychology, and physical activity show that teens who are fit and active enjoy multiple benefits. For example, they perform better in school, have more energy to participate in activities that are important to them, have higher self-esteem, and have less anxiety and depression.

Hyperkinetic Conditions

You've probably heard the saying "too much of a good thing can be bad." This saying can even be true of physical activity. The fact that some physical activity is good does not mean that more activity is always better. In some cases, people experience **hyperkinetic conditions**—health problems caused by doing too much physical activity.

Overuse Injuries

Overuse injuries occur when you do so much physical activity that you suffer damage to a bone, muscle, or other tissue. Examples include stress fractures, shinsplints, and blisters.

Activity Neurosis

Neurosis is a condition in which a person is overly concerned or fearful about something. People with an **activity neurosis** are overly concerned about getting enough exercise. They feel upset if they miss a regular workout and often continue physical activity when they are sick or injured. Activity neurosis is more common among aerobic dance instructors, bodybuilders, and runners than other active groups. Aerobic dance instructors often teach many classes and also take classes to improve their dance skills. Some experts believe this can lead to a compulsive need to exercise. Some bodybuilders seek perfection and continue to do more exercise in pursuit of this ideal. Reasons for activity neurosis

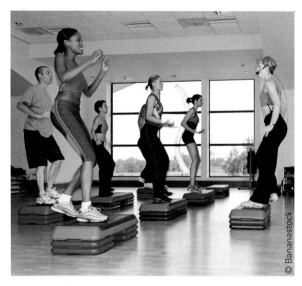

People who are overly concerned about getting enough exercise may have a condition called activity neurosis.

among runners may be the desire to improve running times or distance.

Body Image and Eating Disorders

People with body image disorders try to achieve their idea of an ideal body by doing excessive exercise. This idealized body is unrealistic and distorted. People with this disorder often perform excessive resistance training and sometimes use dangerous supplements or substances such as steroids. Use of steroids and dangerous supplements or substances is most common among teenage boys and young adult men but can occur in both men and women of all ages. Teenage girls and young women, and to a lesser extent young men, often strive for extreme thinness, which is both unhealthy and unrealistic. An extreme desire to be abnormally thin is associated with several kinds of **eating disorders**. People with these conditions have dangerous eating habits and often resort to excessive activity to expend calories for fat loss. Eating disorders that include abuse of exercise are considered to be hyperkinetic conditions. People with body image disorders and eating disorders often need the help of an expert to overcome their problem.

Lesson Review

1. Name and describe at least four hypokinetic conditions. How can physical activity reduce your risk of getting these conditions?
2. What are some health and wellness benefits of physical activity?
3. How is physical activity related to hyperkinetic conditions? Give examples.

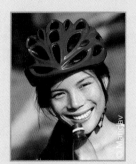

A risk factor is any action or condition that increases your chances of developing a disease. Some risk factors, such as your age and your genetic makeup, are beyond your ability to control or change. But there are also risk factors that you can control—for example, your diet and physical activity. Therefore, your actions can affect the probability that you will get a disease.

Here's an example. Last summer, Brenda's family took a trip to the mountains, where they planned to hike, raft the rivers, and ride bikes and horses. Unfortunately, Brenda's father did not get to enjoy all of the activities. Brenda was surprised: "I never thought my father had any health problems because he was always busy with work and taking care of the house. He never went to the doctor."

But Brenda's father was a smoker. And though he was busy, he didn't actually do much physical activity because he easily became short of breath. On the trip, Brenda's father found that he couldn't keep up with the rest of the family. While hiking, he became so short of breath that he almost fainted. While riding a bike, he fell far behind the others. And in the evening, while the rest of the family did other things, Brenda's father went to bed.

When they returned home, Brenda's father visited his doctor, who recommended that he change his lifestyle. Specifically, his doctor advised him to stop smoking and get more exercise. The doctor also warned that if he continued his present lifestyle, he was at risk for heart disease and other health problems.

For Discussion

What controllable risk factors for heart disease did Brenda's father have? What can Brenda's father do to reduce his risk? Is there anything that Brenda can do to help her father reduce his risk? What can Brenda do now to minimize her own disease risk later in life? Consider the guidelines presented in the following Self-Management feature as you answer these discussion questions.

SELF-MANAGEMENT: Skills for Reducing Risk Factors

Of the 10 leading causes of death, 6 can be considered hypokinetic conditions. Many of these conditions can be prevented if you adopt a healthy lifestyle early in life. You can take the following steps, even in your teen years, to reduce your risk of hypokinetic conditions.

- **Know how to identify important risk factors.** In order to lower your disease risks, you must first identify them. Risk factors for hypokinetic disease that are not in your control include heredity, sex, age, and diseases such as type 1 diabetes (which increases the risk of heart disease). You do have some control over risk factors such as your body fat, blood pressure, and blood fat, but they are also influenced by heredity. Risk factors over which you have more control are diet, physical activity, tobacco and alcohol use, and exposure to stress.

- **Periodically self-assess your risk factors.** You can't change risk factors if you don't know you have them. Doing a self-assessment helps you plan for reducing your risks and lets you know when you need to seek medical help. Because risk increases with age, it becomes even more important to check your risk factors as you grow older.

- **Learn about your family history.** Heredity is a factor over which you have no control. You can, however, check to see what diseases or conditions your parents or grandparents have had—and thus which ones you may inherit a tendency to develop (for example, heart disease, diabetes, and some forms of cancer). You can then pay special attention to controllable risk factors for those diseases.

- **Take steps to change risk factors that are partially in your control.** Some risk factors are influenced by heredity but can also be modified through healthy lifestyle choices. These risk factors include your blood pressure, your blood fat, your body's ability to regulate sugar, and your body fatness. You can influence these factors through choices such as getting regular physical activity, eating properly, and seeking proper medical care. If you have a family history of any of these risk factors, seek medical help and professional advice about how to make lifestyle changes to reduce your risk.

- **Take steps to change risk factors that are fully in your control.** Some risk factors are well within your control—for example, physical activity, what you eat, tobacco and alcohol use, and your stress level.

- **Use the self-management skills you learn in this book to make lifelong changes.** You'll learn many self-management skills throughout this book. Use them to change the risk factors that you identify.

TAKING ACTION: The Warm-Up

As noted in the Science in Action feature in lesson 1, your warm-up should vary depending on the workout you plan to perform. Because *Fitness for Life Canada* includes many types of activities, the type of warm-up you perform will vary from day to day. Before you engage in low- to moderate-intensity activity, no warm-up is typically necessary, though you may choose to do one if you wish. The activities in the warm-up you use before vigorous activity will vary depending on the nature of your workout activity. For vigorous activities that involve strength, speed, and power, you may choose a dynamic warm-up. If you prefer a stretching warm-up before vigorous activities, the stretches should last 15 to 30 seconds. Be sure not to stretch longer than 60 seconds, because that can result in reduced performance in some activities. You will take action here by

trying both a stretching warm-up and a dynamic warm-up. After you've tried them, you can work with your teacher and use the guidelines in the Science in Action feature to create warm-up activities for each type of workout you're planning to do.

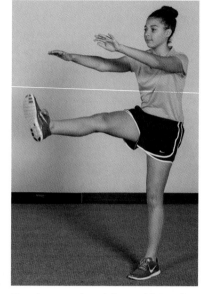

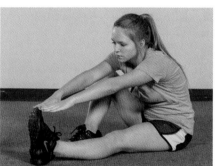

Those who choose a stretching warm-up before vigorous-intensity exercise should hold stretches for 15 to 30 seconds.

For vigorous-intensity activities that involve strength, speed, and power, you can use a dynamic warm-up.

CSEP|SCPE GET ACTIVE WITH CSEP
THE GOLD STANDARD IN EXERCISE SCIENCE AND PERSONAL TRAINING

Used with permission, Canadian Society of Exercise Physiology. www.csep.ca

Who We Are

The Canadian Society for Exercise Physiology (CSEP) is the principal body for physical activity, health. and fitness research and personal training in Canada.

What We Do

We foster the generation, growth, synthesis, transfer. and application of the highest-quality research, education. and training related to exercise physiology and science. We are the gold standard of health and fitness professionals dedicated to getting Canadians active safely by providing the highest-quality customized and specialized physical activity and fitness programs, and guidance and advice based on extensive training and evidence-based research.

Get Involved

Many graduating students seeking to become qualified exercise professionals pursue certification options offered by CSEP. CSEP's rigorous evidence-based certification process is what sets it apart from others. CSEP offers two levels of certification based on candidates' academic background: the CSEP-Certified Personal Trainer (CSEP-CPT) and CSEP Certified Exercise Physiologist (CSEP-CEP) (more advanced than a CSEP-CPT). The CSEP-CPT will have completed some university credits and works with healthy individuals to help them achieve a healthier lifestyle. The CSEP-CEP requires a university degree and works with healthy individuals, elite athletes, those who may have chronic conditions, and others requiring special consideration. To learn more about the CSEP certifications, visit csep.ca, Facebook at www.facebook.com/csep.scpe, Twitter at @CSEPdotCA, and Instagram at #csep.

Used with permission, Canadian Society of Exercise Physiology. www.csep.ca

Reviewing Concepts and Vocabulary

Complete the following in order for you to determine your growing understanding of fitness, health, and wellness. Answer items 1 through 5 by correctly completing each sentence with a word or phrase.

1. The seven questions used to determine readiness for physical activity are called the _____.
2. The two factors used to determine the heat index are _____.
3. The measure used to determine whether it is too cold to exercise is called the _____.
4. Symptoms of frostbite include _____.
5. Hot, dry, flushed skin and rapid pulse and lack of sweating are symptoms of _____.

For items 6 through 10, match each term in column 1 with the appropriate phrase in column 2.

6.	osteoporosis	a. inability to regulate blood sugar
7.	diabetes	b. measure of weight relative to height
8.	air quality index	c. weak and deteriorating bone structure
9.	hypothermia	d. extremely low body temperature
10.	BMI	e. indicator that helps determine whether it is safe to exercise

For items 11 through 15, respond to each statement or question.

11. What is medical readiness and why is it important before engaging in a regular physical activity program?
12. Discuss three ways in which the environment affects people participating in physical activity.
13. Discuss how warm and cold environments affect the choice of clothing.
14. What are the benefits of physical activity in preventing cardiovascular disease?
15. Describe two hyperkinetic conditions and one of the possible consequences with each condition.

Thinking Critically

Write a paragraph to answer the following question.

Why is inactivity a primary risk factor for many diseases?

Project

Your community is providing a $1,000 prize for the best presentation on the health benefits of physical activity. The contest requires that you prepare a 10-minute oral or video presentation on the health benefits of physical activity. You know this will get you closer to your goal of helping to pay for a car, so you decide to enter. Create an oral or video presentation and share it with others.

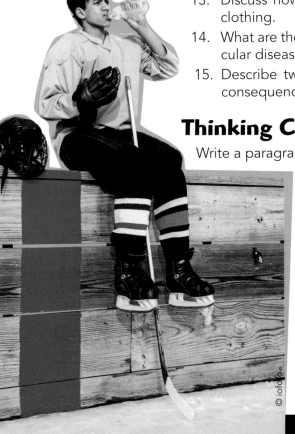

5

Supporting Physical Activity and Healthy Eating

 Student Web Resources
www.fitnessforlife.org/student

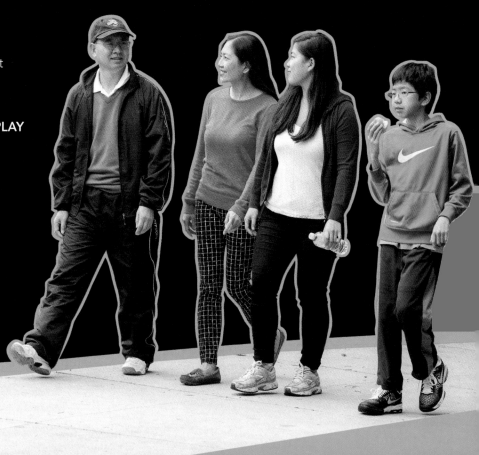

Lesson 5.1
Factors Influencing Physical Activity and Healthy Eating

Lesson Objectives

After participating this lesson, you should be able to

1. list four factors that influence physical activity and healthy eating,
2. list the three individual factors that you have the most control over,
3. describe how individual factors influencing physical activity can affect one another, and
4. provide an example of how communities can influence physical activity and healthy eating.

Lesson Vocabulary

bikeability, built environment, food environment, interpersonal, social–ecological model, social justice, walkability

Do you have people in your life who help you get physically active? Do you have people who encourage you to eat healthfully? Does your school support healthy eating and physical activity? While most people know it is important to participate in physical activity and eat healthy foods, few Canadians meet physical activity and healthy eating guidelines. Why do you think this is the case? Well, there is no easy answer, because there are many factors that affect physical activity and healthy eating. In this lesson you will learn about the factors that influence physical activity and healthy eating. More specifically, this lesson provides a "big picture" of the many factors that affect physical activity and healthy eating, and the next lesson will narrow your focus to the role of social support for physical activity and healthy eating.

What Factors Influence Physical Activity and Healthy Eating?

Physical activity and healthy eating are behaviours, and because there are so many factors that influence human behaviours, behavioural researchers create models to help us organize our thinking. The **social–ecological model** is a popular model used by behavioural health researchers to understand health behaviours. The word "social" indicates the model's

> " Awareness without action is worthless. "
>
> —Dr. Phillip McGaw, PhD psychologist and TV personality

focus on society, and the word "ecological" refers to study of the interactions among living organisms and their environment. So the social–ecological model is a model that illustrates how behaviours are the result of the interactions of living organisms and their environments. Researchers around the world use the social–ecological model to examine all kinds of human and animal behaviours, as well as the behaviours of other living organisms. This lesson uses the social–ecological model to highlight the factors that influence the physical activity and eating behaviours of humans. A version of the social–ecological model for physical activity is presented in figure 5.1. The next lesson focuses on the importance of social support for physical activity and healthy eating. Becoming aware of the factors that influence your physical activity and eating behaviours could help you make positive changes in your life and in the lives of others.

Individual Factors

The individual factors that influence physical activity and healthy eating include a person's knowledge,

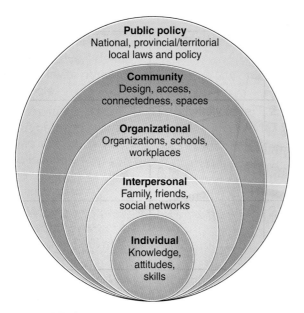

Public policy
National, provincial/territorial
local laws and policy

Community
Design, access,
connectedness, spaces

Organizational
Organizations, schools,
workplaces

Interpersonal
Family, friends,
social networks

Individual
Knowledge,
attitudes,
skills

FIGURE 5.1 Social–ecological model for physical activity. This model can also be applied to healthy eating and many other human behaviours (e.g., driving, smoking, drinking).

Adapted from L. Heise, M. Ellsberg, and M. Gottemoeler, 1999, A social ecological model for physical activity. Available: http://www.activecanada2020.ca/sections-of-ac-20-20/appendix-a/appendix-b/appendix-c-1/appendix-d

skills, and attitudes. From lesson 1.2, you might remember that physically literate persons have the knowledge, skills, and attitudes that support their participation in regular physical activity. It is important to recognize that the individual factors of knowledge, skills, and attitudes influence one another. For example, if you have knowledge about the benefits of regular physical activity participation, you will be more likely to have a positive attitude about physical activity and will participate more. When you participate in more physical activity, you develop your skills in that physical activity. If you have the skills to prepare nutritious foods, you will be more likely to engage in, gain more knowledge about, and value nutritious food preparation. It is beneficial when knowledge, skills, and attitudes affect each other positively; however, a negative interaction between those individual factors is destructive. For example, if a person has a negative experience with physical activity (e.g., being made fun of on the field, getting bullied in physical education), that person might develop a negative attitude toward physical activity and will be less likely to value the skills and knowledge that contribute to successful participation. This results in a lack of motivation to practice the activity, a lack of skill

development, and a lack of motivation to learn more about the activity. This outcome is especially negative because we know how important regular physical activity is to fitness, health, and wellness.

You have a lot of control over the individual factors of knowledge, skills, and attitudes that influence physical activity and healthy eating. You can seek opportunities to learn more, you can practice, and you can change your attitudes. However, there are individual factors that influence physical activity and healthy eating that you have little control over. Individual factors that are not in your control are factors such as your heredity, age, sex, and ability level. Another factor that you might have little control over at this stage in your life could be your income level. As a teenager, the amount of money you have may affect your ability to participate in certain physical activities and to eat healthfully. If you can recognize the individual factors that you have control over and how they support your regular participation in physical activity and healthy eating, you can also figure out how individual factors affect other health behaviours such as sleep, smoking, substance use, and stress management.

FIT FACT

Research has shown that having a positive attitude toward healthy eating results in healthier food purchases and healthier diets.

Interpersonal Factors

Interpersonal factors that influence physical activity and healthy eating are sometimes referred to as "relationship" or "social" factors because they focus on our relationships with family, friends, and the people we interact with. *Inter* means between, and *personal* means individual. So, interpersonal factors are the factors that result from social interactions between individuals. Interpersonal factors are critical for healthy behaviours. The physical activity and the eating behaviours of family and friends have a strong influence on a person's physical activity and eating behaviours. In fact, the best predictors of youth physical activity levels are the physical activity levels of their closest friends and family members. The majority of the food you consume is chosen by your parents. Your eating habits are also influenced by your friends. It is important to acknowledge that both healthy and unhealthy behaviours are affected by interpersonal factors. If your friends smoke or use drugs, this will influence your smoking and drug use behaviours. The strong influence of interpersonal factors on our health behaviours has led health researchers and professionals to focus on the importance of social support for helping people adopt healthy behaviours. The next lesson in this chapter focuses on the importance of social support (i.e., an interpersonal factor) for physical activity and healthy eating.

FIT FACT

If your closest friend is regularly physical active, you are more likely to be physically active.

> " I have been incredibly lucky all my life. I've had a family that has loved me and given me incredible opportunities. I've gone to great schools. I've travelled across the country. "
>
> —Justin Trudeau, 23rd prime minister of Canada

Community Factors

Community factors that influence physical activity and healthy eating behaviours include the cultural and physical environments of schools, workplaces, and communities. The cultural environment is determined by how people act and behave, while the physical environment is determined by the physical structures (e.g., facilities and equipment) in the environment. For example, does your school place a high priority on physical education, physical activity during recess and lunch, and before- and after-school physical activity? If your school promotes physical activity opportunities and the importance of physical activity throughout the school day, then your school has developed a cultural environment where physical activity is a priority. Does your school have facilities and spaces that support physical activity? If so, your school has a physical environment that supports physical activity. Examples of cultural and physical environments that support physical activity and healthy eating in schools, workplaces, and communities are presented in figure 5.2.

Public Policy Factors

Public policy factors that influence physical activity and healthy eating include the global, national, provincial, territorial, and local policies that create the social, cultural, health, and educational environments we live in. For example, in British Columbia, schools are required to provide students with 30 minutes of physical activity each day. While this does not meet the 60-minute recommendation for children's daily physical activity, it does represent a commitment by the Government of British Columbia to support the importance of physical activity for children's healthy development. At the national level, Health Canada created the Trans Fat Task Force in 2007 to ensure that the food industry would limit the amount of trans fats in foods sold to Canadians. The Trans Fat Task Force is an example of a national policy that supports healthy eating. There are numerous examples of how public policy discourages unhealthy behaviours (e.g., smoking, not wearing seat belts, drinking and driving), but it is also important to realize how public policy affects our healthy behaviours (physical activity, sleep, healthy eating, stress management). Consider how

© Alex Brosa/Getty Images

97

Physical activity		Healthy eating	
Cultural environment	Physical environment	Cultural environment	Physical environment
Schools • Promote quality physical education and physical activity at school and outside of school. • Classroom teachers have short activity breaks to energize students' bodies and minds. • Advertise physical activity events for all students on bulletin boards and newsletters. • Make announcements about the importance of physical activity. • Create schoolwide healthy living initiatives (e.g., Terry Fox Walk). • Offer physical activity opportunities for teachers and students together (cooperative or competitive).	• Provide outside and indoor spaces for students to be physically active. • Provide equipment for physical activity. • Provide safe and clean spaces for students to shower and change.	• Promote healthy eating in class, on bulletin boards, through announcements, newsletters, and school/district policy. • Provide opportunities for students to learn how to buy and prepare nutritious foods. • Make announcements and put up posters about community farmer's markets. • Provide opportunities for living gardens where students can grow their own food.	• Provide inexpensive nutritious foods in the cafeteria, at school events, and in vending machines. • Eliminate the amount of empty-calorie snack foods in vending machines and at school events. • Provide spaces for students to prepare nutritious foods. • Provide spaces within and outside of the school for classroom and community gardens.
Workplaces • Support physical activity through social events, teams, reduced fees to physical activity opportunities (e.g., wellness clubs, fitness clubs, pools), and flexible hours that allow employees to work out during the work day. • Promote and support physical activity opportunities in the community.	• Provide onsite spaces, equipment, and classes for physical activity indoors and outdoors. • Allow standing or activity work stations. • Provide transportation to physical activity facilities.	• Promote healthy eating at meetings, on office bulletin boards, and at social events. • Promote and support events/businesses that serve or focus on nutritious foods. • Make announcements and put up posters about community farmer's markets.	• Provide inexpensive nutritious foods in the cafeteria, at meetings, and in vending machines. • Eliminate the amount of empty-calorie snack foods in the workplace and at social events. • Provide spaces for employees to prepare nutritious foods.
Communities • Families in neighbourhood play outside in green spaces and on the streets. • People in the neighbourhood are outside in all seasons (e.g., walking, bicycling, sliding, skating). • Neighbourhood and community physical activity events are planned and advertised.	• Accessible parks with outdoor resistance equipment, swings, climbing structures, sports fields, fitness facilities, recreation centres, walking trails and paths, bicycle trails and paths, skateboard parks, tennis courts, swimming pools, ice rinks, curling rinks, golf courses, and running tracks. • Traffic signs and roads encourage traffic to slow down in neighbourhoods where kids and adults play. • Lighting for safe physical activity participation in outdoor spaces.	• Neighbourhood gatherings that include nutritious foods. • Families prepare nutritious foods together. • Neighbours garden vegetables and fruit on their property or on common property. • Neighbours share excess vegetables and fruit with each other. • Communities advertise and host farmer's markets, recipe sharing, progressive dinners, and potluck dinners with nutritious foods.	• Neighbourhoods have businesses that provide nutritious foods. • Space for community gardens. • Locations for farmer's markets. • City bylaws allow for growing fruits and vegetables on city property.

FIGURE 5.2 Examples of community factors that influence physical activity and healthy eating.

What's the Difference Between Community and Neighbourhood?

"Community" is a word that has different meanings to different people. Community could refer to a neighbourhood where people live, a town, or a city. Community can refer to a geographical area, but it doesn't have to. Community can also refer to a group of people who interact together—for example, a community of drummers who come together in drum circles. It could be a community of coaches, a community of teachers, or a community of First Nations Elders. When communities are defined in this way, members of the community may not occupy the same geographical space.

Neighbourhood is a term that refers to a geographical place. It is often a defined area that includes where a person lives or works—for example, you might say "I work in that neighbourhood" or "I used to live in that neighbourhood." It is positive when people feel a great sense of community in their neighbourhood; however, some people live in neighbourhoods where they are isolated and are not connected to the community in that neighbourhood.

Are you part of the community in your neighbourhood? Are you part of any communities with people who do not live in your neighbourhood?

SCIENCE IN ACTION: The Built Environment Affects Healthy Behaviours

Researchers interested in improving the health of humans through physical activity and healthy eating have identified the importance of the **built environment**. The built environment refers to the physical places where you live and spend time. Researchers examining the built environment are interested in assessing whether or not a community supports physical activity through physical facilities like bike paths, walking paths, parks, and recreation centres. They often look at the amount of free and fee-for-service physical activity resources in a community. Tools have been developed for assessing the **walkability** or the **bikeability** of communities. These tools allow you to score your community on how well it supports walking or biking by simply assessing the physical features of its streets.

In terms of healthy eating, researchers are looking at the community **food environment**. The community food environment refers to the availability of healthy foods in a community and how easily residents can access those foods. Food environments have also been evaluated based on the number of businesses that provide nutritious food in a community relative to the number of

businesses that provide mostly empty calories (e.g., fast food restaurants, convenience stores, gas stations).

Research on physical activity and food environments demonstrates that when people have more access to physical activity resources and nutritious foods, they have increased physical activity levels and increased consumption of fruits and vegetables. People living in poverty, families with single parents, and families with less money are more likely to live in communities that don't support physical activity or healthy eating. This has raised a **social justice** issue and an important question for health researchers and professionals: How can we improve the built environment of communities to support physical activity and healthy eating for the people who most need it?

Student Activity

Take some pictures of your home environment and environments where you spend a lot of time. Do an informal analysis of those pictures and describe how those environments support or hinder healthy behaviours.

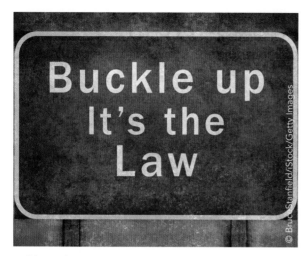

Public policies encourage you to engage in healthy behaviours.

local policies might affect the creation of parks, bicycle lanes, walking paths, and access to nutritious foods in your city and community.

FIT FACT

Canada was the first country to require that the levels of trans fat in prepackaged food be included on the mandatory Nutrition Facts Table. The World Health Organization (WHO) has recommended that the total amount of trans fats consumed per day should be less than 1 percent of your daily energy intake.

Become Aware of the Factors That Influence Your Health Behaviours

Becoming aware of the individual, interpersonal, community, and public policy factors that influence health behaviours is an important step in your learning. If you can understand how individual factors influence healthy behaviours and can identify the factors you have more and less control over, you have taken an important step to becoming more physically literate. If you understand that interpersonal and community factors influence healthy behaviours, you can make choices to create and participate in social and physical environments that positively affect your health and the health of others. In the next lesson you will learn about the importance of social support for participating in healthy behaviours. Finally, if you can recognize that public policy factors influence healthy behaviours, you might become more active in your community or in local, provincial, and national politics.

"
Raising awareness on the most pressing environmental issues of our time is more important than ever. "

—Leonardo DiCaprio, actor and activist

Lesson Review

1. What are the four factors that influence physical activity and healthy eating?
2. What are the three individual factors that you have the most control over?
3. How do the individual factors influencing physical activity affect one another?
4. Provide an example of how you could initiate something in your community to influence physical activity, healthy eating, or both.

SELF-ASSESSMENT: Assessing Social Support

You can assess the level of social support that you receive from others and the level of social support you provide to others. It is important to keep in mind that if you need social support, you should ask for it. If you find that you have a low score on the receiving social support scale, start thinking about the steps you could take to get the social support you need. It may be that you just need to ask a friend, a family member, or a community member.

Assessing Perceived Social Support: Receiving Support

Instructions: This scale is made up of statements that may or may not be true about you. On a separate sheet of paper, record the number of your response to each question. If a statement is always true for you, write the number that corresponds to "definitely true." If you think the statement is probably true for you but you are not sure, write the number that corresponds to "probably true." Write the number that corresponds to "definitely false" if you are sure the statement is always false for you. Finally, if you think the statement is prob-ably false for you but are not sure, write the number that corresponds to "probably false." Instructions for scoring the level of social support that you receive follow the questions.

Scoring instructions: Add up the numbers for all of your responses. For example, the sum of the two responses "1. definitely true" and "4. definitely true" would give you 5. Use the range of scores listed next to assess your perceived level of social support. A higher number means that you believe you have a strong social support network.

1. I would have a hard time finding someone to go with me if I wanted to go for a walk at lunch or after school.	1. definitely true	2. probably true	3. probably false	4. definitely false
2. I feel that there is no one I can talk to about my most private worries and fears related to eating.	1. definitely true	2. probably true	3. probably false	4. definitely false
3. If I were tired and unmotivated to get active, I could easily find someone to help me become motivated and active.	1. definitely false	2. probably false	3. probably true	4. definitely true
4. There is someone I can turn to for advice about handling problems with my level of physical activity.	1. definitely false	2. probably false	3. probably true	4. definitely true
5. If I decide one afternoon that I would like to be active that evening, I could easily find someone to go with me.	1. definitely false	2. probably false	3. probably true	4. definitely true

> continued

> continued

6. When I need suggestions on how to deal with a personal problem, I know someone I can turn to.	1. definitely false	2. probably false	3. probably true	4. definitely true
7. I don't often get invited to do things with others.	1. definitely true	2. probably true	3. probably false	4. definitely false
8. If I had to go out of town for a few weeks, it would be difficult to find someone who would look after my household chores (e.g., plants, pets, garden).	1. definitely true	2. probably true	3. probably false	4. definitely false
9. If I wanted to have a healthy lunch with someone, I could easily find someone to join me.	1. definitely false	2. probably false	3. probably true	4. definitely true
10. If I was stranded 15 kilometres from home, there is someone I could call other than my parents or a family member who could come and get me.	1. definitely false	2. probably false	3. probably true	4. definitely true
11. If a family crisis arose, it would be difficult to find someone who could give me good advice about how to handle it.	1. definitely true	2. probably true	3. probably false	4. definitely false
12. If I needed some help painting my room and moving my furniture around, I would have a hard time finding someone to help me.	1. definitely true	2. probably true	3. probably false	4. definitely false
Total				

41 and above	Excellent! You seem to have strong social support.
31-40	Good! You seem to have support in most situations.
21-30	You might not always have the support you need (could be improved).
12-20	Social support is lacking (needs improvement).

Assessing Perceived Social Support: Providing Support

Instructions: This scale is made up of statements that may or may not be true about you. On a separate sheet of paper, record the number of your response to each question. If a statement is always true for you, write the number that corresponds to "definitely true." If you think the statement is probably true for you but you are not sure, write the number that corresponds to "probably true." Write the number that corresponds to "definitely false" if you are sure the statement is always false for you. Finally, if you think the statement is probably false for you but you are not sure, write the number that corresponds to "probably false." Instructions for scoring the level of social support that you receive are at the end of the questions.

Scoring instructions: Add up the numbers for all of your responses. For example, the sum of the two responses "1. definitely true" and "3. probably false" would give you 4. Use the range of scores listed next to assess your perceived level of social support. A higher number means that you believe you are very supportive of others.

1. If a friend asked me to go for a walk today (for example, at lunch or after school), I would not go.	1. definitely true	2. probably true	3. probably false	4. definitely false
2. My friends feel as if they can't talk to me about their worries and fears.	1. definitely true	2. probably true	3. probably false	4. definitely false
3. I often help motivate my friends to get active and outdoors when they are feeling lazy and bored.	1. definitely false	2. probably false	3. probably true	4. definitely true
4. If a friend was having problems with his or her family, he or she would feel comfortable talking with me about it.	1. definitely false	2. probably false	3. probably true	4. definitely true
5. If a friend texted me in the afternoon to participate in physical activity (e.g., skating, bowling, ice fishing, walking, snowmobiling) that evening, I would make time to go.	1. definitely false	2. probably false	3. probably true	4. definitely true
6. I am a friend who my friends turn to when they need help with a personal problem.	1. definitely false	2. probably false	3. probably true	4. definitely true

> continued

> continued

7. When I make plans to be active, I don't often invite other people.	1. definitely true	2. probably true	3. probably false	4. definitely false
8. If a friend goes out of town, I am the one who gets asked to look after her or his things (e.g., pets, plants, garden).	1. definitely false	2. probably false	3. probably true	4. definitely true
9. When I am invited to eat lunch with someone, I will most often agree.	1. definitely false	2. probably false	3. probably true	4. definitely true
10. If someone I knew was stranded 15 kilometres from home, that person would call me for help.	1. definitely false	2. probably false	3. probably true	4. definitely true
11. When my friends are involved in a family crisis, I am the person they want to talk to and get advice from.	1. definitely false	2. probably false	3. probably true	4. definitely true
12. If a friend asked for help painting or moving furniture around his or her room, I wouldn't make myself available to help.	1. definitely true	2. probably true	3. probably false	4. definitely false
Total				

41 and above	Excellent! You believe you provide others with a lot of social support.
31-40	Good! You believe you will support others in most situations.
21-30	You believe that you might not provide others the support they need. If you want to provide more support to others, how will you work to do this?
12-20	You believe that you don't support others. If you want to provide more support to others, ask someone who supports you (e.g., a teacher, guidance counsellor, friend, family member) how you could change this behaviour.

Lesson 5.2
Social Support for Physical Activity and Healthy Eating

Lesson Objectives

After participating in this lesson, you should be able to

1. provide an example of how social support can influence healthy behaviours and unhealthy behaviours,
2. identify three sources of social support,
3. explain why it is important to give social support,
4. describe three types of social support that you can give or receive, and
5. list three important benefits of giving and receiving social support.

Lesson Vocabulary

colleague, empathy, social support, win–win

Do you like to help others? Do you accept help from others, or are you the type of person who feels as if you can do it all by yourself? What are some of the feelings you get when you help another person succeed? In this lesson, you will learn about the importance of social support for living an active and healthy life.

What Is Social Support?

Social support is having people in your life that care for you and help you. The support you get from family, friends, teammates, coworkers, and members of your community is social support. In chapter 1 you were introduced to the idea that health and wellness have many components, including physical, intellectual, emotional-mental, spiritual, and social (figure 5.3). The positive social component of health and wellness is involvement with family, friends, and your community. In the previous lesson you also learned that social support is an interpersonal factor that influences physical activity and healthy eating.

Social support can help you succeed in school, in relationships, at work, and in sport. Social support can also help you live an active and healthy life. In

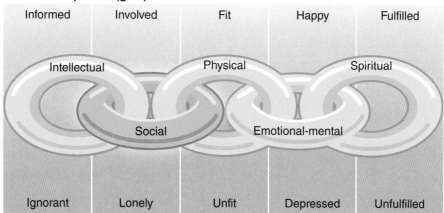

Positive component (goal)

| Informed | Involved | Fit | Happy | Fulfilled |

Intellectual · Physical · Spiritual

Social · Emotional-mental

| Ignorant | Lonely | Unfit | Depressed | Unfulfilled |

Negative component (avoid)

FIGURE 5.3 The social component of health and wellness has both a positive and a negative aspect.

Based on Corbin et al. 2011.

fact having, and giving, social support is associated with living a happier, healthier, and longer life. Unfortunately, the opposite is also true. People who are alone and isolated from family, friends, and community are often more depressed, are less healthy, and live shorter lives.

FIT FACT

The top reason active adults remain physically active is because they have social support. So, go and be that friend who encourages and supports physical activity among those you are close to.

Social Support Influences Health Behaviours

Research conducted by health psychologists clearly demonstrates that social support has a strong influence on health behaviours. This is both good news and bad news. The good news is that social support can positively affect healthy behaviours. The bad news is that social support can negatively affect healthy behaviours. The remainder of this lesson focuses on social support that influences healthy behaviours such as physical activity, healthy eating, and sleep; however, it is important to recognize that social support can play an important role in all areas of our lives, including how we handle stress, how we manage relationships, how we perform in sport, and how we treat others.

Who Provides Social Support?

There are many different sources of social support that people can access. Common sources of social support include family, friends, neighbours, colleagues, and communities. The sources of social support that people access also change throughout life. As children, most people rely heavily on the social support from their family, but as people age they might rely more on social support from friends and colleagues. Common sources of social support are described next.

You

You can provide social support to your friends, family, colleagues, and community members. Your support might change someone's life for the better. Take a minute to think about all of the ways you

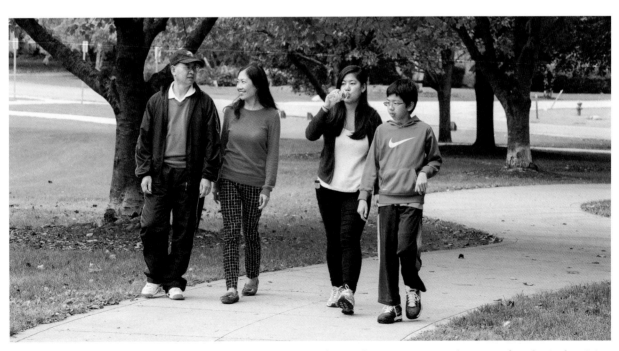

Going for a walk with a friend or family member is one way of providing positive social support for physical activity.

support the healthy behaviours of people in your life. When you support others with regard to living healthy lives, you are being of service to them. Research shows that people who provide service to others have higher levels of self-confidence and self-esteem and a higher quality of life than those who do not. You can support others throughout your life with whatever skills, knowledge, and special gifts you have to share. This is a **win–win** opportunity because you get to help others and help yourself at the same time.

> " The best way to find yourself is to lose yourself in the service of others. "
>
> —Mahatma Gandhi, human rights activist

Family

You often get a lot of social support from your primary caregiver(s) (parents, grandparents, or foster parents) during your childhood and teenage years. Positive social supports can be created through the provision of an environment where physical activity is encouraged, healthy foods are made available, and healthy habits (e.g., tooth brushing, honest communication, sharing, and sleep) are encouraged. You might have been supported in your physical activity pursuits by being walked or driven to sport or dance practice, the skateboard park, a school dance, or a community powwow.

As you age, the social support you seek from your family or primary caregiver might decrease while you seek social support from other sources (e.g., friends). If you get married when you get older, you might receive support from your partner or give support to your partner around healthy behaviours. For example, going for a walk with your partner might support that person's physical activity plan. Preparing a healthy dinner for your partner might support the person's healthy eating plan. If you decide to have children when you get older, you will provide a lot of support to them and might also receive a lot of social support from them as you age.

Friends

Friends provide social support throughout your life. The amount of social support you receive from friends will change throughout life. During your teenage years you might rely heavily on social support from your friends to help you work through stressful situations or challenging relationships. Research shows that teens who have active friends are more physically active, and this serves as a good

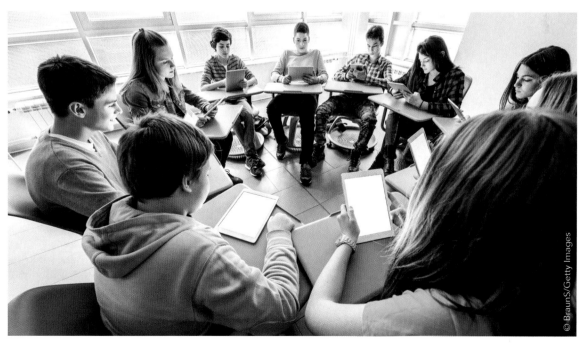

© BraunS/Getty Images

Colleagues can provide you with social support.

example of how friends can support healthy behaviours. Friends can also have a negative impact on healthy behaviours. For example, teens who have friends who smoke are more likely to smoke.

> " My friends and family are my support system. They tell me what I need to hear, not what I want to hear, and they are there for me in the good and bad times. Without them I have no idea where I would be and I know that their love for me is what's keeping my head above the water. "
>
> —Kelly Clarkson, pop singer

Colleagues

While some people work alone at their jobs, most people work with others. **Colleagues** are people you work with at your job, on committees, and in clubs (e.g., student clubs, service clubs, and community clubs). Colleagues can provide a lot of support by sharing their experience, knowledge, and resources that might help you reach a goal or complete a task. Colleagues might have experience with a challenging situation that you are encountering. When a colleague takes the time to listen to you and understand your challenges, that person is providing social support. When a colleague shares ideas, knowledge, and resources that help you address your problem, the person is also providing social support. Colleagues can support healthy

 # FITNESS TECHNOLOGY: Cyber Social Support

Technology has made it easier than ever for people to access social support. You can receive anonymous social support by posting questions to online forums and hearing from people who have had similar experiences. You can ask for social support from friends using popular social media tools. Technology allows you to see the person you are giving social support to or receiving it from. If you are trying to get more active or eat more healthfully, mobile applications (apps) have been created that connect you with personal trainers and registered dieticians who can support your physical activity and healthy eating behaviours. Of course, the reverse is also true. Social media technology can also be used harmfully and lead to unhealthy behaviours.

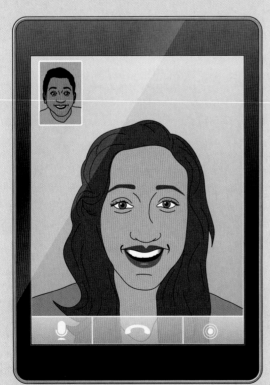

Using Technology

List all of the ways that you use technology to get social support. For each technology, identify whether that technology is supporting physical activity and healthy eating or preventing physical activity and healthy eating. Come up with three ideas for how you could use one technology to get social support for physical activity and healthy eating.

behaviours by keeping the workplace free of empty calories (i.e., high-calorie, low-nutrient foods and beverages), by having walking or standing meetings, and by inviting coworkers to participate in physical activity at lunch or outside of work. If you are in a student club or on a committee, try to promote some of the strategies listed in this section and get feedback from the group. Take in their feedback and keep trying to enhance your health and the health of those you interact with.

Community

Social support can be provided by a variety of communities. Communities that can provide social support include the people who live in your neighbourhood, people who make up your school (students, staff, volunteers, teachers, administrators), people who have similar interests (academic clubs, sport teams, musicians, artists, religious groups), and community organizations (service clubs, community centres, homeless shelters, churches, nonprofit organizations). Communities can support physical activity and healthy eating by actively promoting healthy behaviours, making it easy and safe for people to be physically active and obtain nutritious foods, and helping people find places where they can be physically active and eat healthfully.

What Kinds of Social Support Can You Give and Access?

The four general types of social support include emotional, instrumental, informational, and appraisal. The four types of social support are presented in table 5.1 with a basic description and examples.

Why Is Social Support Important?

Research around the world consistently demonstrates that people who give and seek social support

TABLE 5.1   Types of Social Support

Type of social support	Basic description	Examples
Emotional	Sharing expressions of caring, love, trust, and **empathy**	Listening to a close friend's or family member's challenges; telling a close friend or family member that you love and care for the person; letting friends know that you can understand how they are feeling
Instrumental	Providing resources (e.g., time, money, equipment)	Doing the dishes after dinner so others in your family can go for a walk together; lending your friend the bike you are not using so she or he can ride back and forth from school; doing fund-raising that supports young kids to participate in sports; volunteering your time at a breakfast program
Informational	Providing advice, ideas, and information	Sharing your experiences and knowledge with a friend about how you achieved a healthy weight; giving your friend ideas of how to study more efficiently in order to get more sleep
Appraisal	Providing information that helps a person self-evaluate	Reminding your brother about all of his positive qualities that will help him get better at basketball; reminding a close friend about what she says she wants and how her behaviours could change to better support that goal; recommending that a friend perform a physical activity, fitness, or healthy eating self-assessment

CONSUMER CORNER: Putting Technology Into Action

Advances in technology have limited the amount of physical activity that many people get each day. Often, they get screen time instead. At the same time, however, technological advances have produced wonderful tools for use in almost every part of our lives, and some of these tools can help you implement the Fitness for Life Canada program.

You can use software (apps) for smartphones, tablets, and computers to help you achieve the objectives of the Fitness for Life Canada program. You can also access exercise video clips to see how to perform exercises properly. And you can use devices such as pedometers, accelerometers, and heart rate monitors to help with your self-assessment and self-monitoring.

If you decide to use one or more of these devices, consider the following consumer guidelines.

- **Apps.** Check the app to determine if it adheres to the exercise principles described in this book.
- **Exercise videos.** View the video. Check to see if it includes any risky exercises. Check to see if the video follows exercise principles described in this book.
- **Pedometers.** Check the accuracy of a pedometer with a simple walk test. Set the pedometer to zero, then walk and count exactly 100 steps. Check the pedometer to see if it counted 100 steps; an error of up to 3 steps in 100 is considered acceptable. You may also find that a pedometer counts more accurately in one location on your body than in another. Test the accuracy in different positions on your belt. If the unit does not count accurately in any position, try a different pedometer.

are more likely to be active and eat more healthfully than those without social support. People who give and seek social support also have fewer stress-related health problems, stronger relationships, increased confidence, a higher quality of life, and a longer life.

Some people think that seeking help from others means they are weak or incapable. The opposite is actually true. Seeking support takes courage and results in numerous benefits for you and the person providing support.

Lesson Review

1. How can social support influence both healthy behaviours and unhealthy behaviours?
2. What are three sources of social support?
3. Why is it important to give social support?
4. Describe three types of social support that you can give or receive.
5. What are three important benefits of social support?

Social support involves your family members, friends, teachers, and community members encouraging your physical activities or participating with you. You're more likely to begin or continue an activity if the people you associate with also do it.

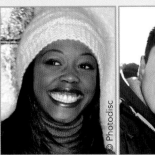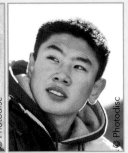

© Photodisc

Shannon's family has always enjoyed bike riding. As a toddler, she would ride in the child's seat behind her mother. Every evening, the family would ride through the neighbourhood. By the time she was in school, Shannon had her own two-wheeler. Now a teenager, Shannon still loves to ride, but school activities sometimes prevent her from riding with her family. She wants to continue riding but doesn't want to do it alone.

Aleem's family has never been very active. Most of his friends tend to watch television, play video games, or just hang out rather than doing anything active. Sometimes Aleem watches while a group of his classmates plays a quick game of volleyball after school. They often invite him to join the game. He has been tempted to join but has hesitated because he is not friends with any of the players. He has enjoyed the activities he has tried in the past but has never continued them for very long.

Both Shannon and Aleem need social support. Shannon needs it to continue an activity she already enjoys. Aleem needs it to encourage him to begin an activity and then reinforce his participation.

For Discussion

Who might Shannon ask to go riding with her? What could Aleem do to become involved in physical activity? What other suggestions can you offer for finding social support? What groups might Shannon and Aleem identify with to get social support? Consider the guidelines presented in the Self-Management feature when you answer the discussion questions.

SELF-MANAGEMENT: Skills for Finding Social Support

Experts indicate that people who experience support from others are more likely to participate in regular physical activity, especially over the course of a lifetime. Social support is also helpful to people in reaching and maintaining a healthy body weight, building muscle fitness, and improving eating habits. Consider the following guidelines to help you gain others' support for your physical activity.

- **Do a self-assessment of your current level of social support.** Ask your teacher about the social support worksheet that can help you do this assessment. Use the self-assessment to determine areas in which you can improve your social support.

- **Birds of a feather flock together.** Find friends who are interested in the activities that interest you, or encourage your current friends to support you or join you in your participation.

- **Join a club or team.** If no club or team exists for your chosen activity, talk to a teacher, family member, or community recreation leader about starting one.

- **Contact local organizations.** Organizations such as the R.E.A.L. (Recreation Experiences and Leisure) program financially support children and teens to join clubs and teams, and they also provide equipment when possible.

- **Discuss your interests with family and teachers.** Ask them for their support. Ask them to help you learn the activity.

- **If possible, take lessons.** In addition to formal lessons, you can also ask teachers and others to support you by helping you learn to perform an activity properly.

- **Family matters.** Encourage your family members to try the activity.

- **Get proper equipment.** Ask for equipment for your birthday or other special occasion.

TAKING ACTION: Accessing Social Support

Staying regularly physically active is hard, and getting physically active can be even tougher. That's what friends are for! If you want to be successful staying or getting physically active, you need to take action to get support from others. If you have an active friend, that's a great place to start. Ask your friend to commit to regular physical activity with you. If you don't have a friend, try participating in community physical activities that are social. Chances are you will find someone with similar interests and the commitment to be active with you. Once you have connected in person, you might want to share your progress on Facebook, share your experiences with a picture on Instagram, or tweet out your successes. Physical activity researchers have clearly demonstrated that getting support from others is one of the best ways to stay active throughout your life. What are you waiting for?

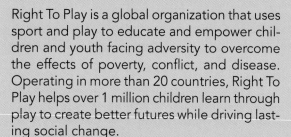

Just completed my 45 min walk

Good for you....btw are we on for yoga tomorrow?

Definitely...cu there

Excited to get my stretch on ;)

Active friends can give you social support to take action.

GET ACTIVE WITH RIGHT TO PLAY

© Right to Play

Who We Are

Right To Play is a global organization that uses sport and play to educate and empower children and youth facing adversity to overcome the effects of poverty, conflict, and disease. Operating in more than 20 countries, Right To Play helps over 1 million children learn through play to create better futures while driving lasting social change.

What We Do

Right To Play leads programs all around the world, but here is an example of the work that we do that is making an impact right here in Canada through the PLAY and Youth to Youth programs.

The Promoting Life-skills in Aboriginal Youth (PLAY) program partners with more than 55 First Nation communities and urban aboriginal organizations across Ontario, Manitoba, British Columbia, and Alberta to deliver programming for children and youth. Guided by an indigenous community development model, Right To Play and its partners create safe and inclusive spaces where children and youth can share their ideas and hopes and fears and learn the skills for becoming positive agents of change. Through activities that are fun and engaging, indigenous children and youth learn about healthy food and lifestyle choices, build skills transferable to school and employment such as communication, teamwork, and planning, and build healthy relationships and connections within their community.

The Youth to Youth program partners with 25 inner-city schools and community centres across Toronto to provide safe, inclusive play-based programming for children and youth in priority neighbourhoods. Schools identify particular students who want the opportunity to develop their leadership skills. Right To Play then partners with teachers to train youth leaders in facilitation skills, behaviour management skills, and the use of games and activities as a vehicle for learning. Youth leaders then plan and lead weekly play-based activities for younger children.

Get Involved

Start your own Right To Play club at your school! Discuss what you can do as a school to stay socially responsible. Visit righttoplay-schools.ca for resources and more information. Follow us on Twitter at @RighttoPlayCan or find us on facebook.com/righttoplaycan.

Reprinted, by permission, from Monica Abdel-Messih. © Right to Play

Reviewing Concepts and Vocabulary

Complete the following in order to determine your growing understanding of fitness, health, and wellness. Answer items 1 through 5 by correctly completing each sentence with a word or phrase.

1. Individual, _____, community, and public policy influence physical activity and healthy eating.
2. The individual factors you have most control over include knowledge, _____, and attitudes.
3. People who seek and provide social support are more _____ and eat more healthfully than those without social support.
4. People who are alone and isolated from family, friends, and community are often more _____, are less healthy, and live shorter lives.
5. When you let friends know that you can understand how they are feeling, you are providing _____ social support.

For items 6 through 10, match each term in column 1 with the appropriate phrase in column 2.

6. emotional support   a. providing information that that helps a person self-evaluate
7. instrumental support   b. providing resources (e.g., time, money, equipment)
8. social support   c. sharing expressions of caring, love, trust, and empathy
9. informational support   d. having people in your life who care for you and help you
10. appraisal support   e. providing advice, ideas, and information

For items 11 through 15, respond to each statement or question.

11. List four factors that influence physical activity and healthy eating.
12. Provide an example of how social support can support healthy behaviours and unhealthy behaviours.
13. Explain why it is important to give social support.
14. Describe three types of social support that you can give or receive.
15. List three important benefits of giving and receiving social support.

Thinking Critically

Create a mind map (e.g., spider web, cloud, bubbles, a brain) to identify behaviours you would like to change and how you might change these behaviours.

Identify a health behaviour you would like to change in order to be healthier (e.g., physical activity, eating, sleep, flossing your teeth, smoking, alcohol or drug use). Use this as the middle of your mind map. As you reflect on that behaviour, add all the factors currently influencing your behaviour. Now add changes you could make to improve those specific behaviours. Consider the impacts of social support, cultural environments, and physical environments in your answer.

Project

Use your phone or a camera to take a picture or series of pictures that illustrate social support or any of the four factors that influence physical activity and healthy eating (i.e., individual, interpersonal, community, public policy). Using the picture(s), write down or record your explanation of how the picture(s) represents an influence on physical activity or healthy eating. An Internet search will help you find tools to support you in this project (e.g., "photo narrative app"; "using photos to tell a story").

6

How Much Physical Activity and Fitness Is Enough?

In This Chapter

 Student Web Resources
www.fitnessforlife.org/student

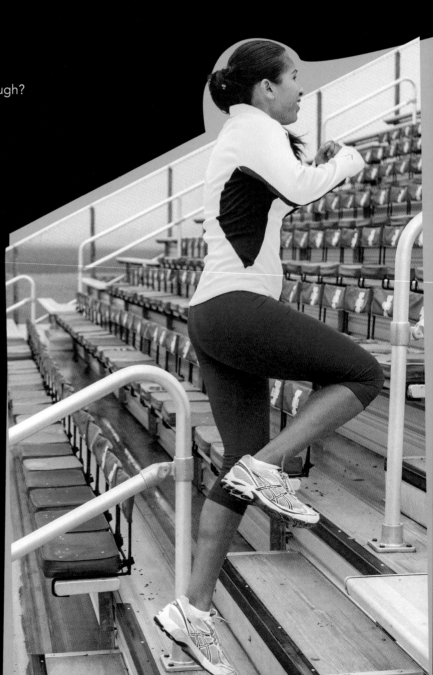

Lesson 6.1
How Much Physical Activity Is Enough?

Lesson Objectives

After participating in this lesson, you should be able to

1. name and describe the three principles of exercise;
2. describe the four parts of the FITT formula and discuss how they relate to threshold of training, target ceiling, and fitness target zone; and
3. describe the five types of physical activity included in the Physical Activity Pyramid.

Lesson Vocabulary

fitness target zone, FITT formula, frequency, hypokinetic disease, intensity, Physical Activity Pyramid, principle of overload, principle of progression, principle of specificity, target ceiling, threshold of training, time, type

How much physical activity is enough? This question might seem very simple, but the answer can be complicated, especially if you're just beginning an activity program. In this lesson, you'll develop an understanding of three basic exercise principles as a good first step in answering the question of how much is enough.

Principles of Physical Fitness

Consider this example. Mia has been exercising for several months. Every day, she does the same physical activities for about 15 minutes. Her activity program has not changed since she started. Initially, Mia saw some positive results from her program: She was no longer tired at the end of her exercise, and a self-assessment showed that her cardiorespiratory endurance had improved. Lately, however, Mia has felt disappointed because her strength and flexibility haven't been improving as much as they did at first. Mia wants to know what she's doing wrong. For some clues to the answer, let's look at the three principles of exercise: overload, progression, and specificity.

Principle of Overload

The most basic law of physical activity is the **principle of overload**, which states that the only way to produce fitness and health benefits through physical activity is to require your body to do more than it normally does. Increased demand on your body—overload—forces it to adapt. Your body was designed to be active, so if you do nothing (underload), your fitness will decrease, and you will increase your risk of **hypokinetic disease**.

Since Mia is no longer overloading when she exercises, she is maintaining but no longer gaining increased fitness and health benefits. If she wants to continue improving her strength and flexibility, she'll have to increase the amount of her physical activity.

Principle of Progression

The **principle of progression** states that the amount and intensity of your exercise should be increased gradually. After a while, your body adapts to an increase in physical activity (load), and the activity gets easier for you to perform. When this happens, you can gradually increase your activity.

Figure 6.1 shows the minimum overload you need in order to build physical fitness. This amount is called your **threshold of training**. Performing activity above your threshold builds your fitness and promotes your health and wellness. Since Mia has exercised for several months at the same level, she may now be exercising below her threshold of training for at least some parts of fitness.

This correct range of physical activity is called your **fitness target zone**, typically shortened to just *target zone*. It begins with the threshold of training and has an upper limit called the **target ceiling**. Exercise below the threshold is not enough to produce benefits. Activities above the target ceiling (excessive exercise) can increase risk of injury and

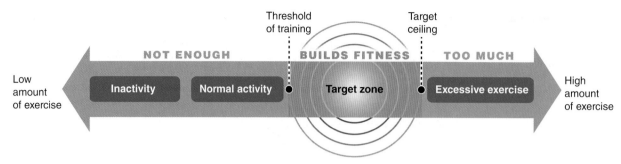

| NOT ENOUGH | | BUILDS FITNESS | TOO MUCH |

Threshold of training

Target ceiling

Low amount of exercise

Inactivity | Normal activity | Target zone | Excessive exercise

High amount of exercise

FIGURE 6.1 The fitness target zone.

soreness and may produce less than optimal benefits. Some people think you have to experience pain in order to gain fitness, but the principle of progression provides the basis for rejecting the theory of "no pain, no gain." If you experience pain when you exercise, you're probably overloading too much or too quickly for your body to adjust.

Principle of Specificity

The **principle of specificity** states that the particular type of exercise you perform determines the particular benefit you receive. Different kinds and amounts of activity produce very specific and different benefits. An activity that promotes health benefits in one part of health-related fitness may not be equally good in promoting high levels of fitness in another part of fitness. For example, Mia jogs on a track several days a week, but she does not do stretching exercises as often as she should. She may also need to use more resistance in her muscle fitness exercises.

In addition, exercises performed for specific body parts, such as the calf muscles, may provide benefits only for those parts. For example, if Mia does exercises only for her calf muscles, she will not build the muscles in her back, shoulders, arms, or other parts of her legs.

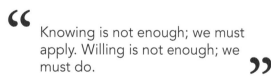

Knowing is not enough; we must apply. Willing is not enough; we must do.

—Johann Wolfgang von Goethe, writer and artist

FITT Formula

You know that you must do more physical activity than normal to build fitness. You also know that

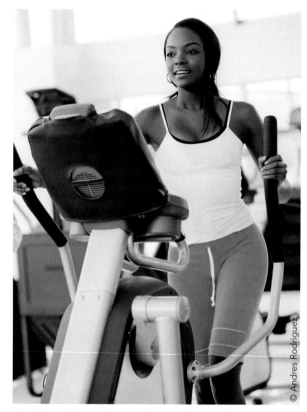

Applying the principle of specificity is important for getting optimal benefits.

you should gradually increase your physical activity in order to stay within your fitness target zone. But how much physical activity do you need?

To help you apply the principles of exercise, you can use the **FITT formula**. Some people refer to it as the FITT *principle,* but we use the term *formula* in this book because a formula refers to a prescription or recipe. In this case, the prescription is for determining the right amount of physical activity for applying the three exercise principles. In fact, each letter in the acronym FITT represents a key factor in determining how much physical activity is enough: **F**requency, **I**ntensity, **T**ime, and **T**ype.

- **Frequency refers to how often you do physical activity.** For physical activity to be beneficial, you must do it several days a week. Optimal **frequency** depends on the type of activity you're doing and the part of fitness you want to develop. To develop strength, for example, you might need to exercise two days a week. To lose fat, you should exercise daily.

- **Intensity refers to how hard you perform physical activity.** If the activity you do is too easy, you will not build fitness or gain other benefits. But remember—extremely vigorous activity can be harmful if you don't work up to it gradually. **Intensity** is determined differently depending on the type of activity you do and the type of fitness you want to build. For example, you can use your heart rate to determine your intensity of activity for building cardiorespiratory endurance, whereas you would use the amount of weight you lift to determine the intensity for building strength.

- **Time refers to how long you do physical activity.** As with frequency and intensity, the length of **time** during which you should do physical activity depends on the type of activity you're doing and the part of fitness you want to develop. For example, to build flexibility you should exercise for 15 seconds or more for each muscle group, whereas to build cardiorespiratory endurance you need to be vigorously active for a minimum of 20 minutes.

- **Type refers to the kind of activity you do to build a specific part of fitness or gain a specific benefit.** One **type** of activity may be good for building one part of fitness but not for building another part. For example, doing vigorous aerobics builds your cardiorespiratory endurance but does little to develop your flexibility. Throughout this book, you'll learn how to apply the FITT formula to different activities that build specific parts of physical fitness. Once you determine the type of activity, you can drop the second "T" in FITT and determine the frequency, intensity, and time (or FIT) for each specific activity. FIT information is given for each type of activity included in the Physical Activity Pyramid (see figure 6.2).

The Physical Activity Pyramid

National physical activity guidelines for youth developed by the Canadian Society for Exercise Physiology in partnership with ParticipAction and the Public Health Agency of Canada recommend at least 60 minutes of moderate- to vigorous-intensity physical activity each day for children and youth ages 5 through 17. The five steps of the **Physical Activity Pyramid** (figure 6.2) help you understand the five kinds of physical activity, which build different parts of fitness and produce different health and wellness benefits (recall the principle of specificity). To meet the recommended 60 minutes of daily activity, you can choose from the different types of activity. For optimal benefits, you should perform activities from all parts of the pyramid each week. As you can see, activities at or near the bottom of the pyramid may need to be done more frequently or for a longer time than those near the top of the pyramid to get the same volume of activity.

Moderate-Intensity Physical Activity

Moderate-intensity physical activity is the first step in the Physical Activity Pyramid, and it should be performed

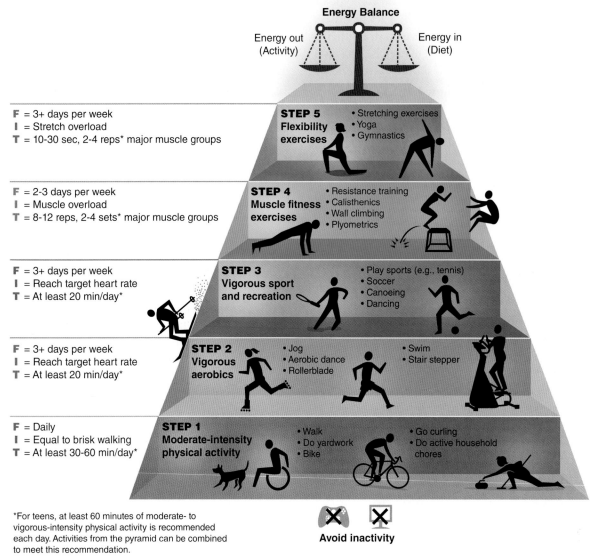

Energy Balance

Energy out (Activity) — Energy in (Diet)

| STEP 5 Flexibility exercises | • Stretching exercises • Yoga • Gymnastics |

F = 3+ days per week
I = Stretch overload
T = 10-30 sec, 2-4 reps* major muscle groups

STEP 5 Flexibility exercises
• Stretching exercises
• Yoga
• Gymnastics

F = 2-3 days per week
I = Muscle overload
T = 8-12 reps, 2-4 sets* major muscle groups

STEP 4 Muscle fitness exercises
• Resistance training
• Calisthenics
• Wall climbing
• Plyometrics

F = 3+ days per week
I = Reach target heart rate
T = At least 20 min/day*

STEP 3 Vigorous sport and recreation
• Play sports (e.g., tennis)
• Soccer
• Canoeing
• Dancing

F = 3+ days per week
I = Reach target heart rate
T = At least 20 min/day*

STEP 2 Vigorous aerobics
• Jog
• Aerobic dance
• Rollerblade
• Swim
• Stair stepper

F = Daily
I = Equal to brisk walking
T = At least 30-60 min/day*

STEP 1 Moderate-intensity physical activity
• Walk
• Do yardwork
• Bike
• Go curling
• Do active household chores

*For teens, at least 60 minutes of moderate- to vigorous-intensity physical activity is recommended each day. Activities from the pyramid can be combined to meet this recommendation.

Avoid inactivity

FIGURE 6.2 The new Physical Activity Pyramid for Teens.

© Charles B. Corbin

daily or nearly every day. Moderate-intensity activity involves exercise equal in intensity to brisk walking. It includes some activities of normal daily living (also called lifestyle activities), such as yard work (for example, raking leaves or mowing the lawn) and housework (for example, mopping the floor). It also includes sports that are not vigorous, such as bowling and golf. Some other sports can be either moderate intensity or vigorous intensity; for example, shooting basketballs is typically a moderate-intensity activity, whereas playing a full-court game is a vigorous-intensity activity. National guidelines recommend 60 minutes of moderate- to vigorous-intensity activity each day for teens. Moderate-intensity activity should account for some of this time each day. It is also associated with many of the health benefits of activity described in this book, such as controlling your level of body fat, and is well suited for people of varying abilities.

Vigorous Aerobics

Step 2 of the Physical Activity Pyramid represents vigorous aerobics, which includes any exercise that you can do for a long time without stopping and that is vigorous enough to increase your heart rate, make you breathe faster, and make you sweat. Thus these activities are more intense than moderate-intensity activities such as brisk walking. Vigorous aerobics, such as jogging and aerobic dance, are typically continuous in nature. Like moderate-intensity activity, they provide many health and wellness benefits, and they're especially helpful for building a high level of cardiorespiratory endurance. You should perform vigorous aerobics (or vigorous sport or recreation) at least three days a week for at least 20 minutes each day in order to meet national activity guidelines.

Vigorous Sport and Recreation

Like vigorous aerobics, vigorous sport and recreation (represented in step 3 of the Physical Activity Pyramid) require your heart to beat faster than normal and cause you to breathe faster and sweat more. As your muscles use more oxygen, your heart beats faster, and you breathe faster and more deeply to meet the oxygen demand. Unlike vigorous aerobics, however, vigorous sport and recreation often involve short bursts of activity followed by short bursts of

rest (as in basketball, football, soccer, and tennis). When done for at least 20 minutes a day in bouts of 10 minutes or more at a time, these activities provide fitness, health, and wellness benefits similar to those of vigorous aerobics. They also help you build motor skills and contribute to healthy weight management. As with vigorous aerobics, you can use vigorous sport and recreation to meet national activity recommendations when you do them for at least 20 minutes a day on three days a week.

Muscle Fitness Exercises

Step 4 in the Physical Activity Pyramid represents muscle fitness exercises, which build your strength, muscular endurance, and power. Muscle fitness exercises include both resistance training (with weights or machines) and moving your own body weight (as in rock climbing, calisthenics, and jumping). This type of exercise produces general health and wellness benefits, as well as better performance, improved body appearance, a healthier back, better posture, and stronger bones. These exercises can be used to meet national activity guidelines and should be performed on two or three days a week.

Flexibility Exercises

Step 5 of the Physical Activity Pyramid represents flexibility exercises. There is some evidence that

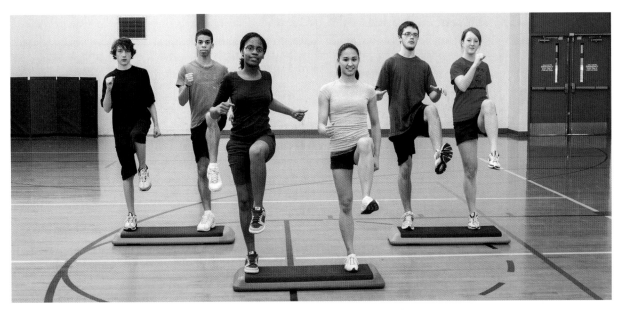

Vigorous aerobic activity helps you build cardiorespiratory endurance.

FITNESS TECHNOLOGY: Activity Trackers

Technology is making it easier to keep track of your physical activity levels. People no longer need pen-and-paper logbooks or calendars to write down how far they have walked or how long they have exercised. Activity trackers are typically wrist-worn devices that use accelerometer (i.e., motion sensing) and global system positioning (GPS) technology to keep track of

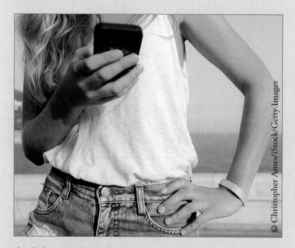

Activity trackers help you monitor your physical activity level.

how many steps you have taken, how far you have traveled, and how much time you spent in physical activity. Using built-in algorithms (i.e., equations that use several variables to predict a score), these devices can also estimate the intensity of your physical activity, estimate the number of calories you burned, and monitor your sleep. Do your homework before you purchase one of these devices, and determine how you will use the device before you spend between $40 and $300 for an activity tracker. Pick a fun colour so that people ask you about it. Starting a conversation about physical activity is positive.

Using Technology

Search the web for "fitness trackers" or "activity trackers." Find an article that compares several trackers, read the article, and present the findings to your class. Focus on the similarities and differences between the various trackers and come up with an opinion on the best tracker value based on cost and function.

flexibility exercises may reduce soreness, prevent injuries, and reduce risk of back pain. Flexibility exercises also improve your performance in activities such as gymnastics and dance. They also are used in therapy to help people who have been injured. Two examples of flexibility exercise are stretching and yoga (figure 6.3). To build and maintain flexibility, you should perform flexibility exercise at least three days a week.

Avoiding Inactivity

Just below the Physical Activity Pyramid (see figure 6.2) you'll notice pictures of a television set and a video game controller with an "X" over them. This illustration emphasizes the fact that being sedentary, or inactive, poses a health risk.

Just as you should do 60 minutes of physical activity each day, drawing from the five types of activity presented in the pyramid, you should also

avoid the inactivity that is common among people who log too much "screen time" on a daily basis. Screen time refers to time spent in front of a TV, computer game, phone screen, or any other device that substitutes inactivity for activities from the pyramid. A survey conducted in Canada revealed that time spent viewing television and using computers was positively associated with obesity, inactive leisure time, and a poor diet. Other research revealed that one in every three Canadian teens spends 40 hours a week watching TV and surfing the net—that averages out to over 5 hours a day! Some teens spend as much as 50 or 60 hours a week on screen time.

We all need to take time to recover from daily stresses and prepare for new challenges, so periods of rest and sleep are important for good health. Some activities of daily living—such as studying, reading, and even a moderate amount of screen time—are appropriate. But general inactivity or sedentary

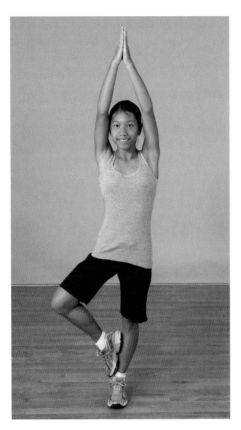

FIGURE 6.3 Yoga is one type of physical activity for improving flexibility.

living is harmful to your health. Your choices from active areas of the pyramid should exceed your choices from the inactivity area.

Balancing Energy

The top of the pyramid presents a balance scale illustrating the need to balance the energy you take in (food) with the energy you put out (activity). Energy balance means that the calories in the food you eat each day are equal to the calories you expend in exercise each day. Balancing your energy in this way is essential to maintaining a healthy body composition.

Patterns of Moderate- and Vigorous-Intensity Activity

A pattern is a schedule you use to accumulate minutes of activity from the pyramid each day and each week. One pattern is continuous activity, in which you do all of your physical activity for the day in one continuous session (for example, 60 minutes of continuous moderate- to vigorous-intensity activity).

The second pattern is accumulated activity, in which you do sessions of 15 minutes or more in order to accumulate your targeted daily total (for example, 15 + 15 + 15 + 15 = 60). Bouts of less than 10 minutes may provide some health benefits but are not recommended for use in accumulating your recommended daily activity time, because bouts of less than 10 minutes are considered below the threshold of training for getting benefits.

The third pattern is that of the "weekend warrior." This pattern is marked by inactivity during most of the week punctuated by relatively long sessions of activity—sometimes for several hours at a time and often all in one day. Adults often do this extended activity on weekends because of their work commitments during the week—thus the name "weekend warrior." This pattern is not recommended and can even be dangerous for people with risk factors because it violates the principle of progression and can lead to soreness and injury. Thus you should do your activity on most days of the week using a continuous or accumulated pattern.

Lesson Review

1. What are the three principles of exercise, and why are they important?
2. How are threshold of training, target ceiling, and fitness target zone related to the parts of the FITT formula?
3. What are some characteristics and examples of each of the five types of activity included in the Physical Activity Pyramid?

121

In this assessment, you'll perform two tests (but it's important to remember that there are other tests we learn about in this text that you could use): one to assess your cardiorespiratory endurance and another to measure the flexibility and fitness of your back and trunk muscles. If you have not done so already, practice each test before performing it for a score. Record your scores and fitness ratings for the two tests as directed by your teacher. Performing these tests will provide information that you can use in your personal needs profile for preparing your personal physical activity plan. If you're working with a partner, remember that self-assessment information is personal and considered confidential. It shouldn't be shared with others without the permission of the person being tested.

PACER (Progressive Aerobic Cardiovascular Endurance Run, or 20-Metre Shuttle Run)

This test of cardiorespiratory endurance was originally developed in Canada and called the 20-metre shuttle run, and that name is still used in many countries. The name PACER, as it is called in FitnessGram, was the winning entry, submitted by Dr. Jack Rutherford, in a contest designed to create a new name for the test that would be easy to remember.

The test is scored differently by different test batteries. In this book, you'll use the number of laps you perform as the score on which your fitness rating is based; laps are also used for scoring in the Alpha-Fit test. Using laps makes it easy for you to see if you improve after performing your personal activity plan.

Directions

1. The test objective is to run back and forth across a 20-metre (almost 22-yard) distance as many times as you can at a predetermined pace (pacing is based on signals from a special audio recording provided by your instructor).

2. Start at a line located 20 metres from a second line. When you hear the beep from the audio track, run across the 20-metre area to the second line, arriving just before the audio track beeps again, and touch the line with your foot. Turn around and get ready to run back.

3. At the sound of the next beep, run back to the line where you began. Touch the line with your foot. Make sure to wait for the beep before running back.

4. Continue to run back and forth from one line to the other, touching the line each time. The beeps will come faster and faster, causing you to run faster and faster. The test is finished when you twice fail to reach the opposite side before the beep.

5. Your score is the number of laps you ran (the number of times you ran the 20-metre distance from one line to the other) before your test was finished. Using laps as your score allows you to easily test yourself to see how you improve over time. This method of scoring provides you with a good indicator of your cardiorespiratory endurance, which is a measure of functional fitness—your ability to function effectively in daily living.

6. Use table 6.1 to determine your rating. Record your score and rating.

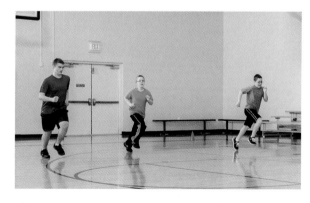

The PACER test assesses cardiorespiratory endurance.

TABLE 6.1 Rating Chart for PACER

| | 13 years old | | 14 years old | | 15 years old | | 16 years old | | 17 years or older | |
	Male	Female	Male	Female	Male	Female	Male	Female	Male	Female
High performance	≥36	≥31	≥45	≥34	≥54	≥38	≥60	≥40	≥67	≥50
Good fitness	29–35	25–30	36–44	27–33	42–53	30–37	47–59	32–39	54–66	38–49
Marginal fitness	23–28	19–24	28–35	21–26	32–41	23–29	36–46	25–31	42–53	30–37
Low fitness	≤22	≤18	≤27	≤20	≤31	≤22	≤35	≤24	≤41	≤29

Scores in this table refer to the number of completed laps.

Based on data provided by G. Welk.

Trunk Lift (Upper Back)

1. Lie facedown with your arms to your sides and your hands under your thighs.

2. Lift the upper part of your body very slowly so that your chin, chest, and shoulders come off the floor. Lift your trunk as high as possible, to a maximum of 30 centimetres (12 inches). Hold this position for three seconds while a partner measures how far your chin is from the floor. Your partner should hold the ruler at least 2.5 centimetres (1 inch) in front of your chin. Look straight ahead so that your chin is not tipped abnormally upward.

3. Do the trunk lift two times (lifting slowly) and record how far from the floor you can lift and hold your chin (for three seconds). Do not record scores above 30 centimetres (12 inches).

Caution: The ruler should not be placed directly under your chin, in case you have to lower your trunk unexpectedly.

4. Use table 6.2 to determine your fitness rating. Record your score and rating.

TABLE 6.2 Rating Chart for Trunk Lift

Rating	Centimetres
High performance	28–30
Good fitness	23–27
Marginal fitness	18–22
Low fitness	≤17

To convert centimetres to inches, multiply centimetres by 0.39. Alternatively, you can use the Internet to find a calculator that converts centimetres to inches.

Data based on *FitnessGram*.

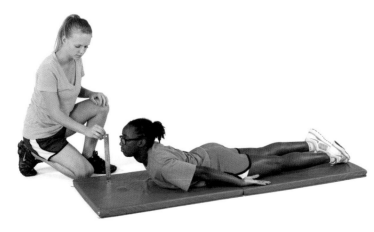

This test measures the flexibility of your back and trunk muscles, as well as the muscle fitness of your back muscles.

Lesson 6.2
How Much Fitness Is Enough?

Lesson Objectives

After participating in this lesson, you should be able to

1. describe the four fitness rating categories and how they apply to your physical activity program,
2. identify factors that contribute to fitness, and
3. explain how a person can attain good health and fitness even if some factors make it difficult to succeed.

 Lesson Vocabulary

criterion-referenced health standards, maturation

You now know that physical activity is necessary to build each part of physical fitness. But exactly how much fitness do you need? In this lesson, you'll learn some ways to decide how much fitness is enough for you.

Fitness Standards and Rating Categories

Sometimes people judge their fitness by comparing themselves with others. If they score higher on a fitness test than most other people, they consider themselves fit. This type of comparison creates several problems. First, it suggests that only a few people can be fit. Second, it suggests that only high test scores are adequate for fitness. In this lesson, you'll learn why neither of these suggestions is true.

Most experts agree that you should judge fitness using **criterion-referenced health standards**. The word "standard" refers to an established amount or quantity. The word "criterion" refers to a marker used to establish the standard (as it relates to health). So a criterion-referenced standard for health-related fitness refers to the amount of fitness you need in order to achieve good health. This type of standard does not require you to compare yourself with others. It does require you to have enough fitness to

- reduce your risk of health problems,
- achieve wellness benefits,
- function effectively in your daily life,
- meet emergencies, and
- enjoy your free time.

As noted in this chapter's Science in Action feature, you'll learn to do many self-assessments for each of the health-related parts of physical fitness. In this book, we use a rating system based on criterion-referenced health standards. It is similar to the rating systems used in test batteries such as FitnessGram, and we use it here so that you can rate your fitness in all of the tests included in this book by means of the same system.

To rate yourself in each of the six parts of health-related physical fitness, you'll use one of the following four fitness rating categories. If you attain a rating of "good fitness" for all six fitness areas, you'll achieve the basic health and wellness standards of physical fitness.

- **Low fitness.** If you have a low fitness rating, you have an above-average risk of developing health problems. You also might not look your best, feel your best, or work and play as efficiently as you could. If you have a low fitness rating, you should work to achieve a marginal fitness rating.

- **Marginal fitness.** Moving from the low to the marginal rating shows important progress in fitness. However, if you have a marginal rating, you should try to get a good fitness rating.

- **Good fitness.** This rating indicates that you have the fitness needed to live a full, healthy life. In fact, achieving a good fitness rating is the goal of most people. To maintain this level of fitness, you'll need to continue being physically active.

SCIENCE IN ACTION: Personal Fitness Assessment

Experts in physical education and exercise physiology have worked together to develop various physical fitness test batteries. A battery is a group of tests designed to assess all parts of physical fitness. As introduced in chapter 2, FitnessGram is one fitness test battery used in many schools throughout the world and is the national fitness test battery in the United States. In Canada, the Canadian Society for Exercise Physiology (CSEP) has a fitness test battery as part of their Physical Activity Training for Health (PATH) program. Alpha-Fit is a fitness test battery widely used in Europe. The three batteries contain some similar tests and some that differ from each other.

In this book, you'll try many fitness tests. The goal is to help you select test items for your own *personal fitness test battery* that you can use throughout your life to self-assess your fitness. You will perform all of the test items in the FitnessGram and Alpha-Fit batteries, some tests from the CSEP-PATH program, as well as several other tests. For all tests in this book, you'll use the Fitness for Life rating system, but you can also learn how to use standards and ratings from other test batteries. What's most important is that you learn to test your own fitness and use your personal self-assessment results to plan your own fitness and physical activity.

Fitness self-assessments are considered personal health information. True fitness self-assessments are performed by you and for you and help you identify your personal fitness needs. The Fitness for Life Canada program will have you complete a number of personal fitness self-assessments. Please respect your classmates' personal fitness information by not sharing any of their results that you might observe.

Of course, you are free to share your own personal fitness assessment results.

Student Activity

Identify three important components of fitness for your favourite activity. Look at the self-assessments provided throughout this textbook, and create your own personal fitness test battery by choosing three tests that would assess the components of fitness you identified for your favourite activity.

- **High performance.** Most experts agree that many health benefits can be achieved without reaching a high performance rating. However, performing the amount of physical activity necessary to reach this rating has additional health benefits because you get more benefits with a greater volume of activity (when not overdone). It should be noted that the fitter you get, the harder it is to improve. Achieving a high performance rating is necessary if you want to be an athlete or perform a physically demanding job, such as firefighter, soldier, or police officer.

Factors Influencing Physical Fitness

Physical activity is the most important thing you can do to improve or maintain your health-related physical fitness. Fortunately, it is also something that you can control. You can choose the kinds of activity you want to do and schedule a regular time to do them. But as figure 6.4 shows, physical activity is not the only factor that contributes to your physical fitness. Other important factors are **maturation**, age, heredity, environment, and lifestyle choices such as nutrition and stress management.

Maturation

Physical maturation means becoming physically full grown and developed. This process begins in your early teen years because of hormones that promote the growth and development of tissues such as muscle and bone. Some people mature earlier than others, and early developers often do better on physical fitness tests than those who mature later. But ultimately, time is the great equalizer. We all develop fully over time, and it is not unusual for those who develop after most of their peers to achieve fitness levels that equal or exceed the fitness levels of those who develop earlier.

Age

Studies show that older teens perform better on fitness tests than younger teens. Even in the same class, those who are older typically do better than those who are younger. This difference results mostly from the fact that the older you are, the more you've grown and the more physically mature you're likely to be. As you learned earlier, age and maturation do not always parallel each other. However, sometimes one person matures earlier than another, and in such cases a younger but more physically mature person could have an advantage in performing physical fitness tests.

 Do not let what you cannot do interfere with what you can do.

—John Wooden, basketball coach

Heredity

Heredity involves the characteristics we inherit from our parents, including the physical characteristics that influence how we perform on physical fitness tests. For example, some people have more fat cells than others because of heredity. Similarly, some people have more of the muscle fibres that help them run fast, whereas others have more of the muscle fibres that help them run a long time without fatigue. Each person's heredity enables better performance in some areas and makes it harder to perform well in others. Fortunately, fitness is composed of many different parts. Your heredity helps determine the parts of fitness in which you do well and the parts in which you may not do as well, but you can also affect this somewhat by applying the FITT formula to become more fit.

Environment

Your fitness is also affected by environmental factors, such as where you live (city, suburbs, country), your school environment, and the availability or unavailability of places to play and do other types

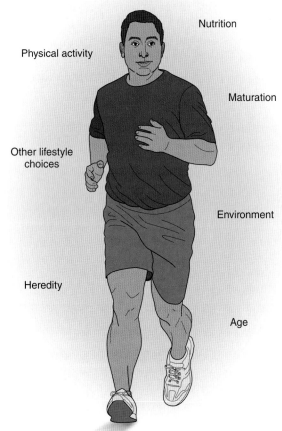

Physical activity

Nutrition

Maturation

Other lifestyle choices

Environment

Heredity

Age

FIGURE 6.4 Various factors influence your physical fitness.

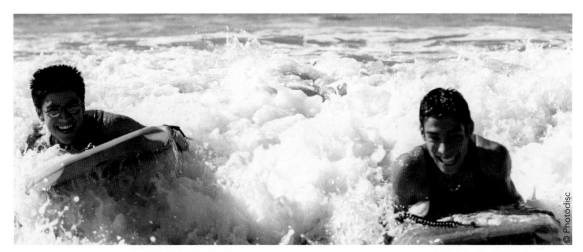

© Photodisc

Compare your fitness with criterion-referenced health standards rather than with your friends' fitness levels.

of physical activity. Even your social environment can affect your fitness, including the friends you choose. For example, people who live near parks and those who have active friends are typically more active than those who don't.

FIT FACT

Teens who walk or ride a bicycle to school are more active overall than those who do not. Specifically, they get an average of 16 minutes more activity each day, and that difference in itself is more than 25 percent of the recommended amount of daily activity.

Anyone Can Succeed

Because many factors contribute to physical fitness, it is possible for some people who do relatively little physical activity to achieve relatively good fitness scores while they are in their teens. These people probably matured early and inherited physical characteristics that help them do well on physical fitness tests. However, they may also be in danger of concluding that they don't need to do physical activity. This may be true enough if they care only about doing well on fitness tests while they're young, but it will not be true for a lifetime. As people get older, they can no longer gain a fitness advantage from early physical maturation or the energy of youth. Sooner or later, physical inactivity will catch up with even those who enjoy a hereditary advantage. Therefore, if you want lifetime fitness, health, and wellness, you need to perform regular physical activity and make healthy lifestyle choices.

Just as some people enjoy fitness advantages because of age, maturation, and heredity, others face disadvantages. For some people, even if they

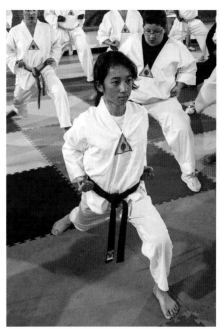

Find an activity that you enjoy and will be able to do later in life.

do physical activity, they still find it hard to get high fitness scores, and they may become discouraged. If this describes you and you find yourself becoming discouraged, remember to avoid comparing yourself with others. Try to achieve a good fitness rating rather than worrying about getting a high performance rating. Good fitness may be harder to achieve for some people than others, but all people can do it. In fact, studies show that people who are good at sports in school but do not remain active later in life are less healthy and die earlier than those who do regular activity throughout their lives—even if they were not especially good performers when they were young.

No matter who you are, physical activity is crucial to your fitness, health, and wellness. With regular physical activity, you can achieve a good fitness rating in all parts of fitness.

Lesson Review

1. What are the four fitness ratings? How do they apply to your physical activity program?
2. What factors contribute to fitness?
3. How can a person attain good health and fitness even if he or she has factors that make it difficult to build a high level of fitness?

TAKING CHARGE: Learning to Self-Monitor

An activity log is a written account of your physical activities during a specified time period. It's a way to keep track of what you do so that you can tell whether you're meeting your activity goals. Self-monitoring refers to any of a variety of techniques for keeping track of your behaviour (for example, a log, diary, or step counter).

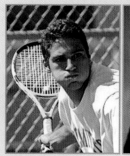 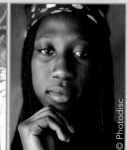

© Photodisc

Drey enjoyed playing tennis on the weekends. He would start out full of energy, but he lacked the endurance to play well for a complete match. His instructor suggested that he do some daily activities to improve his endurance. For several weeks, Drey reported that he faithfully engaged in the activities. But Drey's instructor was a little sceptical based on his level of improvement. Finally, she suggested that Drey keep a log of all the times that he did the activities, and the results were eye-opening: "I was definitely surprised," said Drey. "I usually didn't spend as much time as I thought on each activity. I really thought I was doing well until I saw the results I had written down."

Diya's situation was different. She had knee surgery and was ordered to limit both the kinds and the amount of her activity and to follow a schedule of rehabilitation exercises. She was also supposed to elevate her leg whenever possible. Diya's leg was often swollen and sore at the end of the day, so her physical therapist suggested that she keep a daily log. Diya discovered that she was spending much more time on her feet than she had intended. As a result, she realized that she had to continue doing her rehabilitation exercises but curtail her other activities so that her knee could heal.

For Discussion

How did keeping a log help Drey and Diya? What are some other ways in which a log might help someone? In what other ways might Drey and Diya self-monitor their physical activity levels? Consider the guidelines presented in the following Self-Management feature as you answer these discussion questions.

SELF-MANAGEMENT: Skills for Learning to Self-Monitor

One of the truths of human nature is that adults tend to underestimate how much they eat and overestimate how much physical activity they get. People also make other errors in estimating what they do. For example, we often underestimate how much television we watch and how much money we spend on nonessential items. One term for keeping track of what we do is "self-monitoring." We all self-monitor our behaviour in informal ways, but sometimes it's necessary to make formal assessments if we want accuracy. You can self-monitor your behaviours to help you set goals and make plans—and to evaluate whether you're meeting your goals and fulfilling your plans. Self-monitoring of physical activity is sometimes referred to as "record keeping" or "keeping an activity log." Use the following guidelines to effectively monitor your physical activity.

- **Keep a log.** Make a formal record of your activities by using a written activity log or journal or a free fitness app.

- **Consider using an activity monitor.** Examples include pedometers, heart rate watches, activity trackers, and activity apps for smartphones. A pedometer counts the number of steps you take; it is typically worn on your belt or arm. A heart rate monitor uses a strap around your chest and a watch-like device on your wrist. Either of these devices gives you objective information that you can record in your activity log.

- **Record information as frequently as possible.** The longer you wait before you write down what you do, the more likely you are to make an error. Write things down as soon as possible.

- **Start by self-monitoring your current activity pattern.** To get an accurate picture of your activity level, monitor yourself for at least three days. At least one of the days should be a weekend day, since most people's activity pattern is different on weekends than on weekdays.

- **Use your current activity pattern to help you determine your goals and plans.** People who are already active can set higher goals than those who are less active (or just beginning).

- **Determine how much activity you do in each area of the Physical Activity Pyramid.** For each type of activity included in the pyramid, determine your frequency, intensity, and time (FIT).

- **Write down your goals and plans and keep records to see whether you fulfill them.** Putting your goals and plans in writing can help you self-monitor. Keep records to see whether you did what you planned to do. Keep a diary or an activity chart. Ask your physical education teacher or coach to support you in providing you with equipment or opportunities to reach your goals while you are at school.

You can also use these guidelines to self-monitor other behaviours, such as your eating patterns.

TAKING ACTION: Physical Activity Pyramid Circuit

The Physical Activity Pyramid illustrates how much physical activity you need of different types in order to build fitness, health, and wellness. The Physical Activity Pyramid is a visual presentation of the physical activity guidelines for Canadian teenagers. For example, you need to perform moderate-intensity physical activity (the first step of the pyramid) almost every day to get health benefits, whereas you need to perform muscle fitness activities only two or three times per week. The area below the pyramid represents inactivity or sedentary living. Aside from sleeping, you should minimize your daily sedentary time. A Physical Activity Pyramid circuit is an exercise circuit with stations that provide opportunities for you to take action by performing activities from each step of the Physical Activity Pyramid.

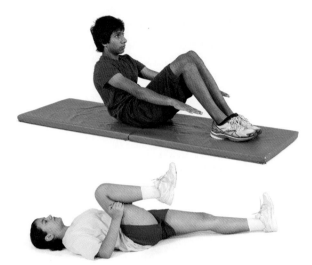

The Physical Activity Pyramid circuit includes activities from each step of the pyramid, including step 4 (muscle fitness) and step 5 (flexibility).

♦ Sport for Life GET ACTIVE WITH SPORT FOR LIFE SOCIETY

©Sport for Life Society

Who We Are

Sport for Life Society is recognized as the international experts on the Canadian Sport for Life (CS4L) movement, long-term athlete development (LTAD), and physical literacy development. The aim of CS4L is high-quality programs for all Canadians based on developmentally appropriate sport and physical activity. LTAD is a seven-stage training, competition, and recovery pathway guiding people's experience in sport and physical activity from infancy through all phases of adulthood. Physical literacy is the motivation, confidence, physical competence, knowledge, and understanding to value and take responsibility for engagement in physical activities for life. CS4L, with LTAD, represents a paradigm shift in the way Canadians lead and deliver sport and physical activity in Canada.

What We Do

Sport for Life Society improves the quality of sport and physical activity in Canada by linking and integrating programs delivered by health, recreation, education, and sport and aligning programming in clubs, provincial, or territorial and national sport and multisport organizations. Sport for Life Society addresses the overarching system and structure of sport and physical activity in Canada, including the relationship between school sport, physical education, and organized sport at all levels, from policy to program delivery.

Get Involved

Are Sport for Life principles embedded in your school sport system? One way to find out is to examine your school's sports and determine whether they are developmentally appropriate and provide meaningful competition, improving the chance to succeed and even win. However, success requires some uncertainty and excitement.

Once you've had a chance to examine your school sport system, answer these questions:

- What percentage of competition at your school is meaningful?
- How developmentally appropriate are the sports in your school?

Share your findings with the Sport for Life Society: info@canadiansportforlife.ca.

If you want to get more involved with the Canadian Sport for Life movement, you can do the following:

- Become a champion: http://canadian sportforlife.ca/become-champion
- Sign up for our newsletters: http:// canadiansportforlife.ca/signup-e-news
- Go to the Sport for Life Society website: http://canadiansportforlife.ca or follow on Twitter: @CS4L_ACSV.

©Sport for Life Society

Reviewing Concepts and Vocabulary

Complete the following in order to determine your growing understanding of fitness, health, and wellness. Answer items 1 through 5 by correctly completing each sentence with a word or phrase.

1. The diagram with five steps that helps you understand the types of physical activity is called the _____.
2. The minimum amount of overload needed to achieve physical fitness is called the _____.
3. Age, maturation, _____, and the environment are factors that affect your physical fitness.
4. If you achieve a _____ fitness rating, you're probably at the level of fitness you need in order to live a full, healthy life.
5. The preferred standard used to rate fitness based on health is called a _____.

For items 6 through 10, match each term in column 1 with the appropriate phrase in column 2.

6. target ceiling   a. how hard you perform physical activity
7. intensity   b. gradual increase of exercise
8. progression   c. upper limit of your physical activity
9. specificity   d. performing more exercise than you normally do
10. overload   e. exercising for one part of fitness

For items 11 through 15, respond to each statement or question.

11. How does the FITT formula help you become healthier? In your answer include (a) what the FITT formula is, (b) what each letter of the acronym represents, and (c) a brief description of each of the components of the formula.
12. Why is it important for you to develop a lifetime physical activity plan even if you're already in the good fitness zone now?
13. Explain why your physical activity program should include activities from all steps of the Physical Activity Pyramid. In your answer include which ones should have the most emphasis and why.
14. What are three guidelines for self-monitoring physical activity?
15. Explain why you shouldn't compare yourself with others when assessing fitness.

Thinking Critically

Your friend says, "It's not good enough to only get a 'good' fitness rating, you have to get a 'high performance' fitness rating to be able to say that you are fit." How would you respond? Write a paragraph to explain your answer.

Project

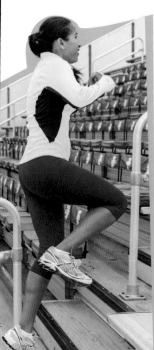

Investigate places in your school and community that offer facilities and equipment for performing activities in the Physical Activity Pyramid. Compile a directory of 10 places that includes the following information for each one:

- address
- phone number
- website
- what is offered (i.e., facilities, equipment, programs, specialities such as women- or men-only locations)
- age restrictions and whether there are reductions in price or special offers for teens

Spread the news by posting it on the bulletin board in class, on a website that other students can access, to social media, or more than one of these.

UNIT III

Being Active and Building Fitness

● ● ● ● ● ● ● ● ● ● ● ● ● ● ● ● ● ●

Self-Assessment Features in This Unit
- Walking Test
- Step Test and One-Mile Run Test
- Assessing Jogging Techniques

Taking Charge Features in This Unit
- Learning to Manage Time
- Self-Confidence
- Choosing Good Activities

Self-Management Features in This Unit
- Skills for Managing Time
- Skills for Building Self-Confidence
- Skills for Choosing Good Activities

Taking Action Features in This Unit
- Your Moderate-Intensity Physical Activity Plan
- Target Heart Rate Workout
- Your Vigorous-Intensity Physical Activity Plan

Canadian Sport and Health Organization Features in This Unit
- Get Active With HALO
- Get Active With Canada Soccer
- Get Active With Canada Basketball

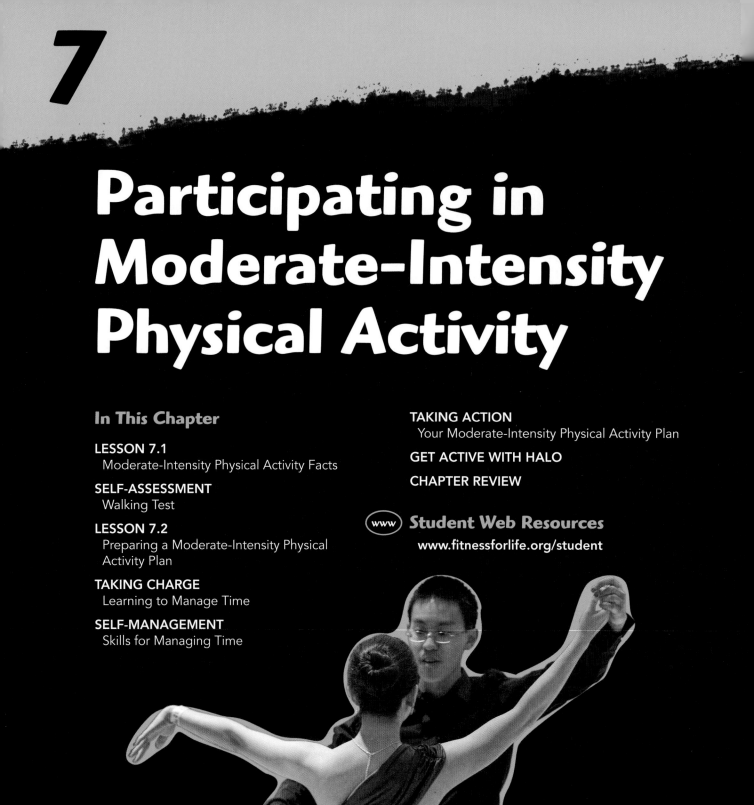

7

Participating in Moderate-Intensity Physical Activity

In This Chapter

LESSON 7.1
Moderate-Intensity Physical Activity Facts

SELF-ASSESSMENT
Walking Test

LESSON 7.2
Preparing a Moderate-Intensity Physical Activity Plan

TAKING CHARGE
Learning to Manage Time

SELF-MANAGEMENT
Skills for Managing Time

TAKING ACTION
Your Moderate-Intensity Physical Activity Plan

GET ACTIVE WITH HALO

CHAPTER REVIEW

www **Student Web Resources**
www.fitnessforlife.org/student

Lesson 7.1
Moderate-Intensity Physical Activity Facts

Lesson Objectives

After participating in this lesson, you should be able to

1. explain the meaning of the term *MET* and why it is important,
2. list three examples of moderate-intensity physical activity,
3. describe the benefits of moderate-intensity physical activity, and
4. describe the FIT formula for moderate-intensity physical activity.

Lesson Vocabulary

accelerometer, lifestyle physical activity, metabolic equivalent (MET), moderate-intensity physical activity, pedometer

Have you ever wondered if you can be healthy without feeling pain and getting sweaty during exercise? Do you know the minimum amount of weekly physical activity you need for good health? While it's good to choose activities from each of the five steps of the Physical Activity Pyramid, public health scientists place a high priority on the first step—moderate-intensity physical activity. The reason is that moderate-intensity physical activities provide many of the health benefits described in this book. These activities are easy to do and can be performed by people of all ages and ability levels. They are sometimes referred to as the foundation of health-enhancing physical activity and thus are appropriately placed at the base of the Physical Activity Pyramid.

What Are Moderate-Intensity Physical Activities?

The term **metabolic equivalent (MET)** comes from the word "metabolism," which refers to the amount of energy (oxygen) necessary to sustain life. You can use the abbreviated term *MET* to help you determine the intensity of any type of exercise. One MET represents the energy expended during

Walking is [our] best medicine.

—Hippocrates, Greek physician and originator of modern medicine

sitting at rest. Physical activities are rated according to their MET value from very light to maximal. The harder the body works, the higher the MET level. For teens, activities requiring less than 2 METs are considered to be very light—for example, eating, reading, and using a computer. Activities that require 2 to 3.9 METs are considered to be light activities; examples include making a bed, washing dishes while standing, preparing food, and walking slowly. These activities are not intense enough to be considered as health enhancing as those presented in the Physical Activity Pyramid (figure 7.1). However, as you've learned, research has shown that some activity is better than none, and performing light or very light activity does expend energy and thus helps you maintain a healthy weight.

Moderate-intensity physical activity requires you to use four to seven times as much energy as being sedentary (thus 4 to 7 METs). For most teens, a good example of moderate-intensity physical activity is brisk walking. Moderate-intensity physical activities are often divided into the following

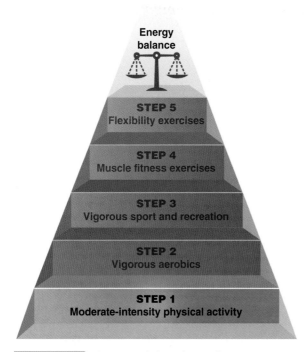

Energy balance

STEP 5
Flexibility exercises

STEP 4
Muscle fitness exercises

STEP 3
Vigorous sport and recreation

STEP 2
Vigorous aerobics

STEP 1
Moderate-intensity physical activity

FIGURE 7.1 Step 1 of the Physical Activity Pyramid, moderate-intensity physical activity, provides a foundation for all other activities.

Adapted from Physical Activity Pyramid for Teens, source: C.B. Corbin.

FIT FACT

The amount of energy (the number of METs) used in an activity depends in part on your fitness level. Fit people use fewer METs than unfit people use for the same activity.

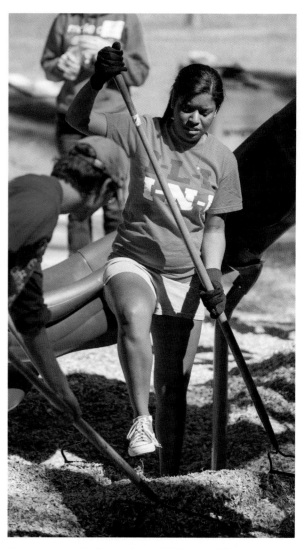

Many moderate-intensity activities are lifestyle activities, such as yard work and housework.

categories: **lifestyle physical activities** done as part of daily life (such as walking to school and doing yard work or housework), moderate sports (such as bowling and golf), moderate recreational activities (such as social dancing and biking slowly), and occupational activities (such as carpentry or landscaping). Curling is considered moderate because there is a lot of standing around, walking, and talking interspersed with some vigorous-intensity sweeping. Table 7.1 presents examples in each of these categories along with the METs for each activity. Some of the activities can require more than 7 METs, and when they are performed at that level they are considered vigorous activities.

Where Do You Get Energy for Moderate Physical Activities?

The human body uses three systems to provide energy for physical activity. For short bursts of very vigorous activity, such as sprinting (for 10 seconds or less), the body uses a high-energy fuel (ATP-PC)

TABLE 7.1 Moderate-Intensity Physical Activities for Teens

Activity type	Description	METs
Lifestyle activities	Walking (brisk)	4.0–5.5
	Yard work	
	Wood chopping	6.0–7.0
	Pushing mower (hand)	6.0–7.0
	Pushing mower (power)	4.0–5.0
	Leaf raking	3.0–4.0
	Shovelling	5.0–7.0
	Housework	
	Floor mopping	3.0–4.0
	Cleaning (heavy)	3.0–4.0
Moderate sports	Bowling	3.0–4.0
	Golf (walking)	3.5–4.5
	Basketball (shooting only)	4.0–5.0
Moderate recreation	Bicycling (slow)	3.0–5.0
	Bicycling (brisk)	5.0–7.0
	Fishing (standing in water)	3.5–4.5
	Social dance	3.0–6.0
Occupational activities	Bricklaying	3.5–4.5
	Carpentry	3.5–5.5
	Heavy assembly work	5.0–6.0

METs for people with low fitness will be higher than those shown in the table; likewise, they will be lower for people with high fitness.

stored in the muscles to provide energy. This system is called the ATP-PC system. When the high-energy fuel is used up, a second system takes over. For vigorous activities that last between 11 seconds and about 90 seconds, such as running up and down a soccer field several times or lifting a heavy weight many times, the body uses the glycolytic system to provide energy. A carbohydrate called glucose is stored in the muscles and liver as glycogen, which provides energy to perform vigorous activity in this second system.

For sustained activity of moderate intensity, such as brisk walking, the body uses the oxidative system (also called the aerobic system) to provide energy. This system allows you to perform activity for many minutes or even hours. Like the glycolytic system, this system uses glucose to provide energy. But since adequate oxygen is available to convert carbohydrate and fat in the body into glucose during moderate-intensity activity, the body does not have to rely primarily on glycogen (glucose) stored in the muscles and liver. More information about energy systems is available in the student section of the Fitness for Life Canada website.

Why Should I Do Moderate-Intensity Physical Activities?

Experts used to think that in order to gain health benefits you had to do vigorous-intensity physical activity (using more than 7 METs). We now know that many health benefits can be achieved by doing moderate-intensity physical activity. Here's a summary of the benefits of moderate-intensity physical activity.

- Reduced risk of hypokinetic disease, such as heart disease, cancer, diabetes, and other chronic diseases

- Improved bone health

- Fitness benefits for people in the low and moderate fitness zones (whereas vigorous activity is required for fitness improvement in people in the good fitness and high performance zones)

- Healthy weight maintenance as a result of adequate energy expenditure

SCIENCE IN ACTION: Sedentary Living

Exercise physiologists have recently learned that extended periods of inactivity can be harmful to your health—the more time people spend sitting, the higher their rate of chronic disease. For this reason, scientists now refer to excessive sedentary living as the "sitting disease." One major reason for sitting among teens today is screen time (whether it be with a television, computer, smartphone, or other device). In fact, teens spend more time sitting now than in the past, and from age 12 to age 16 the amount of sitting and inactivity increases by more than 100 percent.

The danger posed by the sitting disease is the reason that the words "Avoid inactivity" are included under the first step of the Physical Activity Pyramid. In 2016, the Canadian Society of Exercise Physiology (CSEP), along with several other health and physical activity partners, released the first-ever evidence-based, 24-hour movement guidelines for youth (aged 5-17 years). The guide-lines are presented in the shape of the number 4 and communicate the importance of limiting sitting time, accumulating 60 minutes of moderate-to vigorous-intensity physical activity, and getting uninterrupted sleep at consistent times. The clear focus on reducing sitting time reflects the science behind the health risks of sedentary living. Among adults, many companies now offer activity breaks to reduce sitting time, and some companies provide workstations for employees that allow them to stand, walk on treadmills, and even sit and pedal to encourage employees to move while working.

Student Activity

Keep track of the daily time you spend in front of a screen. Do you need to reduce your screen time? If so, how could this be done? How could part of the screen time be replaced with physical activity?

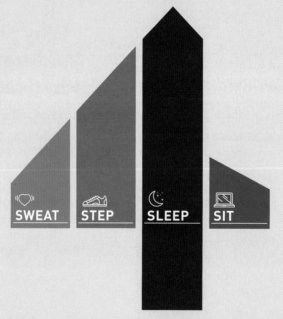

SWEAT
MODERATE TO VIGOROUS PHYSICAL ACTIVITY
An accumulation of at least 60 minutes per day of moderate to vigorous physical activity involving a variety of aerobic activities. Vigorous physical activities, and muscle and bone strengthening activities should each be incorporated at least 3 days per week;

STEP
LIGHT PHYSICAL ACTIVITY
Several hours of a variety of structured and unstructured light physical activities;

SLEEP
SLEEP
Uninterrupted 9 to 11 hours of sleep per night for those aged 5–13 years and 8 to 10 hours per night for those aged 14–17 years, with consistent bed and wake-up times;

SIT
SEDENTARY BEHAVIOUR
No more than 2 hours per day of recreational screen time; Limited sitting for extended periods.

The 24-hour movement guidelines for youth focus on limiting sitting time.

Source: 24-Hour Movement Guidelines for Children and Youth, ©2016. Used with permission from the Canadian Society for Exercise Physiology, www.csep.ca/guidelines.

- Improved wellness and functional fitness, including feeling good, enjoying free time, and doing the things you want to do without undue fatigue
- Improved academic performance (such as improved mental performance resulting from physical activity done before taking a test)

" All the physical comes from the mental. "

—Clara Hughes, Canadian Olympic athlete and mental health awareness advocate

How Much Moderate-Intensity Physical Activity Is Enough?

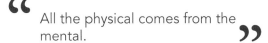

National physical activity guidelines in Canada recommend 60 minutes of moderate- to vigorous-intensity daily activity for teens to gain health benefits. Vigorous activity (e.g., running, in-line skating, soccer) should be performed at least three days a week. Moderate-intensity activity (e.g., walking, skating, bike riding) that promotes muscle fitness and bone building should be performed at least three days a week as well. For adults to achieve health benefits, the recommendation is 150 minutes of moderate to vigorous aerobic activity per week, in bouts of 10 minutes or more. At least two days should be devoted to bone and strengthening activities using major muscle groups. This translates to 30 minutes per day on five days a week. For this reason, many experts recommend that teens get at least 30 minutes of moderate-intensity activity each day so that they develop the habit of meeting the adult activity guideline.

You need to be familiar with the FIT formulas for moderate physical activity for both teens and adults (see table 7.2). The teen guidelines apply, of course, while you're in school, and the adult guidelines will apply for the rest of your life after school.

For teens, the goal is to accumulate at least 60 minutes each day, but more is better. Moderate-intensity

TABLE 7.2   FIT Formulas for Health and Wellness Benefits From Moderate-Intensity Physical Activity

FIT formula	Threshold of training†	Target zone†
Teens		
Frequency	Most days of the week	Daily
Intensity	4 METs Moderate-intensity activity equal in intensity to brisk walking	4–7 METs At least as intense as brisk walking but less intense than normal jogging
Time	60 min of total activity, some of which should be moderate-intensity activity in bouts of ≥10 min*	60 min to several hours of total activity, some of which should be in bouts of ≥10 min*
Adults		
Frequency	Most days of the week	Daily or most days of the week
Intensity	4 METs** Moderate-intensity activity equal in intensity to brisk walking	4–7 METs At least as intense as brisk walking but less intense than normal jogging
Time	30 min in bouts of ≥10 min***	30–60 min in bouts of ≥10 min***

†Threshold is the *minimum* physical activity you need to get health and wellness benefits. Target zone is the correct range of physical activity for health and wellness benefits (see chapter 6).

*Using 30 of the 60 minutes for moderate-intensity activity would meet the teen and adult guidelines.

**Less fit adults may use activities of 3 to 4 METs.

***At least 150 minutes per week, spread over multiple days.

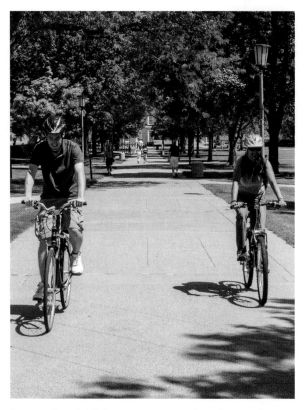

Recreational biking is an example of a moderate-intensity physical activity. It's one of many activities you can choose to accumulate your 60 minutes of daily physical activity.

substitute 75 minutes per week of vigorous exercise for the 150 minutes of moderate-intensity activity; they can also meet the guidelines by combining moderate- and vigorous-intensity activity.

Counting Steps and Movement

Another way to determine how much moderate-intensity physical activity you perform is to count the steps you take each day. You can do so by using a pedometer (see the Fitness Technology feature), which automatically tracks your step count; the disadvantage is that a pedometer counts all steps that you take, regardless of whether they come in very light, light, or even vigorous-intensity activity. Still, wearing a pedometer can help you see how active you really are; you may have the opportunity to wear one in school. The American College of Sports Medicine states that moderate-intensity physical activity requires a step rate of 100 steps per minute.

For adults, some experts believe that taking 10,000 steps each day is necessary to be in the target zone for moderate physical activity. Other experts are concerned about this advice because you can reach 10,000 steps without doing any sustained activity (bouts of 10 minutes or more). On the other hand, some people can do 60 minutes of moderate-intensity activity each day and still not reach a 10,000-step count. Rather than setting an absolute daily step count, most experts recommend monitoring your activity for a full week and then determining your average daily step count. People who want to increase their activity level can then establish a realistic step goal that is 500 to 1,000 steps per day higher than their average step count. Once they reach this goal, they can, if desired, gradually increase their step count to higher levels.

Studies show that Canadian children take between 10,779 and 13,103 steps a day. The national average is 11,607 steps a day; to meet the national physical activity guidelines of 60 minutes a day, most teens would require 12,000 steps. However, if you're just beginning, remember the principle of progression. Instead of starting with a high goal such as 12,000 steps per day, work gradually toward a realistic step goal.

As mentioned previously, you can monitor moderate-intensity physical activity by using devices

activities can be combined with other activities from the pyramid to meet the goal. Experts now agree that it is best to get your 60 minutes in bouts or activity sessions lasting at least 10 minutes each. In other words, you could do six 10-minute bouts, three 20-minute bouts, two 30-minute bouts, or other combinations that total 60 minutes a day. Accumulating 60 minutes in bouts shorter than 10 minutes each is better than doing nothing, but it does not give you optimal benefits.

For adults, the recommendation is 150 minutes per week because this amount provides many health benefits with a minimum of effort. As with teens, moderate-intensity exercise is best done on several days a week (see table 7.2) and in bouts of at least 10 minutes each. Doing more than 30 minutes at a time gives additional benefits and is recommended for maintaining a healthy weight and for achieving good fitness, health, and wellness. Adults can

⬤ FITNESS TECHNOLOGY: Pedometers and Accelerometers

A **pedometer** is a small, battery-powered device that can be worn on your belt. It counts each step you take and displays the running count on a meter. You simply open the face of the pedometer or push a button to see how many steps you've taken. Some pedometers also contain a small computer that allows you to enter the length of your step (your stride length) and your body weight so that the computer can estimate the distance you walk and the number of calories you expend. More expensive pedometers can also track the total time you spend in activity during the day and the number of bouts of activity that you perform lasting 10 minutes or longer. Less expensive pedometers must be reset at the end of the day, but some more expensive ones can store steps for several days. There are also numerous free or inexpensive apps for Apple and Android devices.

Accelerometers are similar to pedometers but measure physical activity in more detail. Specifically, accelerometers can record the *intensity* of your movements (for more about intensity, see the discussion of METs and recall the "I" in the FITT formula), as well as the amount of *time* (the first "T" in the FITT formula) you spend at different intensities. Like a pedometer, an

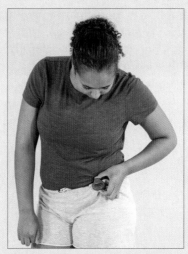

A pedometer counts steps and is a good way to self-monitor moderate activity.

accelerometer is worn on your belt and contains a small computer and a device (the accelerometer itself) that measures the intensity of your movements. Most accelerometers can count your steps taken per day and estimate the calories you expend in activity. There are also numerous free or inexpensive apps for Apple and Android devices. Be sure to check the customer reviews when searching for apps.

Using Technology

Estimate the number of steps you take on a typical weekday and a typical weekend day. Then wear a pedometer to see how many steps you actually take (weekday and weekend day). See if you're as active as you think you are!

FIT FACT

The average person in Canada accumulates 3,500 to 5,000 steps per day. This is considerably less than the averages in some other countries—for example, 9,000 or more in Australia and Switzerland and 7,000 or more in Japan—where obesity rates are much lower.

such as an accelerometer (see the Fitness Technology feature). Heart rate monitors can also be used, and as with the accelerometer, there are heart rate monitor apps. An accelerometer both counts your steps and gives you a better idea of your exercise intensity than a pedometer can. You can determine the distance you've walked by finding out the length of your step (your stride length), then multiplying it by the number of steps you take.

Counting Physical Activity Calories

We know that moderate-intensity activity should be done according to the FIT formula summarized in table 7.2. Another way to determine whether you perform enough moderate-intensity activity is to count the calories you expend in activity. For example, a teen who weighs 68 kilograms (150 pounds) would expend 300 to 400 calories during 60 minutes of moderate-intensity activity, such as brisk walking. Therefore, this number of calories expended per day would be a good goal for moderate activity. You can learn more about counting calories in chapter 14.

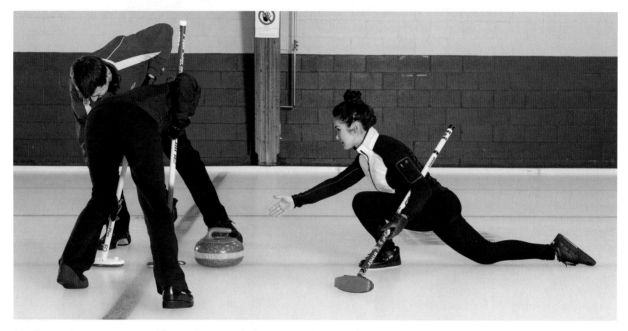

Moderate-intensity sports like curling can help you reach your daily goal for calorie expenditure.

Lesson Review

1. What does the term *MET* mean, and how is it useful?
2. What are some types of moderate-intensity physical activity?
3. What are some benefits of moderate-intensity activity?
4. What is the teen FIT formula for obtaining health and wellness benefits from moderate-intensity physical activity?

Many of the self-assessments you perform in this course require vigorous-intensity physical activity. If you're a very active person and are quite fit, the mile run or PACER may be the best way to estimate your cardiorespiratory endurance, but the walking test is also a good one. The test is especially good for people who are beginners, who haven't done a lot of recent activity, or who are regular walkers but do not regularly get more vigorous-intensity activity. The walking test is also good for older people and for those who cannot do running tests due to joint or muscle problems. Try the walking test and record your scores and fitness ratings. You can then use the information in preparing your personal physical activity plan. If you're working with a partner, remember that self-assessment information is personal and considered confidential. It shouldn't be shared with others without the permission of the person being tested.

1. Walk a mile at a fast pace (as fast as you can go while keeping approximately the same pace for the entire walk).

2. Immediately after the walk, count your heartbeats for 15 seconds. Multiply the result by 4 to calculate your one-minute heart rate.

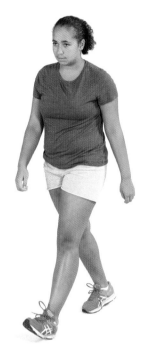

The walking test is a good assessment for beginners or people who don't do a lot of vigorous-intensity physical activity.

3. Use the appropriate chart to determine your walking rating. Locate your heart rate in the left column of the chart and your walking time along the bottom row. Find the point where the row and column intersect to determine your rating.

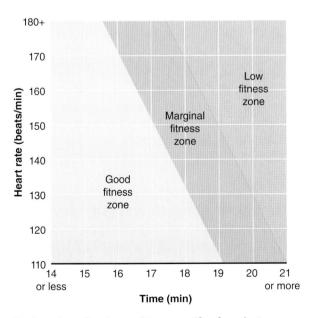

Rating chart for the walking test (for females).

Adapted from the *One Mile Walk Test* with permission of author James M. Rippe, M.D.

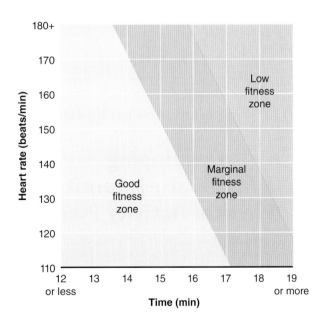

Rating chart for the walking test (for males).

Adapted from the *One Mile Walk Test* with permission of author James M. Rippe, M.D.

Participating in Moderate-Intensity Physical Activity **143**

Preparing a Moderate-Intensity Physical Activity Plan

Lesson Objectives

After participating in this lesson, you should be able to

1. prepare a moderate-intensity physical activity plan using the five planning steps, and
2. carry out your moderate-intensity activity plan for several days.

Lesson Vocabulary

habituate

Have you ever created your own fitness plan? Have you ever tracked your daily activities? In this lesson, you'll use the five steps of program planning to develop a moderate-intensity physical activity plan for yourself. You'll then carry out that plan. Implementing a good plan will help you meet national physical activity guidelines—both now and later in your life. The most popular physical activities among adults are moderate-intensity ones, including walking, biking, yard work, and home calisthenics. If you establish the habit of doing moderate-intensity physical activity early in your life, you're more likely to be active as you grow older. And people who **habituate** to activity get multiple health benefits over the course of a lifetime.

> **"** Walking is the best possible exercise. Habituate yourself to walk very far. **"**
>
> —Thomas Jefferson, U.S. president

Developing a Moderate-Intensity Physical Activity Plan

Javier used the five steps of program planning to prepare a moderate-intensity physical activity program. Because he created the plan as an assignment for his physical education class, it covered only two weeks. Later, he would get the opportunity to prepare a longer plan. Notice that in doing his planning, Javier used steps similar to those for the scientific method. You can prepare a similar plan.

Step 1: Determine Your Personal Needs

To get started, Javier collected some basic information. First, he answered questions about his moderate-intensity physical activity levels in the past week. He also wrote down his fitness test results that related to moderate physical activity. He recorded his results in figure 7.2.

Javier had a good fitness rating for both the PACER and the walking test (see figure 7.2). He also met the national activity guideline of 60 minutes a day on three days of the previous week. His moderate-intensity activity included mostly walking to and from school (20 minutes each weekday) and riding his bike for 10 minutes two days a week (Tuesday and Thursday). He also performed 10 minutes of vigorous calisthenics (Tuesday, Thursday, and Saturday). On Saturday he played tennis in addition to his calisthenics. Still, his physical

FIT FACT

Walking, a moderate-intensity physical activity, is the most popular type of activity in many parts of the world. Men (64 percent) and women (75 percent) have reported walking in their leisure time. People with a dog walk more frequently than people who don't have a dog.

Physical fitness profile			
Fitness self-assessments	**Score**	**Rating**	
Walking test	Time: 15:00 Heart rate: 140	Good fitness	
PACER	41 laps	Good fitness	
Physical activity profile			
Day	**Moderate-intensity activity (min)**	**All activity (min)**	**Met guideline**
Mon.	30	30	
Tues.	30	60	✓
Wed.	30	30	
Thurs.	30	60	✓
Fri.	30	60	✓
Sat.	30	30	
Sun.	0	0	

FIGURE 7.2 Javier's physical activity and fitness profiles.

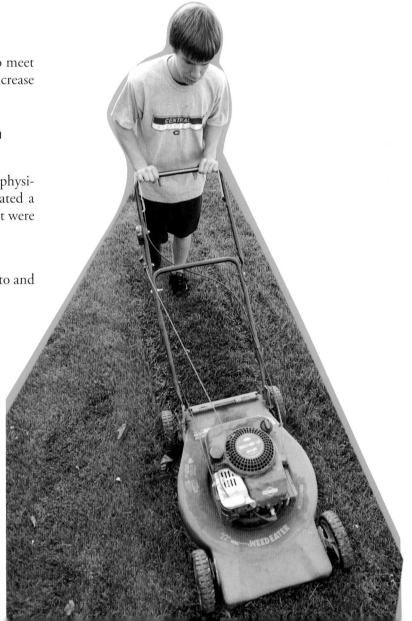

activity profile told him that if he wanted to meet national activity guidelines, he needed to increase his physical activity.

Step 2: Consider Your Program Options

Javier looked at the list of moderate-intensity physical activities presented in table 7.1 and created a list of other moderate-intensity activities that were easily available to him.

Lifestyle Activities
- More walking in addition to walking to and from school
- Yard work at home

Moderate-Intensity Sports
- Bowling
- Shooting baskets

Moderate-Intensity Recreation
- Fishing
- More bike riding

Occupational or School Activity
- Physical education class activities

Step 3: Set Goals

Since two weeks was too short a time for setting long-term goals, Javier developed only short-term goals for his moderate-intensity physical activity plan; as a result, all of his goals were physical activity goals. He did this because he knew that activity goals (process goals) work best as short-term goals. He also knew that if he met his activity goals he would be making progress toward his fitness (product goals). Later, when he prepares a longer plan, he will develop long-term goals, including physical fitness goals. For these first two weeks, Javier decided to focus on moderate-intensity activity through the following goals.

1. Continue to perform the same activities that he has regularly been doing.
2. Walk to school and back three days a week (30 minutes each day).
3. Perform 30 minutes of moderate-intensity activity on three days each week in physical education class.
4. Rake the yard for 30 minutes on one day every two weeks.
5. Shoot baskets for 30 minutes two days a week.
6. Bike with friends for 30 minutes on two days a week.
7. Mow the neighbour's yard once every two weeks (60 minutes).
8. Go fishing one day a week (includes walking for 60 minutes).
9. Walk with family for 15 minutes on two days a week.

Javier remembered to use SMART goals. His goals listed *specific* activities and amounts of time because he wanted to be able to *measure* his progress. He also tried to make his goals challenging but *attainable* and *realistic*. Finally, he wanted his goals to be *timely*—just right for his life at this time and able to be achieved in the time allotted.

Step 4: Structure Your Program and Write It Down

Javier's plan included at least the recommended 60 minutes of moderate-intensity physical activity on each day during the two-week period. On several days, he planned to do more than 60 minutes. As shown in figure 7.3, he wrote down the activities and the times when he planned to perform them.

Week 1				Week 2			
Day	Activity	Time	✓	Day	Activity	Time	✓
Mon.	Walk to school* Walk home* Shoot baskets	7:45–7:55 a.m. 3:30–3:40 p.m. 3:45–4:15 p.m.		Mon.	Walk to school* Walk home* Shoot baskets	7:45–7:55 a.m. 3:30–3:40 p.m. 3:45–4:15 p.m.	
Tues.	Walk to school* PE class activity* Walk home*	7:45–7:55 a.m. 10:00–10:30 a.m. 3:30–3:40 p.m.		Tues.	Walk to school* PE class activity* Walk home*	7:45–7:55 a.m. 10:00–10:30 a.m. 3:30–3:40 p.m.	
Wed.	Walk to school* Walk home* Ride bike	7:45–7:55 a.m. 3:30–3:45 p.m. 3:45–4:00 p.m.		Wed.	Walk to school* Walk home* Ride bike	7:45–7:55 a.m. 3:30–3:45 p.m. 3:45–4:00 p.m.	
Thurs.	Walk to school* PE class activity* Walk home*	7:45–7:55 a.m. 10:00–10:30 a.m. 3:30–3:40 p.m.		Thurs.	Walk to school* PE class activity* Walk home*	7:45–7:55 a.m. 10:00–10:30 a.m. 3:30–3:40 p.m.	
Fri.	Walk to school* PE class activity* Walk home*	7:45–7:55 a.m. 10:00–10:30 a.m. 3:30–3:45 p.m.		Fri.	Walk to school* PE class activity* Walk home*	7:45–7:55 a.m. 10:00–10:30 a.m. 3:30–3:40 p.m.	
Sat.	Mow the grass* Ride bike	9:00–9:30 a.m. 1:00–1:30 p.m.		Sat.	Rake the yard* Ride bike	9:30–10:30 a.m. 1:00–1:30 p.m.	
Sun.	Bowling Family walk	2:30–3:30 p.m. 6:30–6:45 p.m.		Sun.	Bowling Family walk	2:30–3:30 p.m. 6:30–6:45 p.m.	

*Activities that Javier was already doing.

FIGURE 7.3 Javier's two-week written program plan.

Step 5: Keep a Log and Evaluate Your Program

Over the next two weeks, Javier will self-monitor his activities and place a checkmark beside each activity he performs. At the end of the two-week period, he'll evaluate his performance to see whether he met his goals. He can then use that evaluation to help him make another activity plan.

FIT FACT

Canadian laws provide tax incentives for increasing regular physical activity. Families that enrol children and teens in youth activity programs get an income tax break, and people who buy bicycles get a reduction in sales tax.

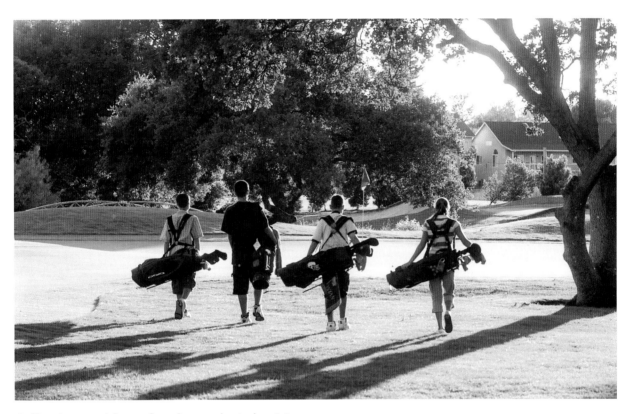

Golfing is a good form of moderate physical activity.

Lesson Review

1. How do you use the five steps in planning to prepare a personal moderate-intensity physical activity plan?
2. How can you best implement your personal plan over a span of several days?

TAKING CHARGE: Learning to Manage Time

Why can some people always find time for an added activity while others barely have time to do their regularly scheduled activities? For a lot of people, the answer is time management. Good time managers know how to make the best use of their time. They efficiently control their daily schedule in order to complete their activities without wasting time. These people are more likely to find time for regular physical activity.

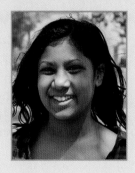

Here's an example of poor time management. Jennifer lives near some good cross-country ski trails. In the winter, her friends spend a few hours skiing every Monday and Wednesday after school; they also go skiing on weekends. Although they always ask her to join their fun, Jennifer usually refuses. Her common excuse is, "I just don't have the time. I really love skiing, but with three honours classes, homework, and my job at the mall, I barely have time to eat, let alone ski. I wish I could go with you, but I can't. It's impossible! I'll ski next year when my schedule is easier. Then I'll have more spare time."

Jennifer's friends are used to her excuses. In fact, she used many of the same ones last year. Her friends have the same classes and work hours that Jennifer has, but they complete their homework assignments and handle their jobs with time to spare. They do not understand why Jennifer can't manage to find the time to go skiing with them but has lots of time for social media and video games.

For Discussion

What can Jennifer do to manage her time better so that she can do things with her friends? What can her friends do to help? What suggestions can you make to help anyone who would like to manage time better? Consider the time management strategies presented in this chapter's Self-Management feature when answering the discussion questions.

SELF-MANAGEMENT: Skills for Managing Time

How many times do you hear yourself and others say, "I don't have the time"? It seems to be a common complaint. If you're one of those who seem to have too little time, how can you remedy the problem? Many experts believe that learning to manage time is a good solution. In this lesson, you'll learn how to manage your time so that you can be more active.

In 1900, the average person worked more than 60 hours a week. Now the average workweek is less than 40 hours. Similarly, in 1900, many young people were not enrolled in school and were already working long hours in factories and on farms. Now most teens are in school, and those who work limit their work hours.

Fewer working hours has made free time much more abundant now than it was years ago. But work and school aren't the only things that take time. Most of us make other time commitments when we aren't working or going to school. For example, you might have to care for a brother or sister, or you might have committed to a school or community activity such as a club, band, chorus, or sport team. And of course you also spend time on necessary activities such as eating, sleeping, dressing, and getting to and from school or work. The time you spend in all of these activities is called committed time.

Free time, on the other hand, is the time left over after accounting for your school and work time and your other committed time. Some people make so many commitments that they have very little free time. Often, people who say they don't have time for physical activity have not planned their time carefully. Active people manage their time effectively so that they can commit regularly to being active. If you're in the group of people who often say, "I don't have time," the following guidelines can help you.

- **Keep track of your time.** The best way to start managing your time more efficiently is to see what you're doing with it now. You can do this by keeping records (self-monitoring your use of time). Write down what you do during the course of each day. Record when you sleep, when you eat, when you're in school, when you're at work, and when you do all of the other things you do. You might use three categories: school and work, other committed time, and free time. Most people who keep records of their time use are surprised by the results. For example, some people who say they don't have time to exercise spend several hours a day watching television. Others find that they spend a lot of time doing nothing.

- **Analyze your use of time.** Once you've tracked your time for several days, review your records to see how many hours you spend in each of the three categories. You can also identify exactly how you spend your committed time and your free time. Doing so will help you decide whether you're using your time in the way you really want to use it.

- **Decide purposefully what to do with your time.** After you determine how much time you spend doing various activities, decide whether you're managing your time efficiently. Efficient time management enables you to do the things you think are most important. To decide what's most important to you, answer the following questions.
  - What activities did you spend more time on than you wanted to?
  - How much less time could you spend on each?
  - Are the activities you would like to change under your control?
  - What activities do you want to spend more time on?
  - How much more time would you like to spend on these activities?

- **Schedule your time.** After you decide how you would like to spend your time, create a schedule to ensure that you make time for the things you identified as most important. If you feel that regular physical activity is important, you will commit time to doing it. Plan a schedule for one day, making sure you have time to do the most important things.

Sometimes good scheduling allows you to do two things at once. For example, since you have to get to school somehow, what if you did so by walking or riding a bicycle? You would be effectively committing that time to two different purposes. Similarly, if you join a sport team or activity club, the time you commit to that group is also committed to doing physical activity.

Prepare a two-week moderate-intensity physical activity plan using the five steps described in this chapter. Like Javier, consider moderate-intensity activities from each activity category: lifestyle activity, moderate-intensity sports, moderate-intensity recreation, and occupational or school activity. The goal is to accumulate at least 60 minutes of activity each day, including a considerable portion that involves moderate-intensity activity. Prepare a written plan and carry it out over a two-week period. Your teacher may give you time in class to do some of the activities in your plan. Consider the following suggestions for taking action and building moderate-intensity activity into your plan.

- **Lifestyle activity.** Walk or bike to school. If driving, park away from your destination and walk the rest of the way. When you have a choice, take the stairs. Walk while talking on the phone. Work in the yard.
- **Moderate-intensity sports.** Consider bowling or shooting baskets with friends.
- **Moderate-intensity recreation.** Walk with friends at lunch or go for a walk in the park.
- **Occupational or school activity.** Do yard work for pay, take an optional physical education class, participate in intramural activities, or start a walking club.

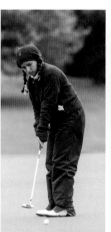
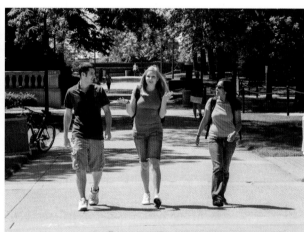

Lifestyle activities can be part of your plan for taking action.

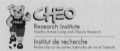

GET ACTIVE WITH HALO

©Healthy Active Living and Obesity Research Group

Who We Are

The HALO Group (Healthy Active Living and Obesity Research Group) is a driven, passionate, innovative, and fun multidisciplinary team of researchers and students who walk the talk of living a healthy, active lifestyle.

What We Do

HALO provides international leadership and research excellence in active living for the promotion of health and wellness in children and youth, including the prevention, management, and treatment of obesity.

Get Involved

Seek ways to HALOize your day! At HALO we find unique ways to be active indoors and outdoors. For example, we have walking meetings. Try walking meetings or lessons to think on your feet and get some fresh air. We also encourage people to stand up as much as possible during meetings or lessons. On lunch break, we play road hockey. We also developed a Fit Club to gather like-minded people to support each other in sitting less and moving more. If you don't already have a Fit Club at school, why not start one? At HALO we find it's easier to be active when it's the norm. With a little creativity, you can create an environment where it's easier to be active. How can you HALOize your day? Visit www.haloresearch.ca/haloize-your-workday for more ideas or contact us at www.haloresearch.ca/contact-us to get involved with our research.

©Healthy Active Living and Obesity Research Group

Reviewing Concepts and Vocabulary

Complete the following in order to determine your growing understanding of fitness, health, and wellness. Answer items 1 through 5 by correctly completing each sentence with a word or phrase.

1. Activity that is equivalent to brisk walking in intensity is considered to be _____ physical activity.
2. An activity done as part of daily life is called a/an _____ activity.
3. A device worn on your belt that counts steps is called a/an _____.
4. Intensity of activity can be expressed in units called _____.
5. Considering your program options is step _____ of the planning process.

For items 6 through 10, match each term in column 1 with the appropriate word or phrase in column 2.

6. excessive inactivity
7. yard work
8. recreational activity
9. occupational work
10. housework

a. mopping
b. carpentry
c. sitting disease
d. bowling
e. mowing

For items 11 through 15, respond to each statement or question.

11. What does *sedentary* mean, and what can be done to reduce sedentary living among teens?
12. Describe several devices that can be used to self-monitor physical activity.
13. How much moderate-intensity physical activity is enough?
14. List and describe the five steps for planning a moderate-intensity physical activity program.
15. Describe several guidelines for managing time effectively.

Thinking Critically

Write a paragraph to answer the following question.

Teens are often more vigorously active than adults. For this reason, some people say that teens should begin to do more moderate-intensity activity to increase their chance of staying active later in life. Do you think you will become more or less active as you grow older? What types of activity do you think you'll do as you grow older? Why do you think you'll choose these activities (e.g., I am good at them and I enjoy them, I like being outdoors, they don't cost money, I can do them with my friends)? What do your activity choices tell you about the factors that support your physical activity participation?

Project

National polling groups regularly conduct surveys to learn people's opinions about various issues, including health and fitness. Assume that you work for a polling company. Develop a list of questions about moderate activity and ask at least six people to answer them. Try to interview people from different age groups. Graph your results. Analyze your results and prepare a brief news article reporting the results.

8

Developing Cardiorespiratory Endurance

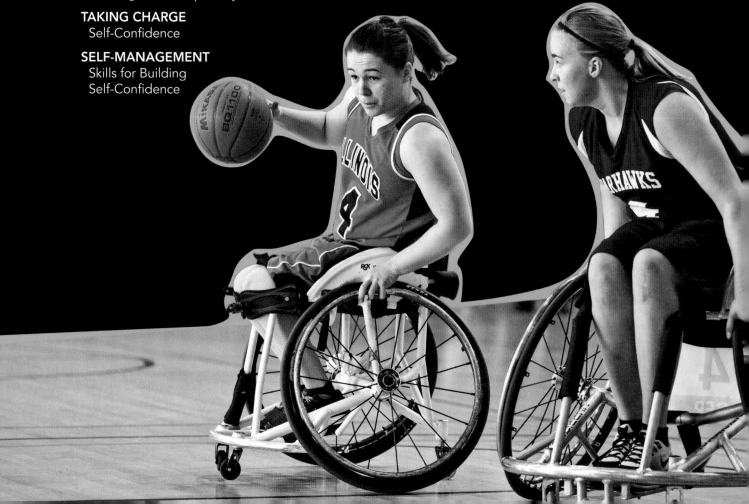

Lesson 8.1
Cardiorespiratory Endurance Facts

Lesson Objectives

After participating in this lesson, you should be able to

1. describe the health and wellness benefits of cardiorespiratory endurance;
2. explain how physical activity benefits the cardiovascular, respiratory, and muscle systems;
3. describe some methods for assessing your cardiorespiratory endurance; and
4. determine how much cardiorespiratory endurance is enough.

Lesson Vocabulary

aerobic capacity, artery, cardiorespiratory endurance, cardiovascular system, cholesterol, fibrin, graded exercise test, high-density lipoprotein (HDL), lipoprotein, low-density lipoprotein (LDL), maximal oxygen uptake, respiratory system, vein

How would you know if you have good cardiorespiratory endurance? What kinds of physical activities will allow you to build good cardiorespiratory endurance? Of the 11 parts of fitness, cardiorespiratory endurance is the most important because it gives you many health and wellness benefits, including a chance for a longer life. In addition, the activity that you do to improve your cardiorespiratory endurance helps you look your best. As shown in figure 8.1, cardiorespiratory endurance requires fitness of your heart, lungs, blood, blood vessels, and muscles. In this lesson, you'll learn how proper physical activity improves your cardiorespiratory endurance. You'll also learn how to assess your cardiorespiratory endurance.

Cardiorespiratory endurance is the ability to exercise your entire body for a long time without stopping. It requires a strong heart, healthy lungs, and open blood vessels to supply your large muscles with oxygen. Examples of activities that require good cardiorespiratory endurance are distance running, swimming, and cross-country skiing. Cardiorespiratory endurance is sometimes referred to by other names, including cardiovascular fitness, cardiovascular endurance, and cardiorespiratory fitness. The term *aerobic capacity* is also used to refer to good cardiorespiratory function, but it is not exactly the same as cardiorespiratory endurance (see this chapter's Science in Action feature).

This book uses the term *cardiorespiratory endurance.* The first word in the term is "cardiorespiratory" because two vital systems are involved. Your

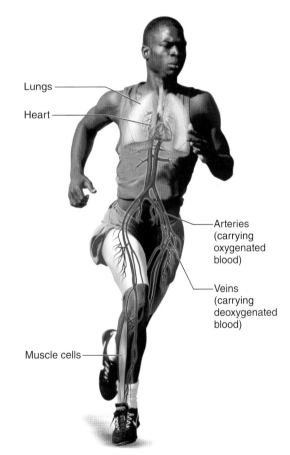

FIGURE 8.1 Cardiorespiratory endurance requires fitness of many parts of the body, including heart, lungs, muscles, and blood vessels.

cardiovascular system is made up of your heart, blood vessels, and blood. Your **respiratory system** is made up of your lungs and the air passages that bring air, including oxygen, to your lungs from outside your body. In your lungs, oxygen enters your blood, and carbon dioxide is eliminated. Your cardiovascular and respiratory systems work together to bring your muscle cells and other body cells the materials they need and to rid the cells of waste. Together, the two systems help you function both effectively (with the most benefits possible) and efficiently (with the least effort).

The second word in the term *cardiorespiratory endurance* refers to the ability to sustain effort. Together, then, these two words—"cardiorespiratory" and "endurance"—refer to the ability to sustain effort, which hinges on fitness of the cardiovascular (cardio) and respiratory systems.

Benefits of Physical Activity and Cardiorespiratory Endurance

Doing regular physical activity can help you look better by controlling your weight, strengthening your muscles, and helping you develop good posture. Regular physical activity also produces changes in your body's organs, such as making your heart muscle stronger and your blood vessels healthier. These changes improve your cardiorespiratory endurance and wellness and reduce your risk of hypokinetic diseases, especially heart disease and diabetes.

Physical activity provides benefits for both your cardiovascular and respiratory systems. In this lesson, you'll learn how each part of these systems

FIT FACT

In the early 1900s, medical doctors referred to an enlarged heart as "athlete's heart" because athletes' hearts tended to be large, and enlarged hearts were associated with disease. By midcentury, medical research showed that trained athletes' hearts are typically large on the left side, which is a sign of health, not disease. Inactive adults with heart problems typically have hearts that are large on the right side, which is a sign of disease.

benefits and how all the parts work together to promote optimal functioning and good health.

Heart

Because your heart is a muscle, it benefits from exercise and activities, such as jogging, swimming, and long-distance hiking. Your heart acts as a pump to deliver blood to cells throughout your body. When you do vigorous-intensity physical activity, your muscle cells need more oxygen and produce more waste products. Therefore, your heart must pump more blood to supply the additional oxygen and remove the additional waste. If your heart is unable to pump enough blood, your muscles will be less able to contract and will fatigue more quickly.

Your heart's capacity to pump blood is crucial when you're doing physical activity, especially for an extended length of time. Your heart has two ways to get more blood to your muscles—by beating faster and by sending more blood with each beat (this is called stroke volume).

To determine your resting heart rate, you count the number of heartbeats per minute when you're relatively inactive. A person who does regular physical activity might have a resting heart rate of 55 to 60 beats per minute, whereas a person who does not exercise regularly might have a resting heart rate of 70 or more beats per minute. As a result, a very fit person's heart beats approximately 9.5 million fewer times each year than that of the average person. As you can see in figure 8.2, a fit person's heart works more efficiently by pumping more blood with fewer beats.

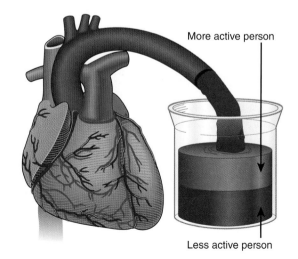

FIGURE 8.2 The heart muscle of a fit, active person pumps more blood per heartbeat than that of a less active person.

Lungs

When you inhale, air enters the lungs, causing them to expand. In the lungs, oxygen is transferred from the air to the blood for transport to the tissues of the body. When you exhale, air leaves the lungs. The diaphragm (a band of muscular tissue located at the base of your lungs) and abdominal muscles (which help move the diaphragm) work to allow you to breathe in and out (figure 8.3*a*). Fit people can take in more air with each breath than unfit people because they have more efficient respiratory muscles. As shown in figure 8.3*b*, a fit person gets more air into the lungs with each breath and therefore can transport the same amount of air to the lungs in fewer breaths. Healthy lungs also have the capacity to easily transfer oxygen to the blood. Together, healthy lungs and fit respiratory muscles contribute to good cardiorespiratory endurance.

Blood

Although your body needs a certain amount of fat, excessive amounts trigger formation of fatty deposits along your artery walls. **Cholesterol**—a waxy, fat-like substance found in meat, dairy products, and egg yolk—can be dangerous because high levels can build up in your body without your noticing it.

Cholesterol is carried through your bloodstream by particles called **lipoproteins**. One kind, **low-density lipoprotein (LDL)**, is often referred to as "bad cholesterol" because it carries cholesterol that is more likely to stay in your body and contribute to atherosclerosis. An LDL count below 100 is considered optimal for good health. Another kind of lipoprotein, **high-density lipoprotein (HDL)**, is often referred to as "good cholesterol" because it carries excess cholesterol out of your bloodstream and into your liver for elimination from your body. Therefore, HDLs appear to help prevent atherosclerosis. An HDL count above 60 is considered optimal for good health.

In addition to being free of fatty deposits, healthy arteries are free from inflammation, which contributes to arterial clogging. Blood tests can pick up markers of inflammation.

Regular physical activity helps you improve your health and resist disease by reducing your LDL (bad cholesterol) and increasing your HDL (good cholesterol). It also helps reduce inflammation in your arteries and can help prevent the formation of blood clots by reducing the amount of **fibrin** in your blood. Fibrin is a substance involved in making your blood clot, and high amounts of fibrin can contribute to the development of atherosclerosis.

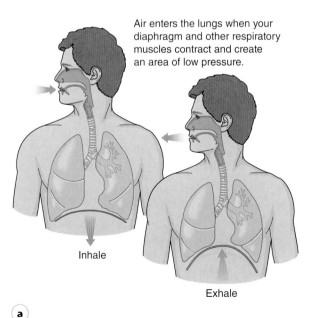

Air enters the lungs when your diaphragm and other respiratory muscles contract and create an area of low pressure.

Inhale

Exhale

a

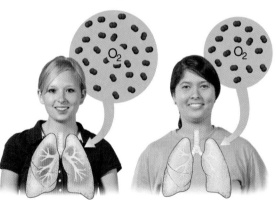

The average lung holds 3 to 5 litres of air.

O₂ O₂

Trained individuals take bigger breaths, thus requiring fewer breaths to get the same amount of oxygen.

Untrained individuals take shallow breaths and thus need more breaths to get sufficient oxygen.

b

FIGURE 8.3 *(a)* The lungs and diaphragm during inhalation and exhalation; *(b)* fit people can breathe more efficiently than unfit people.

Arteries

Each **artery** carries blood from your heart to another part of your body. The beating of your heart forces blood through your arteries. Therefore, a strong heart and healthy lungs are not very helpful if your arteries are not clear and open. As you now know, fatty deposits on the inner walls of an artery lead to atherosclerosis. An extreme case of atherosclerosis can totally block the blood flow in an artery. The hardened deposits can also allow the formation of blood clots, severely blocking your blood flow. In either case, your heart muscle does not get enough oxygen, and a heart attack occurs.

Regular physical activity also provides other cardiovascular benefits. Scientists have found that people who exercise regularly develop more branching of the arteries in the heart. Figure 8.4 shows that the heart muscle has its own arteries (coronary arteries), which supply it with blood and oxygen. People who exercise regularly develop extra coronary arteries. The importance of this richer network of blood vessels can be shown in two examples.

- After astronaut Ed White died in a fire while training for a mission, an autopsy was performed. Doctors found that one of the major arteries in his heart was completely blocked due to atherosclerosis. However, because of all the physical training that astronauts perform, scientists think that White's body had developed an extra branching of arteries in his heart muscle. Therefore, he didn't die of a heart attack when a main artery was blocked. Instead, he had been able to continue a high level of physical fitness training without signs of heart trouble.

- Like White, professional hockey player Richard Zednik had very good cardiorespiratory endurance. This fact became crucial to his survival during a hockey game when his carotid artery was cut by an opponent's skate. For most people, this would be a deadly injury. However, the doctor who performed the rescue surgery reported that because of Zednik's fitness level, he had very healthy and elastic arteries that were large and easy to repair. Zednik made a full recovery.

Veins

Each **vein** carries blood filled with waste products from the muscle cells and other body tissues back to the heart. One-way valves in your veins keep the blood from flowing backward. Your muscles squeeze the veins to pump the blood back to your heart. Regular exercise helps your muscles squeeze your veins efficiently. Lack of physical activity can cause the valves, especially those in your legs, to stop working efficiently, thereby reducing circulation in your legs.

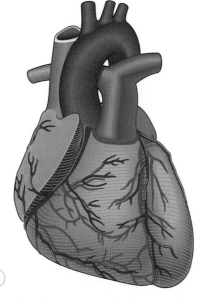
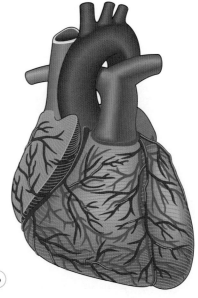

(a) (b)

FIGURE 8.4 Blood vessels on the heart: *(a)* the heart of a typical person; *(b)* the heart of a person who exercises regularly.

If you don't do what's best for your body, you're the one who comes up on the short end.

—Julius Erving (Doctor J),
Hall of Fame basketball player

Nerves of Your Heart

Your heart muscle is not like your arm and leg muscles. When your arm and leg muscles contract, nerves in them are responding to a message sent by the conscious part of your brain. In contrast, your heart is not controlled voluntarily; it beats regularly without your consciously telling it to do so. Instead, your heart rate is controlled by a part of it called a pacemaker, which sends out an electrical current telling it to beat regularly. People who do regular vigorous-intensity aerobic exercise often develop a slower heart rate because the heart pumps more blood with each beat—meaning that it has greater stroke volume—and therefore can beat less often. Thus, if you exercise properly, your heart works more efficiently because each heartbeat supplies more blood and oxygen to your body than if you did not exercise. You can also function more effectively during an emergency or during vigorous-intensity physical activity.

Muscle Cells

In order to do physical activity for a long time without getting tired, your muscle cells must also function efficiently and effectively. Regular physical activity helps your cells be effective in their use of oxygen and in getting rid of waste materials. Physical activity also helps your muscle cells use blood sugar, with the aid of the hormone called insulin, to produce energy. This function is important for good health.

 FITNESS TECHNOLOGY: Heart Rate Monitors

One way to count your heart rate is to use your wrist or neck pulse. But it's difficult to do so while you're exercising, so pulse is typically counted after exercise.

To count your pulse during activity, you can use a high-tech device called a heart rate monitor. One type requires you to wear a band around your chest. The band contains sensors that detect electrical stimulation from your heart's nervous system (similarly to how an electrocardiogram works). A transmitter in the chest band sends a signal to a receiver located in a special watch worn on your wrist. The receiver picks up the signal and displays your heart rate on the watch. Another type of monitor counts your pulse and displays your heart rate on a watch located on your arm. It does not require the band around your chest.

You can set a heart rate watch to tell you whether you're exercising in your heart rate target zone. You can also set it to keep track of how many minutes you stay in your target zone. Heart rate monitors vary in cost, and some are better than others, so consult with your teacher or another reliable source before buying one. If your school has heart rate watches, you might want to use one to monitor your heart rate during vigorous-intensity activity.

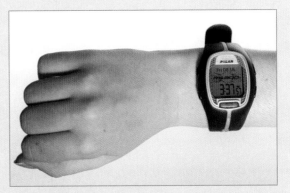

A heart rate watch is helpful for counting your pulse during activity.

Using Technology

Use a variety of sources to evaluate several heart rate monitors. Consider cost, reliability, and ease of use; then decide which monitor would be the best buy. For instance, there are free heart rate monitor apps for both Apple and Android devices, but be sure to check customer ratings and that the app does what you need it to do. A little research on what are considered to be the best heart rate monitor apps will help you make an informed decision.

Summary of Benefits

As noted in the previous sections, regular physical activity benefits many different body systems. A summary of these benefits is presented in figure 8.5.

Cardiorespiratory Assessment

You might be curious about your own cardiorespiratory endurance. How good is it? Several tests can help you find the answer.

You can assess the fitness of your cardiorespiratory systems in two settings: in the laboratory and in the field (for example, in a gym or on an athletic field). Two types of laboratory tests are the **maximal oxygen uptake** test (also referred to as the $\dot{V}O_2$max test) and the **graded exercise test**.

The maximal oxygen uptake test is considered the best for assessing fitness of the cardiovascular and respiratory systems. It measures how much oxygen you can use when you're exercising very vigorously. To take the test, you run on a treadmill while connected to a special gas meter (figure 8.6).

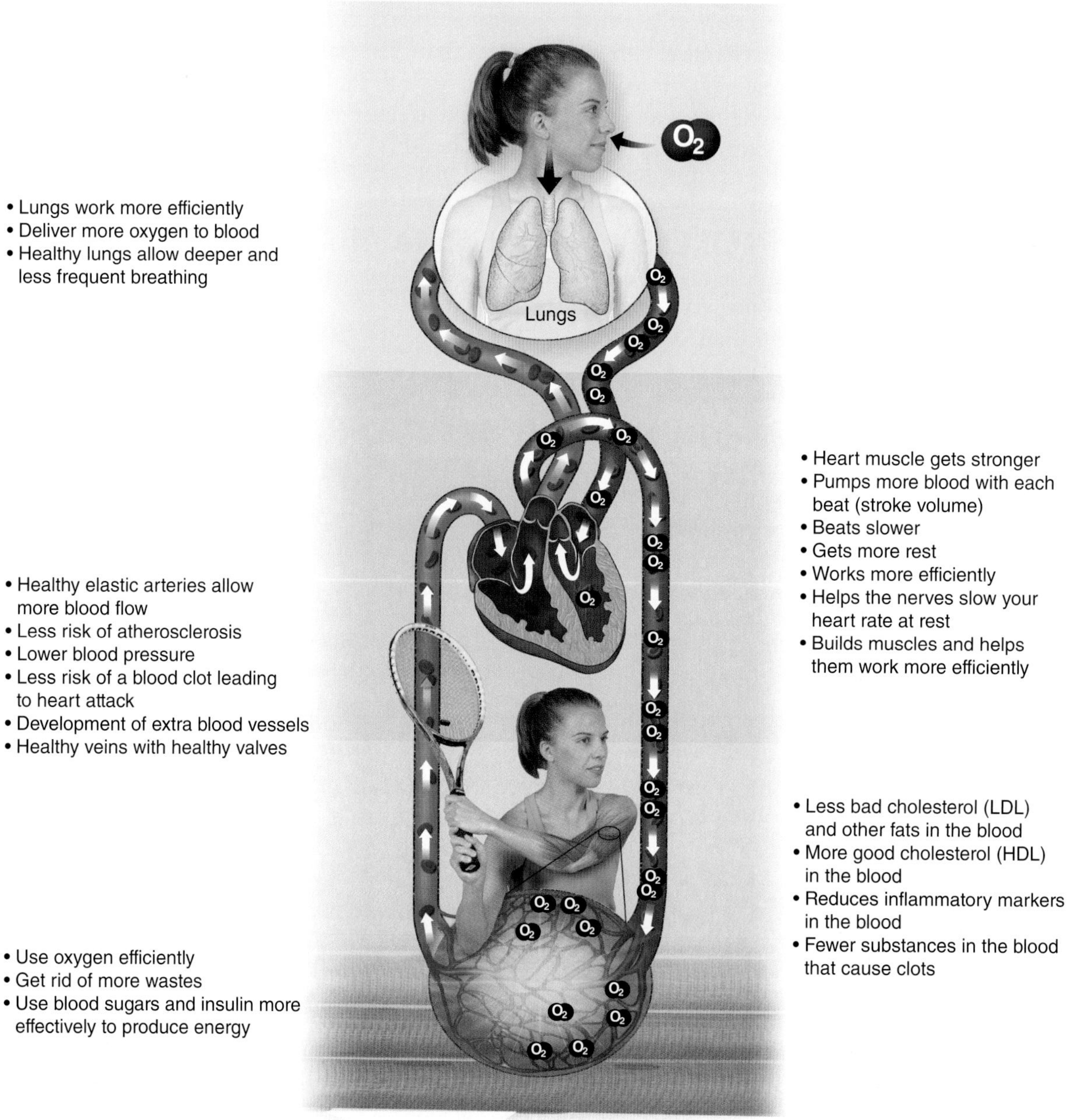

- Lungs work more efficiently
- Deliver more oxygen to blood
- Healthy lungs allow deeper and less frequent breathing

- Healthy elastic arteries allow more blood flow
- Less risk of atherosclerosis
- Lower blood pressure
- Less risk of a blood clot leading to heart attack
- Development of extra blood vessels
- Healthy veins with healthy valves

- Use oxygen efficiently
- Get rid of more wastes
- Use blood sugars and insulin more effectively to produce energy

- Heart muscle gets stronger
- Pumps more blood with each beat (stroke volume)
- Beats slower
- Gets more rest
- Works more efficiently
- Helps the nerves slow your heart rate at rest
- Builds muscles and helps them work more efficiently

- Less bad cholesterol (LDL) and other fats in the blood
- More good cholesterol (HDL) in the blood
- Reduces inflammatory markers in the blood
- Fewer substances in the blood that cause clots

FIGURE 8.5 Benefits of physical activity for the cardiovascular and respiratory systems.

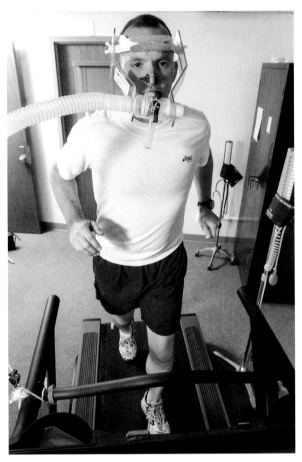

FIGURE 8.6 The maximal oxygen uptake test measures the amount of oxygen you use while running on a treadmill.

The difficulty increases as the treadmill goes faster and you begin to run uphill. As you exercise, the gas meter measures the amount of oxygen you use each minute. The amount (volume) of oxygen you can use during the hardest minute of exercise is considered your $\dot{V}O_2$max score (see Science in Action).

Medical doctors and exercise physiologists sometimes use another laboratory test called a graded exercise test (or an exercise stress test). This test is used to detect potential heart problems. During the test, your heart is monitored by means of an electrocardiogram while you run on a treadmill.

Both the graded exercise test and the maximal oxygen uptake test are done in a laboratory and require special equipment and people who are trained to administer them. Most people, however, assess their cardiorespiratory endurance using practical nonlaboratory tests called field tests. These tests require little equipment and can be done at home or at school. Scores are determined based on your ability to function (your functional fitness)

rather than on the amount of oxygen you can use. Examples include the PACER, the walking test, the step test, and the one-mile run test.

FIT FACT

Studies show that endurance athletes—such as cross-country skiers, cyclists, and distance runners—typically have very high aerobic capacity and score well on field tests of cardiorespiratory endurance.

Interpreting Self-Assessment Results

Self-assessments are not as accurate as laboratory tests of fitness; therefore, you should perform more than one self-assessment for cardiorespiratory endurance. However, self-assessments do give a good estimate of your fitness level, and each assessment has its own strengths and weaknesses. For example, the results of the PACER and the one-mile run are influenced by your motivation; if you don't try very hard, you won't get an accurate score. Because these tests require a high level of exertion, they may not be the best tests for people who have not been exercising regularly or who have low fitness.

The walking test, on the other hand, is a good indicator of fitness for most people but is not best for assessing very fit people. It would be a good test for a beginner. The step test (included in this chapter) uses heart rate; therefore, motivation does not influence the results as much as it does some other assessments. But step test results can be distorted if you've done other exercise that might elevate your heart rate before doing the assessment. Your heart rate can also be influenced by emotional factors (e.g., stress) and nutritional factors (e.g., caffeine) that cause it to be higher than normal. Finally, your results may vary depending on the time of day the assessment is done. For example, fatigue associated with daily activities may result in poorer scores late in the day.

Regardless of which tests you do, practice them before using them to assess your fitness. Practice allows you to pace yourself properly during the test and enables you to perform the tests properly so that you get accurate assessments. Because you may get different ratings on different tests of cardiorespiratory endurance, consider the strengths and weaknesses of each test when making decisions

SCIENCE IN ACTION: Aerobic Capacity

After extensive research, the Institute of Medicine recommended the use of the term *cardiorespiratory endurance* for performance on field tests such as the PACER. Because of this recommendation, we use the term *cardiorespiratory endurance* in this book rather than some of the other commonly used terms (such as *cardiovascular fitness* or *aerobic fitness*). Cardiorespiratory endurance reflects a person's functional fitness—the ability to perform tasks of daily life such as leisure-time activities and the ability to meet emergencies without undue fatigue.

As noted earlier, the term **aerobic capacity** is similar to, but not exactly the same as, cardiorespiratory endurance. The only true measure of aerobic capacity is your score on a laboratory-based maximal oxygen uptake test. Your score on the maximal oxygen uptake test ($\dot{V}O_2$max test) is recorded in litres of oxygen per minute. You may want to adjust your aerobic capacity score (in litres) to account for body size because big people use more litres of oxygen simply because of their size. So aerobic capacity scores are commonly reported as millilitres of oxygen per kilogram of body weight per minute (mL/kg/min).

You can also get an idea of your aerobic capacity in other ways. For example, when used with FitnessGram, your cardiorespiratory endurance score is converted to an estimated aerobic capacity score. You can find more information and tables for estimating aerobic capacity from PACER scores in the student section of the Fitness for Life Canada website.

> **Student Activity**
>
> Estimate your aerobic capacity score in millilitres of oxygen per kilogram of body weight per minute (mL/kg/min) using your PACER score. Tables for converting PACER scores to aerobic capacity scores are available in the student section of the Fitness for Life Canada website.

about which score best represents your fitness. After you've done regular exercise over time, test yourself again to see how much you've improved.

How Much Cardiorespiratory Endurance Is Enough?

To get the health and wellness benefits associated with cardiorespiratory endurance, you should achieve the good fitness zone in the rating charts that accompany each self-assessment in this book. Health benefits are associated with moving out of the low and marginal zones and into the good fitness zone. The risk of hypokinetic diseases is greatest for people in the low fitness zone.

Some people aim for especially high cardiorespiratory endurance because they want to perform at a high level in a sport or a physically demanding job—for example, as a soldier or a police officer. To be properly fit for such challenges, you must train harder than most people. Achieving the high performance zone will be difficult for some people, and doing so is not necessary in order to get many of the health benefits of fitness. Nevertheless, the higher your cardiorespiratory endurance score, the lower your risk of hypokinetic disease.

Lesson Review

1. What are some health and wellness benefits of cardiorespiratory endurance?
2. How does physical activity affect the various parts of your cardiovascular and respiratory systems?
3. What are some methods for assessing cardiorespiratory endurance and aerobic capacity, and how are they done?
4. How much cardiorespiratory endurance is enough?

As you've learned, the maximal oxygen uptake test is the best test of fitness of the cardiovascular and respiratory systems. But if you want a quicker, easier, and less expensive test, try the step test or the one-mile run test. Then, after you've done regular exercise over time, test yourself again to see how much you've improved. Try the tests and record your scores and fitness ratings for either test (or both). You can then use the information in preparing your personal physical activity plan. If you're working with a partner, remember that self-assessment information is personal and considered confidential. It shouldn't be shared with others without the permission of the person being tested.

Step Test

1. Use a bench that is 30 centimetres high. Step up with your right foot. Step up with your left foot.
2. Step down with your right foot. Step down with your left foot.
3. Repeat this four-count pattern (up, up, down, down). Step 24 times each minute for three minutes.
4. Immediately after stepping for three minutes, sit and count your pulse. Begin counting within five seconds. Count for one minute.
5. Use table 8.1 to determine your cardiorespiratory endurance rating. Record your heart rate, minutes of stepping, and rating.

Note: The height of the bench and the rate of stepping are both crucial to getting an accurate test result. Sit calmly for several minutes before the test to ensure that your resting heart rate is normal.

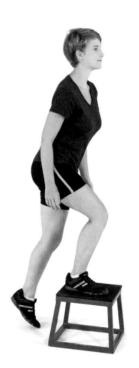
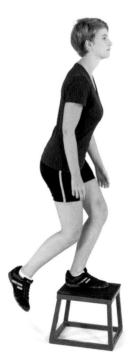

The step test assesses cardiorespiratory endurance.

TABLE 8.1 Rating Chart: Step Test (Heartbeats per Minute)

	13 years old		14–16 years old		17 years or older	
	Male	Female	Male	Female	Male	Female
High performance	≤90	≤100	≤85	≤95	≤80	≤90
Good fitness	91–98	101–110	86–95	96–105	81–90	91–100
Marginal fitness	99–120	111–130	96–115	106–125	91–110	101–120
Low fitness	≥121	≥131	≥116	≥126	≥111	≥121

Those who cannot step for three minutes receive a low fitness rating.

One-Mile Run

An alternative test of cardiorespiratory endurance is the one-mile run. Remember that this test is for your own information; it's not a race. Your goal is a good fitness rating, which indicates reduced risk of hypokinetic disease and enough fitness to function effectively. Some people may strive to achieve the high performance zone, which provides additional health benefits and allows you to perform sports and jobs requiring strong cardiorespiratory endurance.

1. Run or jog for one mile (1.6 kilometres) in the shortest possible time. A steady pace is best. Try to set a pace that you can keep up for the full run. If you start too fast you might not be able to run the entire distance. It is important to run the entire mile to get an accurate estimate of your cardiorespiratory fitness. You can use target heart rate or ratings of perceived exertion (explained later in this chapter) to help you set a good pace. Another indicator is the talk test. If you are unable to talk comfortably while running (for example, talking with a friend), then you are probably running too fast.

2. Your score is the amount of time it takes you to run the full distance. Record your time in minutes and seconds.

3. Find your rating in table 8.2 and record it.

TABLE 8.2 Rating Chart: One-Mile Run (min:sec)

	13 years old		14 years old		15 years old		16 years old		17 years or older	
	Male	Female	Male	Female	Male	Female	Male	Female	Male	Female
High performance	≤7:45	≤8:40	≤7:30	≤8:25	≤7:15	≤8:10	≤7:00	≤7:45	≤6:50	≤7:35
Good fitness	7:46–10:09	8:41–10:27	7:31–9:27	8:26–10:15	7:16–9:00	8:11–9:58	7:01–8:39	7:46–9:46	6:51–8:26	7:36–9:31
Marginal fitness	10:10–12:29	10:28–13:03	9:28–11:51	10:16–12:48	9:01–11:14	9:59–12:27	8:40–10:46	9:47–12:11	8:27–10:37	9:32–11:54
Low fitness	≥12:30	≥13:04	≥11:52	≥12:49	≥11:15	≥12:28	≥10:47	≥12:12	≥10:38	≥11:55

Based on data provided by G. Welk.

Lesson 8.2

Building Cardiorespiratory Endurance

Lesson Objectives

After participating in this lesson, you should be able to

1. define *vigorous aerobic activity* and give several examples,
2. describe the FIT formula for developing cardiorespiratory endurance,
3. describe how to count your resting heart rate and determine your maximal heart rate, and
4. explain how to use two methods for determining your threshold of training and your target zone for building cardiorespiratory endurance.

Lesson Vocabulary

aerobic activity, heart rate reserve (HRR), maximal heart rate, vigorous aerobics

You now know that physical activity is important to your cardiorespiratory endurance. But how much physical activity do you have to do to improve your cardiorespiratory endurance? In this lesson, you'll learn about the best types of activity for building cardiorespiratory endurance. You'll also learn to determine how much physical activity you need in order to build your own cardiorespiratory endurance.

> " To keep the body in good health is a duty; otherwise, we shall not be able to keep our mind strong and clear. "
>
> —The Buddha

Physical Activity and Cardiorespiratory Endurance

The term *aerobic* means "with oxygen," and **aerobic activity** is activity that is steady enough to allow your heart to supply all the oxygen your muscles need. Moderate-intensity physical activities are considered to be aerobic because you can do them for a long time without stopping. Moderate-intensity activities provide many health benefits and can build cardiorespiratory endurance in low-fit people, but they are not intense enough to build cardiorespiratory endurance for most people.

Vigorous aerobics, represented on the second step of the Physical Activity Pyramid for Teens, is the most effective way to build cardiorespiratory endurance. Vigorous aerobic activities are intense enough to elevate your heart rate above your threshold of training and into your target zone for cardiorespiratory endurance. National physical activity guidelines for teens recommend doing vigorous-intensity activity on at least three days a week because they promote benefits beyond those provided by moderate-intensity activity.

Vigorous sport and recreation activities, represented on the third step of the Physical Activity Pyramid for Teens (figure 8.7), also build cardiorespiratory endurance. Vigorous sports (e.g., soccer, basketball, and tennis) often involve quick bursts of vigorous-intensity activity followed by rest, and for this reason they are not totally aerobic. However, they offer the same benefits as vigorous aerobic activity. To be considered vigorous intensity, sports and recreation activities must be intense enough to elevate your heart rate above your threshold of training and into your target zone for cardiorespiratory endurance.

How Much Vigorous-Intensity Activity Is Enough?

As you're already aware, teens should accumulate 60 minutes of physical activity each day of the week. Some of that recommended activity should be vigorous in intensity. Specifically, you should perform vigorous-intensity activity at least three days a week

The FIT formula for building cardiorespiratory endurance is shown in table 8.3. As you can see, both the threshold of training and the target zone are different for people who are sedentary than for people who are regularly active. Sedentary people exercise at a lower intensity and use a different target heart rate zone than more active people.

When using table 8.3, first find your current physical activity level among the options listed in the first row. Rows below indicate frequency and length of exercise in days and minutes. The intensity of your exercise is determined by one of two methods of counting heart rate; these two methods are described in the next section of this chapter. Once you learn how to count your heart rate using one of the two methods, you can use table 8.3 to determine your exercise intensity.

FIT FACT

Another way (besides heart rate) to determine intensity is to use rating of perceived exertion (RPE). In this method, you estimate the intensity of your exertion during exercise using numbers from 0 (sitting; no exertion) to 10 (sprinting up a hill; maximal exertion). An RPE of 5 to 8 is typically equal to the target zone for cardiorespiratory endurance (see table 8.3). Rating of perceived exertion can be used to help you determine your pace during vigorous aerobic activity.

Energy
balance

STEP 5
Flexibility exercises

STEP 4
Muscle fitness exercises

STEP 3
Vigorous sport and recreation

STEP 2
Vigorous aerobics

STEP 1
Moderate-intensity physical activity

FIGURE 8.7 Vigorous-intensity activities from steps 2 and 3 are best for building cardiorespiratory endurance.

Adapted from Physical Activity Pyramid for Teens, source: C.B. Corbin.

in exercise sessions totalling at least 20 minutes per day. Vigorous-intensity activity should be of a high enough intensity that it increases your heart rate above your threshold level and into your target zone.

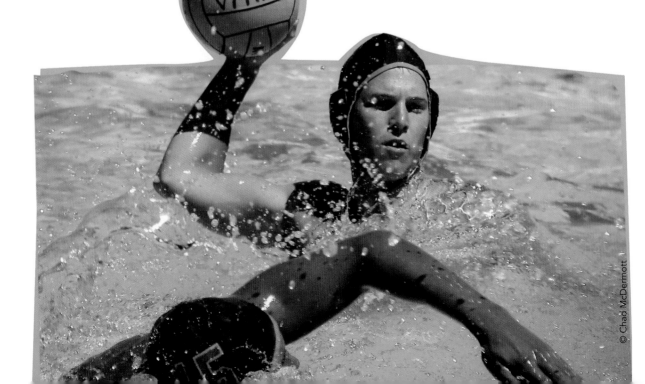

© Chad McDermott

TABLE 8.3   Threshold of Training and Target Heart Rate Zones (FIT Formula) for People With Different Activity Levels

	Threshold of training			Target heart rate zone		
Current activity level	No regular vigorous activity	Some vigorous activity	Regular vigorous activity	No regular vigorous activity	Some vigorous activity	Regular vigorous activity
Frequency	3 days a week for all fitness levels			3–6 days a week for all fitness levels		
Intensity	Percentage			Percentage		
HRR*	50	60	70	50–70	60–80	70–89
% max HR**	70	80	84	70–85	80–91	84–95
Time	20 min for all activity levels***			20–90 min for all activity levels***		

*HRR indicates heart rate reserve.

**% max HR indicates percent of maximal heart rate.

***Sessions of at least 10 minutes can be combined to meet time recommendations.

Based on *ACSM exercise prescription guidelines*.

Heart Rate and Intensity of Physical Activity

Monitoring heart rate is a common technique for determining exercise intensity. This is because taking a pulse count to determine your heart rate is relatively easy to do. But what exactly are we looking for when we take a pulse count? In order to build cardiorespiratory endurance, you need to overload the cardiovascular and respiratory systems. Calculating a target heart rate zone, including your threshold of training and target ceiling, is the scientific approach to providing optimal overload. Once you know your target heart rate zone, you know how high you need to elevate your heart rate to pace your exercise for building cardiorespiratory endurance. The Canadian Society of Exercise Physiology (CSEP) and the American College of Sports Medicine (ACSM) recommend two methods for determining your target heart rate zone. The first is the percent of heart rate reserve (% HRR) method, and the second is the percent of maximal heart rate (% max HR) method.

In this lesson, you'll learn how to use both of these methods to calculate your threshold target heart rate zone. After learning both methods, you'll choose one to use. You can then count your heart rate during or right after exercise to determine whether you're exercising at the right intensity for your target zone.

Counting Resting Heart Rate

To determine your target heart rate zone, you first need to determine your resting heart rate, which is the number of times your heart beats when you're relatively inactive. Use the following instructions.

1. Sit and take your heart rate by using the first and second fingers of your hand to find a pulse at the opposite wrist (your radial pulse) (figure 8.8*a*). Do not use your thumb. Practice so that you can locate your pulse quickly.

2. Count the number of pulses for one minute. Record your one-minute heart rate.

3. Take your resting (seated) heart rate again, this time counting the pulse at your neck (figure 8.8*b*). This is your carotid pulse. Use two fingers (index and middle) of either hand. Start with your two fingers at the side of your nose and move your fingers straight downward to your neck. Move until you locate the pulse. Press only as hard as necessary to feel the pulse; be careful not to press too hard.

4. Now take both your wrist and your neck pulse while you are standing. Repeat the pulse count (both wrist and neck) while sitting. Compare your results. Usually, your standing pulse is faster than your sitting pulse.

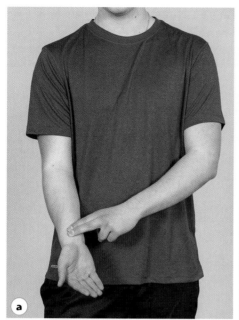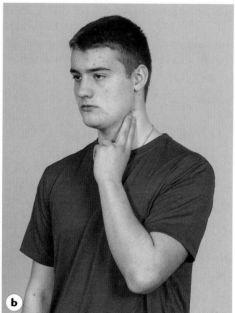

FIGURE 8.8 Use your first and second finger to find a pulse *(a)* at your wrist and *(b)* at your neck.

5. Take a partner's pulse while your partner takes your pulse (both standing). Compare your self-counted heart rate with your heart rate as determined by your partner. You can use different methods of counting, but use the same one as your partner when making comparisons.

6. As directed by your teacher, record your resting heart rate using the methods just described.

Determining Maximal Heart Rate (Max HR)

Maximal heart rate (max HR) is the highest heart rate that a person can reach during the most vigorous-intensity exercise. To estimate your max HR, you can count your heart rate after a very vigorous-intensity exercise session; or, to determine a more accurate max HR, you can wear a heart rate monitor to see how high your heart rate gets during very vigorous-intensity exercise. Be aware, however, that people who are unfit or are not regularly active should not complete an exercise session vigorous enough to determine max HR.

Because determining a true max HR requires very vigorous activity that isn't appropriate for some people, exercise physiologists have developed several formulas for estimating max HR without doing exercise. Five different formulas are listed by the ACSM for estimating max HR. Each has advantages and disadvantages. Here we use the formula that is most commonly employed by exercise experts. It's simple to use, and the estimated max HRs from the formula are very similar to those calculated using a more complex formula for young people including teens. You can use the following formula or estimate your max HR by using table 8.4.

220 – age in years = maximal heart rate

Example for 16-year-old: 220 – 16 = 204

Before your next activity or exercise, record your estimated max HR. You'll use it when determining your heart rate target zone.

Counting Exercise Heart Rate

It can be difficult to count your pulse during activities such as jogging, but you can get a good estimate of your heart rate during a physical activity by determining your heart rate immediately after exercising. To estimate your heart rate during exercise based on your after-exercise pulse count, use the following instructions.

1. Immediately after exercise, locate your pulse (within five seconds).

2. Use either your wrist or neck pulse to count your heart rate for 15 seconds. Multiply your 15-second count by 4 to get your one-

minute heart rate, or take your pulse count for 10 seconds and multiply by 6 to get your one-minute heart rate. This method is useful because you can do it quickly and because your heart rate slows down quickly when you stop exercising, which means that longer counts (e.g., 30 seconds) may underestimate what your heart rate was during the exercise. On the other hand, counting for a shorter time (e.g., five seconds) can result in error because a single counting mistake is multiplied. You can use table 8.5 to help you determine your one-minute heart rate from your 15-second count.

3. While you count your heart rate, you may want to continue to walk slowly because slow walking can help you recover faster. If you have trouble counting your heart rate while walking, stand still when you count, then begin moving.

Percent of Heart Rate Reserve Method for Determining Target Heart Rate

To build cardiorespiratory endurance, you must elevate your heart rate above your threshold of

training and into your target zone (see table 8.3). The percent of heart rate reserve (% HRR) is one of two methods for determining target heart rate. This method is considered the most accurate, but it is a bit more difficult to calculate than the other method. To use this method, you must know your resting and maximal heart rates and your **heart rate reserve (HRR)**. Table 8.6 provides an example of the calculations for a 16-year-old who has a resting heart rate of 67 and is in the good fitness zone for cardiorespiratory endurance.

1. Begin by determining your resting and max HR as described earlier in this chapter. In the example, the resting HR is 67 and the max HR is 204.

2. Next, determine your heart rate reserve by subtracting your resting heart rate from your maximal heart rate (max HR). In the example, the resting heart rate is 67, so the heart rate reserve is 137.

3. To calculate the threshold heart rate, multiply the heart rate reserve (HRR) by a percentage of the max HR—60 percent (0.6) in the example. As shown in table 8.3, different percentages are used for people of different activity levels; use the percentage that fits

TABLE 8.4 Estimated Maximal Heart Rates

Your age (years)	12	13	14	15	16	17	18	19
Max HR	208	207	206	205	204	203	202	201

Find your age in the top row, then find your estimated max HR immediately below your age.

TABLE 8.5 Heart Rate in 15-Second and 1-Minute Intervals

15-sec rate	1-min rate	15-sec rate	1-min rate	15-sec rate	1-min rate
15	60	27	108	39	156
16	64	28	112	40	160
17	68	29	116	41	164
18	72	30	120	42	168
19	76	31	124	43	172
20	80	32	128	44	176
21	84	33	132	45	180
22	88	34	136	46	184
23	92	35	140	47	188
24	96	36	144	48	192
25	100	37	148	49	196
26	104	38	152	50	200

Find your 15-second heart rate in a shaded column; your one-minute heart rate is in the white column to the immediate right of it.

your current activity level. This number is then added to the resting heart rate. In the example, the threshold is 149.

4. The target ceiling heart rate is calculated by repeating steps 1 through 3, but in step 3 you multiply by a higher percentage—80 percent (0.8) in the example. Refer to table 8.3 to find the percentage you should use for your target zone based on your current activity level. Then add your resting heart rate. In the example, the target ceiling heart rate is 177.

5. Thus the target heart zone is 149 to 177 (60 to 80 percent of HRR) in the example of the 16-year-old who is in the good fitness zone.

Percent of Maximal Heart Rate Method for Determining Target Heart Rate

The second method, percent of maximal heart rate (% max HR), is not quite as accurate as the HRR method but is easier to calculate. In this method,

you do not use your resting heart rate. Table 8.7 provides an example using the % max HR method for a 16-year-old in the good fitness zone for cardiorespiratory endurance.

1. Estimate your maximal heart rate. In the example, the maximal heart rate is 204.

2. In this example, the max HR (204) was multiplied by 80 percent (0.8) to find the threshold heart rate. As noted in table 8.3, different percentages are used for people of different activity levels; use the percentage that fits your current activity level. In the example, the threshold is 163.

3. To calculate the target ceiling rate, repeat steps 1 and 2, but in step 2 multiply by 91 percent (0.91). This number will vary based on your activity level (see table 8.3). In the example, the ceiling rate is 186.

4. Thus the target heart rate zone is 163 to 186 (80 to 91 percent of max HR) in the example of the 16-year-old in the good fitness zone

TABLE 8.6   Calculating Heart Rate Target Zone (% HRR Method)

Threshold HR	Step 1:	204 (max HR)*
	Step 2:	− 67 (resting HR)
		137 (HRR)
	Step 3:	× 0.6 (threshold %)
		82
		+ 67 (resting HR)
		149 (threshold HR)
Target ceiling	Step 1:	204 (max HR)*
	Step 2:	− 67 (resting HR)
		137 (HRR)
	Step 3:	× 0.8 (ceiling %)
		110
		+ 67 (resting HR)
		177 (target ceiling HR)
Target HR zone	149–177 beats per minute	

*The example is for a 16-year-old with a resting HR of 67 with cardiorespiratory endurance in the good fitness zone.

TABLE 8.7   Calculating Heart Rate Target Zone (% max HR Method)

Threshold HR	Step 1:	204 (max HR)*
	Step 2:	× 0.8 (threshold %)
		163 (threshold HR)
Target ceiling rate	Step 1:	204 (max HR)*
	Step 2:	× 0.91 (ceiling %)
		186 (target ceiling rate)
Target HR zone	163–186 beats per minute	

*The example is for a 16-year-old with a resting HR of 67 and cardiorespiratory endurance in the good fitness zone.

for cardiorespiratory endurance. Note that these numbers are slightly higher than those generated with the % HRR method.

Exercise for Ellen

Ellen is a high school sophomore. She took the PACER and the walking test and got a marginal fitness rating in both. She was not surprised, because she only participated in vigorous-intensity exercise occasionally, but she did want to improve her cardiorespiratory endurance. To do so, she knew that she had to start doing more vigorous-intensity activity each week.

Specifically, based on information presented in table 8.3, Ellen learned that she needed to do vigorous-intensity exercise at least three (and up to six) days a week. She decided to begin with three, and she chose to jog for 20 minutes on each of the three days because table 8.3 recommends sessions of 20 minutes.

In class, Ellen learned how to use the % HRR and % max HR methods for determining her target heart rate zone. She decided to use the % HRR method. She first determined her maximal heart rate (204 beats per minute) and resting heart rate (67 beats per minute). She then determined that her heart rate reserve (HRR) was 137 by subtracting her resting heart rate from her maximum heart rate (204 – 67 = 137).

Next, she calculated her target heart rate zone, and she did so with the 50 percent to 70 percent range shown in table 8.3 for someone who does no regular vigorous-intensity activity. Specifically, she did the following calculations: 50 percent of 137 (her heart rate reserve) is 69, and 70 percent of 137 is 96. Ellen then added 67 (her resting heart rate) to each of these figures to get her threshold heart rate (69 + 67 = 136) and her target ceiling heart rate (96 + 67 = 163). Thus she determined that her target heart rate zone was 139 to 163 beats per minute.

Immediately after each jogging session, Ellen counted her heart rate to see if it was in her target heart rate zone. On a few days, it was below the zone, so she ran a bit faster the next time. Over time, Ellen expects to improve her cardiorespiratory endurance so that she will be in the good fitness zone.

Lesson Review

1. What is vigorous aerobic activity? Give several examples.
2. What is the FIT formula for developing cardiorespiratory endurance?
3. How can you determine your resting heart rate and estimate your max HR?
4. How can you determine your threshold of training and your target heart rate zone for building cardiorespiratory endurance? Describe two methods.

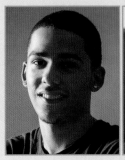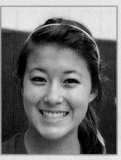

Self-confidence involves believing that you can be successful in an activity. If you think you'll succeed, you have more confidence than if you're unsure about how well you'll do. You're more likely to participate in an activity if your self-confidence is high. An important component of physical literacy is moving with confidence in a variety of activities and environments (e.g., land, air, water, snow).

Tony rarely takes part in any physical activity. He went through an awkward stage in his pre-teen years and thinks that people laugh at the way he runs: "My arms and legs don't seem to work together when I run. I think I look foolish."

Mei, on the other hand, loves any kind of physical activity. Every day, she shoots baskets or rides her bike, and she is a member of multiple teams. Even though she excels in sport, she would like to socialize more, but she feels shy around strangers: "I can't think of anything witty or even halfway intelligent to say. When I try to talk, I get tongue-tied. It's easier for me to just avoid talking."

Tony and Mei both lack self-confidence but in two different situations. Tony wants to participate in physical activity, and Mei wants to socialize; but they both avoid situations in which they might get involved because they feel uncomfortable. Both need to find a way to build their self-confidence so they can succeed in these situations.

For Discussion

For different reasons, people like Tony may avoid trying new activities or may quit an activity prematurely. People like Mei who lack confidence in social situations may avoid them. What are some reasons that people lack self-confidence? How can they increase their self-confidence? What advice can you give Tony to get him to try new activities and stick with them? What advice can you give Mei to help her be more comfortable in social situations? Also consider the guidelines presented in the Self-Management feature when answering the discussion questions.

 SELF-MANAGEMENT: *Skills for Building Self-Confidence*

A recent study of teenagers found that one of the best indicators of who will be physically active is self-confidence. A person is self-confident if he or she thinks *I can do that* rather than *I don't think I can*. Some people are not very confident when it comes to physical activity because they think they are not very good at it or that others are better than they are. Does it surprise you to learn that self-confident people are not always the best performers and that some good performers lack self-confidence? In fact, research involving teenagers in schools shows that all students can find some type of activity in which they can be successful, regardless of physical ability. In addition, people who think they can succeed in activity are nearly twice as likely to be active as people who don't think they can succeed.

Building self-confidence is a self-management skill that you can learn. You may want to assess your self-confidence using the worksheet supplied by your teacher. Then, if necessary, you can use the following guidelines to improve your self-confidence.

- **Learn a new way of thinking.** One major reason some people lack self-confidence is that they think their own success depends on how they compare with others. Practicing a new way of thinking means setting your own standards of success rather than comparing yourself with others. These guidelines are designed to help you build self-confidence by developing a new way of thinking.

- **Set your own personal standards for success.** Assess yourself and set standards for success related to your own improvement. Comparing yourself with others is not necessary for your success, and it can contribute to low self-confidence.

- **Avoid competition if it causes you a problem.** Some people like to compete, but others don't. If competition makes you feel less confident in a physical activity, try to find noncompetitive activities (such as walking, jogging, and swimming) that allow you to feel good about yourself.

- **Set small goals that you're sure to reach.** Setting goals that are a bit higher than your current level is a good idea, but don't set them too high. As you reach one small goal, you can set another. Reaching several small goals builds your self-confidence, whereas not reaching one unrealistic goal can make you less confident.

- **Think and act on positive—not negative—ideas.** When you're involved in a physical activity, think of how you can improve. Talk to yourself about what you did well and what you can practice to improve in the future. Avoid negative self-talk, such as berating yourself for what you didn't do well or referring to yourself in negative terms.

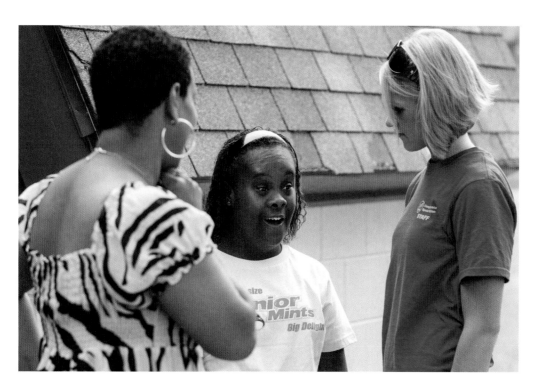

Setting a personal standard of success and getting reinforcement from others can help a person build self-confidence.

Cardiorespiratory endurance is important for living a long and healthy life. It's also essential for competing, participating in your favourite physical activities, and maintaining a healthy body weight. As you've learned in this chapter, you must do vigorous-intensity physical activity above your threshold of training and in your target zone to build cardiorespiratory endurance. Take action by doing vigorous-intensity activity that fulfills the FIT formula: at least three days each week (addressing "F" for frequency in the FIT formula), in your target heart rate zone (addressing "I" for intensity), and for at least 20 minutes each session (addressing "T" for time). Consider the following tips as you take action by performing a target heart rate workout.

- Determine your target heart rate by using either the percent of

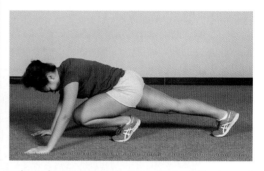

heart rate reserve method or the percent of maximal heart rate method.

- Before choosing vigorous-intensity activities, consider your level of fitness.
- Before doing vigorous-intensity activity, perform a five-minute cardiorespiratory general warm-up.
  - Check your pulse rate or RPE periodically to make sure you're maintaining the intensity of your workout in your target heart rate zone.
  - After your vigorous-intensity workout, perform a cool-down.

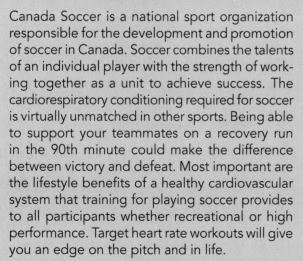

Take action by doing a workout that elevates your heart rate into the target zone.

 ## GET ACTIVE WITH CANADA SOCCER

©Canada Soccer

Who We Are

Canada Soccer is a national sport organization responsible for the development and promotion of soccer in Canada. Soccer combines the talents of an individual player with the strength of working together as a unit to achieve success. The cardiorespiratory conditioning required for soccer is virtually unmatched in other sports. Being able to support your teammates on a recovery run in the 90th minute could make the difference between victory and defeat. Most important are the lifestyle benefits of a healthy cardiovascular system that training for playing soccer provides to all participants whether recreational or high performance. Target heart rate workouts will give you an edge on the pitch and in life.

What We Do

In association with our provincial member associations we provide leadership and direction on player, coaching, and referee development; field men's, women's, and youth teams in domestic, regional, and international competitions; and support opportunities for all Canadians to participate in the beautiful game.

Get Involved

Whether you're a fan looking for information on Canada's path to the FIFA World Cup, a potential referee looking to find information on training and registration, a youth player looking to discover the development pathway to strive for the next level, or a budding young coach looking for an opportunity to help develop the younger generation of stars, Canada Soccer can help you fulfill your soccer dreams. Visit CanadaSoccer.com.

©Canada Soccer

Reviewing Concepts and Vocabulary

Complete the following in order to determine your growing understanding of fitness, health, and wellness. Answer items 1 through 5 by correctly completing each sentence with a word or phrase.

1. Vessels that carry blood from the muscles back to the heart are called _____.
2. The body system that includes your heart, blood vessels, and blood is the _____ system.
3. The substance in your blood that helps it clot is called _____.
4. The method for determining exercise intensity by estimating it without measuring it is called rating of _____.
5. The highest your heart rate ever gets is called your _____.

For items 6 through 10, match each term in column 1 with the appropriate phrase in column 2.

6. carotid
7. cholesterol
8. high-density lipoprotein
9. low-density lipoprotein
10. maximal oxygen uptake

a. waxy, fatlike substance in blood
b. neck pulse
c. bad cholesterol
d. aerobic capacity
e. carries bad cholesterol out of the bloodstream

For items 11 through 15, respond to each statement or question.

11. Explain how cardiorespiratory endurance helps your cardiovascular and respiratory systems work more efficiently and thus helps to prevent cardiovascular disease.
12. Define *aerobic capacity*. How does it relate to cardiorespiratory endurance?
13. Describe the two field tests of cardiorespiratory endurance discussed in this chapter.
14. Describe two methods for determining your target heart rate zone.
15. Describe several guidelines for building self-confidence.

Thinking Critically

Write a paragraph to answer the following question.
   Sue has a resting heart rate of 76 beats per minute. Bill has a resting heart rate of 54. Assuming that neither has a disease or illness, what are three to five possible reasons that their resting heart rates differ so much? Explain each.

Project

Create a poster, an online poster (e.g., Glogster), a slide presentation (e.g. PowerPoint, Prezi), or a video describing the benefits of physical activity for the cardiovascular and respiratory systems.

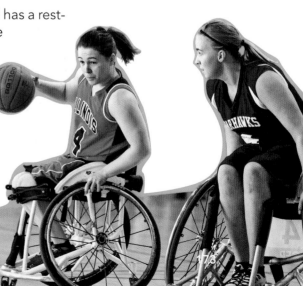

9

Engaging in Vigorous-Intensity Physical Activity

In This Chapter

LESSON 9.1
Vigorous Aerobics, Sport, and Recreation

SELF-ASSESSMENT
Assessing Jogging Techniques

LESSON 9.2
Preparing and Performing a Safe and Vigorous-Intensity Physical Activity Program

TAKING CHARGE
Choosing Good Activities

SELF-MANAGEMENT
Skills for Choosing Good Activities

TAKING ACTION
Your Vigorous-Intensity Physical Activity Plan

GET ACTIVE WITH CANADA BASKETBALL

CHAPTER REVIEW

(www) **Student Web Resources**
www.fitnessforlife.org/student

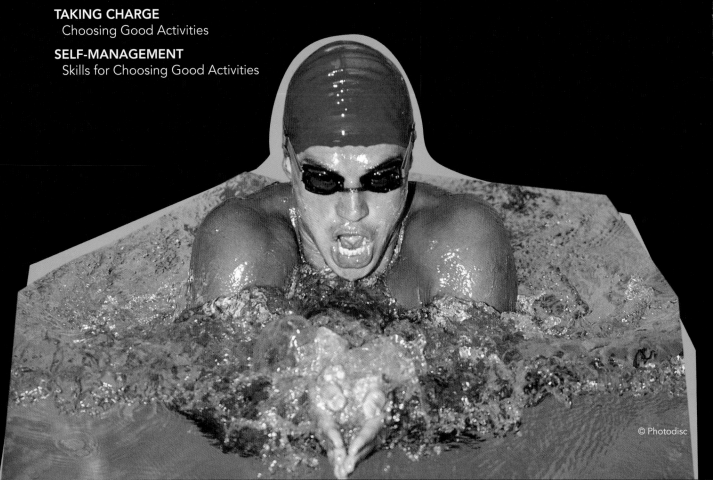

© Photodisc

Lesson 9.1

Vigorous Aerobics, Sport, and Recreation

Lesson Objectives

After participating in this lesson, you should be able to

1. list and describe the three types of vigorous-intensity physical activity (one from step 2 and two from step 3 of the Physical Activity Pyramid),
2. list and describe several types of vigorous aerobic activity (pyramid step 2),
3. describe the four categories of vigorous sport (pyramid step 3),
4. define *recreation* and *leisure*, and
5. list three types of vigorous recreation (pyramid step 3).

Lesson Vocabulary

aerobic, anaerobic activity, anaerobic capacity, circuit training, leisure time, lifetime sport, recreation, sport, vigorous aerobics, vigorous recreation, vigorous sport

How often do you engage in activities that make you breathe hard and sweat? Did you know that building fitness increases your chances of living longer? Vigorous-intensity physical activities are activities that make you breathe hard and sweat. The Physical Activity Pyramid shows two types of vigorous-intensity physical activity: vigorous aerobics (step 2) and vigorous sport and recreation (step 3) (figure 9.1). Activities included in these steps are more vigorous (requiring 7 METs or more) than the moderate-intensity activities included in step 1 (which require 4 to 7 METs) and are especially good for building cardiorespiratory endurance. (As discussed in chapter 7, 1 MET represents the energy you expend when at rest.) The MET count increases as activity becomes more vigorous. Research shows that vigorous-intensity physical activity (7+ METs) provides the health benefits of moderate activity—and more. In this lesson, you'll learn more about the many types of vigorous-intensity activity.

Vigorous Aerobic Activity

Most activities included in the Physical Activity Pyramid (including moderate activities) can be considered **aerobic**. But only activities that are intense enough to elevate your heart rate above your threshold of training and into your target zone are considered **vigorous aerobics**. Aerobic activities—such as jogging, aerobic dancing, cycling,

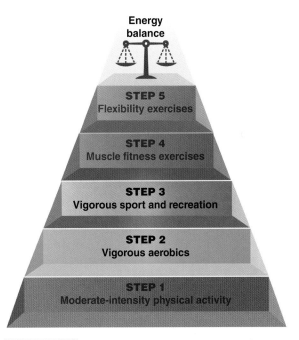

FIGURE 9.1 Vigorous aerobics, sport, and recreation (steps 2 and 3) build cardiorespiratory fitness and have many other health benefits.

Adapted from Physical Activity Pyramid for Teens, source: C.B. Corbin.

and swimming—are among the most popular and most beneficial of all the activities included in the Physical Activity Pyramid. They are popular for the following reasons.

- They often do not require high levels of skill.
- They frequently are not competitive.
- They often can be done at or near home.
- They often do not require a partner or group.

There are many types of vigorous aerobic activity. Some of the most popular are described in the following sections. Some activities could be classified in more than one section of the Physical Activity Pyramid. For example, swimming is a sport, a type of vigorous aerobic activity, and a type of vigorous recreation; in this book, it is classified as a vigorous aerobic activity. Each activity is described only once in this chapter even if it could fit in multiple places.

Aerobic Dance

Aerobic dance involves continuously performing various dance steps to music. Unlike social dancers, aerobic dancers typically dance by themselves, often following a leader or a video. This activity first became popular in the 1970s and remains one of the most popular forms of aerobic exercise. Forms of aerobic dance include low-impact, high-impact, and step aerobics. Low-impact aerobics is typically done with one foot staying on the ground at all times. This form is best for beginners because it leads to fewer injuries than other forms. High-impact aerobics is typically more vigorous and involves jumping. Step aerobics involves dance steps done on a step or box. Some types of aerobic dance use light weights, rubber bands, and other types of exercise equipment, as well as movements from other activities such as martial arts.

Aerobic Exercise Machines

Types of aerobic exercise machines include treadmills, stair steppers, elliptical trainers, exercise bicycles, rowing machines, and ski machines. You can purchase these machines for use in your own home or use them in health clubs and schools. They can be effective if used properly, but some people do not find exercise on machines to be as enjoyable as activities that allow them to move more freely. For example, skiing may be more enjoyable than using a ski machine. On the other hand, exercise machines are often convenient and efficient.

Cycling

Cycling is a sport because some people compete in it and a recreational activity because some do it for fun. If done slowly, it can also be considered a form of moderate physical activity. It is included here because it is often done continuously at a consistent speed that elevates the heart rate. Some forms of cycling, such as BMX and downhill mountain biking, are considered extreme sports.

Circuit Training

Circuit training involves performing several different exercises one after another. The performer does one exercise for a period of time, then moves to the next with only a brief time between exercises. The goal is to keep the heart rate in the target zone. Circuit training can use exercise machines, small equipment such as jump ropes or rubber bands, free weights, or no equipment at all (for example, calisthenics). Doing different activities helps build muscle fitness as well as cardiorespiratory endurance and can increase your enjoyment because of the variety. Sometimes people use music to determine how much time to spend on each exercise. A break in the music signals that it's time to move to the next exercise.

Dance

Dance is one of the oldest art forms and has been a means of expression in many cultures. Some dance forms are not only enjoyable but also excellent forms of vigorous aerobic exercise. More traditional dance activities include modern, ballet, folk, and square dance. Another category of dance is social dance, which includes both more traditional types (such as the waltz, country dancing, and Latin dancing) and newer forms (such as hip-hop and stepping). Some dance activities have been altered so that traditional steps are used in ways that make the activity similar to aerobic dance. For example, Zumba uses Latin music and Latin dance steps in ways that resemble aerobic dance. All can be good forms of vigorous aerobics if you do them vigorously enough to elevate your heart rate.

Jogging and Running

Jogging and running consistently rank among the most popular forms of vigorous aerobic activity. Jogging is generally considered to be noncompetitive, whereas running is a faster movement than jogging and is a competitive activity for some people. Runners often participate in competitive events such as 5K and 10K races. Jogging and running are combined into one category here because they are very similar. You'll learn more about them in the self-assessment that follows this lesson.

Martial Arts Exercise

Judo and karate are just two of the several hundred martial arts practiced around the world. Different countries throughout the world have different forms. Martial arts can build various parts of fitness, but they are not always good at building cardiorespiratory endurance because they may not involve enough continuous activity to keep the heart rate elevated. Some forms of martial arts, however, have been combined with aerobic dance to create martial arts exercises; examples include Tae Bo and cardio karate. These forms of exercise can build cardiorespiratory endurance but may not be as effective for learning self-defence as more traditional techniques.

Rope Jumping

Rope jumping has long been used by boxers and other athletes as a method of training. Because it requires moving the arms and legs, as well as the entire body, it can be quite vigorous. For this reason, people sometimes alternate rope jumping with other forms of exercise, such as calisthenics (e.g.,

 FITNESS TECHNOLOGY: Global Positioning System

The global positioning system (GPS) is a satellite-based system that communicates precise location information to places around the world. Satellites send signals to a receiver, which sends the signal to a computer that analyzes the information. The GPS was developed by the U.S. government to aid in national defence, but the technology is now available for consumer use. Global positioning system technology is quite accurate and has been used in automobiles to help drivers find their way. It is now being used to help bikers, joggers, hikers, and others who perform outdoor physical activities. The GPS can also provide information about how fast you're moving, the distance you've traveled, the altitude you've gained or lost, and the average pace for your total workout. The first GPS systems for use in physical activity were complicated and required arm or leg straps with a receiver, as well as a watch-like device worn on the arm. Others required a computer chip built into

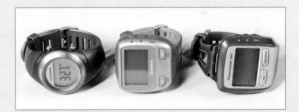

Global positioning system technology can help track your physical activity—for example, these watches can track how far a jogger has run.

shoes to pick up the satellite signal. Technology changes rapidly, however, and now GPS devices for use in physical activity are more advanced.

Using Technology

Research GPS technology for use in physical activity. Identify the device that you think would be the best buy and give reasons for your choice.

push-ups, sit-ups, planks). Practitioners have developed many rope-jumping moves. Rope jumping is inexpensive and can easily be done at home or in your neighbourhood. You can also easily transport the needed equipment when traveling.

Swimming

Swimming is both a sport and a form of recreation. It is included here because it is one of the most popular fitness activities among adults and can serve as a good way to improve cardiorespiratory endurance for almost all people. Like water aerobics, it is a good choice for people who are overweight, elderly, or suffering from joint problems. For swimming to be an effective aerobic exercise, however, your heart rate must be elevated, which means that you must swim continuously for many minutes. Many people who swim do not meet either of these standards.

Water Aerobics

Water aerobics, sometimes called aqua dynamics, involves doing calisthenics or dance steps in a swimming pool. This form of aerobic exercise is especially good for people who are overweight, elderly, or suffering from arthritis or other joint problems because the water reduces stress on the joints. For stronger exercisers, water can also be used to provide resistance and thus increase the intensity of exercise.

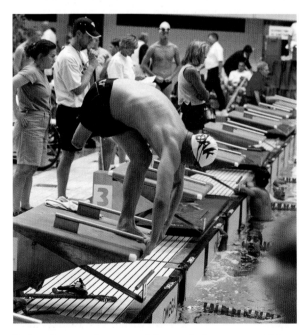

Swimming can be a good form of vigorous aerobics.

Vigorous Sports

Sport involves physical activity that is competitive (has a winner and loser) and follows well-established rules. Some sports, such as golf and bowling, are classified as moderate physical activity (step 1 of the Physical Activity Pyramid). **Vigorous sports** (step 3 of the pyramid) elevate the heart rate above the threshold level and into the target zone for cardiorespiratory endurance.

There are so many vigorous sports that it is impossible to mention them all here. We can, however, mention general categories: team sports; dual sports; individual sports; and outdoor, challenge, or extreme sports. Certain other sports are not considered here either because they are not among the most popular or because they have little relevance to a personal physical activity program (for example, auto racing and horse racing).

Team Sports

Team sports such as football, hockey, soccer, volleyball, and basketball are among the most popular for high school students and for adult spectators. These activities can be very good for helping participants build fitness (though of course they do little for the fitness of spectators!). Team sports can be harder to do after your school years are completed because they require other participants (teammates), as well as special equipment and facilities. Even though baseball and softball involve some vigorous-intensity activity and training for these sports often requires vigorous-intensity physical activity, they are usually considered to be moderate activities.

Golf, primarily an individual sport, is the most widely practiced sport in Canada. The next five most widely practiced sports are team sports (ice hockey, soccer, baseball, volleyball, and basketball); numbers 7 through 10 are dual or partner sports (downhill skiing, cycling, swimming, badminton). No team sport is among the 10 most popular types of physical activity performed by adults in Canada, but basketball, soccer, volleyball, hockey, and baseball are listed among the top 20. The 10 most popular activities are mostly either moderate physical activities or vigorous aerobics. Because relatively few people who play team sports when they are young continue to pursue them for a lifetime, it will be important for you to actively seek opportunities if you want to play team sports as you grow older.

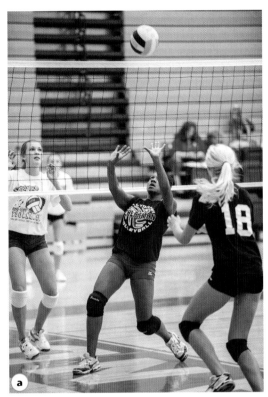 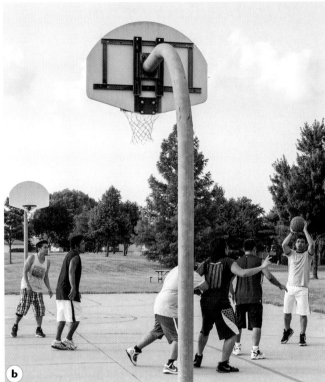

Team sports: *(a)* Volleyball and *(b)* basketball are two of the most practiced sports in Canada.

Another way to stay active is to begin learning an individual sport, a dual sport, or an aerobic activity that you can enjoy later in life.

Dual or Partner Sports

Dual sports are those you can do with just one other person (the person you are playing against) or with a partner against another set of partners (for example, tennis doubles). Examples include tennis, badminton, fencing, and judo. Because they require fewer people than team sports, dual sports are often referred to as **lifetime sports** in that they are easier to continue throughout your life. Badminton is often included in the top 10 participation activities in Canada partly because it can be done with just one other person and is easy to set up in backyards and on beaches.

Some dual sports are not activities that many people do as adults. For example, wrestling is considered a dual sport but is not often done as a lifetime sport, even though it does develop many important parts of health-related fitness. Dual sports that are not done by many adults are not considered lifetime sports.

Individual Sports

Individual sports are those that you can do by yourself. Golf (as mentioned earlier, the most widely practiced sport in Canada), gymnastics, and swimming are truly individual sports because you do not have to have a partner or a team to perform them. Many of these sports are also lifetime sports because they are more likely to be done throughout life, although some, such as gymnastics, are not done by many people later in life (and gymnastics often requires a spotter). Skiing and skating are two forms of vigorous recreation that are also sometimes classified as individual sports.

Outdoor, Challenge, or Extreme Sports

Many types of vigorous recreation can also be classified as sports. Certain vigorous recreation activities are sometimes referred to as outdoor or challenge sports, such as mountain biking, rock climbing, sailing, and water skiing. Some other activities may be referred to as extreme sports, such as snowboarding, skateboarding, surfing, and BMX cycling.

Vigorous Recreation Activities

Vigorous recreation includes activities that are fun and, typically, noncompetitive. **Recreation** is something you do during your free time; therefore, recreational activities are sometimes called leisure activities.

Many types of vigorous recreation are done outdoors because participants feel that the beauty of the setting and the fresh air help rejuvenate them. Examples of vigorous recreation are discussed next.

Backpacking and Hiking

Hiking is particularly enjoyable because it takes place outdoors and can be done either independently or in a group. Most municipalities and national parks offer scenic trails for hikers of all levels of experience. Hiking usually involves a one-day trip, whereas backpacking often involves a multiday venture that requires you to carry food, shelter, and other supplies on your back.

> " [Leave] all the afternoon for exercise and recreation, which are as necessary as reading; I will rather say more necessary, because health is worth more than learning. "
>
> —Thomas Jefferson, U.S. president

Boating, Canoeing, Kayaking, and Rowing

Boating can be done in various forms that offer the enjoyment of water and the outdoors, free from the hassles of normal daily life. When performed at a vigorous intensity, these activities also help you build fitness and promote good health. Kayaking and rowing can be especially vigorous, and they require considerable skill to perform well and safely. When not done at a vigorous intensity, boating activities can be relaxing and refreshing.

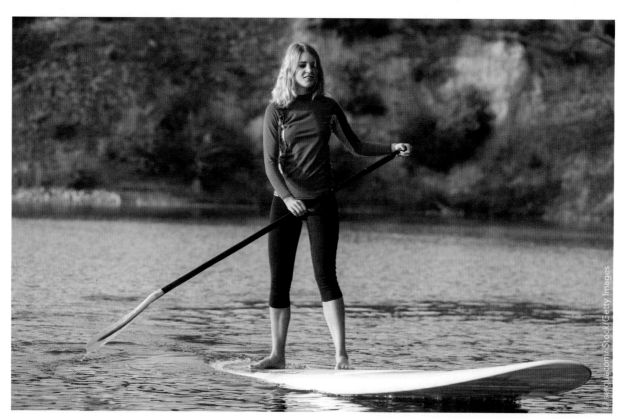

Paddleboarding can be a vigorous recreational activity that builds cardiorespiratory endurance and provides other health benefits.

Surfing and Stand-Up Paddleboarding

Surfing and stand-up paddleboarding (SUP) are increasing in popularity. These board sports can get participants outdoors and require good balance. Surfing requires upper body strength to paddle out to the waves, as well as flexibility and power to get from lying down on the board to standing up and surfing. Stand-up paddleboarding can be a vigorous recreation activity when you are paddling for speed and distance, or it can be a moderate-intensity physical activity when you are taking a relaxing paddle in calm water.

Orienteering

Orienteering combines walking, jogging, and skilled map reading. It is usually done in a rural area and might include hiking through rugged terrain. Participants depart from a starting point in staggered fashion every few minutes so that no participant can simply follow another. Each participant uses a compass (compass apps are available) and a map that describes a course up to 16 kilometres long. The compass is used to help locate several checkpoints marked by flags or other identifiers. At each checkpoint, the participant marks a card to indicate that he or she has located it. The activity can be competitive if the goal is to cover the course as fast

FIT FACT

Leisure time is more than free time. It involves an attitude of declaring freedom from doing things you have to do. Similarly, the word "recreation" suggests refreshing or re-creating yourself. Thus a recreational activity is one that you do during your leisure or free time to refresh or re-create yourself. Recreational activities are done for fun and enjoyment. They need not be vigorous or purposeful. They can include watching TV, reading a book, playing chess, creating art, making music, and doing many other relatively inactive pursuits. Some leisure activities—such as fishing, camping, and some forms of boating—can be considered moderate activities.

as possible. Urban orienteering uses the same ideas and skills but in inner-city areas rather than rural settings.

Rock Climbing and Bouldering

Many schools now teach rock climbing on climbing walls. Learning on a climbing wall allows you to get proper instruction with good spotting (protection against falling). More advanced climbers are skilled in using special safety ropes and equipment. Beginners and intermediate climbers should always climb with the help of an expert. When rock climbing is done properly with proper equipment, it is a relatively safe activity. It's also a good type of activity for building muscle fitness.

Bouldering is a type of rock climbing in which the climber tries to reach the top of a boulder using only gloves and special shoes (no special ropes or other equipment). Bouldering is most often done outside, but some clubs have artificial boulders for indoor climbing. The height of climbs is typically limited to about 9 metres (30 feet). As with rock climbing, bouldering requires specials skills, so instruction is recommended for beginners.

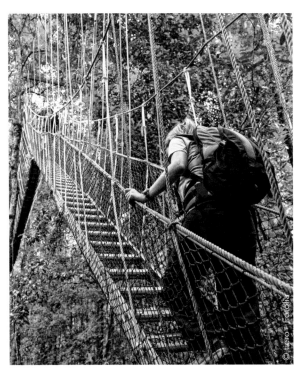

Outdoor vigorous recreational activities have health benefits and help you meet national activity guidelines.

⚛ SCIENCE IN ACTION: Anaerobic Physical Activity

Unlike aerobic activity that can be sustained for long periods of time, **anaerobic activity** is activity that is so intense your body cannot supply adequate oxygen to sustain performance for more than a few seconds. Very vigorous anaerobic activity, such as an all-out sprint, can be sustained for only about 10 seconds and relies on high-energy fuel stored in the muscles (ATP-PC). Some vigorous activities (also anaerobic) are not "all-out" but are still very intense (they can be sustained for 11 to 90 seconds), and for those activities, the glycolytic system is used. Glucose (glycogen) stored in the muscles and liver provides the energy. Anaerobic activities are typically done in short bursts followed by rest periods. During anaerobic activities your body builds up an oxygen debt because it can't take in enough oxygen to replenish the fuel needed to continue performance. After the activity is completed, oxygen is available to replenish the fuel stores—it "repays" the oxygen debt.

Your ability to perform anaerobic activity is referred to as **anaerobic capacity**. One of the most common tests of anaerobic capacity is the Wingate Test, which is done on a bicycle ergometer (stationary bicycle) and requires an all-out effort to pedal as fast as possible. This test is typically reserved for people interested in high-level anaerobic performance.

Sports such as basketball, football, and soccer involve sprints up the court or down the field. These sprints are anaerobic because they often require short but maximal effort. Sports allow time for recovery after these anaerobic bursts. This pattern means that players' heart rates may exceed the target zone during anaerobic sprints, then drop below the threshold of training during rest intervals (for example, when a free throw is taken in basketball). In fact, vigorous sports are not true aerobic activities, but when they are done for similar amounts of time they can be considered similar to vigorous aerobics. This is because they provide health benefits and improve cardiorespiratory endurance.

These sports offer the added advantage of building anaerobic capacity (also called *anaerobic power* and *anaerobic fitness*). Anaerobic capacity allows you to recover more quickly from anaerobic bursts and therefore improve your performance in certain sport activities. Some vigorous recreation activities, such as kayaking, are similar to vigorous sport activities in that they require good cardiorespiratory endurance as well as anaerobic fitness.

People who train for vigorous sport and recreation activities often use special anaerobic training techniques, such as interval training. Interval training involves repeated high-intensity exercise alternated with rest periods or bouts of lower-intensity exercise. There are many different kinds of interval training, including high-intensity interval training (HIIT) that alternates bouts of exercise at various intensities and lengths. The FIT formula for the most commonly used type of interval training is as follows.

- **F**requency = three to six days a week
- **I**ntensity = upper level of the target heart rate zone (because your exercise bouts are short)
- **T**ime = multiple exercise bouts of 10 to 60 seconds alternated with 1- to 2-minute rest periods or bouts of moderate exercise (totalling at least 10 minutes of exercise)

Depending on your goal, the length of exercise may vary from the durations given in the preceding formula. This type of training is appropriate for people who have already achieved the good fitness zone for cardiorespiratory endurance and who have regularly been doing vigorous-intensity physical activity. Before beginning this type of training, consult your doctor, teacher, or coach or other qualified expert in kinesiology.

Student Activity

While participating in an intermittent activity—such as basketball, soccer, or tennis—count your heart rate right after several vigorous bursts of activity. Determine whether the intensity of the activity is near the upper level of your target heart rate zone for aerobic activity.

Skateboarding

As you probably know, skateboarding is a popular recreational activity among teens. Competitive skateboarding is now considered an extreme sport. Therefore, it can be considered both a recreational activity and a sport (for high-level competitors). Like in-line skating, skateboarding is a risky activity, so you should use proper safety equipment and seek proper instruction. You also need to find a proper place to perform skateboarding, and many cities offer planned skate parks to provide safe places to skate.

Skating

Types of skating include in-line, roller, and ice. In-line skating was originally developed as a method of training for cross-country skiers in the summer, but its popularity has grown, and in-line sports (for example, hockey) have been developed. One study by a sports medicine group found that in-line skating was the most risky of the many participation activities studied, possibly because people fail to use proper safety equipment or because they try advanced skills too soon. The risk involved in skating activities makes it especially important for you to follow the safety guidelines described later in this chapter.

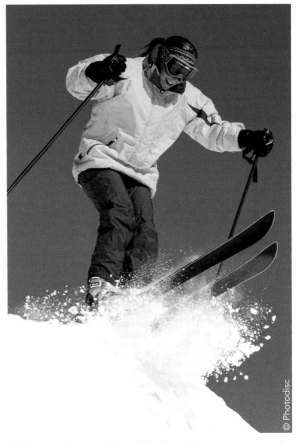

Skiing can be considered both a vigorous sport and a form of vigorous recreation.

Skiing

Kinds of skiing include cross-country skiing (a type of Nordic skiing), downhill skiing, snowboarding, and ski jumping. Cross-country skiing is typically done at a steady pace over a relatively long distance. For this reason, it could be considered a vigorous aerobic activity. Downhill skiing typically involves faster skiing, sometimes over moguls (bumps) and jumps. Snowboarding is like skateboarding on snow and has become extremely popular. It has joined the other forms of skiing as an Olympic sport, and some forms of snowboarding (halfpipe, superpipe, and slopestyle) can also be considered extreme sports. Ski jumping is also an Olympic sport, involving skiing down a ramp and jumping, trying to land as far down the hill as possible. All types of skiing could be considered sports, but they are included here because so many people do them just for fun and recreation, although ski jumping isn't typically a recreational activity for most people.

Lesson Review

1. What are the three major categories of vigorous-intensity physical activity (one from step 2 and two from step 3 of the Physical Activity Pyramid)?
2. What are three types of vigorous aerobic activity? Thinking about each activity individually, why would you consider each a vigorous-intensity aerobic activity?
3. What are four categories of vigorous sport? Give an example of each.
4. Define *recreation* and *leisure*.
5. What are three examples of vigorous recreation?

SELF-ASSESSMENT: Assessing Jogging Techniques

If you're looking for an excellent vigorous-intensity physical activity that requires little skill and no equipment—except for a good pair of running shoes and proper clothing—then jogging might be for you. Millions of people jog (that is, run recreationally and noncompetitively), and millions more run competitively (and are called runners rather than joggers). Learning to jog properly can help you make the activity safe and fun. Guidelines for jogging have been developed on the basis of the principles of biomechanics and exercise physiology. Look over the two sets of principles, and then study table 9.1 to learn about jogging guidelines.

Biomechanical Principles

- Changing velocity (acceleration) is less efficient than maintaining a constant velocity.
- Applying force in the direction of movement is more efficient than moving to the side.
- Friction is necessary in order to apply force and to prevent slipping.
- Action (foot striking) results in a reaction (impact to the sole of the foot or heel).
- Stability requires a wide base of support.
- Proper leverage increases efficiency.
- Proper posture increases efficiency.

Exercise Physiology Principles

- Muscle contractions not used to produce movement are inefficient.
- You must do more than normal to improve (this is the overload principle).

Work With a Partner

- Jog about 90 metres (100 yards) while your partner stands behind you and checks your technique.
- Have your partner answer the questions in table 9.1 after watching you jog. Your instructor may provide a worksheet that contains the questions.
- Now have your partner jog while you evaluate her or his technique.
- Discuss the assessment with your partner.
- Keeping in mind what you just discussed, both you and your partner can perform the jog a second time.
- Try to correct your technique and have your partner check you again. Do the same for your partner.

The partner assessment will help you jog more efficiently and can also reduce your risk of injury. Improper jogging technique can cause injuries such as sore shins, sore calves, and even a sore back. Having your feet and legs out of alignment can cause unnecessary strain on your joints and muscles.

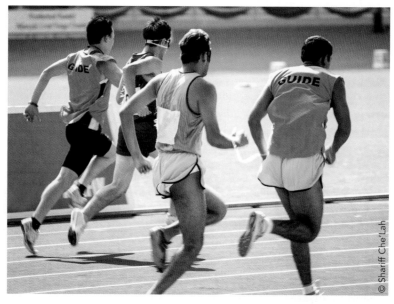

© Shariff Che'Lah

Proper technique is important for everyone, from beginning joggers to elite runners.

TABLE 9.1 Jogging Self-Assessment Guidelines and Checklist

Guideline	Principle	Checklist	✔
Use proper foot action. Land on your heel or your entire foot. Then rock forward and push off with the ball of your foot and your toes.	Leverage	Do you land on your heel or whole foot? Do you push off with the ball of your foot and toes?	
Swing your legs and feet forward. Do not let your feet turn out to the sides.	Force application	Do your legs and feet swing and land straight ahead?	
Swing your arms forward and backward. Do not swing them across your body or to the sides.	Force application	Do your arms swing straight forward and backward?	
Keep your trunk fairly erect. When jogging, do not lean forward as you would when starting to run fast. Keep your head and chest up.	Proper posture	Is your body erect or leaning forward only slightly? Are your head and chest up?	
Use a longer step than your normal walking step.	Leverage	Is your jogging stride longer than your walking stride?	
Keep your arms bent at the elbow and your hands relaxed. Try to keep your shoulders relaxed. Avoid jogging with a clenched jaw to allow your upper body to relax more.	Efficient muscle use	Are your elbows bent properly (90°) with your hands relaxed? Is your jaw relaxed?	
Jog at a steady pace. Avoid speeding up and slowing down. Correct jogging pace can vary from person to person. Find your own pace that elevates your heart rate into your target zone. If you are panting or gasping for breath, you are jogging too fast.	Velocity Overload	Is your pace steady? Is your heart rate in your target zone after several minutes of jogging? Is your pace slow enough to prevent gasping for breath?	
Wear shoes with a wide sole and heel, good heel cushions, and outer soles designed for running.	Stability Friction	Do your shoes have a wide heel and sole and good tread?	

Beginner's Jogging Workout

This workout helps you learn about how fast to jog in order to get a fitness benefit (by reaching your target heart rate). Try this workout after you've practiced your jogging technique.

1. Determine your target heart rate.

2. Jog for five minutes, trying to get your heart to the target level. Keep track of how long you run—how long you run is more important than how far. By using time instead of distance, you can jog anywhere. Set your own course. Try to jog half the time moving away from your starting point and the other half returning to your starting point. If you are not near your starting point at the end of five minutes, walk the rest of the way back.

3. Focus on using the jogging techniques that you learned earlier in the partner assessment.

4. At the end of five minutes, determine your one-minute exercise heart rate. Determine whether your rate was in your target heart rate zone.

5. Jog for five minutes again. If your exercise heart rate was lower than your target heart rate on the first jog, jog faster this time. If your exercise heart rate was higher than your target rate on the first jog, jog more slowly this time. If your exercise heart rate was in the target zone on the first jog, jog at the same speed this time. After your second run, count your exercise heart rate again.

6. Record your results.

Lesson 9.2

Preparing and Performing a Safe and Vigorous-Intensity Physical Activity Program

Lesson Objectives

After participating in this lesson, you should be able to

1. describe several guidelines for participating safely in vigorous-intensity physical activity,
2. collect information about your personal needs and build a fitness and activity profile,
3. set goals for vigorous-intensity physical activity, and
4. select vigorous-intensity activities and write a plan for a safe and vigorous-intensity activity program.

Lesson Vocabulary

compendium, overexercising

Are you prepared to do regular vigorous-intensity physical activity? In this lesson, you'll learn why it's important to be well prepared before you begin. You'll also use the five steps of program planning to prepare your personal plan for vigorous-intensity physical activity. Creating your plan will help you meet national physical activity guidelines both now and later in life. Vigorous-intensity activities can be some of the most enjoyable, and they also offer many health benefits.

Fitness for Vigorous Aerobics, Sport, and Recreation

Just as vigorous-intensity physical activity contributes to good fitness, you also must stay fit in order to participate in vigorous-intensity activity. Some people mistakenly assume that fitness is not necessary for certain sports, especially if the sport itself does little to build fitness. For example, softball is not particularly good for developing fitness, but it does require good fitness. Similarly, some people snow ski only once or twice a year and otherwise do not exercise regularly. Nevertheless, they believe they are fit enough to ski. In reality, these people should exercise regularly for at least several weeks before skiing in order to get ready for the activity and to reduce their chance of injury.

Participating in vigorous-intensity activity involves greater risk of injury than doing no activity or doing light or moderate-intensity activity. Even vigorous aerobics, which is relatively safe compared to other vigorous sport and recreational activities, can result in injury if overdone. Jogging (or running) is one of the top five activities in terms of injury to participants, and regular participants in high-impact and step aerobics are also often injured. Unlike common sport injuries such as ligament sprains and muscle strains, the injuries typically experienced by joggers and aerobic dancers involve overuse—for example, heel bruises, sore shins, stress fractures in the legs and feet, and sometimes knee or back injury. Long-distance runners and aerobic dance instructors also have a higher than normal rate of injury. More generally, the people most prone to injury are those who train every day or who participate in several vigorous aerobic activity sessions in a day.

Safety Tips for Vigorous-Intensity Physical Activity

- **Warm up before your workout.** Use a low- to moderate-intensity general warm-up for 5 to 10 minutes, a series of dynamic exercises, or a stretching warm-up, depending on the activity to be performed (see the Science in Action feature in chapter 4). For a stretching warm-up, remember to hold stretches no more than 30 seconds before doing strength, power, and speed activities.

- **Cool down after the workout.** A cool-down helps you recover more quickly.

- **Wear proper safety equipment.** For example, bikers and skaters should wear helmets, and skaters should also wear hand and knee pads. Dress appropriately for the weather.

- **Use safe equipment.** Bikes should have lights and reflectors. Backpacking equipment should fit your body size, and loads should not be too heavy. Skis and other equipment should be in good repair, properly sized, and equipped with proper releases or other safety features. Boaters should wear life preservers. Rock climbers should use appropriate safety equipment. When doing any vigorous-intensity activity, especially in the heat, drink water regularly.

- **Get proper instruction.** Whether you're skiing, in-line skating, boating, rock climbing, or doing some other activity, you should get proper instruction before participating. Performing an activity improperly has caused many people to get injured or have an accident.

- **Perform within the limits of your current skills.** Many injuries occur because people try to perform beyond their skill limits; for example, beginning skiers should not attempt to ski advanced slopes. For all activities, start with simple skills and then gradually attempt to perform more difficult skills as your abilities improve.

- **Don't overdo it.** Taking at least one day a week to rest can help you avoid injury, especially if you're participating in a vigorous aerobic activity such as aerobic dance or running. Most injuries can be prevented simply by not **overexercising** (doing so much exercise that you increase your risk of injury or soreness).

- **Plan ahead.** If you're going on a hike, make sure that you have a map and know where you're going. Carry an emergency phone. If you're going skiing, make sure that the trail is open, and don't ski in restricted areas. When backpacking, carry enough food and water to supply you if you get lost. When traveling in an unfamiliar area, stay with your group.

For most vigorous sport and recreation activities, you must have good fitness in order to perform well. For example, a baseball player must sprint between bases, slide into bases, and jump to catch the ball. Each of these actions could result in an injury if the player is not physically fit. Good or high performance fitness is especially necessary for activities with the following characteristics:

- Physical contact (football, ice hockey, martial arts such as judo or tae kwon do, lacrosse, rugby, wrestling)

- Sprinting (baseball, soccer, softball, Ultimate)

- Sudden fast starts and stops (basketball, badminton, volleyball, track)

- Vigorous jumping (basketball, dance, gymnastics, high jumping, soccer)

- Danger of falling (skiing, skating, judo)

- Danger of overstretching muscles (football, tennis, squash, gymnastics)

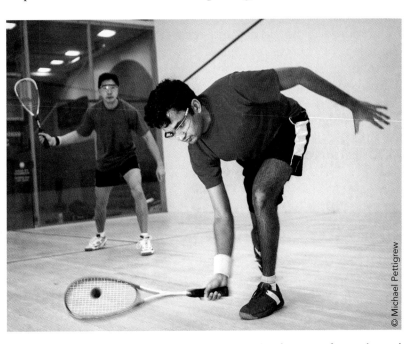

Exercise helps you get fit, but you must also be fit to perform physical activities safely.

© Michael Pettigrew

Engaging in Vigorous-Intensity Physical Activity **187**

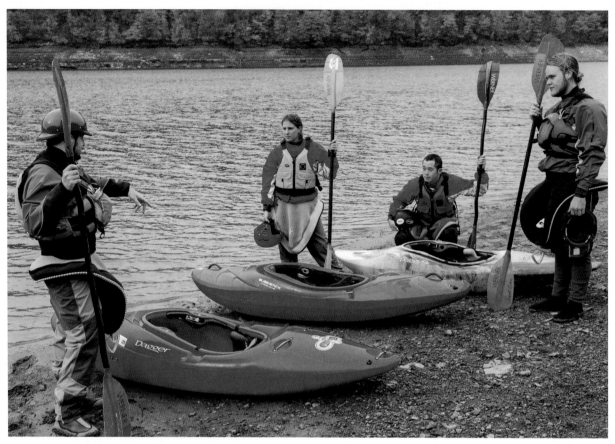

Important safety tips for vigorous-intensity physical activity include using safe equipment and getting proper instruction.

FIT FACT

In Canada, cycling injuries are the most common summer sport and recreational injuries. In the winter, skiing and snowboarding are responsible for the most sport and recreation injuries. Medical groups state that you can dramatically decrease your risk of injury by following simple safety tips when participating in physical activity.

Finding the Best Vigorous-Intensity Activities for You

In this class, you'll get the opportunity to try many types of vigorous-intensity activities, such as aerobic dance, step aerobics, line dancing, jogging, exercise circuits, and rope jumping. Try a variety of activities to discover which ones you like best. For any given activity, try it more than once before you decide whether to do it in the future. It takes time to decide what you like and don't like. If you're going to stick with an activity over the long term, it must be enjoyable. To help you enjoy an activity, consider finding good instruction, wearing appropriate clothing, getting good equipment (if necessary), and finding others with whom you can participate.

Preparing a Vigorous-Intensity Physical Activity Plan

Lin Su used the five steps of program planning to prepare a vigorous-intensity physical activity plan. She had been doing some regular moderate activity but wanted to do more vigorous-intensity activity. Her program is described in the following sections of this chapter.

FIT FACT

Teen boys are more likely than teen girls to do vigorous-intensity activity at least three times a week, and high school girls are especially likely to become less active as they grow older. Health experts are interested in finding ways to help teen girls be more physically active.

Step 1: Determine Your Personal Needs

To get started, Lin Su wrote down her fitness test results that related to vigorous-intensity physical activity. She also made a list of the vigorous-intensity physical activities that she had performed over the past week. Her results are shown in figure 9.2.

Lin Su's cardiorespiratory endurance ratings showed that she was in the marginal category for each of the self-assessments that she performed. She met the national activity guideline of 60 minutes per day on two days of the previous week. She did vigorous-intensity activity for 20 minutes on Tuesday and Thursday in her physical education class. On Friday she jogged for 20 minutes with her friend Eric, but she didn't do that regularly. She

had also walked to and from school (20 minutes each way), and this moderate-intensity activity combined with her physical education activities and jogging totalled 60 minutes. On the other days, she did only moderate activity (walking to and from school) totalling less than 60 minutes, except on Tuesday and Thursday when she had physical education class. Lin Su knew that she needed to be more active and especially wanted to do more vigorous-intensity activity.

Step 2: Consider Your Program Options

Lin Su wanted to include activities that would help her build her cardiorespiratory endurance and that offered other health and fitness benefits. She also wanted to focus on activities that she thought she would enjoy. To select vigorous-intensity activities, she used table 9.2, which illustrates the health-related fitness benefits of a wide variety of vigorous-intensity activities. Even this list, however, includes only a sample of the most popular vigorous aerobics, sport, and recreation activities; it was adapted from a larger **compendium** of activities. A link to the compendium can be found in the student section of the Fitness for Life Canada website.

Physical fitness profile			
Fitness self-assessment	**Score**	**Rating**	
Walking test	Time: 18:30 Heart rate: 150	Marginal	
PACER	37 mL/kg/min	Marginal	
Step test	Heart rate: 104	Marginal	
One-mile run (1.6 km)	No score	No rating	
Physical activity profile			
Day	**Vigorous-intensity activity (min)**	**All activity (min)**	**Met 60-min guideline?**
Mon.	0	40	
Tues.	20	60	✔
Wed.	0	40	
Thurs.	20	60	✔
Fri.	20	40	
Sat.	0	20	
Sun.	0	20	

FIGURE 9.2 Lin Su's vigorous-intensity physical activity and fitness profiles.

TABLE 9.2 Health-Related Benefits of Selected Vigorous-Intensity Physical Activities

Activity	Develops cardiorespiratory endurance	Develops strength	Develops muscular endurance	Develops flexibility	Helps control body fat
Aerobic dance*+	Excellent	Fair	Good	Fair	Excellent
Aerobics machine+	Excellent	Fair	Good	Poor	Excellent
Backpacking+	Fair	Fair	Excellent	Poor	Good/Excellent
Badminton+	Fair	Poor	Fair	Fair	Fair/Good
Baseball/Softball*	Poor	Poor	Poor	Poor	Poor/Fair
Basketball, half-court*+	Fair	Poor	Fair	Poor	Poor/Fair
Basketball, full-court*+	Excellent	Fair	Good	Poor	Excellent
Biking+	Good	Fair	Good	Poor	Good/Excellent
BMX cycling	Good	Good	Excellent	Fair	Good
Canoeing+	Fair	Fair	Fair	Poor	Fair/Good
Circuit training+	Good	Good	Good	Fair	Good/Excellent
Football*	Fair	Good	Fair	Poor	Fair
Gymnastics	Fair	Excellent	Excellent	Excellent	Fair
Handball/Racquetball*+	Good/Excellent	Fair	Good	Poor	Good/Excellent
Hiking	Fair	Fair	Fair/Good	Poor	Good
Hip-hop dance	Good/Excellent	Fair	Good	Fair	Good/Excellent
Ice hockey*	Excellent	Good	Good	Fair	Excellent
Kayaking*+	Good	Good	Good	Fair	Good
Lacrosse*	Excellent	Good	Good	Fair	Excellent
Martial arts*+	Good	Fair	Fair	Fair	Fair
Mountain or rock climbing*+	Good	Good	Good	Poor	Good
Racquetball*+	Good/Excellent	Fair	Good	Poor	Good/Excellent
Rowing (crew)*	Excellent	Fair	Excellent	Poor	Excellent
Sailing+	Poor	Poor	Poor	Poor	Poor
Skating (roller or ice)*+	Good	Fair	Good	Fair	Good
Skiing (cross-country)*+	Excellent	Fair	Good	Poor	Excellent
Skiing (downhill)*+	Fair/Good	Fair	Good	Poor	Fair/Good
Snowboarding*+	Fair/Good	Fair	Good	Fair	Fair/Good
Soccer*	Excellent	Fair	Good	Fair	Excellent
Social dance+	Fair	Poor	Fair	Fair	Fair
Surfing*+	Fair	Poor	Good	Fair	Fair/Good
Swimming+	Good	Fair	Good	Fair	Good/Excellent
Table tennis*+	Poor	Poor	Poor/Fair	Poor	Poor/Fair
Tennis*+	Good/Excellent	Fair	Good	Poor	Good/Excellent
Volleyball*+	Fair	Fair	Good	Poor	Fair/Good
Waterskiing*+	Fair	Fair	Good	Poor	Fair/Good

*Fitness needed to prevent injury.

+Lifetime activity.

After reviewing the list of activities, Lin Su wrote down her preferred activity options.

Continue Current Activities

- Walking to and from school
- Jogging
- Physical education class activities

Vigorous Aerobics

- More jogging
- Aerobic dance

Vigorous Recreation

- Hiking
- In-line skating

Vigorous Sport

- Tennis
- Badminton

School

- Before-school recreation
- After-school sports

Step 3: Set Goals

For this vigorous-intensity activity plan, Lin Su chose a time period of two weeks. Because this was too short to accommodate long-term goals, she developed only short-term physical activity goals for the plan. Later, she will develop long-term goals, including some physical fitness goals, when she prepares a longer plan. For now, in developing her short-term goals for vigorous-intensity physical activity, she referred to her activity preferences decided in step 2. She also reviewed her work to be sure that she was setting SMART goals. She set the following goals.

1. Continue to jog one day a week for 20 minutes.
2. Continue to do vigorous-intensity activity in physical education class two days a week (20 minutes).
3. Play tennis for 60 minutes of moderate-intensity activity one day every other week.
4. Do aerobic dance for 30 minutes one day a week.
5. Go hiking for 60 minutes one day every other week.

Step 4: Structure Your Program and Write It Down

Lin Su's written two-week plan for vigorous-intensity physical activity is shown in figure 9.3. Lin Su included most of the activities from her list. She didn't include badminton or in-line skating, and she didn't participate in before-school recreation or after-school sports. Her plan met the national activity guideline of vigorous-intensity activity three days a week. In fact, her plan called for more than 20 minutes of vigorous-intensity activity on five days of the week. Lin Su decided to take a break from vigorous-intensity activity on Sunday and Monday. She also kept walking to and from school daily. Although this was moderate-intensity activity, she planned to keep doing it to help her meet the national activity goal of 60 minutes of moderate- to vigorous-intensity physical activity each day.

Week 1				Week 2			
Day	**Activity**	**Time**	**✔**	**Day**	**Activity**	**Time**	**✔**
Mon.	No planned activity			Mon.	No planned activity		
Tues.	Physical education class	10:30–11:15 a.m.*		Tues.	Physical education class	10:30–11:15 a.m.*	
Wed.	Aerobic dance	4:00–4:30 p.m.		Wed.	Aerobic dance	4:00–4:30 p.m.	
Thurs.	Physical education class	10:30–11:15 a.m.*		Thurs.	Physical education class	10:30–11:15 a.m.*	
Fri.	Jog	4:00–4:20 p.m.		Fri.	Jog	4:00–4:20 p.m.	
Sat.	Tennis	9:00–10:00 a.m.		Sat.	Hiking	9:00–10:00 a.m.	
Sun.	No planned activity			Sun.	No planned activity		

*Only 20 minutes of the 45-minute class included vigorous-intensity activity.

FIGURE 9.3 Lin Su's written plan.

blank
off

 CONSUMER CORNER: Using the Web for Fitness, Health, and Wellness Information

Health is the most common subject of web searches, and 75 percent of all teens and young adults seek health information on the web. But many websites, including popular web encyclopaedias, contain incorrect information about health, which can result in injury, illness, failure to get adequate care, and loss of money spent on products and treatments that don't work. With all this in mind, one of the most important goals of Fitness for Life Canada is to help you become a critical consumer of fitness, health, and wellness information. Consider the following guidelines when you search the web.

- Consider using websites provided by government agencies. They contain information supplied by experts based on scientific research. Most government website addresses end with the extension "gc.ca". In the United States, most government website addresses end with the extension ".gov". Health Canada and the U.S. Centers for Disease Control and Prevention are two reliable sources for health information.

- Consider using websites provided by universities and professional organizations (such as the Canadian Medical Association and the Canadian Society for Exercise Physiology). Professional organizations' website addresses typically end with the extension ".org", and universities' addresses typically end with the extension ".edu".

- Beware of websites with names intended to fool you. When the web was first developed, only a few extensions (such as .gov, .org, .edu, and .com) were available for use at the end of a web address. Now, many more extensions are in use, and some people take advantage of this variety to create copycat websites intended to fool you into thinking you're choosing a reliable site when in fact you're not. They do this by using the same name as a reliable website (or a similar name) but a different extension—for example, reliablewebsite.xyz instead of reliablewebsite.gov.

Step 5: Keep a Log and Evaluate Your Program

Over the next two weeks, Lin Su will self-monitor her activities and place a checkmark in her written plan beside each of the activities that she performs. At the end of two weeks, she will evaluate her activity to see whether she met her goals, then use the evaluation to help her create another activity plan.

In the Taking Action activity later in this lesson, you will get to use the same planning steps that Lin Su used to create a two-week personal plan

 We are what we repeatedly do.

—Aristotle, Greek philosopher

for vigorous-intensity physical activity. Use tables similar to those used by Lin Su to help you in your planning. Then try out your program and see if you can meet your goals. The same steps can be used in the future to plan health goals or prepare for a special event, such as running a 10K race or participating on the cross-country team.

Lesson Review

1. What steps can you take to make vigorous-intensity activity safe and fun?
2. How can you assess personal needs and build a fitness and activity profile?
3. What are some factors to consider in setting goals for vigorous-intensity physical activity?
4. How can you best select vigorous-intensity activities and write a plan for vigorous-intensity activity?

TAKING CHARGE: Choosing Good Activities

You can help yourself be active by choosing activities you're likely to do both now and throughout your life. One way to evaluate an activity is to find out the number of people who participate and how long they tend to stay involved. Here's an example.

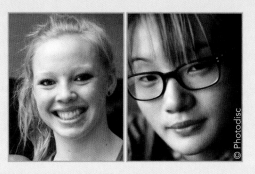

At a recent high school reunion, the graduates enjoyed seeing their former classmates again. Everyone remembered Nischelle as an athlete. She had played soccer, basketball, and softball. What a surprise when her classmates discovered that 10 years later Nischelle was doing very little physical activity! The closest she got to participating in any sport was to watch her son's tee ball games. According to Nischelle, "It is just too hard to find people who want to play the team sports I used to enjoy."

Kim Lea was just the opposite. In high school, she had always gone to the games and cheered for the teams, but she had never dreamed of taking part in a sport. In fact, she would have been the first to admit that she was sedentary. Now, Kim Lea was biking with her two children and organizing her neighbourhood aerobics class. She described it this way: "Every Tuesday and Thursday morning, we all get together and talk while we work out. No one cares how we dress or how good we are at doing the exercises. We all just seem to be energized as we go on to our next activities."

For Discussion

Why did Nischelle feel that it was no longer feasible to continue participating in the sports she played in high school? What might help her get involved in a physical activity again? Why do you think Kim Lea started to participate in activities? What advice would you have for other people who want to get active later in life? Consider the guidelines presented in the Self-Management feature as you answer the discussion questions.

SELF-MANAGEMENT: Skills for Choosing Good Activities

Research shows that the most active people in society are those who have identified specific activities that they enjoy. For example, many people love tennis, golf, or running and participate in their chosen activity on a regular basis. Others prefer variety, so they choose several activities. In both cases, these people might not have become so active if they were not doing activities that they especially enjoyed. Use the following guidelines to help you find a physical activity (or activities) especially good for you.

- **Consider your physical fitness.** How well you do in an activity depends on all parts of fitness—both health related and skill related. Choose activities that match your abilities in both kinds of fitness. Also consider activities that help you build health-related fitness (see table 9.2).

- **Consider your interests.** Don't avoid an activity that you really enjoy or have always wanted to do just because it doesn't match your fitness profile. Do be aware, however, that even with practice it may take you longer than others to learn the activity. But finding an activity that is fun for you is very important, so consider a variety of activities.

- **Consider an activity that you can do with others.** Try to find others of your own ability so that you won't be discouraged if you don't learn the activity as quickly as you'd like.

- **Consider the activity's benefits.** As you progress through this book, you'll learn about the benefits of various activities. If you want to get optimal fitness, health, and wellness benefits, select activities

Engaging in Vigorous-Intensity Physical Activity **193**

from each area of the Physical Activity Pyramid.

- **Practice, practice, practice.** Becoming skilled in a sport or activity increases your enjoyment. If you choose an activity that is new to you, there is no substitute for practice. To make your practice more productive, consider taking lessons.

- **Consider activities that do not require high levels of skill.** Some activities do not require high levels of any part of skill-related fitness. Of the activities included in the Physical Activity Pyramid, sport provides the most benefit for skill-related fitness, but it also requires relatively high levels of both sport skill and skill-related fitness in order to play. Sport skills such as throwing, catching, hitting, and kicking are different from skill-related fitness abilities such as agility, balance, and coordination—though these do help you learn sport skills more easily. Learning sport skills requires a lot of practice in order to perform them well. Generally speaking, fewer skills are required for moderate and vigorous aerobic activities than for sport. As a result, even people with relatively low scores on most or all parts of skill-related fitness can find a moderate-intensity or vigorous-intensity aerobic activity to enjoy—for example, jogging, walking, or cycling. Because these activities don't require high skill levels, they also tend not to require extensive practice. Therefore, you might want to consider one of these activities if you're not willing to put in the necessary time to learn a more complicated one.

TAKING ACTION: Your Vigorous-Intensity Physical Activity Plan

Prepare a vigorous-intensity physical activity plan using the five steps described in the second lesson in this chapter. Like Lin Su, consider activities from all three categories: vigorous aerobics, vigorous sport, and vigorous recreation. Your goal should be to accumulate at least 20 minutes of vigorous-intensity physical activity on at least three days each week.

Prepare a written plan and carry it out over a two-week period. Your teacher may give you time in class to do some of the activities included in your plan. Consider the following suggestions for taking action.

- Before you do vigorous-intensity physical activity, perform a dynamic warm-up, stretching exercises, or both.
- Consider the tips presented in this chapter for safe vigorous-intensity activity.

- Consider the guidelines presented in this chapter for making good activity selections.
- Progress gradually. Don't try to do too much too soon.
- After your workout, perform a cool-down. Many safe cool-downs can be found through web searches.

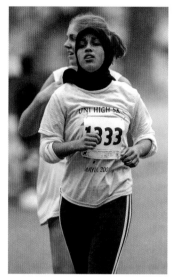

Take action by performing your vigorous-intensity physical activity plan.

GET ACTIVE WITH CANADA BASKETBALL

CANADA
BASKETBALL
©Canada Basketball

Who We Are

Canada Basketball is the national sporting organization for the sport of basketball in Canada. Canada Basketball is respected throughout the world and is recognized by the International Amateur Basketball Federation (FIBA) and the Government of Canada as the sole governing body of the sport of amateur basketball in Canada.

Canada Basketball represents all basketball interests and provides leadership, coordination, and direction in all areas of the sport. We are a not-for-profit organization run under a sound business model by a volunteer board of directors with full-time professional staff members to run the affairs of the organization.

What We Do

Under the umbrella of a national sport organization, we are responsible for coaching and technical leadership, domestic development, marketing, and high-performance development. We work closely with our provincial

and territorial partners to ensure all athletes, coaches, and officials are able to train and play in an optimal environment.

Canada Basketball is responsible for the preparation of national teams that complete in world championships and the Olympics. Steve Nash Youth Basketball is a grassroots program that develops fundamental skills, sportsmanship, and a love of the game. National Coach Certification Program (NCCP) is a series of workshops that prepare coaches for their level of athletes. Whether you're a community coach or a national team coach, there are courses for you.

Get Involved

Clubs, community programs, and school programs are all across Canada. If you want to play, coach, or officiate, there is a place for everyone. Canada Basketball also has a coach education website that allows coaches to track their progress, plan their practice, view videos, and find the optimal drill in the library. To learn more about Canada Basketball, visit www.basketball.ca or follow on Twitter: @CanBball.

©Canada Basketball

Reviewing Concepts and Vocabulary

Complete the following in order for you to determine your growing understanding of fitness, health, and wellness. Answer items 1 through 5 by correctly completing each sentence with a word or phrase.

1. Vigorous-intensity physical activity is exercise that raises your heart rate above the _____.
2. Activities that are competitive and have rules are called _____.
3. Activities so intense that you can perform them for only a few seconds are called _____ activities.
4. Free time, or time free from work, is called _____.
5. A _____ is a list that tells you the intensity of various activities.

For items 6 through 10, match each term in column 1 with the appropriate phrase in column 2.

6. water aerobics   a. aqua dynamics
7. orienteering   b. several exercise stations
8. in-line skating   c. done for fun during free time
9. recreational activity   d. uses map-reading skills
10. circuit training   e. has relatively high injury risk

For items 11 through 15, respond to each statement or question.

11. What is the difference between individual and dual sports?
12. What are some examples of outdoor, challenge, and extreme sports? Why are these sports popular?
13. What is interval training and what are the best frequency, intensity, and time (FIT) for performing it?
14. What are several safety tips for vigorous-intensity physical activity?
15. What are some guidelines for making good physical activity selections?

Thinking Critically

Write a paragraph to answer the following question.

You have a friend who wants to avoid vigorous-intensity physical activity because of having suffered frequent injuries in the past. What advice would you give your friend to help him or her avoid such problems in the future while also still being able to participate in vigorous-intensity activities that the person seems to thoroughly enjoy?

Project

Create a vigorous aerobics exercise routine. Choose music paced at about 100 to 120 beats per minute and plan for the routine to last two to three minutes. You can do an aerobic dance routine, a hip-hop routine, or some other form of continuous exercise. Work with a group to perform a routine (yours or another group member's) in class. Remember, you don't have to "reinvent the wheel"; there are examples of routines on the Internet that you could use to build your routine.

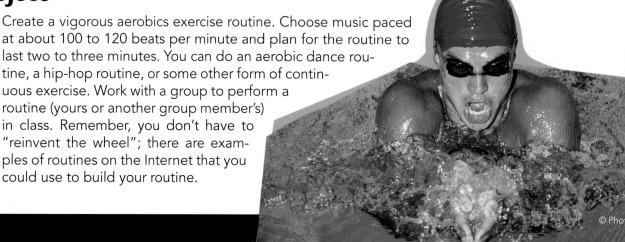

© Photo

UNIT IV

Building Muscle Fitness and Flexibility

● ● ● ● ● ● ● ● ● ● ● ● ●

Self-Assessment Features in This Unit
- Muscle Fitness Testing
- Healthy Back Test and Assessing Posture
- Arm, Leg, and Trunk Flexibility

Taking Charge Features in This Unit
- Overcoming Barriers
- Preventing Relapse
- Building Positive Attitudes

Self-Management Features in This Unit
- Skills for Overcoming Barriers
- Skills for Preventing Relapse
- Skills for Building Positive Attitudes

Taking Action Features in This Unit
- Resistance Machine Exercises
- Your Muscle Fitness Exercise Plan
- Your Flexibility Exercise Plan

Canadian Sport and Health Organization Features in This Unit
- Get Active With canfitpro
- Get Active With Hockey Canada
- Get Active With Canada Snowboard

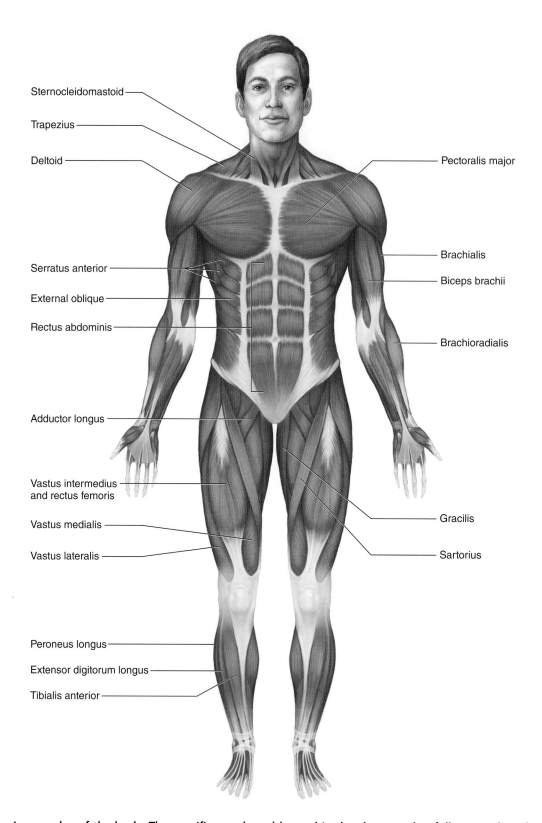

Sternocleidomastoid

Trapezius

Deltoid

Serratus anterior

External oblique

Rectus abdominis

Adductor longus

Vastus intermedius
and rectus femoris

Vastus medialis

Vastus lateralis

Peroneus longus

Extensor digitorum longus

Tibialis anterior

Pectoralis major

Brachialis

Biceps brachii

Brachioradialis

Gracilis

Sartorius

The major muscles of the body. The specific muscles addressed in the chapters that follow are described with each exercise. Refer to these two illustrations for exact muscle locations.

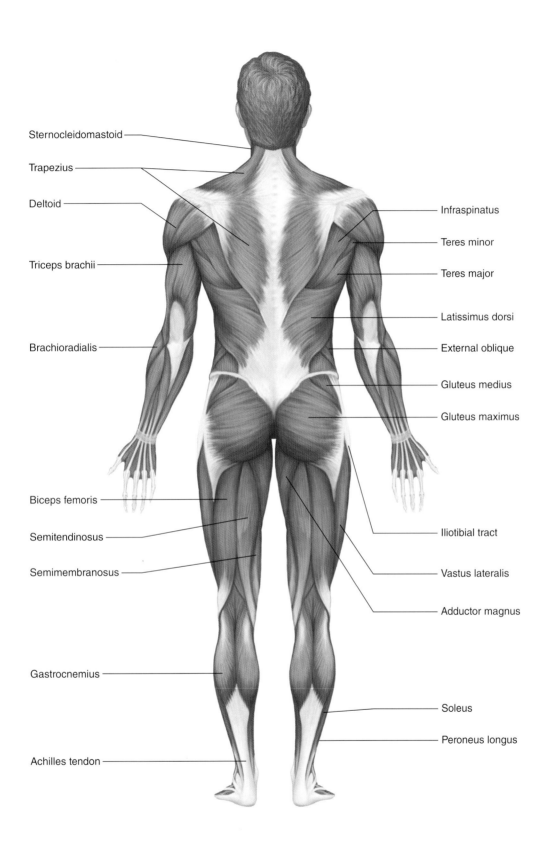

Sternocleidomastoid

Trapezius

Deltoid

Triceps brachii

Brachioradialis

Biceps femoris

Semitendinosus

Semimembranosus

Gastrocnemius

Achilles tendon

Infraspinatus

Teres minor

Teres major

Latissimus dorsi

External oblique

Gluteus medius

Gluteus maximus

Iliotibial tract

Vastus lateralis

Adductor magnus

Soleus

Peroneus longus

10

Building Muscle Fitness: The Basics

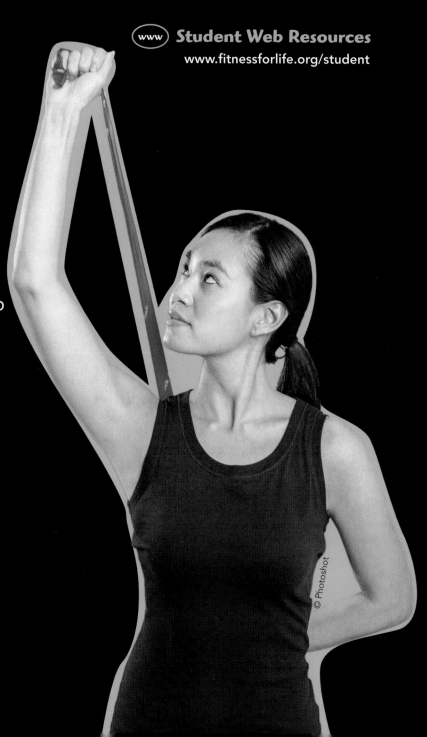

In This Chapter

(www) **Student Web Resources**
www.fitnessforlife.org/student

© Photoshot

Lesson 10.1
Muscle Fitness Facts

Lesson Objectives

After participating in this lesson, you should be able to

1. explain the differences between strength, muscular endurance, and power;
2. describe how exercise principles apply to muscle fitness;
3. describe the types of muscle fitness exercise; and
4. describe several methods for assessing muscle fitness.

Lesson Vocabulary

1-repetition maximum (1RM), absolute strength, calisthenics, concentric, dynamometer, eccentric, fast-twitch muscle fibre, hypertrophy, intermediate muscle fibre, isokinetic exercise, isometric contraction, isometric exercise, isotonic contraction, isotonic exercise, plyometrics, principle of rest and recovery, progressive resistance exercise (PRE), relative strength, reps, set, slow-twitch muscle fibre

Does your favourite activity require muscle fitness? Do you have enough muscle fitness? Muscle fitness is made up of three health-related parts of physical fitness: strength, muscular endurance, and power.

FIT FACT

Together strength, muscular endurance, power, and flexibility are referred to as *musculoskeletal fitness* because all four of these parts of fitness are associated with the muscular and skeletal systems. In this book, *muscle fitness* is used as a general term to describe the three parts of musculoskeletal fitness that require the muscles to produce force (strength, muscular endurance, and power).

Strength is the amount of force that a muscle can exert. The amount of weight that a group of muscles can lift one time is called a **1-repetition maximum (1RM)**, which is a good indicator of force exerted. This is considered the best measure of strength. Having good strength enables you to apply effective force in sports (such as football) and in tasks that require heavy lifting (figure 10.1*a*).

Muscular endurance is the ability to contract muscles many times without tiring or to hold a muscle contraction for a long time without fatigue. Muscular endurance allows you to resist muscle fatigue in recreational activities such as backpacking and to persist in work activities such as carrying a mailbag for hours at a time (figure 10.1*b*).

The third part of muscle fitness is power. Power is the ability to use strength (produce force) quickly; thus it involves both strength and speed. It is often referred to as explosive strength. Examples of power include jumping high or far and throwing objects a great distance. Research has shown that power is especially important to bone health and that bone health built in the teen years provides lifelong benefits (figure 10.1*c*).

All three components of muscle fitness—strength, muscular endurance, and power—are important to both health and good performance. This chapter includes exercises from step 4 of the Physical Activity Pyramid (figure 10.2) to develop muscle fitness.

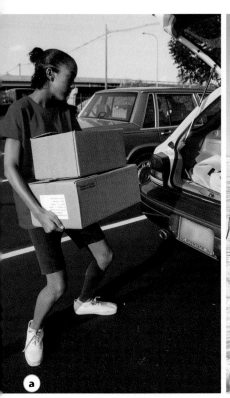
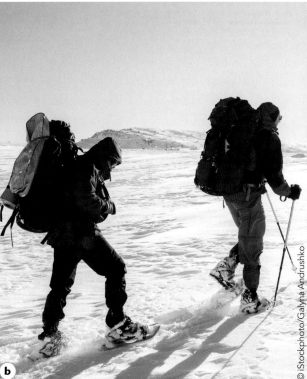
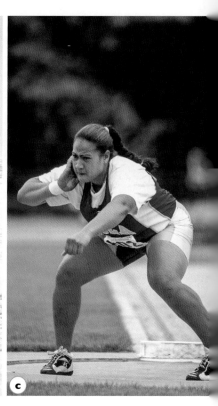

FIGURE 10.1 The parts of muscle fitness: *(a)* Lifting a heavy object requires strength; *(b)* using your muscles for a long time requires muscular endurance; and *(c)* doing activities that involve fast application of force requires power.

Energy balance

STEP 5
Flexibility exercises

STEP 4
Muscle fitness exercises

STEP 3
Vigorous sport and recreation

STEP 2
Vigorous aerobics

STEP 1
Moderate-intensity physical activity

FIGURE 10.2 Activities from step 4 of the Physical Activity Pyramid build muscle fitness.

Adapted from Physical Activity Pyramid for Teens, source: C.B. Corbin.

Muscle Fitness Terminology

You may have heard the terms *reps* and *sets* in relation to muscular fitness, and figure 10.3 can help you understand them. The term **reps** (short for *repetitions*) refers to the number of consecutive times you do an exercise. A **set** is one group of repetitions. For example, suppose you do an exercise eight times, then rest; repeat it eight times, then rest again; and repeat it another eight times. You have just done three sets of eight repetitions each.

The Muscular Endurance–Strength Continuum

The exercises used to develop muscular endurance and strength differ only in the number of repetitions and the amount of resistance. The relationship between endurance and strength can be represented on a continuum such as the one shown in figure 10.4, which presents kilograms of resistance on one edge and number of repetitions on the other.

The continuum shows the resistance and repetitions that a person might use to build muscle fitness.

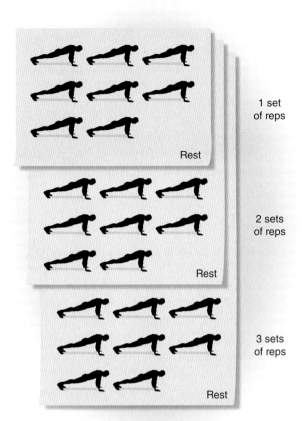

FIGURE 10.3 Muscle fitness exercises are typically done in reps and sets.

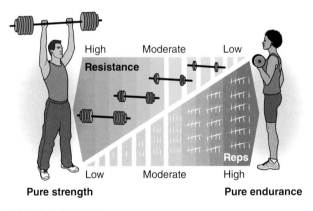

FIGURE 10.4 Muscular endurance–strength continuum.

To develop strength, you would use high resistance with fewer repetitions; to develop endurance, you would use low resistance with more repetitions; and to develop both strength and endurance, you would use the resistance and repetitions shown in the middle of the continuum. This continuum also shows that usually when you train for strength you will also develop some endurance, and when you train for endurance you will also develop some

strength. When starting a muscle fitness program, it is recommended that muscular endurance be developed first. Starting with lower resistance and higher repetitions allows you to develop the proper resistance training techniques with less risk of injury (see the principles of overload and progression further on).

Cardiorespiratory Endurance and Muscular Endurance

Muscular endurance is one part of muscle fitness, and it is different from the other parts (strength and power). It is also different from cardiorespiratory endurance, which depends on your cardiovascular and respiratory systems to supply oxygen. Cardiorespiratory endurance is general (not specific to one area of the body), and good cardiorespiratory endurance allows your entire body to function.

Muscular endurance, on the other hand, is the ability to contract your muscles many times without tiring or to hold one contraction for a long time. Muscular endurance depends on the ability of your muscle fibres to keep working without getting tired. You can have good muscular endurance in one part of your body (such as your legs) without having it in another part of your body (such as your arms).

Strength and Power

For years, power was considered to be a skill-related part of fitness. Sometimes it was referred to as a combined part of fitness because it involves both strength (the ability to exert force) and speed (the ability to cover a distance in a short time). Because it involves a strength component, power is often referred to as explosive strength. There is no doubt that both power and strength are important for performance, but today we understand that both are also important for your health. The Institute of Medicine reports that adults who lack power have a higher than normal risk of chronic disease, reduced life span, and poor functional health as they grow older. Exercise physiologists have also demonstrated that power, and activities that produce power, are very important in building healthy bones in youth. Because of these links to health, power is now classified as a health-related part of fitness.

> " I have arm-wrestled here and there . . . guys seem to want to test my strength. "
>
> —Shania Twain,
> country music singer/songwriter

Fitness Principles and Muscle Fitness

The three basic fitness principles can be applied to muscle fitness exercise. These principles—overload, progression, and specificity—have been covered elsewhere in this book. They are discussed again in this chapter to show how they relate specifically to muscle fitness.

Principle of Overload

To improve muscle fitness, a muscle must contract harder than normal. In other words, the muscle must work against a greater load than it normally bears in regular daily activity. High overload (high resistance) builds strength, whereas more moderate overload repeated many times builds muscular endurance. Exercises for power require overload for speed and strength. Muscle fitness overload also increases bone density and the strength of tendons (i.e., connective tissue that connects muscle to bone) and ligaments (i.e., connective tissue that connects bone to bone). The reverse of the overload principle also applies—if you don't use your muscles, you'll lose muscle fitness. "Use it or lose it!"

Principle of Progression

The principle of progression holds that you should gradually increase load or resistance over time in order to best improve your muscle fitness. If you try to use too much resistance too soon, you can injure yourself. Exercise that increases resistance (overload) until you reach the desired level of muscle fitness is referred to as **progressive resistance exercise (PRE)** or progressive resistance training (PRT). Many kinds of progressive resistance exercise—for example, weight training, resistance machine exercises, and plyometrics—are described later.

⚛ SCIENCE IN ACTION: Resistance Exercise Among Youth

Exercise scientists have developed recommendations to help youth, including preteens and teens, use PRE to build their muscle fitness. The guidelines were developed by a variety of experts—including exercise physiologists, medical doctors, and exercise professionals (such as athletic trainers and strength coaches)—who worked with the Canadian Society of Exercise Physiology (CSEP).

Not so long ago, some experts felt that muscle fitness exercises were unsafe and inappropriate for preteens and teens. CSEP experts now provide evidence that, when done properly, PRE provides health benefits for teens similar to those for adults. These benefits include reduced risk of chronic disease, reduced risk of injury and muscle pain or soreness, improved muscle fitness and sport performance, and psychological well-being. Muscle fitness exercise also builds bone fitness, reduces the risk of osteoporosis (porous and weak bones), reduces the risk of back pain, enhances posture, and increases your ability to work and play without fatigue. In addition, well-developed muscles help you look your best. Muscle is more dense than fat, so it takes up less space. Muscle also uses more calories than fat, so increasing muscle mass helps the body to burn calories.

Keys to keeping PRE safe for youth include using proper technique and safe and appropriate equipment, following sound exercise principles, and seeking and accepting good supervision. Much of this chapter focuses on giving you the information you need in order to meet the safe exercise recommendations for PRE.

Student Activity

Progressive resistance exercise can be safe for teens when done properly but carries risks when done improperly. Create a list of the most important ways to make PRE safe for teens. Consider making a sign to be posted in a fitness room used by teens.

Principle of Specificity

Strength, muscular endurance, and power each have their own FIT formula. The specific type of training that you perform determines which part of muscle fitness you build. In addition, you build specific muscles by doing exercises specifically for those muscles. To build your arm muscles, you must overload your arm muscles. To build your leg muscles, you must overload your leg muscles. Examples of types of PRE for each part of muscle fitness and the basic exercises for specific muscle groups are discussed later in this chapter.

Principle of Rest and Recovery

The **principle of rest and recovery** holds that you need to give your muscles time to rest and recover after a workout. This is why muscle fitness exercises are typically performed on only two or three days per week. Because you need to perform exercises to build all of the important muscles of your body, some people choose to work out every day but do exercises for different muscle groups on different days. For example, they might perform upper body exercises one day and lower body exercises the next. For optimal results, you should also rest between sets of exercise (more information about rest is given throughout this chapter).

> " Be strong in body, clean in mind, lofty in ideals. "
>
> —James Naismith, physical educator and inventor of basketball

Muscles and Muscle Biomechanics

Your body's muscles create the movement that allows you to do the activities described in this book. There are hundreds of muscles in the human body. Some of the most frequently used muscles in physical activity are illustrated in figure 10.5. This section helps you learn more about how your muscles work.

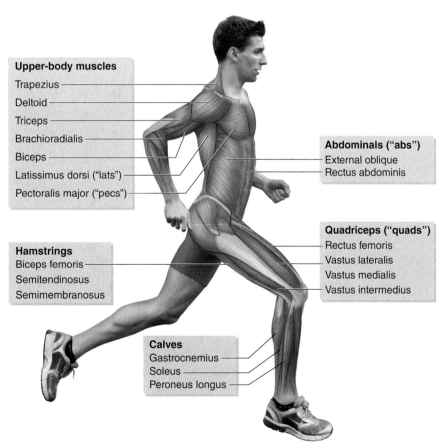

Upper-body muscles
Trapezius
Deltoid
Triceps
Brachioradialis
Biceps
Latissimus dorsi ("lats")
Pectoralis major ("pecs")

Abdominals ("abs")
External oblique
Rectus abdominis

Quadriceps ("quads")
Rectus femoris
Vastus lateralis
Vastus medialis
Vastus intermedius

Hamstrings
Biceps femoris
Semitendinosus
Semimembranosus

Calves
Gastrocnemius
Soleus
Peroneus longus

FIGURE 10.5 Some of the major muscles used in physical activity.

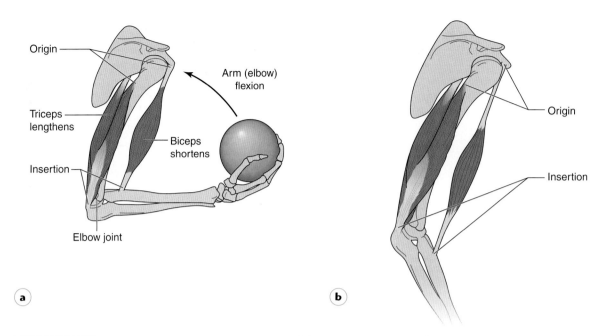

Origin

Arm (elbow) flexion

Triceps lengthens

Biceps shortens

Insertion

Elbow joint

Origin

Insertion

a

b

FIGURE 10.6 The origin, insertion, and action of the arm muscles: *(a)* flexion; *(b)* extension.

Muscle Contraction and Joint Movement

Your skeletal muscles are attached to your bones and make your movements possible. You use these muscles to do physical activity. They are called voluntary muscles because you consciously control them. Your muscles work together to allow your body parts to function efficiently and effectively. For example, when you contract your biceps muscle (see figure 10.6*a*), your arm bends at the elbow, bringing your hand closer to your shoulder. At the same time, your triceps muscle relaxes to allow your biceps to do its work.

The tendons of each muscle connect with bone in two places, the origin and the insertion. The origin is typically connected to the bone that is stationary during a movement, and the insertion is typically connected to the bone that moves. In figure 10.6, the origin of the biceps is at the shoulder, and the insertion is on the bone of the lower arm that moves during flexion and extension.

Type of Muscle Fitness Exercise

As figure 10.6 shows, your skeletal muscles are attached to your bones on either side of a joint; your bones act as levers to which your muscles apply force. When stimulated by a nerve, muscle fibres are activated to apply force. Muscle contractions can be isotonic or isometric. **Isotonic contractions**

pull on your bones to produce movement of your body parts. **Isotonic exercises** are those that use muscle contractions to move body parts. The two types of isotonic muscle contractions are **concentric** (shortening contraction) and **eccentric** (lengthening contraction). Figure 10.6*a* shows the biceps muscle doing a concentric contraction in which the muscle shortens to cause the elbow to flex. In figure 10.6*b*, as the arm is slowly straightened, the biceps is doing an eccentric, or lengthening, contraction that causes the elbow to extend.

In contrast, an **isometric contraction** (sometimes called a static contraction) occurs when muscles contract and pull with equal force in opposite directions so that no movement occurs. **Isometric exercises** involve isometric contractions, and body parts do not move in these exercises. One example of an isometric contraction involves pushing your hands and arms together in front of your body. You push hard with each hand, applying force against the other, but no movement occurs. You can also do isometric calisthenics, such as holding your body still in the push-up position.

Plyometrics is a type of muscle fitness exercise that is especially useful in building power. This type of activity involves doing isotonic muscle contractions explosively (as in jumping). You'll learn more about all forms of muscle fitness exercise later in this chapter.

Isokinetic exercise is a type of isotonic exercise in which the velocity of movement is kept constant through the full range of motion. As noted in the Fitness Technology feature, isokinetic exercise requires special machines.

FIT FACT

An eccentric contraction is sometimes called a braking contraction because the lengthening of a muscle works against gravity to slow the lowering of a weight (see figure 10.6). For example, in a biceps curl after using a concentric contraction to flex the elbow and lift a weight, you lower the weight using an eccentric contraction. The lengthening of the biceps slows the weight down (or "puts on the brakes") so that the weight does not drop too quickly.

Muscle Fibres

Muscle fibres are long, thin, cylindrical muscle cells. Skeletal muscles (such as those in your arms and legs) are made of many muscle fibres (figure 10.7). The strength and endurance of skeletal muscles depend on whether the muscles are made of slow, fast, or intermediate fibres and on how much exercise they get.

Slow-twitch muscle fibres contract slowly and are usually red because they have a lot of blood vessels delivering oxygen to the muscle. These fibres generate less force than **fast-twitch muscle fibres**

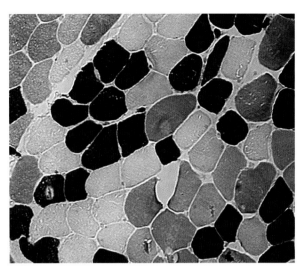

FIGURE 10.7 This photomicrograph shows slow-twitch (black) and fast-twitch (gray and white) muscle fibres.

Reprinted, by permission, from W.L. Kenney, J.H. Wilmore and D.L. Costill, 2004, *Physiology of sport and exercise*, 5th ed. (Champaign, IL: Human Kinetics), 37. By permission of D.L Costill.

but are able to resist fatigue. For this reason, a muscle with many slow-twitch fibres has good muscular endurance, and slow-twitch fibres are involved in activities such as running for distance. Fast-twitch muscle fibres contract quickly and are white because they have less blood flow delivering oxygen. They generate more force when they contract, and for this reason muscles with many fast-twitch fibres are important for strength activities.

FITNESS TECHNOLOGY: Isokinetic Exercise Machines

In recent years, tremendous technological advances have been made in resistance exercise machines. Innovations include adjustable benches and chairs so that machines fit people of all sizes, systems for changing resistance that make the machines easier to use, and the creation of isokinetic resistance machines. These machines use special hydraulics or electronics to regulate movement velocity and allow full exertion at all angles of joint movement during an exercise. In contrast, with traditional free weights or resistance machines, resistance is often greater during the first part of a movement than at the end of the movement, and the speed of the movement may also be greater at one point than at another. Isokinetic exercise allows the muscle to

be developed equally at all joint angles and can be used to develop power by using fast (high speed) movements. Isokinetic machines are considered quite safe and are often used by researchers and people who are rehabilitating injuries. Their disadvantages include being expensive and often not allowing eccentric contractions, which are used frequently in sport performance.

Using Technology

If your school has an isokinetic machine, ask for a demonstration and try it out. If not, see if you can find a machine locally or on the Internet (for a visual demonstration).

Intermediate muscle fibres have characteristics of both slow- and fast-twitch fibres. These fibres support muscle fitness and cardiorespiratory endurance activities.

Your muscle capabilities are determined in part by heredity. People who inherit a large number of fast-twitch muscle fibres are especially likely to be good at activities requiring sprinting and jumping, whereas people who inherit a large number of slow-twitch muscle fibres are likely to be good at activities requiring sustained performance such as distance running and swimming. Although heredity and genes play an important role, we now know that training can also affect muscle fibre function. So, regardless of your genes, you can increase your muscle strength, endurance, and power with proper training.

FIT FACT

Birds, like humans, have both fast-twitch and slow-twitch muscle fibres. The flying muscles (breast muscles) of a duck or goose are dark coloured because they contain many slow-twitch fibres (which are typically red) that are needed for long-distance flights. In contrast, the breast of a chicken is made up of mostly fast-twitch fibres (typically white) because chickens typically don't fly long distances.

Muscle Hypertrophy

Muscle **hypertrophy** refers to growth in the size of muscles and muscle fibres. Hypertrophy is affected not only by overloading but also by several other factors. You've already learned that we each inherit a unique pattern of muscle fibre types and that this inheritance makes a difference in how your body responds to training. But age, maturation, and sex also play a role.

As we age, our muscles grow, as do other tissues in the body. For preteens and young teens, who are not yet fully mature, the body does not produce enough hormones to build big muscles (hypertrophy), even with PRE. These hormones are not fully present until a person reaches full maturity, which occurs at various ages for various people, though typically earlier for girls than for boys. Before maturity, PRE can improve strength but may not noticeably increase muscle size; in fact, the strength gains are

typically due to increased skill in performing the exercises or an increase in the number of muscle fibres called upon for a movement during exercise. In most exercises, only some of the available muscle fibres contract to cause a movement; but with regular PRE, more fibres are called upon, increasing the number of exercises you can perform.

Because preteens and older teens who are late developers may not see big gains in muscle size with training, they may get discouraged and feel that PRE doesn't work. They may want to focus instead on gains in performance skills and accept the fact that noticeable muscular changes will occur when the body begins to produce more of the hormones that stimulate growth in muscle size.

Some people think that only males can build muscle fitness and increase muscle hypertrophy. This notion is false. Both males and females need strength in order to be healthy, avoid injury, look good, and be able to help themselves or others in an emergency.

Some girls and women fear that strength training will cause their body to look masculine. However, the hormones that promote muscle hypertrophy are not as prevalent in the bodies of females. In addition, females at maturity have a lower relative percent of muscle as compared with total body weight than males do. For this reason, most girls and women find it difficult to develop large, bulky muscles even when their exercise amounts are similar to those described in this book. Even so, women and girls who perform strength exercises do develop strong muscles. And both men and women look more attractive with strong muscles because they are more likely to have good posture and a firm body. Building good strength can also help build your self-confidence.

Muscle Fitness Assessment

You can assess muscle fitness in many ways. It is generally agreed that the best test for strength is the 1RM test (see the Self-Assessment feature at the end of this lesson). The 1RM test requires you to determine the amount of weight you can lift or the resistance you can overcome in one repetition. For example, if a person can lift 45 kilograms once, but not twice, 45 kilograms is the 1RM for the muscle group being tested. You can use the 1RM test for each of your major muscle groups, and you can use the results both to get a good idea of your strength and to determine how much weight or resistance to use when you perform exercises.

The true 1RM test is commonly used by athletes and adults. Done properly, it can also be safe for teens, but most experts recommend that teens use a modified self-assessment. The modified 1RM self-assessment gives you a good estimate of your true 1RM but does not require you to lift maximal weight or use maximal resistance. Teens are advised to use only a percentage of 1RM, both in testing their strength and in performing strength exercises. In the Self-Assessment feature included in this chapter, you'll estimate your 1RM by performing the modified 1RM test that uses multiple repetitions and lower than maximal weight (or resistance). This self-assessment is safe for teens when performed properly. You can do a 1RM test for many muscle groups, but two are used most often—one for the upper body (arm press) and one for the lower body (leg press).

Another 1RM test is the grip dynamometer test (figure 10.8), which tests isometric rather than isotonic strength. This grip test is easy to do but does require a grip **dynamometer**. People who score well on the isotonic 1RM test often score well on the grip test as well. This test is used in Canadian Society of Exercise Physiology Physical Activity Training for Health (CSEP-PATH) in Canada for people who are 15 years or older and the Alpha-Fit battery that is often used in Europe. Dynamometers are also available for testing other muscle groups, such as leg muscles, but they are more expensive and harder to use than grip dynamometers and thus are used less frequently.

You've already tried several self-assessments for muscular endurance and power that are used in common fitness test batteries. Muscular endurance tests typically require you to repeat the performance of **calisthenics**; examples include push-ups, curl-ups, and trunk lifts. Common tests of leg power include the long jump and vertical jump, and one common test of upper body power is the medicine ball throw. In the Self-Assessment feature in this lesson, you'll learn how to do tests of strength, muscular endurance, and power beyond those you've already tried.

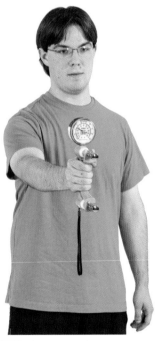

FIGURE 10.8 The grip dynamometer test measures isometric strength.

Absolute Versus Relative Strength

Your 1RM score is an example of **absolute strength**, which is measured by how much weight or resistance you can overcome regardless of your body size. Big people typically have more absolute strength than smaller people, and because males are generally larger than females, their average absolute strength is higher. **Relative strength**, on the other hand, is adjusted for body size. The most common method for determining relative strength is to divide your weight into your absolute strength score to get a score for your strength per kilogram of body weight. Relative strength scores are considered to be fairer assessments of strength for those who do not have large bodies; thus relative strength is used for the ratings in this chapter's Self-Assessment feature.

Lesson Review

1. What are the differences between strength, muscular endurance, and power?
2. What are the basic exercise principles of muscle fitness, and why are they important?
3. What are the types of muscle fitness exercise?
4. What are some methods for assessing muscle fitness?

Self-assessment of any part of fitness—including muscle fitness—is important because it allows you to establish your baseline level of fitness, determine your fitness needs, set goals, and determine whether you've met your goals. Certified personal trainers who know their stuff have their clients perform a baseline fitness test (a pretest) and, after they go through a fitness program, a follow-up fitness test (a posttest) to see if the program was effective. In this class, you are learning to become your own personal trainer.

Before performing these tests, consider doing a general and dynamic warm-up. If the 1RM test causes fatigue that keeps you from doing your best on the muscle fitness tests in part 3 of this sequence, repeat that assessment on another day. As directed by your instructor, record your scores and ratings for the three parts of this self-assessment. If you're working with a partner, remember that self-assessment information is personal and considered confidential. It shouldn't be shared with others without the permission of the person being tested.

Part 1: Estimating Your 1RM

To review, 1RM means 1-repetition maximum—the maximum weight a muscle or group of muscles can lift (or the maximum resistance they can overcome) one time. Because beginners should start gradually (without heavy lifting), a modified method has been developed that allows you to determine your 1RM without overexerting. Your results indicate how strong you are.

The modified 1RM can be done with free weights or machines, but the instructions that follow are for machine use. Resistance machines are recommended for these self-assessments, especially for beginners, because they are safer. Two tests are used most often, and the ones performed in this self-assessment activity are for your upper body (arm press) and your lower body (leg press).

Use the following directions for each of the two self-assessments.

- Choose a weight (resistance) that you think you can lift (move) 5 to 10 times. Do not use a weight that you can lift fewer than 5 times or more than 10 times.

- Using correct technique, lift the weight as many times as you possibly can. Count your lifts and write the total on your record sheet. If you were able to do more than 10 lifts, wait until another day before you try a heavier weight for that assessment. Go to the next muscle group assessment.

- If you can tell that you will not be able to lift the weight at least five times, stop and choose a lighter weight.

- If you were able to do 5 to 10 lifts (no fewer and no more), refer to table 10.1 and find the weight you lifted. Now find the number of reps you did. Your 1RM score is the number in the box where your horizontal weight row and your vertical rep column intersect.

- Divide each of your two 1RM scores (arm press and leg press) by your body weight to get your score for strength per kilogram of body weight. This score adjusts for body size to indicate your relative strength. For example, a person who weighs 68 kilograms and has a 1RM of 45 kilograms on the arm press has a score of 0.67 kilograms lifted per kilogram of body weight. After figuring your relative strength score, use tables 10.2 and 10.3 to determine your fitness rating. Record your 1RM scores, relative strength scores, and ratings.

- Tables 10.2 and 10.3 do not show high performance ratings for the 1RM. For now, focus on getting into the good fitness zone. Athletes should consult coaches in their sport to get more information about appropriate 1RM scores.

Safety tip: Proper form is essential for safety. Before you do the 1RM test, read the descriptions of the exercises and the directions that follow. Before performing each assessment, practice the exercise and have a teacher check your form. Work with a partner to get feedback about proper lifting technique.

TABLE 10.1 Predicted 1RM Based on Reps to Fatigue

Weight (kg)	Repetitions 5	6	7	8	9	10	Weight (kg)	Repetitions 5	6	7	8	9	10
14	34	35	36	37	38	39	64	157	163	168	174	180	187
16	40	41	42	43	44	45	66	163	168	174	180	186	193
18	46	47	49	50	51	53	68	169	174	180	186	193	200
20	51	53	55	56	58	60	70	174	180	186	192	199	207
23	56	58	60	62	64	67	73	180	186	192	199	206	213
25	62	64	66	68	71	73	75	186	192	198	205	212	220
27	67	70	72	74	77	80	77	191	197	204	211	219	227
30	73	75	78	81	84	87	80	197	203	210	217	225	233
32	79	81	84	87	90	93	82	202	209	216	223	231	240
34	84	87	90	93	96	100	84	208	215	222	230	238	247
36	90	93	96	99	103	107	86	214	221	228	236	244	253
39	96	99	102	106	109	113	88	219	226	234	242	251	260
41	101	105	108	112	116	120	91	225	232	240	248	257	267
43	107	110	114	118	122	127	93	231	238	246	254	264	273
45	112	116	120	124	129	133	95	236	244	252	261	270	280
48	118	122	126	130	135	140	98	242	250	258	267	276	287
50	124	128	132	137	141	147	100	247	255	264	273	283	293
52	129	134	138	143	148	153	102	253	261	270	279	289	300
54	135	139	144	149	154	160	104	259	267	276	286	296	307
57	141	145	150	155	161	167	107	264	273	282	292	302	313
59	146	151	158	161	167	173	109	270	279	288	298	309	320
61	152	157	162	168	174	180	111	276	285	294	304	315	327

To convert kilograms to pounds, multiply kilograms by 2.2. Alternatively, you can use the Internet to find a calculator that converts kilograms to pounds.

Adapted from M. Brzycki, 1993, "Strength testing - predicting a one-rep max from reps-to-fatigue," *JOPERD* 64(1): 89. www.informaworld.com

Seated Arm Press

1. Sit on the stool of a seated press machine and position yourself so that the handles are even with your shoulders. Grasp the handles with your palms facing away from you. Tighten your abdominal muscles.

2. Push upward on the handles, extending your arms until your elbows are straight.
   Caution: Do not arch your back. Do not lock your elbows.

3. Lower the handles to the starting position.

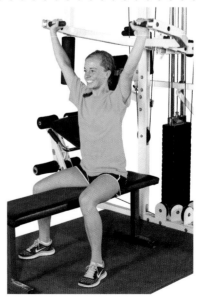

This test evaluates the strength of your triceps and pectoral muscles.

TABLE 10.2 Rating Chart: Relative Strength for Arm Press

	15 years or younger		16 or 17 years old		18 years or older	
	Male	Female	Male	Female	Male	Female
Good fitness	≥0.80	≥0.60	≥1.00	≥0.70	≥1.10	≥0.85
Marginal fitness	0.67–0.79	0.50–0.59	0.75–0.99	0.60–0.69	0.80–1.09	0.67–0.84
Low fitness	≤0.66	≤0.49	≤0.74	≤0.59	≤0.79	≤0.66

Relative strength is calculated by dividing 1RM by body weight.

Seated Leg Press

1. Adjust the seat position on a leg press machine for your leg length. Sit with your feet resting on the pedal.

2. Push the pedal until your legs are straight.
   Caution: Do not lock your knees.

3. Slowly return to the starting position.

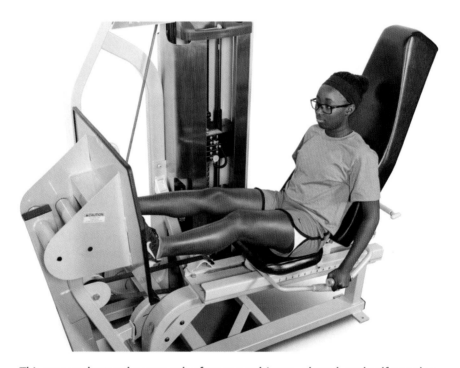

This test evaluates the strength of your quadriceps, gluteal, and calf muscles.

TABLE 10.3 Rating Chart: Relative Strength for Leg Press

	15 years or younger		16 or 17 years old		18 years or older	
	Male	Female	Male	Female	Male	Female
Good fitness	≥1.50	≥1.10	≥1.75	≥1.30	≥1.90	≥1.40
Marginal fitness	1.35–1.49	0.95–1.09	1.50–1.74	1.10–1.29	1.65–1.89	1.30–1.39
Low fitness	≤1.34	≤0.94	≤1.49	≤1.09	≤1.64	≤1.29

Relative strength is calculated by dividing 1RM by body weight.

Part 2: Muscular Endurance Tests

Many tests can help you evaluate muscular endurance, but the best ones assess your body's large muscles. In this self-assessment, you'll perform several isotonic and some isometric tests. For each, check "yes" if you could do the test as long or as many times as indicated. Check "no" if you could not. Look up your rating in table 10.4. As directed by your teacher, record your results.

TABLE 10.4   Rating Chart: Muscular Endurance

Fitness rating	Number of tests passed
Good fitness	5
Marginal fitness	3 or 4
Low fitness	0–2

Side Stand (Isometric)

1. Lie on your side.
2. Use both hands to get your body in position so that it is supported by your left hand and the side of your left foot. Keep your body stiff.
3. Raise your right arm and leg in the air. Hold this position. Record 1 point if you meet the standard (30 seconds if you are male or 20 seconds if you are female).
4. Return to the starting position and repeat the test on your right side.

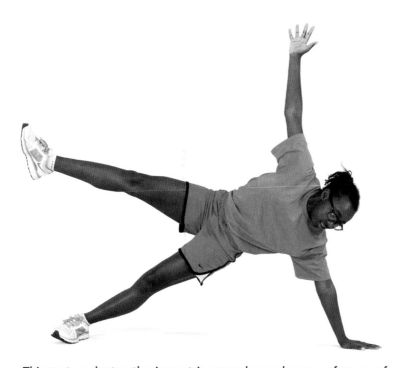

This test evaluates the isometric muscular endurance of some of your leg and arm muscles as well as your trunk-stabilizing muscles.

Trunk Extension (Isotonic)

1. Lie facedown on a stable weight bench or the end of a bleacher that is 38 to 51 centimetres (about 15 to 20 inches) high. The top of your hips should be even with the end of the bench, and your upper body should hang off the end of the bench. If the surface is hard, cover it with a mat or a towel.

2. Have a partner hold your calves using one hand on each leg 30 centimetres (12 inches) above your ankles. Overlap your hands and place them (palms away) in front of your chin.

3. Start with your upper body bent at the hip so that your chin is near the floor with the palm of your lower hand against the floor. Place a small mat on the floor below your hands and chin.

4. Keeping your head and neck in line with your upper body, slowly lift your head and upper body off the floor until your upper body is in line with your lower body.

    Caution: Do not lift your upper trunk higher than horizontal (in line with your lower body).

5. Lower to the starting position so that the palm of your lower hand touches the floor.

6. Perform one lift every three seconds. You may want to have a partner say "up, down" to help you. Record 1 point if you can meet the standard (20 reps if you are male or 15 reps if you are female).

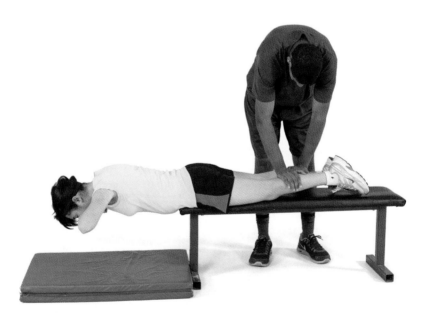

This test evaluates the isotonic muscular endurance of your upper back muscles.

Sitting Tuck (Isotonic)

1. Sit on the floor with your knees bent and your arms outstretched.
2. Lean back (to about a 45-degree angle) and balance on your buttocks. Keep your knees bent near your chest (feet off the floor).
3. Straighten your knees so your body forms a "V." You may move your arms sideways for balance.
4. Bend your knees to your chest again. Repeat the exercise as many times as you can. Count each time you push your legs out. Record 1 point if you can meet the standard (25 reps if you are male or 20 reps if you are female).

Safety tip: Avoid arching your lower back repetitively.

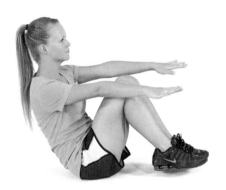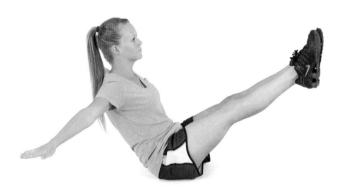

This test evaluates the isotonic muscular endurance of your abdominal muscles and some of your hip and leg muscles.

Leg Change (Isotonic)

1. Assume a push-up position with your weight on your hands and feet.
2. Pull your right knee under your chest, and keep your left leg straight.
3. Change legs by pulling your left leg forward and pushing your right leg back.
   Caution: Do not let your lower back sag.
4. Continue changing legs (about one change with each leg every two seconds).
5. Count the number of leg changes performed in one minute. Record 1 point if you can meet the standard (25 changes for both males and females).

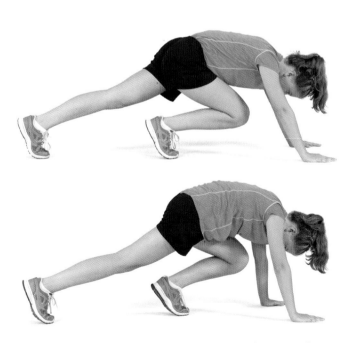

This test evaluates the isotonic muscular endurance of your hip and leg muscles.

Flexed-Arm Hang (Isometric)

1. Hang from a chinning bar with your palms facing away from your body.

2. Standing on a chair, or with help from a partner, lift your chin above the bar.

3. At the start signal, your partner lets go or removes the chair so you are hanging by your own power. Count how long you can hang. The time count begins when the support is removed and ends when your chin touches or goes below the bar or your head tilts backward. Record 1 point if you can meet the standard (hold for 16 seconds if you are male or 12 seconds if you are female).

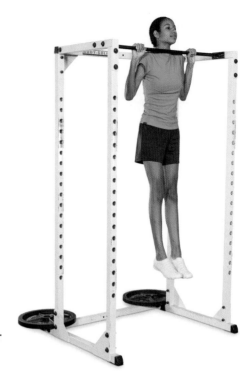

This test evaluates the muscular endurance of your arm, shoulder, and chest muscles (isometric).

Part 3: Tests of Power

In this self-assessment, you'll test the power of your lower body by performing the standing long jump and of the upper body by performing the medicine ball throw.

Standing Long Jump

1. Use masking tape or another material to make the necessary line on the floor.

2. Stand with your feet shoulder-width apart behind the line on the floor. Bend your knees and hold your arms straight in front of your body at shoulder height.

3. Swing your arms downward and backward, then vigorously forward as you jump forward as far as possible, extending your legs.

4. Land on both feet and try to maintain your balance on landing. Do not run or hop before jumping.

5. Perform the test two times. Record the better of your two scores, then find your rating in table 10.5 and record it.

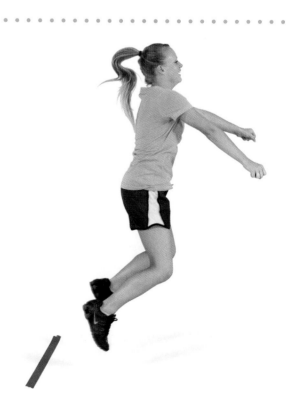

This test evaluates the power of the lower body.

TABLE 10.5 Rating Chart: Standing Long Jump in Centimetres

	13 years old		14 years old		15 years old		16 years old		17 years or older	
	Male	Female	Male	Female	Male	Female	Male	Female	Male	Female
High performance	≥185	≥150	≥203	≥152	≥216	≥155	≥224	≥157	≥231	≥173
Good fitness	170–184	145–149	185–202	147–151	198–215	150–154	208–223	152–156	218–230	160–172
Marginal fitness	155–169	137–144	170–184	140–146	185–197	142–149	196–207	145–151	203–217	147–159
Low fitness	≤154	≤136	≤169	≤139	≤184	≤141	≤195	≤144	≤202	≤146

To convert centimetres to inches, multiply centimetres by 0.39. Alternatively, you can use the Internet to find a calculator that converts centimetres to inches.

Medicine Ball Throw

1. Sit on a chair positioned against a wall. Sit back as far as possible so that your lower and upper back are against the back of the chair.
2. Hold a 6.5-kilogram medicine ball (about 14 pounds) with both hands so that it rests against the middle of your chest.
3. Push with both hands to throw the medicine ball as far as possible. Throw as you would for a basketball chest pass. Keep your back against the chair.
4. Measure the distance from the wall (behind the chair) to the spot on the floor where the ball landed. Measure in centimetres.
5. Measure the distance from the wall to the end of your fingers (that is, your arm length) in centimetres. Your score is the distance the ball was thrown minus the length of your arm.
6. Perform the test two times and use the better of your two scores.

Based on your better score, use table 10.6 to determine your rating. Record your score and your rating.

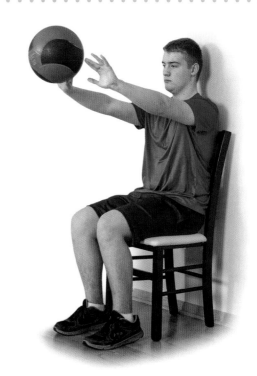

The medicine ball throw test evaluates power in your upper body.

TABLE 10.6 Rating Chart: Medicine Ball Throw in Centimetres

	15 years or younger		16 or 17 years old		18 years or older	
	Male	Female	Male	Female	Male	Female
Good fitness	≥368	≥249	≥394	≥259	≥419	≥274
Marginal fitness	330–367	229–248	356–393	239–258	381–418	249–273
Low fitness	≤329	≤228	≤355	≤238	≤380	≤248

To convert centimetres to inches, multiply centimetres by 0.39. Alternatively, you can use the Internet to find a calculator that converts centimetres to inches.

Lesson 10.2
Building Muscle Fitness

Lesson Objectives

After participating in this lesson, you should be able to

1. explain the FIT formula for developing muscle fitness with isotonic PRE,
2. describe the double progressive system for using PRE,
3. describe several free weight and resistance machine exercises and their advantages and disadvantages,
4. describe several other forms of exercise for building muscle fitness,
5. describe basic guidelines for doing PRE safely, and
6. name some myths about strength and explain why they are wrong.

 ### Lesson Vocabulary

bodybuilding, body dysmorphia, double progressive system, interval training, muscle bound, powerlifting, weightlifting

Do you know the health benefits of PRE (progressive resistance exercise) and muscle fitness? Have you ever wanted to increase your muscle fitness? Are you familiar with the types of resistance training? In this lesson, you'll learn some of the health benefits associated with achieving muscle fitness through PRE. You'll also learn how to apply the FIT formula for the most popular methods of building muscle fitness. And you'll learn about recommended guidelines for properly performing PRE and about some common misconceptions concerning muscle fitness.

Health Benefits of PRE and Muscle Fitness

Many of the health benefits described throughout this book are associated with doing muscle fitness exercises and achieving good muscle fitness. Most people know that muscle fitness helps reduce back problems, improves posture, reduces risk of muscle injury, and increases working capacity. They may not know that muscle fitness exercises are very important to bone health (preventing osteoporosis), prevention of heart disease and diabetes, and rehabilitation from chronic diseases such as cancer. Muscle fitness exercises can also reduce your risk of becoming overweight or obese. In addition, they provide mental health benefits such as looking and feeling your best and experiencing a high quality of life. Among older people, muscle fitness also helps

reduce the risk of falling and improves a person's ability to do tasks of daily life.

Building Muscle Fitness With Isotonic PRE

In this section, you'll learn about the FIT formula for isotonic PRE. You'll also learn some of the advantages and disadvantages of resistance machine and free weight exercises and some general guidelines for performing isotonic PRE.

The FIT Formula for Isotonic PRE: Resistance Machines and Free Weights

Table 10.7 provides FIT formula information for isotonic exercises using resistance machines and free weights, such as those described later in this lesson. The same FIT formula can be used for isokinetic exercises. As indicated in the table, beginners use lower resistance, do more reps, and perform fewer sets than people who are more advanced.

The Canadian Society of Exercise Physiology (CSEP) recommends taking a two- or three-minute rest between sets. In general, you should use longer rests between high-resistance exercises and shorter rests between low-resistance exercises. To make your workout more efficient, you can alternate arm and leg exercises. That way, when your arms are working, your legs are resting, and vice versa.

TABLE 10.7 Fitness Target Zones for Muscle Fitness (Isotonic)

	Beginner		Intermediate		Advanced	
	Threshold	Target	Threshold	Target	Threshold	Target
Frequency (days per week)	2	2 or 3	2	2 or 3	3	3 or 4
Intensity (% of 1RM)	50	50–70	60	60–80	70	70–85
Time	1 set of 10–15 reps	1 or 2 sets of 10–15 reps	2 sets of 8–12 reps	2 or 3 sets of 8–12 reps	3 sets of 6–10 reps	3–4 sets of 6–10 reps

The FIT formula for muscle fitness for teens differs somewhat from the formula for adults, especially for exercise intensity. The CSEP recommends a FIT formula similar to the one shown in the table for teens. For adults, beginners can start at 60 percent of 1RM rather than 50 percent for teens, and advanced exercisers can use 80 to 90 percent of 1RM rather than 70 to 85 percent. Adult beginners can start with two sets rather than one set, which is what is recommended for teens.

The Double Progressive System of PRE

You already know that in order to achieve optimal development of your muscle fitness, you need to progress gradually. The most commonly used method for applying the principle of progression to muscle fitness is the **double progressive system**. The first part of the system involves increasing repetitions (reps). For example, as shown in table 10.7, a beginner starts with one set of 10 reps at 50 percent of 1RM, then gradually increases the number of reps until he or she can easily perform 15 reps.

The second part of the system involves increasing resistance or weight. The number of reps is dropped back to 10, and the resistance is increased by 5 to 10 percent of 1RM; for teens, this often means an increase of about 0.9 to 2.3 kilograms (2 to 5 pounds). This double progression—increasing reps and resistance—continues until the person can do the maximum percent of 1RM in the beginner category. At that point, he or she can add a second set. It may be necessary to drop back to a lower number of reps and a lower percent of 1RM to perform two full sets of 10 to 15 reps.

When doing multiple sets, longer rest intervals between sets allow you to lift a higher percent of

1RM than shorter rest intervals. So it is important to use rest intervals of a consistent length of time.

Once a person can perform two sets of 15 reps at 70 percent of 1RM (a goal that may take several months to attain), he or she is ready to move to the intermediate stage. Here, the double progression sequence begins again. The person follows the double progressive system at the moderate stage until he or she can perform three sets of 8 to 12 reps at 80 percent of 1RM. It may take a year or longer to progress to this point.

Some exercisers choose to stay at the intermediate level because many health benefits can be achieved using the FIT formula for this stage (moderate sets and reps and moderate resistance). Because the FIT formula for advanced exercisers focuses more on low reps and higher resistance, it builds more pure strength than the FIT formula for beginners and intermediates. Therefore, the advanced FIT formula offers benefits for people who plan to do sports or jobs requiring high levels of strength and for people especially interested in muscle hypertrophy. However, the FIT formula for intermediates provides many benefits and is appropriate for regular use by most teens.

Resistance Machines Versus Free Weights

Resistance machine and free weight exercises require considerable equipment but are among the most popular forms of isotonic PRE because they are two of the most effective methods for building muscle fitness. They allow you to build both strength and muscular endurance and isolate most of the major muscle groups in your body with specific exercises. To help you consider these forms of PRE, compare their advantages and disadvantages as outlined in table 10.8. Some basic exercises using free weights and resistance machines are described at the end of this lesson; for each exercise, the muscles used are listed and illustrated.

 FIT FACT

In addition to the CSEP and the NSCA (see the first lesson in this chapter), several other groups of experts have now prepared statements indicating that resistance training can be safe for teens when performed properly. These groups include the Canadian Paediatric Society (medical doctors who specialize in treating children and youth), the American College of Sports Medicine, the Mayo Clinic, and the American Orthopaedic Society of Sports Medicine (medical doctors who specialize in bone problems associated with sport and activity). The self-assessments and muscle fitness exercises described in this book follow the guidelines of these organizations.

" There may be people that have more talent than you, but there's no excuse for anyone to work harder than you do. "

—Derek Jeter, Major League Baseball MVP and five-time World Champion

Progressive Resistance Exercise

When performed correctly, resistance training is safe and improves your muscle fitness while helping you feel and look your best. Stick to the following guidelines created especially to help teens use PRE safely and effectively.

- **Warm up** with recommended dynamic exercises or perform low-resistance sets before doing your regular workout.
- **Learn proper technique.** From the beginning, get good instruction from an expert. Start with little or no weight as you're learning the fundamentals. Use the following tips for good technique.
  ○ **Use moderate-velocity movements—** not too slow and not too fast.
  ○ **Use both concentric and eccentric contractions through a full range of motion.** For example, when doing the biceps curl, lift the weight all the way up (this uses a concentric contraction) and lower the weight all the way down (this uses an eccentric contraction).
  ○ **Avoid sudden or quick movements.** Stop briefly at the beginning and end of each repetition. Use your muscles, not the movement of your body, to do the exercise (for example, don't rock forward and backward with the upper body during a biceps curl).

TABLE 10.8 Resistance Machines Versus Free Weights

	Resistance machines	Free weights
Safety	Safer because weights cannot fall on lifter Spotter often not needed	Greater chance of injury from falling weights Easy to lose control of—spotter needed
Cost	Very expensive to own If not owned, club membership required for use	Relatively inexpensive
Versatility	Easy to isolate specific muscle groups	More balance, muscle coordination, and concentration required More muscles used, movements more like moving heavy loads in daily life
Convenience	Much floor space needed Must be used where installed	Little space needed Some weights small enough to carry around Easily scattered, lost, or stolen

○ **Do not hold your breath when you exercise.** Holding your breath can cause you to black out. Some resistance trainers recommend exhaling when applying resistance and inhaling on the return movement.

○ **Use good biomechanics.** Avoid body positions and movements that cause your joints to move in ways they are not intended to move or that put your muscles at risk of injury.

• **Make sure that your workout area is safe.** Use equipment in good working order. Keep free weights on weight racks rather than scattered on the floor. Clean the machine after you're done by wiping it with a towel—or even before you use it, if it wasn't cleaned by the previous user.

• **When working with free weights, always use spotters.** You might be tempted to work on your own, but working with a partner is much safer. Spotting means supporting a partner by being ready to help if she or he loses control of the weight or gets off balance.

• **Progress gradually.** Young teens, and all people no matter their age with little PRE experience, should exercise with the FIT formula for beginners for several months before moving to the intermediate level. Do not let the word "beginner" be a reason for violating the principle of progression. And remember that the advanced FIT formula is typically reserved for people with at least one year of experience and for older teens who have reached physical maturity.

• **Select exercises for all major muscle groups.** Experts recommend that you perform 8 to 10 muscle fitness exercises to be sure that you build all of the major muscle groups. Performing only a few exercises can lead to unbalanced muscle development. In this book, 8 to 10 exercises are provided for many types of PRE.

• **Rest between sets.** For building pure strength, allow two to three minutes between sets; for muscular endurance, allow one to two minutes between sets.

• **Allow rest days between exercise sessions.** For best results, do not perform PRE for the same muscle group on consecutive days. You can, however, exercise daily if you alternate muscle groups to avoid exercising the same muscle group on consecutive days.

• **Vary your program to keep it interesting.** The CSEP points out the importance of progression and volume when exercising. Using the double progressive method to progress gradually provides variety while helping you get optimal benefits. You can also get variety while keeping your volume (total amount of exercise) constant by varying repetitions and resistance (for example, many reps with low resistance can result in the same volume of exercise as fewer reps with higher resistance).

• **Avoid overhead lifts with free weights.** If possible, use machines for these lifts. If you must use free weights, always use a trained spotter.

• **Master single-joint exercises before attempting multiple-joint exercises or sport movements.** For example, a biceps curl is a single-joint exercise because the only joint it moves is the elbow. Most of the exercises needed to build good health, as shown in this book, are single-joint exercises. Multiple-joint lifts, such as the clean and jerk in the sport of **weightlifting**, require

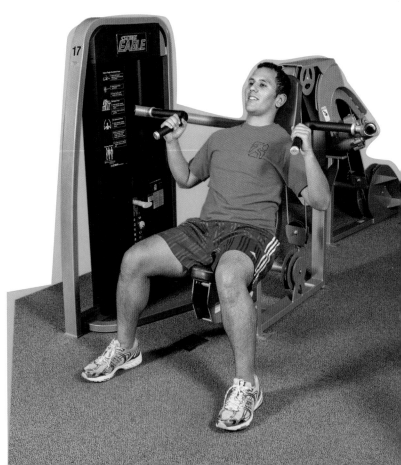

good muscle fitness that results from PRE consisting of single-joint exercises. Multiple-joint exercises also involve a high level of skill that requires special training to ensure good technique.

- **Never use weights carelessly.** Concentrate on your technique and on what you're doing. Use care when changing free weights, and put them away properly when you're finished.

- **Never compete when you do resistance training.** For example, do not have a contest to see who can lift the most weight. Genetic differences have a lot to do with how strong a person can be. Concern yourself only with trying to improve your own strength gradually and enjoying the exercise—not lifting more than someone else.

PRE Using Resistance Machines and Free Weights

Experts recommend doing 8 to 10 basic exercises to build all of your major muscle groups. At the end of this lesson, 9 free weight exercises and 10 resistance machine exercises are described. Before performing these exercises, practice each exercise and the spotting techniques described in the next section. Spotting means supporting a partner by being ready to help if he or she loses control of the weight or gets off balance. Your instructor will help you practice these techniques.

Practicing Proper Exercise and Spotting Technique

Performing and spotting exercises properly require practice. Before you begin your PRE program, practice by moving through the four levels described in this section. Start with level 1 for each exercise until you achieve mastery. Then move to the next level. The specific techniques for performing exercises and spotting properly are explained in this lesson in the individual descriptions of exercises using free weights and resistance machines. Some experts use the phrase "feel is not real" to emphasize that just feeling as if you're doing an exercise properly does not necessarily mean that you really are. In many facilities, mirrors are provided so that you can check your form. A partner can also help you determine whether you're using correct spotting and lifting techniques (figure 10.9).

- **Level 1.** Focus on lifting technique, not weight. Perform each exercise without any weight by using a wand or stick instead of a barbell. When you're practicing a lift, concentrate on correct form (placement of your body parts). When you're watching a partner, give useful coaching.

- **Level 2.** Focus on spotting technique, not weight. While your partner performs the rep with the wand, you and another partner practice correct spotting technique. Pay particular attention to your leg and hand positions.

- **Level 3.** At this level, you combine lifting and spotting with light weights. Perform each exercise by doing five repetitions with light weight. Practice your lifting and spotting techniques and continue to give each other coaching about both lifting and spotting.

- **Level 4.** At this level, you perform a normal workout using free weights. Select the appropriate percentage of your 1RM and the appropriate number of sets and repetitions (see table 10.7). Perform each of the basic exercises.

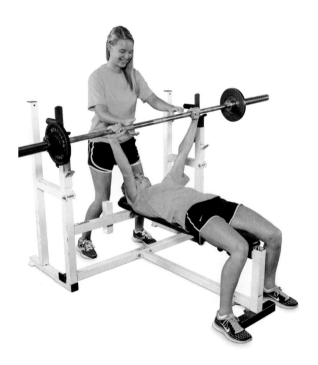

FIGURE 10.9 Having a spotter is essential when using free weights.

Clarifying Progressive Resistance Training Terms

As you now know, PRE is a method of building muscle fitness. It differs from three sports that involve elements of PRE.

Olympic-Style Weightlifting

In this Olympic sport, athletes use free weights to try lifting a maximum load. The sport includes only two lifts: the snatch and the clean and jerk. For those who train with weights but do not participate in Olympic-style weightlifting, the preferred term is *weight training*.

Powerlifting

Powerlifting is another competitive sport using free weights. It includes only three exercises: the bench press, the squat, and the deadlift. Athletes in this sport try to do one maximal lift for each type of lift.

Bodybuilding

Bodybuilding participants are concerned primarily with the appearance of their body, and judges rate them based on how large, well-defined, and symmetrical their muscles are rather than how much they can lift. This sport can also be done competitively.

Other Types of Isotonic PRE

Resistance machine and free weight exercises are popular and effective, but they are not the only types of isotonic PRE. The following sections describe some other frequently used forms, including calisthenics, elastic band exercises, and exercise with homemade equipment.

FIT FACT

The top two fitness trends of 2015 identified by the American College of Sports Medicine were body weight training (i.e., calisthenics) and high-intensity interval training (HIIT). The ability to perform body weight training almost anywhere and at any time for free makes body weight training very popular. High-intensity interval training involves working out at maximal or near-maximal intensity for a short period of time, followed by a short, sometimes active, period of rest. Examples of HIIT are P90X and CrossFit.

Calisthenics

Calisthenic exercises use all or part of your body weight to provide resistance; examples include push-ups, curl-ups, burpees, and triceps dips. Because only your body weight is used for resistance, this type of PRE is better for building muscular endurance than for building strength. The lower resistance also means that you can do calisthenics more frequently. The FIT formula for isotonic calisthenics is shown in table 10.9. Calisthenics are good for both home use and travel because you can do them almost anywhere with little equipment.

Exercising With Elastic Bands, Homemade Weights, Partner Resistance, and Balls

These types of PRE are similar to resistance machine and free weight exercises but use various other means to provide resistance. Like calisthenics, elastic band exercises require little equipment and are easy to do both at home and when traveling. Exercises using a stability ball can also be effective in building core fitness. All of these types of PRE use the

TABLE 10.9 Target Zone for Calisthenics (Isotonic)

	Threshold	Target zone
Frequency (days per week)	3	3–6
Intensity	Moving the weight of parts of the body	Moving the weight of parts or all of the body
Time	1 set of 10 reps	1–4 sets of 11–25 reps

Rest for two minutes between sets.

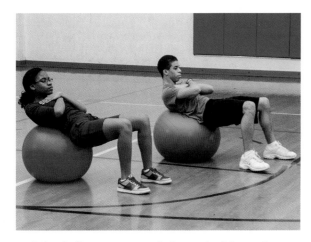

Stability ball exercises can help you build core fitness.

FIT formula described in table 10.7. Some exercises using partner resistance and homemade weights are described in the student section of the Fitness for Life Canada website.

Building Muscle Fitness With Isometric PRE

Isometric exercises can be done easily at home or when you travel because they require little or no equipment and can be done in a confined space—even a space as small as an airplane seat. A disadvantage of isometric PRE is that it's sometimes hard to tell when you're doing a maximum contraction, and this uncertainty can affect your motivation to work hard. In isotonic exercise, on the other hand, you can see your movement and you know how much effort you're giving. In addition, experts do not consider isometric exercise to be as effective in building muscle fitness as isotonic PRE. As with all PRE, when doing isometric exercise, breathe rather than hold your breath while you're performing exercises. The FIT formula for isometric exercises is presented in table 10.10. Some basic isometric exercises are illustrated and described at the end of this lesson. The muscles used in each exercise are also listed and illustrated.

Building Power

As you may recall, power is a combination of strength and speed. Exercise physiologists have shown that power is related to bone development in children and teens and offers health benefits similar to those provided by other parts of muscle fitness. It's also important for good performance in various activities, including soccer (kicking the ball very hard), surfing (paddling into a wave and getting to your feet), and rock climbing (exploding with legs and hands to a handhold; also called a "dyno"). For this reason, athletes often want to improve their power not only for their health but also for improved performance.

One of the most frequently used methods of building power is plyometrics (plyometric exercise). Plyometrics was pioneered by Olympic track and field coaches from the former Soviet Union. Plyometric exercise involves a rapid eccentric contraction of a muscle followed by a concentric contraction of the muscle. For example, one common low-resistance form of plyometric exercise is rope jumping. Landing after a jump requires your calf muscle to do an eccentric, or lengthening, contraction, and the next jump into the air requires a concentric contraction of the calf muscle. Resistance is provided by body weight. Plyometrics often uses more vigorous jumping activities.

Like other forms of muscle fitness exercise, plyometrics was previously thought to be dangerous for teens. However, recent evidence suggests that when performed properly and progressively with good supervision, plyometrics can be safe for teens, enhance athletic performance, increase both power and speed, and actually reduce athletic injuries. Nevertheless, plyometric and other power-building techniques have resulted in injury when performed excessively. The FIT formula for plyometrics is

TABLE 10.10   Target Zone for Isometric Progressive Resistance Exercise

	Threshold	Target zone
Frequency (days per week)	3	3–6
Intensity	Contracting muscle as tightly as possible or holding part or all of body weight	Contracting muscle as tightly as possible or holding part or all of body weight
Time	3 reps (1 rep = hold for 7 sec)	3–4 reps (1 rep = hold for 7–10 sec)

TABLE 10.11   Target Zone for Plyometrics

	Threshold	Target zone
Frequency (days per week)	2 (nonconsecutive)	2 or 3 (nonconsecutive)
Intensity (jumps of varying intensity based on age)	Age 12: low intensity (in place) Age 13: medium intensity (moving jumps and hops) Ages 14 and 15: medium intensity (box and obstacle jumps) Age ≥16: high intensity (bounding—multiple jumps over distance and drop jumping)	Same as threshold
Time	1 set of 6–10 repetitions Rest for 1–3 min between sets	1–3 sets of 6–10 repetitions Rest for 1–3 min between sets

outlined in table 10.11; the formula, developed by experts, shows a progression based on age and fitness level. Fit athletes may do advanced plyometrics or other forms of training, but you should consult with a parent or guardian and an instructor or certified exercise leader before performing them.

Beginners should start at low intensity and progress to higher intensity regardless of age. Youth who have been regularly active and have high fitness may move to more advanced levels at ages lower than suggested with proper supervision by a qualified expert who has evaluated the maturational and fitness status of the exerciser.

Interval Training

Interval training uses bouts of high-intensity exercise followed by rest periods. For example, runners and swimmers often use a series of high-intensity sprints (exercise intervals) followed by rest intervals. This type of training was developed to improve anaerobic performance in activities such as sprinting and fast swimming and in the short bursts of vigorous activity typical of soccer, hockey, football, and basketball. Now, interval training is regularly used by endurance athletes as well. For more information about interval training, check with your physical education teacher or coach.

Myths and Misconceptions

The amount of muscle fitness you need in order to stay healthy and do what you want depends on your personal situation and interests. For example, people who do jobs requiring a lot of lifting need more strength than people who work at a desk. Despite the fact that muscle fitness exercise offers

many benefits, many people still hold misconceptions about it.

No Pain, No Gain

Some people still cling to the myth that exercise must hurt in order to be effective. Some of the worst offenders are people who are hooked on strength-building exercises. In reality, you should listen to your body. If you feel pain, your body is telling you something. When doing PRE, it's true that you'll become quite fatigued and feel a sensation sometimes called the exercise "burn," and you need to learn the difference between this feeling and pain. If in doubt, back off to avoid injury.

Muscle Bound

Some people think that strength training will cause them to be **muscle bound**—to have tight, bulky muscles that reduce range of motion (i.e., flexibility) and prevent them from moving freely. However, inflexibility is caused not by resistance training but by incorrect training. Two kinds of incorrect exercise that can cause a muscle-bound condition are training muscles on only one side of a joint and failing to stretch muscles. Another example of incorrect training is failure to move the joints through their full range of motion when lifting weights or doing other resistance exercises. For example, your elbow joint can bend to allow your hand to reach your shoulder and to let your arm straighten completely. Therefore, when you do a biceps curl with weight, bring the weight all the way to your shoulder, then straighten your elbow each time you lower the weight. *Caution: Do not bend your elbow or any other joint backward beyond its full range of motion. You can damage a joint if you move it in a way in which it was not designed*

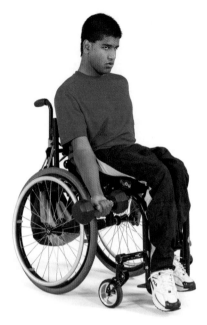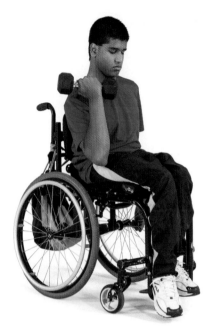

Moving a joint through the full range of motion is important for optimal functioning.

to move. Recent research suggests that when done properly, PRE can actually enhance flexibility.

Muscle Fitness for Females

As noted earlier, some people think that girls and women cannot build muscle fitness. Others think that PRE will cause girls and women to look masculine. Both of these statements are false.

Muscle Tone

Advertisers often promise that a product or program can build something they call muscle tone. However, the word "tone" used in this way is considered a quack word because it does not refer to anything that can be measured in the same way as strength, muscular endurance, or power. Inspecting or feeling a muscle cannot objectively measure it; therefore, "tone" is not a good word to use to define muscle fitness, and any claim based on it is suspect.

Body Dysmorphia

The term **body dysmorphia** refers to a mental disorder that causes people to have a distorted image of their body to the point where it interferes with their life. Body dysmorphia among males might look like an unhealthy obsession with building muscle. This psychological disorder, sometimes referred to as "reverse anorexia," often begins with a reasonable amount of exercise to build muscle fitness. At some point, however, a person with this problem gets carried away in wanting to build more and more muscle. The disorder is an obsessive–compulsive one and often requires treatment by a professional. In more than a few cases, people with this disorder have engaged in unhealthy behaviours, such as taking drugs and doing unhealthy exercises. People with this condition experience high injury rates. Doing reasonable PRE can enhance your health. Becoming obsessed with fitness can hurt it.

Lesson Review

1. What is the FIT formula for developing muscle fitness with isotonic PRE?
2. What is the double progressive system, and how is it helpful in using PRE?
3. What are some basic free weight and resistance machine exercises, and what are their advantages and disadvantages?
4. What are several other forms of exercise for building muscle fitness?
5. What are some of the basic guidelines for doing PRE safely?
6. What are some muscle fitness myths?

The following basic exercises use free weights to work the major muscle groups. The exercises that use barbells (bar and weights) can also be performed with dumbbells (small bar and weights or fixed-weight dumbbells). The last two exercises require dumbbells. You can determine your 1RM for the various muscle groups using some of these exercises, but because resistance machines exercises are safer, they are the preferred method.

SEATED OVERHEAD PRESS

Weights: barbell

This exercise requires two spotters, standing by the lifter's shoulders on either side of the bench. If you are serving as a spotter, keep your hands under the bar with your palms up. Be ready to take the bar if the lifter loses control (especially at the top of the lift), if the barbell begins to move backward, or if the lifter begins to tremble.

1. Sit on the end of a bench in front-stride (split-foot) position.
2. Hold the barbell at chest height in preparation for pushing the bar vertically. Grasp the barbell with your hands facing away from your body and positioned slightly more than shoulder-width apart.
3. Tighten your abdominal, back, and arm muscles. Tip your head back slightly.
4. Push the bar straight up, directly overhead.

Caution: Do not let the bar go forward or backward. Do not lock your elbows. Do not arch your back.

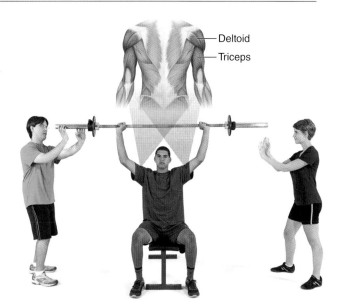

Deltoid
Triceps

This exercise uses the muscles at the top of your shoulders, between your shoulder blades, and on the back of your arms.

BENCH PRESS

Weights: barbell

This exercise requires two spotters, who stand by the lifter's shoulders on either side of the bench. If you are serving as a spotter, place the bar into the lifter's hands. During the exercise, keep your hands under the bar with your palms up. Be prepared to take the bar if the lifter loses control.

1. Lie on your back on a bench with your feet on the floor and your lower back flat. Extend your arms into the up position (perpendicular to the floor).

2. Grasp the bar with a palms-up grip and your hands slightly farther than shoulder-width apart, your elbows straight, and the bar approximately over your collarbones.

3. Lower the bar until it touches your chest just below your armpits. When the bar touches your chest, your forearms should be perpendicular to the floor and your elbows should point neither toward your feet nor out to the sides but halfway between (at 45 degrees).

4. Tighten your abdominal, back, and arm muscles. Tip your head back slightly.
   Caution: Do not lock your elbows.

5. Push the bar up to the starting position with your arms perpendicular to the floor. The bar follows a slightly curved path.

Caution: Do not lock your elbows or bounce the bar off of your chest. Do not arch your back or lift your hips. If the weight gets in front of or behind your arms, you may lose control.

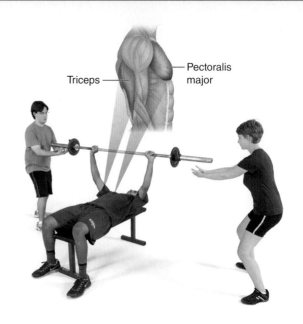

This exercise uses the muscles on the front of your chest (pectoral) and the back of your upper arms (triceps).

KNEE EXTENSION

Weights: weighted boot or ankle weight
   One person can help the lifter put on the boot or ankle weight.

1. Put the weight on one foot or ankle. Sit on a bench with your lower leg hanging over the edge. Grasp the bench with your hands.

2. Lift the weighted boot by extending your knee until your leg is straight.
   Caution: Lift slowly. Do not lock your knee when you extend, and do not kick your leg upward.

3. Repeat the exercise with your other leg.

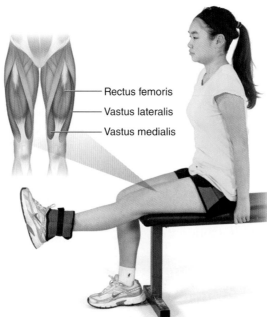

This exercise uses the muscles at the top of your thighs (quadriceps). The fourth quadriceps muscle, the vastus intermedius, lies beneath the rectus femoris and therefore is not shown in the illustration.

HALF SQUAT

Weights: barbell
Note: This exercise can be done only if a squat rack is available.

1. Stand in a side-stride position with your feet shoulder-width or slightly farther apart. Your toes should point straight ahead or be slightly turned out. Keep your head up and your back straight.

2. Hold the barbell across the back of your shoulders at the base of your neck with your hands slightly farther than shoulder-width apart and your palms facing forward. Point your elbows toward the floor with your forearms perpendicular to the floor.

3. Squat until your knees are at a right angle, then rise. Keep your heels flat on the floor. Do not let your knees get in front of your toes. Focus on a spot on the wall slightly higher than your standing height. Look at this spot for the duration of the lift—when lowering and when straightening.

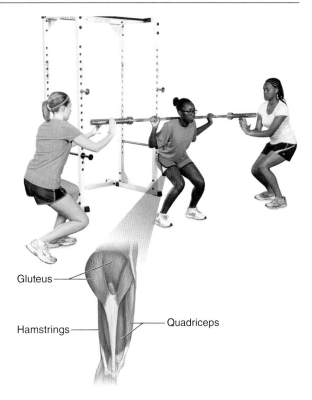

This exercise uses the muscles on the front of your thighs (quadriceps) and your buttock muscles (gluteal).

Caution: Do not round your back. Do not lean too far forward at your hips or let your knees get in front of your toes. Do not squat too deeply.

HAMSTRING CURL

Weights: weighted boot or ankle weight
One person can help the lifter put on the boot or ankle weight.

1. Put the weight on one foot or ankle. Lie facedown on a bench, with your kneecaps hanging over the edge. Grasp the bench with your hands.

2. Lift the weighted boot by flexing your knee to a right angle.
Caution: Do not lock your knee when you extend.

3. Repeat the exercise using your other leg. To determine your 1RM for this exercise, use the hamstring curl on the resistance machine.

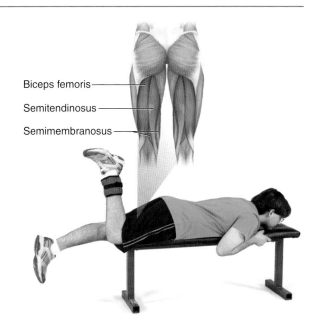

This exercise uses the muscles on the back of your thighs (hamstrings).

BICEPS CURL

Weights: barbell

Spotters are not required, but they can place the barbell in the lifter's palm-up hands.

1. Stand erect with your feet in side-stride position. Tighten your abdominal and back muscles.

2. Grasp the bar with your palms up and your hands slightly more than shoulder-width apart. The arms are fully extended.

3. Keep your elbows close to your sides and lift the weight by bending your elbows only. Raise the weight to near your chin, then return to the starting position.

    Caution: Do not move other joints, especially in your back.

4. You can also perform this exercise with your palms down.

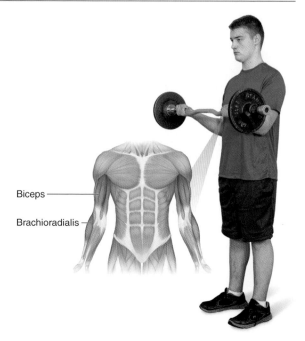

This exercise uses the muscles on the front of your upper arms (biceps) and other elbow flexor muscles.

HEEL RAISE

Weights: barbell

This exercise requires two spotters, who stand by the lifter's shoulders, one on each side.

1. If the weight is manageable, lift the bar above your head as you would in an over-head press (with spotters). Then lower the bar to your shoulders. If the weight is heavier than you can easily press, have spotters lift the weight to your shoulders.

2. Once the bar is on your shoulders, stand with the balls of your feet on a 5-centimetre board and your toes turned in slightly.

3. Rise onto your toes, then lower to the starting position.

    Caution: Keep your spine straight.

4. Advanced lifters may also try this exercise with their toes pointing straight ahead (more difficult) or with their toes turned outward (even more difficult). To determine your 1RM for this exercise, use the heel raise on the resistance machine.

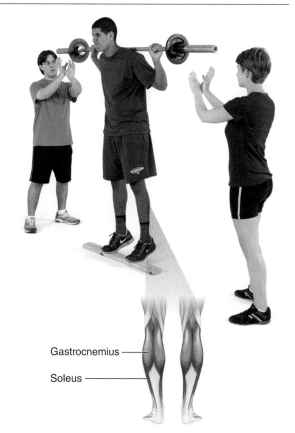

This exercise uses your calf muscles.

SEATED FRENCH CURL

Weights: dumbbell
This exercise requires one spotter.

1. Sit on the end of a bench with your arms extended overhead and your palms facing up.
2. Hold one end of a dumbbell in both hands above and behind your head. Tighten your abdominal and back muscles. Slowly lower the weight toward the back of your neck until your arms are fully flexed at the elbows. Keep your elbows high.
3. Slowly return to the starting position, moving only your elbow joints. To determine your 1RM for this exercise, use the triceps press.

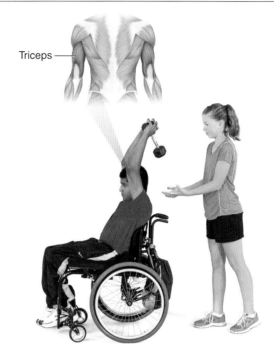

This exercise uses the muscles on the back of your upper arms (triceps).

BENT-OVER DUMBBELL ROW

Weights: dumbbell
This exercise requires no spotters.

1. Hold the dumbbell in one hand and rest your opposite hand and knee on a bench to support the weight of your trunk and protect your back.
2. Pull the dumbbell upward until it touches the side of your chest near your armpit and your upper arm is parallel to the floor.
3. Slowly lower the weight.
4. Repeat the exercise with your other arm. To determine your 1RM for this exercise, use the seated row.

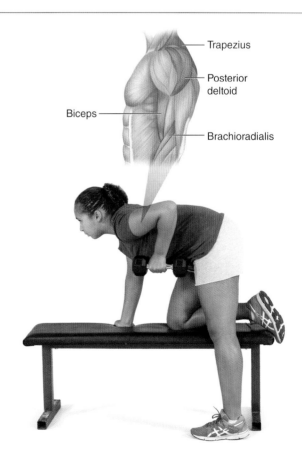

This exercise uses your biceps muscles, your shoulder muscles, and the muscles between your shoulder blades.

RESISTANCE MACHINE EXERCISES

The following basic exercises use resistance machines to work the major muscle groups. They can be used to determine your 1RM for each muscle group just as you determined your 1RM for the seated arm press and leg press in the self-assessment.

SEATED ARM PRESS

1. Sit on the stool of a seated press machine and position yourself so that the handles are even with your shoulders. Grasp the handles with your palms facing away from you. Tighten your abdominal muscles.

2. Push upward on the handles, extending your arms until your elbows are straight.
    Caution: Do not arch your back. Do not lock your elbows.

3. Lower the handles to the starting position.

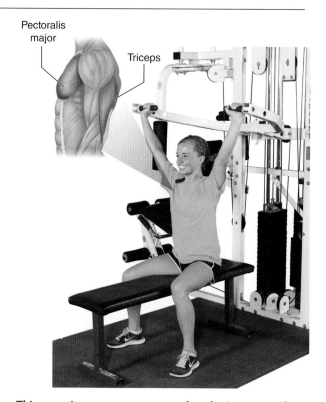

This exercise uses your pectoral and triceps muscles.

BENCH PRESS

1. Lie on your back on the bench with your feet flat on the floor. Grasp the handles with your palms facing away from your body. Flatten your back. If possible, place your feet on the floor to help flatten your back and avoid arching it. If your feet do not reach the floor easily, bend your knees and place your feet on the bench to accomplish the same purpose.
    Caution: Do not place your feet on the bench if it so narrow that your feet might slip off the bench or if the bench is unstable.

2. Push upward on the handles, extending your arms completely.
    Caution: Do not lock your elbows. Do not arch your back.

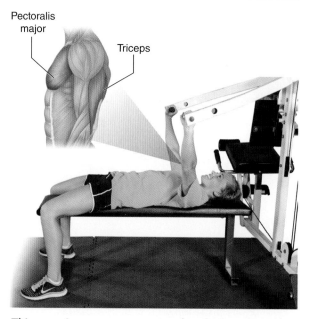

This exercise uses your pectoral and triceps muscles.

3. Return to the starting position.

4. You may choose either this exercise or the seated arm press. You may substitute this exercise in the self-assessment if you have a bench press machine and do not have a seated press machine.

SEATED LEG PRESS

1. Adjust the seat position on a leg press machine for your leg length. Sit with your feet resting on the pedal.

2. Push the pedal until your legs are straight.
   Caution: Do not lock your knees.

3. Slowly return to the starting position.

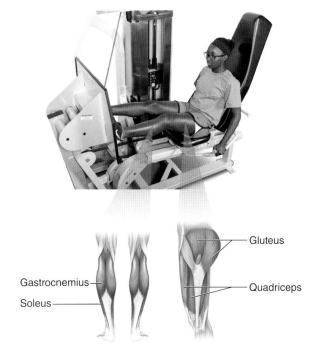

Gluteus

Gastrocnemius

Soleus

Quadriceps

This exercise uses the quadriceps, gluteal, and calf muscles.

KNEE EXTENSION

1. Sit on the bench and hook one of your ankles under the pad. Grasp the handles on the bench.

2. Extend your knee through its full range of motion.

3. Return to the starting position. Repeat the exercise with your other leg.

4. You may choose either this exercise or the seated leg press.

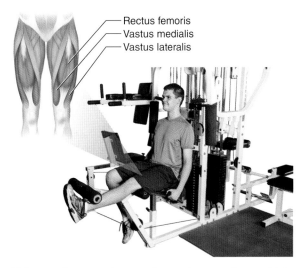

Rectus femoris
Vastus medialis
Vastus lateralis

This exercise uses the muscles at the top of your thighs (quadriceps). The fourth quadriceps muscle, the vastus intermedius, lies beneath the rectus femoris and therefore is not shown in the illustration.

HAMSTRING CURL

1. Lie facedown on the bench with your kneecaps extending over the edge of the bench. Hook your heels under the cylindrical pads. Grasp the handles on the bench.

   Caution: Do not lock your knees when putting your heels under the pads. If necessary, have a partner lift the pads so that you can avoid locking.

2. Bend your knees so that you can lift the cylindrical pads. Bend your knees through their full range of motion. At the top of the lift, the pads will almost touch your buttocks.

3. Lower to the starting position.

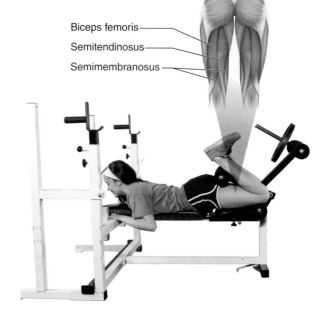

Biceps femoris
Semitendinosus
Semimembranosus

This exercise uses your hamstring muscles.

BICEPS CURL

1. Stand in front of the station and grasp the handle of the low pulley with your palms up. Tighten your abdominal muscles and buttocks (gluteal muscles).

2. Pull the handle from thigh level to chest level. Bend your elbows but keep them close to your sides.

   Caution: Do not move other body parts.

3. Return to the starting position.

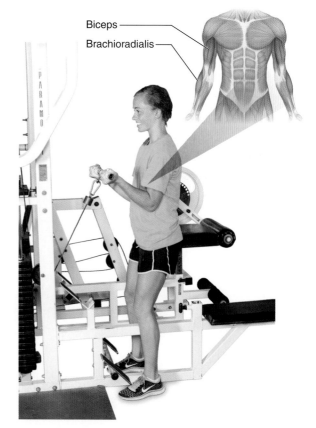

Biceps
Brachioradialis

This exercise uses your biceps and other elbow flexor muscles.

HEEL RAISE

1. Place a board that is 5 centimetres thick on the floor. Stand with the balls of your feet on the board and the handles even with your shoulders.
2. Grasp the handles with your palms facing away from your body. Keep your hands and arms stationary during the lift.
3. Rise onto the balls of your feet, then lower to the starting position.

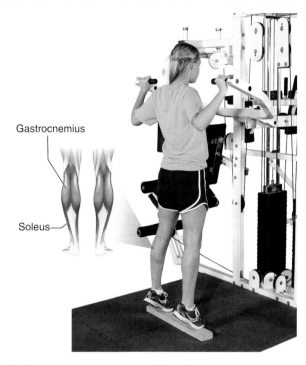

This exercise uses your calf muscles.

LAT PULL-DOWN

1. Sit on the bench (or floor, depending on the machine). Adjust the seat height so that your arms are fully extended when you grab the bar.
2. Grab the bar with your palms facing away from you. Your arms should be at least shoulder-width apart.
3. Pull the bar down to chest level.
4. Return to the starting position.

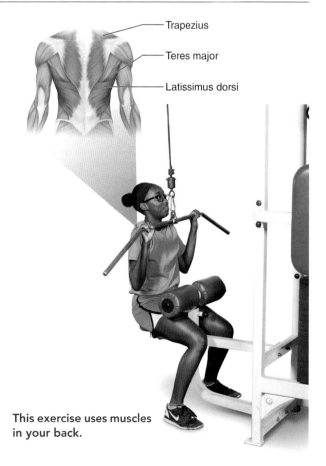

This exercise uses muscles in your back.

TRICEPS PRESS

1. With your palms facing away from you, grab the handles.

   Note: If performed while sitting, adjust the seat height so that your hands are on the handles just above shoulder height.

2. Keep your elbows by your sides, and avoid leaning forward with your body.

3. Keeping your back straight, push forward and down with your arms until they are straight.

4. Return to the starting position.

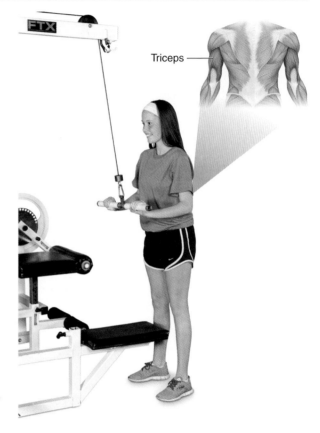

Triceps

This exercise uses the muscles on the back of your arms (triceps).

SEATED ROW

1. Adjust the machine so that your arms are almost fully extended and are parallel to the ground.

2. Grab the handles with your thumbs up.

3. Keeping your back straight, pull straight back toward your chest.

4. Return to the starting position.

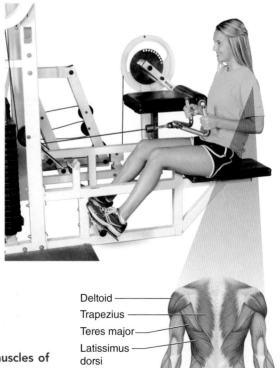

Deltoid
Trapezius
Teres major
Latissimus dorsi

This exercise uses the muscles of your back and shoulders.

ISOMETRIC EXERCISES

The following basic isometric exercises work your major muscle groups.

HAND PUSH

1. Sit in a sturdy chair, on a bench, or on the floor with your back straight. You may cross your legs if you prefer. Place the palms of your hands together.

2. Raise your hands and elbows to shoulder height. Push your hands against each other as hard as you can. Hold the position for 7 seconds; rest for 30 seconds.

3. Do two or three reps as time allows.

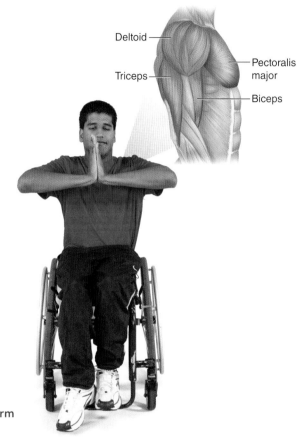

This exercise uses your arm and shoulder muscles.

BACK FLATTENER

1. Lie on your back with your knees bent.

2. Pull in your abdomen by contracting your abdominal muscles as tightly as possible. Flatten your lower back against the floor. Hold the position for 7 seconds; rest for 30 seconds.

3. Do two or three reps as time allows.

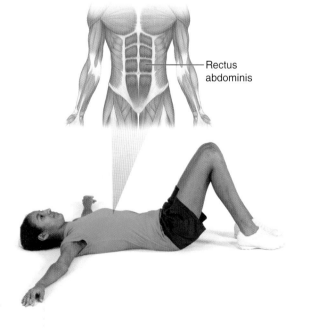

This exercise uses your abdominal muscles.

KNEE EXTENDER

1. Hold on to something for support and stand on your left foot. Lift your right foot behind you, bending your knee to a 90-degree angle.

2. Loop a towel under your right ankle; hold the ends of the towel in your right hand.

3. Push downward with your foot, trying to straighten your leg against the resistance of the towel.

4. Repeat the exercise two or three times with each leg as time allows.

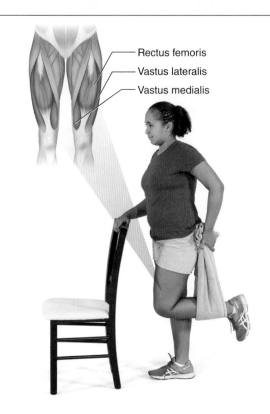

Rectus femoris
Vastus lateralis
Vastus medialis

This exercise uses the muscles on the front of your thighs (quadriceps). The fourth quadriceps muscle, the vastus intermedius, lies beneath the rectus femoris and therefore is not shown in the illustration.

WALL PUSH

1. Stand with your back against a wall.

2. Move your feet out as you lower yourself into a half squat. Keep your thighs parallel to the floor.

3. Push your back against the wall by pushing with your legs as hard as you can. Hold the position for 7 seconds; rest for 30 seconds.

4. Do two or three reps as time allows.

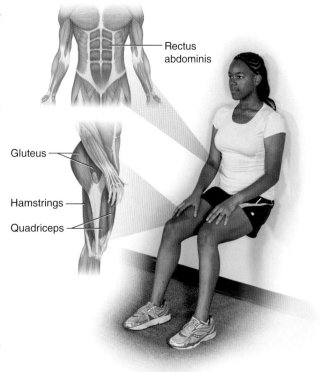

Rectus abdominis

Gluteus

Hamstrings

Quadriceps

This exercise uses the muscles of your legs and abdomen.

BICEPS CURL WITH TOWEL

1. Stand with your back straight and your knees slightly bent.
2. Loop a towel under the back of your thighs.
3. Grasp the towel ends with your palms up. Keep your elbows against your sides.
4. Pull up on the towel as hard as possible. Hold the position for 7 seconds; rest for 30 seconds.
5. Do two or three reps as time allows.

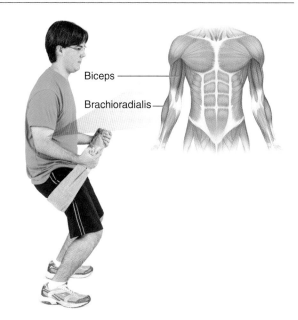

This exercise uses the muscles on the front of your upper arms (biceps).

TOE PUSH

1. Sit on the floor using good posture.
2. Hold the end of a jump rope or towel in each hand. Loop it over the balls of your feet so that it is tight against your soles.
3. Push with the balls of your feet as you pull on the rope or towel. Keep your back straight. Hold the position for 7 seconds; rest for 30 seconds.
4. Do two or three reps as time allows.

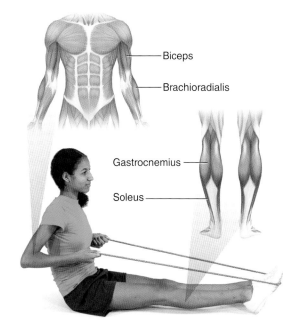

This exercise uses the muscles of your arms and lower legs.

LEG CURL

1. Stand on your left leg. Hold on to a chair or wall for balance.
2. Loop a towel behind your right ankle and stand on the ends of the towel with your left foot.
3. Keeping your posture erect and your back straight, try to bend your knee against the resistance of the towel. Hold the position for 7 seconds; rest for 30 seconds.
4. Do two or three reps with each leg as time allows.

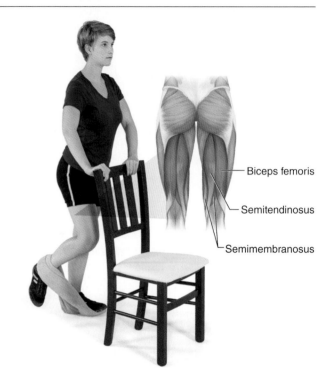

Biceps femoris

Semitendinosus

Semimembranosus

This exercise uses your hamstring muscles.

BOW EXERCISE

1. Stand in a position that an archer would take when shooting a bow.
2. Hold a towel with your right arm as if you were holding a bow.
3. Hold the other end of the towel with your left hand near your chin as if you were holding the string of the bow.
4. Push with your right hand and pull with your left hand. Hold the position for 7 seconds; rest for 30 seconds.
5. Do two or three reps with each arm forward as time allows.

Safety tip: Breathe normally while doing these exercises. Do not hold your breath. Holding your breath can cause dizziness and possibly a blackout.

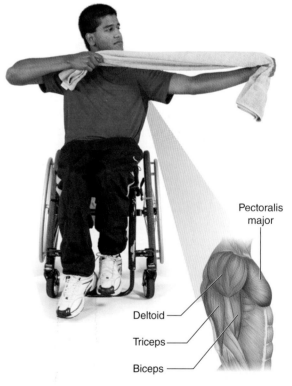

Pectoralis major

Deltoid

Triceps

Biceps

This exercise uses the muscles of your arms and shoulders.

TAKING CHARGE: Overcoming Barriers

When people face a problem beyond their control, they sometimes use it as an excuse for not being physically active. Someone might say, "I'm too short to be a basketball player, so I'm not going to try out for any sports." To be physically active, focus not on what you can't change but on what you *can* do.

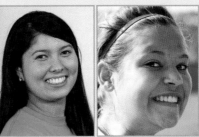

Connie stood at the window. "It's pouring out there! How can we go hiking?"

Bridgette sighed. "I guess we're stuck spending the afternoon here."

Yesterday it was too hot to go hiking; now it was too rainy. It seemed as if they were never going to have good weather. But the weather was not the only problem. The last time they tried hiking, it was sunny, but the paths were too crowded.

"I bet Alonzo is at the athletic club right now," Bridgette said. "He can exercise no matter what the weather is. I wish we could afford to go there!"

Connie glanced down at her sweats. "I'd need to buy more than a membership to go there. They wear expensive exercise clothes at that club. I'd get laughed out of the place in these clothes."

Bridgette smiled. "You don't look so bad—and the rain's starting to let up now. What if we put on older clothes, take rain gear, and hike around the park for a while?"

"You're right! So what if we get a little damp?"

For Discussion

What reasons do Connie and Bridgette give for not being active? Which of these problems can they control? They eventually decide not to let the weather stop them; what other strategies could they use to cope with the problems they've identified? Consider the guidelines in the Self-Management feature when answering the discussion questions.

SELF-MANAGEMENT: Skills for Overcoming Barriers

People face many barriers to becoming and staying active. Some barriers involve the environment (such as areas unsafe for exercise, lack of nearby exercise facilities, bad weather, expense); some involve personal physical characteristics (lack of physical size or skill); and some are psychological (low self-confidence, perceived lack of time). People who are active throughout life overcome such barriers, and programs have been developed to help people overcome barriers. Use the following strategies to overcome the barriers you face.

- **Find a way to exercise at home or at school.** If parks, fitness clubs, and other places for exercise are too expensive, too far away, or unsafe, find another way to exercise. Buy some equipment that you can use at home. If possible, use school facilities to exercise before or after school. Start a fitness club at school and ask school officials to help you find facilities and equipment.

- **Develop alternate plans.** Make multiple plans for activity. That way, for example,

if you plan to play tennis and it rains, you can switch to your alternate plan, which might be an indoor activity. If something interferes with your planned exercise time, find another time.

- **Get active in community or school affairs.** Many communities have developed community centres; trails for biking, walking, and jogging; and other recreational facilities, such as tennis courts, basketball courts, and sport fields. If these options are not available in your community, write to your city or county officials or contact school officials and see what you can help create.

- **Use self-management skills to develop realistic plans that you will stick with.** Practice skills such as goal setting, program planning, self-monitoring, and time management.

- **Develop a new way of thinking.** Accept yourself as you are. If negative self-talk is an issue, use the strategies presented in this book to adjust your self-perceptions and boost your self-confidence.

If you're just starting a muscle fitness program, you may want to begin by using resistance machines at your school or local recreation centre. Developing muscle fitness through resistance training will build your muscle mass and bone density and can help you develop a healthy body composition. Muscle fitness can also help you look your best and make it easier for you to perform everyday tasks, such as climbing stairs, opening food jars, and carrying your backpack. In addition, developing muscle fitness through resistance training helps you perform your best at your favourite sport and other physical activities.

Take action by trying some resistance machine exercises that you've learned in this chapter. Be sure to follow the guidelines for PRE described in the chapter.

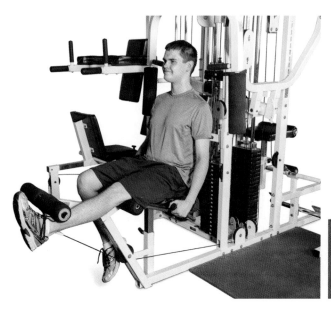
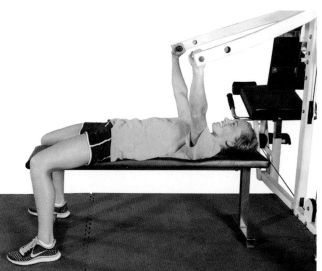

You can take action by doing PRE on resistance machines.

canfitpro GET ACTIVE WITH CANFITPRO

©canfitpro

Who We Are

Canfitpro is the largest provider of education in the Canadian fitness industry and inspires healthy living through fitness education. Founded in 1993, canfitpro delivers accessible, high-quality education, certifications, conferences, trade shows, and membership services. Canfitpro's more than 100,000 members include some of the world's finest fitness professionals, health club operators, industry suppliers, and fitness consumers.

What We Do

Canfitpro is a member-based fitness education organization, delivering cutting-edge experiences to individuals and groups. We provide affordable and attainable fitness education to help you begin your journey into fitness as well as continue it as your experience grows. From membership to our foundational certification programs to the canfitpro world fitness expo held every summer in Toronto, canfitpro has grown to be the largest and most successful fitness education organization per capita in the world, and we want you to be part of our growing family.

Get Involved

You can become a student member of canfitpro and work toward your certification as well as attend one of our live events held in almost every major city across Canada. Visit www.canfitpro.com or find us on social media to get started. Fitness is your passion, so make it your career and join us in inspiring healthy living through fitness education!

Reprinted, by permission, from Rod Macdonald, canfitpro.

Reviewing Concepts and Vocabulary

Complete the following in order for you to show your growing understanding of fitness, health, and wellness. Answer items 1 through 5 by correctly completing each sentence with a word or phrase.

1. _____ is the amount of force a muscle can exert.
2. _____ refers to an increase in muscle fibre size.
3. A person can become _____ if he or she does strength training improperly by developing some muscles while ignoring others.
4. When you do calisthenics to develop strength, you use your body weight as the _____.
5. The _____ system refers to altering reps, sets, and weight as muscle fitness improves.

For items 6 through 10, as directed by your teacher, match each term in column 1 with the appropriate phrase in column 2.

6. isokinetic exercise
7. Olympic-style weightlifting
8. 1RM
9. plyometrics
10. isotonic exercise

a. a sport, not an exercise program
b. the maximum weight that a person can lift once
c. exercise that requires a special machine
d. muscle fitness exercise that involves movement
e. exercise that builds power

For items 11 through 15, respond to each statement or question.

11. How do strong muscles help you look better and prevent health problems?
12. Describe several methods for testing muscle fitness discussed in this chapter.
13. Describe two myths about muscle fitness exercise.
14. Describe several guidelines for overcoming barriers.
15. Discuss the guidelines for using PRE effectively and safely.

Thinking Critically

Go to the student section of the Fitness for Life Canada website for this chapter. The address is on the first page of this chapter. Using information provided there and in this chapter, write a short article about muscle fitness for high school students. You can find additional information on the CSEP website by clicking on the Position Stands link under the Education tab. Look for the position stand on resistance training in children and adolescents. Share your article with your class or submit it to the school newspaper for publication.

Project

Some schools provide wellness programs for teachers and other school employees. Typical offerings include exercise classes before and after school, fitness assessments, and classes in nutrition and stress reduction. Plan a special activity for teachers or some family members and friends addressing one of these topics as it relates to muscle fitness. Prepare a written plan and work with other students to carry it out.

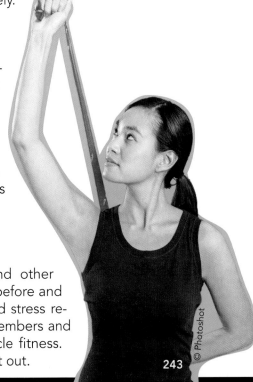

© Photoshot

11

Muscle Fitness Applications

In This Chapter

LESSON 11.1
Core Fitness, Posture, and Back Care

SELF-ASSESSMENT
Healthy Back Test and Assessing Posture

LESSON 11.2
Ergogenic Aids and Preparing a Muscle Fitness Plan

TAKING CHARGE
Preventing Relapse

SELF-MANAGEMENT
Skills for Preventing Relapse

TAKING ACTION
Your Muscle Fitness Exercise Plan

GET ACTIVE WITH HOCKEY CANADA

CHAPTER REVIEW

 Student Web Resources
www.fitnessforlife.org/student

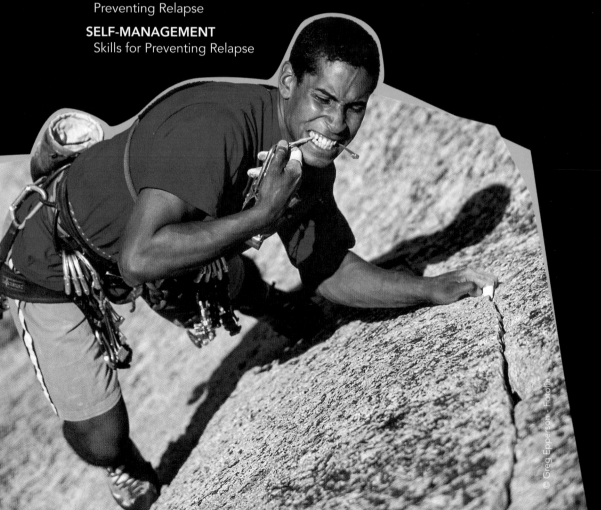

© Greg Epperson—Fotolia

Lesson 11.1

Core Fitness, Posture, and Back Care

Lesson Objectives

After participating in this lesson, you should be able to

1. name several core muscles and types of core muscle exercises and explain why they are important,
2. describe some common back and posture problems, and
3. list some biomechanical principles that can help you improve your posture and avoid back problems.

Lesson Vocabulary

force, kyphosis, laws of motion, lordosis, Pilates, ptosis

Do you know what core fitness is? Do you know what level your core fitness is at and how to improve it? In this lesson, you'll learn about your core muscles and why they are important for good health and functioning. You'll also learn about exercises, including core muscle exercises that you can perform to improve your posture and reduce your risk of back pain and injuries in other muscles.

Core Muscles

Your core muscles support your spine, keep your rib cage and pelvis stable, and help you maintain a healthy posture while standing, sitting, and moving in a variety of body positions. They also are the muscles that connect the upper and lower parts of your body. They include the muscles of your back, hips and pelvis, and abdominal area (see figure 11.1).

It's not uncommon for people to neglect their core muscles and focus more on muscles in their arms, legs, and shoulders because these muscles are easily seen and are considered to be important especially by young people. But you need fit core muscles—not only for healthy living and performing the tasks of daily life but also for performing sport- and work-related activities and preventing injury. Core fitness allows you to keep your trunk stable while performing lifting and movements of all types. Some basic core exercises are presented at the end of this lesson.

Exercises that use resistance machines or free weights often do not build your abdominal muscles and some other core muscles. Because core exercises are an important part of a total muscle fitness

program, they are performed in addition to other progressive resistance exercises (PRE).

Many core exercises can be done without special equipment, and others can be done with inexpensive equipment. For example, you can improve core muscle fitness by exercising with large balls inflated with air. Exercises done with these balls are sometimes called stability ball exercises because physiotherapists use them to help people build muscles that stabilize the body. You can also build your core muscles by doing medicine ball exercises.

FIT FACT

Pilates is a form of training designed to build core muscle fitness that has become quite popular in recent years. It is named for Joseph Pilates, who described core exercises and developed special exercise machines for building the core muscles. However, a recent U.S. court ruling declared that the term "Pilates" is a generic name like yoga and karate, which means that anyone can call him- or herself a Pilates expert even without special training. As a result, although many Pilates instructors may be quite knowledgeable about exercises, others may not. Some Pilates programs have been modified in ways that are inconsistent with Pilates' original principles. When done properly, Pilates is a good way to build and maintain core muscle fitness.

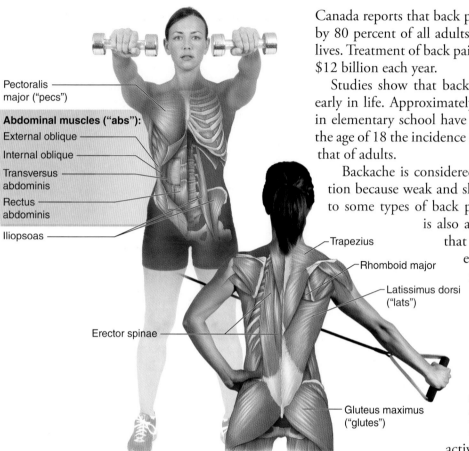

Pectoralis
major ("pecs")

Abdominal muscles ("abs"):

External oblique

Internal oblique

Transversus
abdominis

Rectus
abdominis

Iliopsoas

Erector spinae

Trapezius

Rhomboid major

Latissimus dorsi
("lats")

Gluteus maximus
("glutes")

FIGURE 11.1 The core muscles.

Back Problems

Have you ever had a sore back after sitting for a long time or lifting heavy objects? These are two contributing factors to back pain. Another factor is poor core fitness. Back pain is one of the most common chronic conditions in Canada. Statistics Canada reports that back pain will be experienced by 80 percent of all adults at some point in their lives. Treatment of back pain costs between $6 and $12 billion each year.

Studies show that back problems often begin early in life. Approximately one-third of children in elementary school have had back pain, and by the age of 18 the incidence rate of back pain is near that of adults.

Backache is considered a hypokinetic condition because weak and short muscles are linked to some types of back problems. Poor posture is also associated with muscles that are not strong or long enough. By building fit muscles to improve your posture, you can help reduce your risk of back pain and look your best. Even if you never experience back pain, a healthy back and good posture help you function more efficiently in your daily activities.

How does good fitness help your back operate efficiently? Good biomechanics are important. Your body parts are balanced like blocks on your legs. Your chest hangs from your spine and is balanced over your pelvis. Your head sits on top of your spine, balanced over the other blocks in the stack. Because your spine is flexible and can move back and forth, the pull of your muscles keeps your body parts balanced. If your muscles on one side are weak and long but your muscles on the

---

 FITNESS TECHNOLOGY: Exercise Machines With Memory

Computer technology now allows exercise machines at fitness clubs to "memorize" your exercises. The machine stores your resistance amount for each exercise, making it easy to quickly prepare for each exercise. The machine also stores the number of sets and repetitions you perform for each exercise. You can also install fitness apps on a cell phone, tablet, or other personal computer to help you keep your own record of your exercises that do not require machines (for example, core exercises).

Using Technology

Identify and describe an exercise machine or app that can be used to self-monitor muscle fitness exercise.

opposite side are strong and short, your body parts are pulled off balance.

One back problem that often occurs among teens is **lordosis**, in which the lower back has too much arch. Also called swayback, lordosis results when the core muscles, particularly the abdominal muscles, are weak and the hip flexor muscles (iliopsoas) are too short (see figure 11.2). Lordosis can lead to backache.

Even people who are relatively fit in other areas can lack fitness in the muscles related to back problems. One reason for this lack of fitness is that sports and games often overdevelop some muscles and neglect others. As a result, it is not unusual for basketball players, gymnasts, band members, and other active people to have weak back and abdominal muscles (core muscles) and short hamstrings and hip flexors.

Posture Problems

Figure 11.2*a* illustrates some of the common posture problems associated with poor core fitness. Some of the most common are lordosis, **ptosis** (protruding abdomen), and **kyphosis** (rounded back and shoulders). You might recognize these problems in your own posture or that of someone you know. In figure 11.2*b,* you can see which muscles contribute to posture problems if they are too short or weak. Figure 11.2*c* shows you what good posture looks like and illustrates how it depends on long, strong muscles. Just as strong, long muscles contribute to a healthy back, they also are important for good posture.

Knowing what constitutes good posture can help you improve your own posture. And good posture helps you look good, helps prevent back problems, and helps you work and play more efficiently.

Back and Posture Improvement and Maintenance

You can take several steps to help yourself enjoy good back health. First, you can perform self-assessments to determine your current back health and posture status. You can then identify exercises that will help you develop or maintain the muscle fitness and flexibility necessary for good back health and good posture. You can also use key principles of biomechanics to prevent back pain and injury.

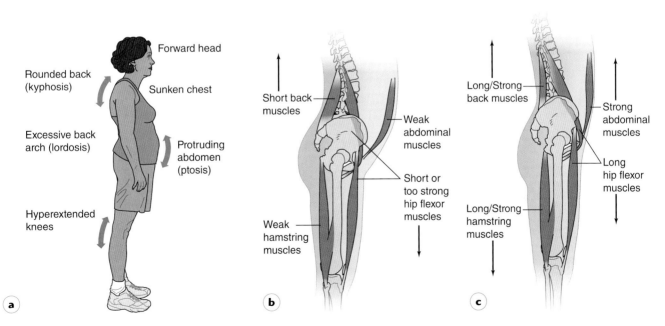

FIGURE 11.2 *(a)* Problems associated with poor posture; *(b)* core muscles in poor posture; *(c)* core muscles in good posture.

FIT FACT

Many teens wear backpacks. To carry a backpack effectively, you need adequate strength and muscular endurance. In a typical year, the U.S. Consumer Product Safety Commission reports more than 6,000 backpack-related injuries, mostly among youth. Improving your muscle fitness can help you reduce your risk of injury from wearing a backpack.

Healthy Back Test

In the Self-Assessment feature at the end of this lesson, you'll get the opportunity to take the healthy back test. This will help you determine what you can do to keep your back fit and healthy. Core exercises are especially good for back health and for maintaining good posture. Stretching exercises are also commonly recommended.

As shown in figure 11.2c, strong and long muscles help you avoid posture problems. The problems shown in figure 11.2a and 11.2b are not present in a healthy posture. The head is centred over the shoulders, the shoulders are back and balanced, the low back has a gentle curve, the abdomen does not protrude, and the knees do not bend backward.

In this chapter's self-assessment you can work with a partner and evaluate your posture to see whether problems exist and whether your body is in proper alignment.

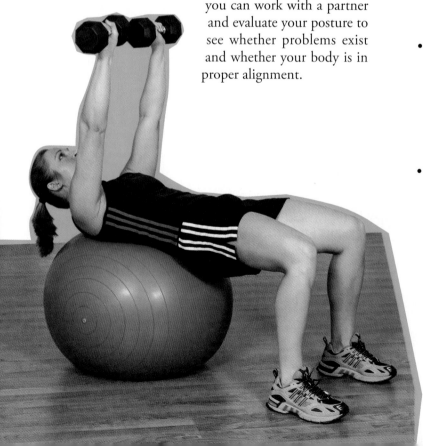

Biomechanical Principles for Lifting, Carrying, and Moving Objects

For good health and safety, avoid exercises that violate the principles of biomechanics. As shown in the Science in Action feature, these principles and **laws of motion** apply when you use your body's levers—the bones of your arms and legs—to apply **force** in lifting, carrying, and moving objects. The most frequent use of these levers occurs when you walk or run or perform skills such as throwing, jumping, kicking, and striking. Using your body levers efficiently is also important in applying force when you perform resistance exercises. Use the following biomechanical principles to help you avoid injury and back problems.

- **Use your large muscles when lifting.** Let your strong leg muscles—not your relatively weak back muscles—do the work.

- **Keep your weight (hips) low.** To make lifting safer, keep your weight low by squatting (bending your knees) with your back straight and your hips tucked.

- **Keep your core muscles firm when lifting.** Tighten your abdominal and back muscles to stabilize your body.

- **Use a wide base of support for balance.** Keep your feet spread about shoulder-width apart for stability when lifting.

- **Avoid a bent-over position when sitting, standing, or lifting.** Your body's levers, such as your spine, do not work efficiently when you are bent over. When sitting in a chair, sit back in the seat and lean against the backrest. Do not work for long periods of time in a bent-over position.

- **Divide a load to make it easier to carry.** For example, carrying two small suitcases, one in each hand, is easier than carrying one larger suitcase in one hand. A backpack is an efficient way to carry books. It's best to carry the backpack using both straps rather than over one shoulder. Avoid overloading your backpack or book bag. If you must carry your books in your arms, carry some in each arm. If you do carry your books in one arm, change arms from time to time.

SCIENCE IN ACTION: The Mechanics of Lifting

Kinesiology experts who study biomechanics have shown that lifting with your back rather than with your legs is inefficient and can be dangerous. The most efficient way to lift is to use your leg muscles and keep the weight near your body (see figure 11.3*a*). When you bend at your waist while lifting, you use your back muscles rather than your stronger leg muscles, and you greatly increase the amount of force necessary to lift the object (figure 11.3*b*). The same is true when you reach while lifting (figure 11.3*c*). These points are illustrated in the following example.

In figure 11.3*a*, a weight is held near the body. When the weight is lifted by using the leg muscles with the back straight, the force needed to do the lifting is only slightly more than the weight of the load itself because the load is held near the body. In figure 11.3*b*, lifting the same weight requires up to 50 times as much force because the lifter has to lift the weight of the upper body and because the necessary force is magnified when the weight is positioned at the end of a long lever. The longer the lever, the more the force is magnified. If a person reaches to lift (figure 11.3*c*), the necessary force is even greater because of the increased length of the lever.

The extra force needed for incorrect lifting puts unnecessary stress on the muscles and causes compression of the discs and bones, especially in the lower back. Incorrect lifting (figure 11.3, *b* and *c*) also requires the lifter to use the back muscles rather than the stronger leg muscles, thus increasing the risk of injury. To reduce your risk of injury due to incorrect lifting, follow the principles described in the section on biomechanics.

As previously mentioned, it is best to use the stronger leg muscles rather than the weaker back muscles when lifting. It's also important to avoid bending at the waist when lifting. However, you need to improve fitness of the back muscles (back extensors) for back health and normal functioning in daily life. To build the back muscles, exercises such as the trunk lift and some forms of the leg lift are appropriate even though they use inefficient movements. The key is to perform the exercises in a controlled manner with appropriate resistance. To remind you how to perform these exercises safely, caution statements are provided for these exercises.

Student Activity

What are some real-life actions that could put you at risk of injury due to movements that use your body's levers poorly? After listing at least three actions that could put you at risk of injury, discuss in detail what you could do to prevent this risk when performing these movements.

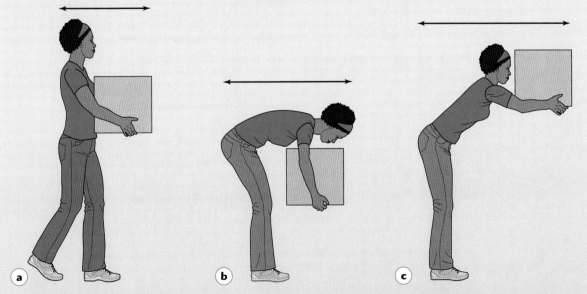

Figure 11.3 For efficiency, *(a)* lift with the weight close to the body. *(b)* Avoid bending forward at the waist or *(c)* reaching while lifting because the longer levers increase stress on the back.

• **Avoid twisting while lifting.** If you have to turn while lifting, change the position of your feet. It's especially important to avoid twisting your spine as you are straightening or bending it.

• **Push or pull heavy objects.** Heavy lifting can cause injury. Pushing or pulling an object is more efficient than lifting it.

Stretching

Healthy back care and good posture also depend on flexibility. Several good exercises are the knee to chest, the hip stretch, the back-saver sit and reach, and the back and hip stretch. Your instructor can show you these exercises when you study flexibility.

Calisthenics

Calisthenics are exercises that use all or part of your body weight to provide resistance—for example, the core exercises illustrated at the end of this lesson. Calisthenics for muscle fitness in your limbs are presented at the end of this lesson. Calisthenics build strength, and because they use body weight and typically involve multiple repetitions, they also build muscular endurance. As well, because they require your body weight you can do them anywhere and without equipment. This is the FIT formula for calisthenics:

• **F:** three to six days a week
• **I:** lift part or all of the body weight
• **T:** one to three sets of 10 to 25 reps

Calisthenics that involve explosive movement such as jumping build power and should adhere to the FIT formula for plyometrics (table 10.11).

Progressive Resistance Exercise and Injury

Experts have now determined that when PRE is performed properly and with good supervision, it is safe for teens. However, even when done properly, there is a risk of injury when you are performing both PRE and lifting sports such as weightlifting. The most frequent injury among school athletes performing PRE is back injury, especially in the low back. However, the National Strength and Conditioning Association indicates that "this risk is no greater than [the risk in] many other sports and recreational activities in which children and adolescents regularly participate." For example, studies show that the average injury rate in youth sports, especially contact sports, is much higher than for PRE. The risk of injury from PRE performed at home is much higher than the risk of PRE done in schools, primarily because of better supervision, better equipment, and required use of spotters at school.

Preventing a back injury is much easier than repairing one.

—U.S. Occupational Safety and Health Administration (OSHA)

Some injuries associated with PRE are not immediately noticeable. As a result, when cautioned about improper lifting or using incorrect biomechanics, people might say, "I've done that before and it didn't cause a problem." But we know that repeated small injuries (microtraumas) can lead to big injuries later. Many people who ignore biomechanical guidelines eventually experience injuries and say "I wish I hadn't done that."

Lesson Review

1. Name three areas of the body that contain core muscles. Name five or more core muscles and describe three or more types of exercises for building core muscles. Explain why it is important to keep those muscles fit.

2. What are some common back and posture problems? What can you do to prevent or correct these problems in yourself or others?

3. What are some biomechanical principles that can help you improve your posture and avoid back problems?

CORE MUSCLE FITNESS EXERCISES

CURL-UP

The curl-up is considered to be among the best abdominal exercises because it isn't risky like some other abdominal exercises. The curl-up is sometimes referred to as the crunch, and it's a good substitute for the straight-leg sit-up and hands-behind-the-head sit-up.

1. Lie on your back with your knees bent at 90 degrees and your arms extended.
2. Curl up by rolling your head, shoulders, and upper back off the floor. Roll up only until your shoulder blades leave the floor.
3. With a controlled motion, slowly return to the starting position and repeat.

Caution: Do not hold your feet while doing a trunk curl. Do not clench your hands behind the head or neck.

Variations

- **Arms across chest or hands by face (more difficult):** Fold your hands across your chest rather than keeping them

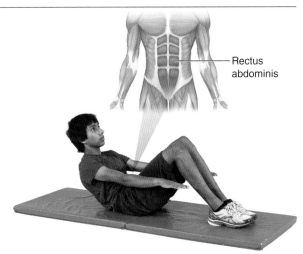

Rectus abdominis

This exercise uses your abdominal muscles.

straight, or place your hands on your face by your cheeks (not behind your head or neck).

- **Twist curl (builds oblique muscles):** Fold your arms across your chest, turn your trunk to the left, and touch your right elbow to your left hip. Repeat to the opposite side.

TRUNK LIFT (BENCH)

1. Lie facedown on a padded bench (or a bleacher with a towel on it) that is 41 to 46 centimetres (16 to 18 inches) high. Your upper body (from your waist up) should extend off the bench.
2. Have your partner hold your calves just below the knees.
3. Place one hand over the other on your forehead with your palms facing away and your elbows held to the side at the level of your ears.
4. Start with your upper body lowered. Lift slowly until your upper body is even with the bench (in line with your legs).
   Caution: Do not lift the trunk higher than horizontal.
5. With a controlled movement, lower to the beginning position and repeat.

Safety tip: As you do these exercises, lift slowly, move only as far as the directions specify, and use slow, controlled movements to return to the starting position. This exercise is appropri-

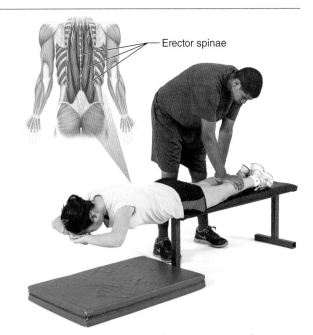

Erector spinae

This exercise uses your back extensor muscles.

ate when performed properly; but as noted earlier, using the trunk muscles for lifting or carrying is not recommended.

TRUNK LIFT (FLOOR)

1. Lie facedown with your hands clasped behind your neck.

2. Pull your shoulder blades together, raise your elbows off the floor, and then lift your head and chest off the floor. Arch your upper back until your breastbone (sternum) clears the floor. You may need to hook your feet under a bar or have someone hold your feet down.

   Caution: Do not lift your chin more than 30 centimetres (12 inches) off the floor. This exercise is appropriate when performed properly; but as noted earlier, using the trunk muscles for lifting or carrying is not recommended.

3. Lower your trunk and repeat the exercise.

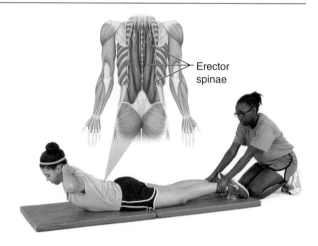

This exercise develops the muscles of your upper back and helps prevent "humpback."

ARM AND LEG LIFT

1. Lie facedown with your arms stretched in front of you.

2. Raise your right arm, then lower it. Raise your left arm, then lower it. Finally, raise both arms, then lower them.

3. Raise your right leg, then lower it. Raise your left leg, then lower it.

4. Raise your right arm and right leg, then lower them. Raise your left arm and left leg, then lower them.

5. Raise your left arm and right leg, then lower them. Raise your right arm and left leg, then lower them.

Caution: Do not arch your back during this exercise.

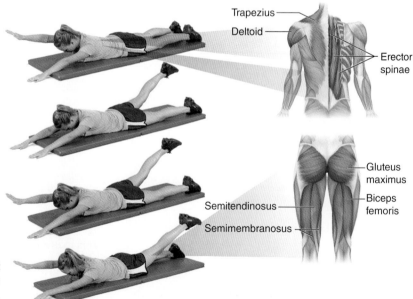

This exercise helps prevent rounded shoulders, sunken chest, and rounded upper back.

BRIDGING

1. Lie on your back with your knees bent and your feet close to your buttocks.
2. Contract your gluteal muscles. Lift your buttocks and raise your back off the floor until your hip joint has no bend.
   Caution: Do not overarch your lower back.
3. Lower your hips to the floor and repeat the exercise.

This exercise develops the muscles of your buttocks (gluteal) and the muscles on the back of your thighs (hamstrings).

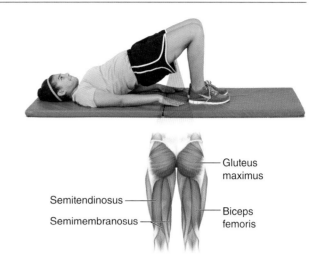

Gluteus maximus
Semitendinosus
Semimembranosus
Biceps femoris

SIDE PLANK

1. From a right-facing, side-lying position on a mat or carpet, lift your body into a side support position, supporting your body weight on your right forearm and your feet. Your left is arm bent and on your left hip. Tighten your abdominal and back muscles.
2. Keep your hips in line with your body. Hold this position for 7 to 10 seconds.
3. Repeat facing to the left.

This exercise develops the abdominal muscles and back muscles.

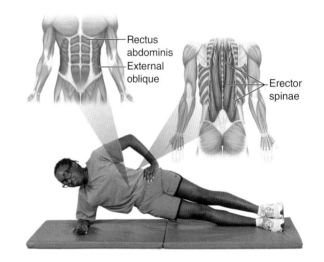

Rectus abdominis
External oblique
Erector spinae

REVERSE CURL

1. Lie on your back. Bend your knees, placing your feet flat on the floor. Place your arms at your sides.
2. Lift your knees to your chest, raising your hips off the floor.
3. Return to the starting position. Repeat the exercise up to 10 times.

This exercise develops your abdominal muscles.

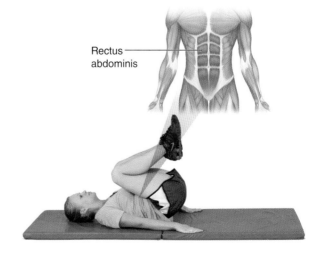

Rectus abdominis

FRONT PLANK

1. On a mat or carpet, support your body with your forearms and toes.
2. Keep your head in line with your body. Hold this position for 7 to 10 seconds.

Variations

- **Less difficult:** Support your body with your knees rather than your feet.
- **More difficult:** Perform the same exercise in the full push-up position.

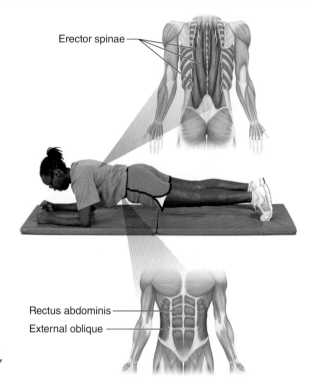

Erector spinae

Rectus abdominis

External oblique

This exercise develops the abdominal, buttock, and back muscles.

DOUBLE-LEG LIFT (BENCH OR TABLE)

1. Lie facedown on a bench (or table that will safely support your body weight and movements) with your legs extending off the end. With a partner holding your upper body, lower your legs to the ground. If you have no partner, grasp under the edge of the table.
2. Lift your legs slowly until they are even with the top of the table.
   Caution: Do not lift any higher. If necessary, lift one leg at a time until you are able to lift both legs at once.
3. Lower to the starting position.

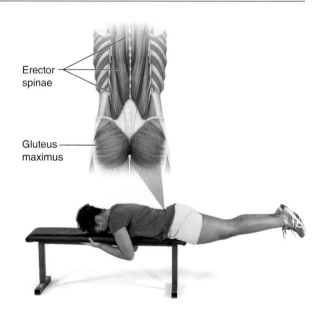

Erector spinae

Gluteus maximus

This exercise strengthens your lower back and gluteal muscles.

PUSH-UP

1. Lie facedown on a mat or carpet with your hands under your shoulders, your fingers spread, and your legs straight. Your legs should be slightly apart and your toes should be tucked under.

2. Push up until your arms are straight. Keep your legs and back straight. Your body should form a straight line.

3. Lower your body by bending your elbows until your upper arms are parallel to the floor (elbows bent at a 90-degree angle). Then push up until your arms are fully extended. Repeat, alternating between the fully extended and the 90-degree arm positions.

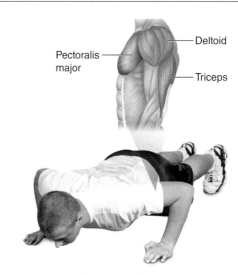

This exercise develops your chest muscles (pectorals) and the muscle (triceps) on the back of your upper arms.

KNEE PUSH-UP

1. If you cannot complete 20 reps of the 90-degree push-up, try this version. Lie facedown with your hands placed under your shoulders.

2. Push up, keeping your body rigid, until your arms are straight, but keep your knees on the floor.

3. Keep your body rigid (i.e., contract abdominal muscles throughout the motion), and lower it until your chest touches the floor.

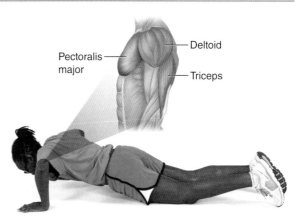

This exercise develops your chest muscles (pectorals) and the muscle (triceps) on the back of your upper arms.

PRONE ARM LIFT

1. Lie facedown on the floor with your arms extended and held against your ears.

2. Keep your forehead and chest on the floor and lift your arms so that your hands are 15 centimetres (6 inches) off the floor.

3. Lower your arms, then repeat the exercise. Keep your arms touching your ears and keep your elbows straight.

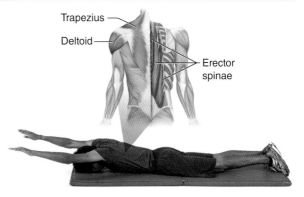

This exercise develops the muscles of your back and shoulders.

STRIDE JUMP

1. Stand with your left leg forward and your right leg back. Hold your right arm at shoulder height straight in front of your body and your left arm straight behind you.

2. Jump and move your right foot forward and your left foot back. As your feet change places, your arms switch positions. Keep your feet 45 to 60 centimetres (about 18 to 24 inches) apart.

3. Continue jumping, alternating your feet and arms. Count one rep each time your left foot moves forward.

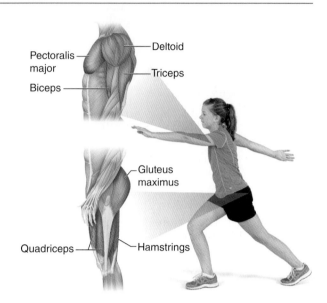

This exercise develops the muscles of your legs and arms as well as cardiorespiratory endurance and power.

SIDE LEG LIFT

1. Lie on your right side. Use your arms for balance.

2. Lift your top (left) leg 45 degrees. Keep your kneecap pointing forward and your ankle pointing toward the ceiling. If your leg rotates so that your knee points upward, you will work the wrong muscles.

3. Lower your leg. Repeat the movement. To increase intensity, you can use an ankle weight.

4. Roll over and repeat the exercise with your right leg.

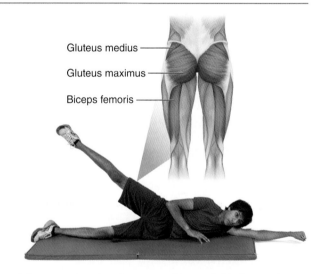

This exercise develops your hip and thigh muscles.

KNEE TO NOSE

1. Kneel on all fours.
2. Pull your right knee toward your nose.
3. Extend your right leg until it is in line with the back and shoulders (parallel to the floor). Keep your head in line with the shoulders, back, and extended leg.

   Caution: Do not lift your leg higher than your hips. Do not hyperextend your neck or lower back.
4. Return to the starting position. Repeat the exercise with your left leg.

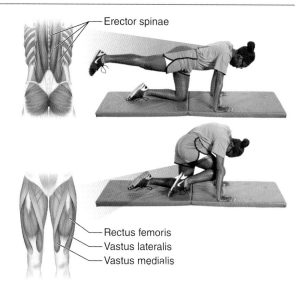

Erector spinae

Rectus femoris
Vastus lateralis
Vastus medialis

This exercise develops the gluteal, lower back, and quadriceps muscles. The fourth quadriceps muscle, the vastus intermedius, lies beneath the rectus femoris and therefore is not shown in the illustration.

HIGH-KNEE JOG

1. Jog in place. Try to lift each knee so that your upper leg is parallel with the floor.
2. Count one rep each time your right foot touches the floor. Try to do one or two jog steps per second.

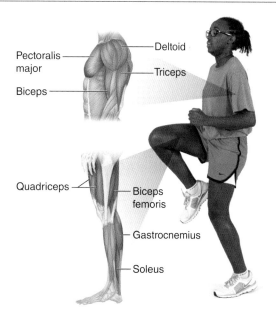

Deltoid
Pectoralis major
Triceps
Biceps

Quadriceps
Biceps femoris

Gastrocnemius

Soleus

This exercise develops the muscles of your arms and legs and is also good for cardiorespiratory endurance.

Back problems are common among adults. In fact, nearly 90 percent of adults experience backache in their lifetime. Poor posture can contribute to backache, and a lot of the work that is completed on desktop computers, laptop computers, tablets, and cell phones contributes to poor posture. Maintaining a healthy back and good posture will help you as you move into and through adulthood. Use these two self-assessments to evaluate your back health and posture.

Healthy Back Test

Backache is often caused by weak muscles and by muscles that are too short. Test your back muscles by using the following self-assessment. Each part focuses on a certain muscle group. If you do well on this assessment, you're likely to have a healthy back. If not, it's especially important that you do exercises to improve your back health. In doing the test, work with a partner. Your partner will anchor your body for certain tests and can help in recording scores. Add your scores for the individual test items to get your total score. Then use table 11.1 to determine your risk of back problems. Record your results. Remember that self-assessment information is personal and considered confidential. It shouldn't be shared with others without the permission of the person being tested.

Test Item 1: Single-Leg Lift (Supine)

1. Lie on your back on the floor. Lift your left leg off the floor as high as possible without bending either knee.
2. Repeat using your right leg. Score 1 point for each leg (i.e., right and left) you can lift to a 90-degree angle with the floor.

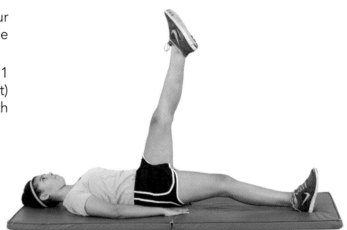

Test Item 2: Knee to Chest

1. Lie on your back on the floor. Make sure your lower back is flat on the floor.
2. Grasp the back of your thigh to bring your right knee up until you can hold it tightly against your chest. Keep your left leg straight. The left leg may lift off the floor to allow the right knee to reach your chest.
3. Repeat using your left leg.
4. Score 1 point if you can keep your left leg touching the floor while holding your right leg against your chest. Score an additional point if you can keep your right leg touching the floor while holding your left leg against your chest.

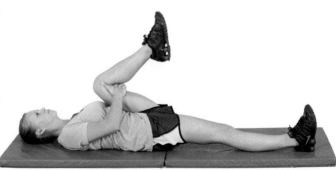

Test Item 3: Single-Leg Lift (Prone)

1. Lie facedown on the floor. Lift your straight right leg as high as possible. Hold the position for a count of 10. Then lower your leg.
2. Repeat using your left leg.

3. Score 1 point if you can hold your right leg 30 centimetres (12 inches) off the floor for a count of 10. Score an additional point if you can do the same with your left leg.

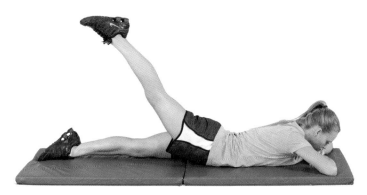

Test Item 4: Curl-Up

1. Lie on your back with your knees bent at 90 degrees and your arms extended.
2. Curl up by rolling your head, shoulders, and upper back off the floor. Roll up only until your shoulder blades leave the floor.

3. Score 1 point if you can curl up with your arms held straight in front of you and hold the position for 10 seconds without having to lift your feet off the floor.
4. Score an additional point if you can curl up with your arms across your chest and hold the position for 10 seconds without your feet leaving the floor.

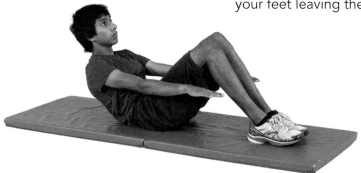

Test Item 5: Trunk Lift and Hold

1. Lie facedown on a padded bench (or a bleacher with a towel on it) that is 41 to 46 centimetres (16 to 18 inches) high. Your upper body (from your waist up) should extend off the bench.

2. Have your partner hold your calves just below the knees.

3. Place one hand over the other on your forehead with your palms facing away and your elbows held to the side at the level of your ears.

4. Start with your upper body lowered. Lift slowly until your upper body is even with the bench. Hold the position for a count of 10.

5. Score 1 point if you can lift your trunk even with the bench. Score an additional point if you can hold your upper body even with the bench for a count of 10.

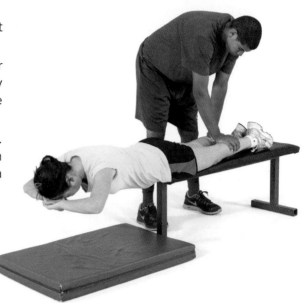

Test Item 6: Front Plank

1. On a mat or carpet, support your body with your forearms and toes.

2. Keep your head in line with your body and hold this position for 10 seconds.

3. Score 2 points if you can hold your body straight for the full 10 seconds.

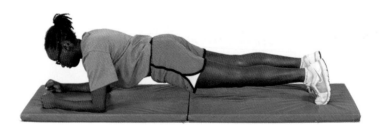

TABLE 11.1 Rating Chart: Healthy Back Test

Rating	Score
Good fitness	11 or 12
Marginal (some risk)	9 or 10
Low (greater risk)	6–8
High risk	≤5

Assessing Your Posture

You can use the following self-assessment to determine whether your posture is as good as it should be. If you find that improvements are needed, you can work at applying proper biomechanics when sitting, standing, and walking.

For this self-assessment, wear exercise clothing. If your shirt is really loose, tuck it into your shorts or exercise pants so that your partner can clearly see your upper and lower back. Work with a partner to determine each other's scores. Record your results.

1. Stand sideways next to a string hanging from a point at least 30 centimetres (12 inches) above your head. The string should be weighted at the bottom so that it hangs straight and reaches nearly to the floor. Position yourself so that the string aligns with the side of your ankle bone.

- Head: Is the ear in front of the line?
- Shoulders: Are the shoulders rounded? Are the tips of the shoulders in front of the chest?
- Upper back: Does the upper back stick out in a hump?
- Lower back: Does the lower back have excessive arch?
- Abdomen: Does the abdomen protrude beyond the pelvic bone?
- Knees: Do the knees appear to be locked or bent backward?

   Now stand with your back to the string so that the string is aligned with the middle of your back.

- Head: Is more than half of the head on one side of the string?
- Shoulders: Is one shoulder higher than the other?
- Hips: Is one hip higher than the other?

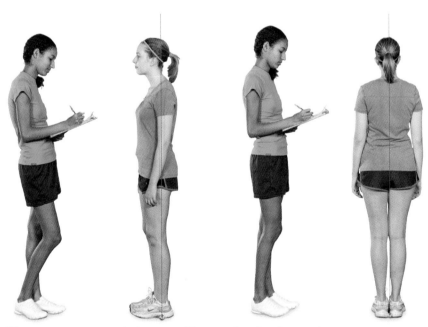

The posture test can help you achieve and maintain good posture.

2. Add the number of yes answers to get a total score. Then determine your rating on table 11.2.

What did you notice by doing this test? With a partner, discuss ways that you can improve your posture, or if you have good posture, discuss ways that you can maintain good posture.

TABLE 11.2 Rating Chart: Posture Test

Score (yes answers)	Rating
0 or 1	Good posture
2–4	Can use some improvement
≥5	Needs considerable improvement

Lesson 11.2

Ergogenic Aids
and Preparing a Muscle Fitness Plan

Lesson Objectives

After participating in this lesson, you should be able to

1. list three ergogenic aids and supplements and the risks associated with their use,
2. collect information about your personal needs and build a muscle fitness and activity profile,
3. set goals for muscle fitness exercise,
4. select muscle fitness exercises and prepare a written muscle fitness exercise plan, and
5. describe periodization and explain why it is used.

Lesson Vocabulary

anabolic steroid, androstenedione, creatine, ergogenic aid, ergolytic, human growth hormone (HGH), periodization, rhabdomyolysis

 Do you know someone who takes pills with the hope of finding an easy way to get muscle fitness? Do the pills really work? Would you like to improve your muscle fitness? Are you among the nearly 50 percent of teens who do no regular muscle fitness exercise? In this lesson, you'll learn about products advertised as muscle builders—and the problems associated with them. You'll also learn how to prepare a personal muscle fitness exercise plan that is safe and effective. Carrying out a good plan is the surest way to build your muscle fitness, which will help you meet national guidelines for physical activity both now and later in your life.

 Fitness—if it came in a bottle, everyone would have a great body.

—Cher, singer and actress

Ergogenic Aids

For centuries, people, especially those interested in high-level performance, have tried to find methods of enhancing performance—including methods other than the exercise training presented in this book. *Ergo* relates to work, and *genic* relates to the word "generate." Thus an **ergogenic aid** helps you generate work or increases your ability to do work, including performing vigorous exercise. Some ergo-

genic aids, or products thought to be ergogenic aids, are classified as drugs, whereas others are classified as food supplements. In Canada, drugs are tightly regulated under the Controlled Drugs and Substances Act. Supplements, however, are regulated as Natural Health Products (NHPs) and fall under NHP regulations enforced by Health Canada's Canadian Food Inspection Agency. Natural Health Products are substances you eat or drink and can be vitamins, minerals, herbs or other plants, amino acids, or parts of these substances.

Many products advertised as ergogenic aids can be dangerous. They can be detrimental to health and performance and are better referred to as **ergolytic** (*ergo* again meaning work and *lytic* meaning destructive). Examples of ergolytic substances include alcohol, tobacco, and marijuana. Some of the products marketed as ergogenic aids are described in the following pages.

Anabolic Steroids and Their Dangers

Many types of steroids are used by doctors to treat disease. **Anabolic steroids** are synthetic drugs that resemble the male hormone testosterone and produce lean body mass, weight gain, and bone maturation. For certain diseases, doctors legally prescribe anabolic steroids in small doses. However, some people illegally buy and use anabolic steroids

CONSUMER CORNER: Health and Fitness in a Bottle

Many products sold as ergogenic aids are classified as NHPs. Natural Health Products are substances you eat or drink; they can be vitamins, minerals, herbs or other plants, amino acids, or parts of these substances. The general public refers to NHPs as "supplements." Health Canada's Canadian Food Inspection Agency (CFIA) is responsible for ensuring the safety, effectiveness, and quality of NHPs. If a product has an eight-digit Natural Product Number, the product has been reviewed and approved by Health Canada. However, so many supplements are sold in Canada that the CFIA has not been able to review all of them for safety, effectiveness, and quality. As a consumer you need to protect yourself from false and misleading claims and ineffective or even dangerous products. Be aware of the following facts about supplements in Canada.

- **Regulation.** Health Canada's CFIA provides an eight-digit Natural Product Number for products that have been reviewed for safety, effectiveness, and quality. Products that have not been fully evaluated by Health Canada can legally be sold in Canada. If a product does not have an eight-digit number, you need to gather information about the product from reliable sources in order to protect yourself.

- **Claims.** Beware of health claims made for supplements. Manufacturers are not supposed to make unsubstantiated health claims for their products, but many do it anyway.

- **Contents.** Many supplements contain too little or too much of the key substance they are supposed to contain. Some have been shown to contain substances that they are not supposed to contain. These problems have led to health risks for some users.

- **Advisories, warnings, and recalls.** Health Canada does provide advisories, warnings, and recalls. You can also report side effects to Health Canada directly.

- **Dose or amount.** Because limited research has been done for supplements, very little is known about appropriate doses (amounts) required for health benefits or the doses that can lead to health problems.

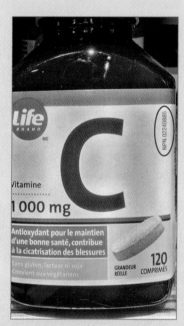

The eight-digit National Product Number (circled in red) means the product has been reviewed and approved by Health Canada.

Courtesy of Douglas Vincer

to increase muscle size and strength. Anabolic steroids are not only illegal when used without a doctor's prescription but also dangerous. Steroid use is prohibited by the International Olympic Committee (IOC) and most other athletic associations because of the potential dangers and the competitive advantage it can provide athletes. Some of the harmful effects of steroids are illustrated in figure 11.4.

Teenagers are at high risk for harm from steroids because their bodies are still growing. Anabolic steroids can damage the growth centres of bones, causing the long bones of the body to stop growing. This condition can prevent people from growing to their full height. Many side effects do not go away when use of the drug is discontinued; examples include hair loss, acne, deepening voice, and dark

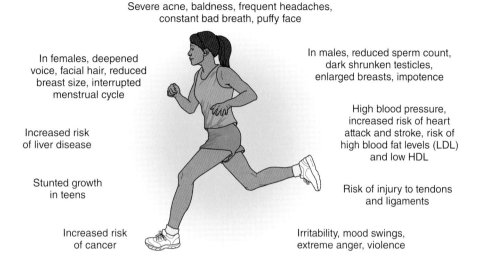

Severe acne, baldness, frequent headaches, constant bad breath, puffy face

In females, deepened voice, facial hair, reduced breast size, interrupted menstrual cycle

In males, reduced sperm count, dark shrunken testicles, enlarged breasts, impotence

Increased risk of liver disease

High blood pressure, increased risk of heart attack and stroke, risk of high blood fat levels (LDL) and low HDL

Stunted growth in teens

Risk of injury to tendons and ligaments

Increased risk of cancer

Irritability, mood swings, extreme anger, violence

FIGURE 11.4 The dangers of using anabolic steroids.

facial hair growth in women. For athletes, another major problem is the increased risk of injury to tendons and ligaments, which become less elastic with steroid use.

Some athletes also use other drugs (e.g., growth hormone, adrenaline, erythropoietin) in an attempt to enhance their performance, and sport officials develop tests to detect these drugs. Like steroids, they can be dangerous and illegal, and most are banned by sport governing bodies.

Steroid Precursors

A precursor is a substance from which another substance is formed. A steroid precursor is a nonsteroid substance that leads to the formation of a steroid once it is ingested. Some supplements are marketed as precursors, and they can cause the body to form its own anabolic steroids. Examples are **androstenedione**, DHEA, and androstenediol.

Androstenedione, often referred to as "andro," is considered a steroid precursor because it is converted into anabolic steroids such as testosterone (male hormone) after it enters the body. The use of steroid precursors such as androstenedione results in side effects similar to those associated with illegal steroid use. As a result, the Canadian Centre for Sports Ethics (CCSE), the World Anti-Doping Agency (WADA), the International Olympic Committee (IOC), and other sport organizations have banned the use of androstenedione, androstenediol, DHEA, and other steroid precursors. Cautions against the use of steroid precursors have also been issued by Health Canada and the CCSE, as well as several medical associations, including the American Medical Association and the American Academy of Pediatrics. It is illegal to purchase androstenedione in Canada without a prescription.

FIT FACT

Some athletes push beyond healthy limits after taking supplements that they think will give them the ability to do extreme training. This practice can result in problems such as rhabdomyolysis. **Rhabdomyolysis** is a condition in which muscle fibres break down, causing the bloodstream to absorb muscle fibre elements (such as myoglobin), which can damage the kidneys. Symptoms include muscle weakness and aching, fatigue, joint pain, and, in severe cases, seizure. Causes of this condition include exercising in the heat, lack of water replacement, and severe exertion. In several reported instances, high school and college athletes have been hospitalized for rhabdomyolysis due to excessive calisthenics and training drills.

Human Growth Hormone

Human growth hormone (HGH) is an illegal drug that is exceptionally dangerous, especially for teens. It causes the bones to stop growing properly, and its effects can be deforming and even life threatening. Like anabolic steroids, HGH is banned by virtually all high school, college, national, and international sport organizations. Testing is now possible to detect HGH, and many sport organizations now do mandatory testing. Many high-profile athletes have destroyed their reputations and careers by using HGH and other substances described in this lesson.

Creatine

Creatine is a natural substance manufactured in the bodies of meat-eating animals, including humans. It is needed for the body to perform anaerobic exercise, including many types of PRE. Creatine can also be taken as a food supplement. Taking extra creatine as a supplement allows your body to store more of it. Medical and kinesiology experts who have studied creatine indicate that it may be effective in improving performance in high-intensity exercise, such as sprinting, possibly because it allows training with shorter rest periods. It does not seem to improve aerobic or endurance performance or to improve performance among older people or highly trained athletes. Doctors use it to treat some medical conditions.

There is some evidence that creatine "loading"—using 20 grams daily for five days—may be more effective than continuous use. But remember, there is still some uncertainty about exactly who can benefit from creatine and at what dose. Studies to date have included only a small number of people (all have involved fewer than 40 participants), and it is not possible to draw firm conclusions from such small numbers.

Some products marketed as creatine may not be creatine or may contain substances other than creatine. There is also some concern about possible increased risk of dehydration among athletes who use creatine. Experts agree that before teens consider using any supplement, including creatine, they should consult with their parents or guardians and a qualified expert such as a medical doctor.

Other Supplements

Athletes and bodybuilders hoping to enhance their appearance or sport performance sometimes use one or more of many other supplements. Sport organizations and Health Canada have banned more than a few of these substances due to health problems associated with them. Ephedra is one example of a substance that was included in many supplements alleged to improve athletic performance and aid in weight loss. It was shown to cause several problems, including irregular heart rate and other potentially dangerous effects on the heart and the nervous system. For this reason, it is considered to be an ergolytic substance.

Protein supplements are also used very commonly among athletes because they are legal and easy to obtain. Indeed, your body needs protein for growth and development of most tissues. Because protein is a major part of the muscles, many people believe that taking extra protein builds extra muscle. However, most people eat more protein in their regular diet than they really need. Health Canada suggests that a healthy diet should contain between 10 and 35 percent protein. This range of protein intake allows for dietary differences among individuals.

Athletes and very active people do need to consume more calories of protein than inactive people; but because they take in many more total calories, experts agree that 12 to 15 percent of their diet is adequate to meet their body's protein needs. Taking more than 15 percent of the diet as protein does not result in greater gains in muscle. If not taken in excess, extra protein in the diet is relatively safe, but too much protein can cause kidney problems. Protein supplements in the form of pills, powders, and protein bars are very expensive, costing as much as 50 cents per gram of protein. In contrast, the protein in foods such as meat, poultry, fish, beans, and eggs is much cheaper, costing only a few cents per gram (figure 11.5). The calories in extra dietary

FIT FACT

Using a Canadian-developed chemical analysis technique called DNA bar coding, University of Guelph researchers showed that nearly 60 percent of herbal products analyzed contained unlabeled plant ingredients, and more than 20 percent contained "fillers" such as rice and wheat, also not listed on the labels.

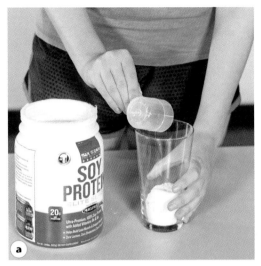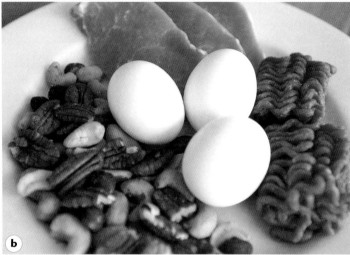

FIGURE 11.5 *(a)* Protein supplements can be expensive; *(b)* foods with protein are generally less expensive than supplements.

protein (in excess of body needs) are stored as fat, as are calories from extra dietary fat and carbohydrate.

Planning a Muscle Fitness Exercise Program

Molly is 15 years old and has used the five steps of program planning to prepare a muscle fitness exercise program. Her program is described here.

Step 1: Determine Your Personal Needs

To get started, Molly made a list of the muscle fitness exercises and activities she had performed over the last week. She also wrote down her fitness test results that related to vigorous physical activity. Her results are shown in figure 11.6.

Molly met the Canadian Physical Activity Guidelines for youth ages 12 to 17 by participating in activities that strengthen muscle and bone at least three times per week. But when she was not in physical education class, she did no muscle fitness exercise. In addition, Molly's fitness test scores were mostly in the marginal zone, indicating that she needed improvement. Molly wanted to try out for the softball team, and she now knew that she needed to improve her muscle fitness in order to be the best player she could be.

Step 2: Consider Your Program Options

Molly wanted to consider all of the various types of muscle fitness exercise, so she made a list of the types of PRE that she had to choose from. Her list is included here.

- Resistance machine exercises
- Free weight exercises
- Core exercises
- Calisthenics
- Elastic band exercises
- Ball exercises
- Homemade weights
- Isometric exercises
- Isokinetic machine exercises
- Pilates
- Plyometric exercises (jump rope)

Step 3: Set Goals

For this muscle fitness plan, Molly set a time period of two weeks—too short for long-term goals—so she developed only short-term physical activity goals. Later, she'll develop long-term goals, including some muscle fitness improvement goals, when

Physical activity profile		
Day	**Muscle fitness exercise(s)**	**How much?**
Mon.	Curl-up Knee push-up	1 set, 10 reps 1 set, 10 reps
Tues.	None	
Wed.	Curl-up Knee push-up	1 set, 10 reps 1 set, 10 reps
Thurs.	None	
Fri.	Curl-up Knee push-up	1 set, 10 reps 1 set, 10 reps
Sat.	None	
Sun.	None	

Physical fitness profile		
Fitness self-assessment	**Score**	**Rating**
1RM arm press (score divided by body weight) 1RM leg press (score divided by body weight)	0.55 (strength per kilogram of body weight) 1.10 (strength per kilogram of body weight)	Marginal Good fitness
Grip strength	48 kg (106 lb)	Marginal
Muscle endurance test	4 points	Marginal
Back test	9 points	Marginal
Standing long jump	150 cm (59 in.)	Marginal
Medicine ball throw	241 cm (95 in.)	Marginal

FIGURE 11.6 Molly's muscle fitness exercise (physical activity) and fitness profiles.

she prepares a longer plan. For now, she wanted to try some new exercises to get started and improve her chances of making the softball team.

Molly used the information she put together in step 2 to help develop her short-term goals for muscle fitness exercise (PRE). She had many choices but decided on resistance machines, core exercises, and plyometrics (jump rope). Before writing down her goals, Molly made sure that she chose SMART goals. Here they are:

1. Continue to perform two calisthenics in physical education class (one set of 10 reps).

2. Perform five resistance machine exercises two days a week (one set of 10 reps at 50 percent of 1RM).

3. Perform four core exercises three days a week (hold 10 seconds or do one set of 10 reps).

4. Perform jump rope two days a week (five minutes).

Step 4: Structure Your Program and Write It Down

Molly's fourth step was to write down her two-week muscle fitness plan (see figure 11.7). Molly chose resistance machine exercises because she could use the school's exercise room on Tuesdays and Thursdays after school and she thought these exercises would be good for preparing for softball. She decided to do them just two days a week because she was just beginning this type of exercise. She decided to do her jump rope (plyometrics) on Tuesday and Thursday as well. She scheduled core exercises because they were good for back health and good posture and she could do them at home. She listed the exercises she did in physical education class because she expected to keep doing them for the two weeks of her plan. Molly's plan met the Canadian Physical Activity Guidelines for youth ages 12 to 17 through participation in activities that strengthen muscle and bone at least three times per week.

| Day | Week 1 | | ✔ | Week 2 | | ✔ |
	Exercises	Time, sets, reps		Exercises	Time, sets, reps	
Mon.	Curl-up* Knee push-up* **Core exercises** Front plank Side plank (left) Side plank (right) Reverse curl	1 set, 10 reps 1 set, 10 reps Hold 10 sec Hold 10 sec Hold 10 sec 1 set, 10 reps		Curl-up* Knee push-up* **Core exercises** Front plank Side plank (left) Side plank (right) Reverse curl	1 set, 10 reps 1 set, 10 reps Hold 10 sec Hold 10 sec Hold 10 sec 1 set, 10 reps	
Tues.	Jump rope **Resistance machine** Arm press Knee extension Hamstring curl Biceps curl Heel raise	3:30–3:35 p.m. 3:35–4:30 p.m. 1 set 10 reps 50% 1RM for each exercise		Jump rope **Resistance machine** Arm press Knee extension Hamstring curl Biceps curl Heel raise	3:30–3:35 p.m. 3:35–4:30 p.m. 1 set 10 reps 50% 1RM for each exercise	
Wed.	Curl-up* Knee push-up* **Core exercises** Front plank Side plank (left) Side plank (right) Reverse curl	1 set, 10 reps 1 set, 10 reps Hold 10 sec Hold 10 sec Hold 10 sec 1 set, 10 reps		Curl-up* Knee push-up* **Core exercises** Front plank Side plank (left) Side plank (right) Reverse curl	1 set, 10 reps 1 set, 10 reps Hold 10 sec Hold 10 sec Hold 10 sec 1 set, 10 reps	
Thurs.	Jump rope **Resistance machine** Arm press Knee extension Hamstring curl Biceps curl Heel raise	3:30–3:35 p.m. 3:35–4:45 p.m. 1 set 10 reps 50% 1RM for each exercise		Jump rope **Resistance machine** Arm press Knee extension Hamstring curl Biceps curl Heel raise	3:30–3:35 p.m. 3:35–4:45 p.m. 1 set 10 reps 50% 1RM for each exercise	
Fri.	Curl-up* Knee push-up* **Core exercises** Front plank Side plank (left) Side plank (right) Reverse curl	1 set, 10 reps 1 set, 10 reps Hold 10 sec Hold 10 sec Hold 10 sec 1 set, 10 reps		Curl-up* Knee push-up* **Core exercises** Front plank Side plank (left) Side plank (right) Reverse curl	1 set, 10 reps 1 set, 10 reps Hold 10 sec Hold 10 sec Hold 10 sec 1 set, 10 reps	
Sat.						
Sun.						

*Performed in physical education class.

FIGURE 11.7 Molly's written plan.

Step 5: Keep a Log and Evaluate Your Program

Over the next two weeks, Molly self-monitored her activities and placed a checkmark on her plan beside each activity she performed. Then she evaluated to see whether she met her goals.

Periodization

Variety and enjoyment are important because they can help you stick with your exercise plan. Experts have found that if you change your program from time to time, you'll find it more interesting and feel more motivated to continue. **Periodization** is a systematic approach to scheduling your muscle fitness training and is used for long-term fitness programs (months to years). When you periodize a training program, you use variations in your exercise routines based on your needs for the given phase of training.

For example, over 15 weeks of training, a person might do three periods of 5 weeks each. In one period, you might focus on muscular endurance exercises with relatively high repetitions and relatively low resistance. In another period, you might focus more on strength using higher resistance and fewer repetitions. Your third period might focus on combining strength and muscular endurance training or on using plyometrics to develop power. Many periodization options exist, so the three periods might look different for different people.

Periodization is used by competitive athletes to gradually increase performance so that they peak, or reach their best performance level, at the right time. For example, an Olympic athlete would want to reach peak performance at the Olympic Games, whereas a high school athlete might want peak performance for a key game or meet. Recreational athletes use periodization more to provide variety and continued interest than for peaking to prepare for a specific sporting event.

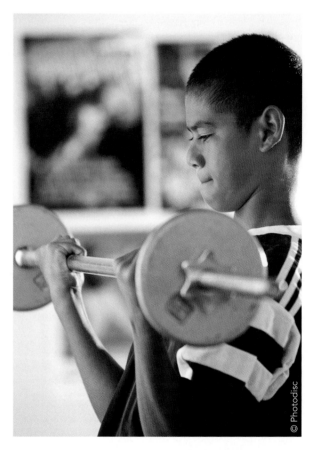

Varying your schedule for resistance training can help keep it interesting.

Lesson Review

1. List three ergogenic aids or supplements, and identify the risks associated with using each.
2. Discuss ways you can assess your personal needs and build a muscle fitness and activity profile.
3. What should you consider in setting goals for muscle fitness exercise?
4. How do you select muscle fitness exercises and prepare a written muscle fitness exercise plan?
5. What is periodization and why is it used, for both competing and noncompeting athletes?

TAKING CHARGE: Preventing Relapse

Anyone can begin a program to increase physical fitness, but just beginning a program is not enough. Some people are active for a while, then drop out for a while. This behaviour is called a relapse. Those who stay active all of their lives learn how to avoid relapses that can lead to becoming sedentary.

Luis missed his old school, especially his old friends. Now he usually came straight home after school instead of heading for the neighbourhood court to play a little three-on-three basketball with his buddies. For the first month after he moved, Luis ate dinner, did his homework, and then clicked on the television to fill the time.

Early one evening, his mom said, "Luis, why are you lying around? You like to be active. Get up and get moving!"

Luis yawned and said, "Where am I going to go? Who am I going to go with? I don't have any friends here."

"What about that boy who lives down the hall? I saw him leave with a gym bag the other day. He must have been going somewhere you'd like to go."

"Well, maybe," Luis said. "But maybe he was going to do weight training or something like that—something I don't know how to do."

"Maybe it wouldn't kill you to learn more about weight training. It might help you be better in basketball, right?"

Luis smiled up at his mom. "Maybe. What's his apartment number?"

"3B—and while you're there, ask his mom whether she knows about any exercise classes around here for old people like me, okay?"

For Discussion

What caused Luis to relapse into inactivity? What could he do if it turns out that the boy down the hall hates basketball? What are some other things that cause relapse? What can be done to avoid them? What other suggestions do you have to help Luis? Consider the guidelines presented in the Self-Management feature as you answer the discussion questions.

SELF-MANAGEMENT: Skills for Preventing Relapse

People who relapse stop doing something that they want to keep doing or think they should keep doing. For example, you might start a PRE program but then stop doing it because you feel you can't take the time. Use the following guidelines to help you stick with something once you've started it.

- **Do an activity self-assessment.** It may help you see whether you're likely to stick with an activity, and it may give you ideas for how to stick with it if you've had relapse problems in the past.

- **Use the information from your self-assessment to determine areas in which you can improve.** Self-assessments help you learn about your current status (for fitness, activity, or nutrition, for example). If you are to improve, you first need to know where you need improvement.

- **Write down your goals for doing the activity.** Put them on the refrigerator or in another place where you'll see them every day. You have good reasons to accomplish these goals or you would not have started to make a change in the first place. Stay focused on your goals.

- **Monitor your behaviour by keeping a log or chart, then use it to reinforce or reward yourself.** Tell yourself that you've stuck with it so far and you can keep it up.

- **Tell other people what you're trying to accomplish.** Ask them to encourage you regularly.

- **Select a regular exercise time.** If you're trying to stick with exercise or another similar behaviour, select a time of day and try to do the behaviour at the same time every day.

- **Do not let one setback be a reason for a long-term relapse.** If you miss a day, tell yourself, "It's okay to take a day off once in a while." Repeat this to yourself periodically.

- **Consider a variety of activities.** Consider trying different physical activities from time to time.

TAKING ACTION: Your Muscle Fitness Exercise Plan

Prepare an exercise plan for muscle fitness using the five steps described in the second lesson of this chapter. Like Molly, consider activities from a variety of types of PRE. The goal is to perform the exercises on at least two days per week for beginners and as many as three days per week for more advanced exercisers. Carry out your written plan over a two-week period. Your teacher may give you time in class to do some of the activities included in your plan. Consider the following suggestions for taking action.

- Before your PRE, perform a dynamic warm-up (see chapter 4).

- Follow the tips for safe PRE.
- Progress gradually—don't try to do too much too soon.
- After your workout, perform a cool-down.

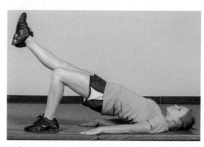
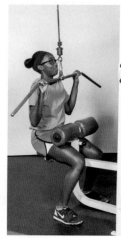

Take action by performing your muscle fitness plan.

©Hockey Canada

GET ACTIVE WITH HOCKEY CANADA

Who We Are

Hockey Canada is the national governing body for hockey in the country. The organization works in conjunction with its 13 provincial members, the Canadian Hockey League, and Canadian Inter-university Sport in growing the game at all levels.

What We Do

Hockey Canada oversees the management of programs in Canada from entry-level to high-performance teams and competitions, including IIHF and IPC world championships, and the Olympic Winter Games. It is also Canada's voice within the International Ice Hockey Federation.

Hockey Canada runs a number of development programs, many in conjunction with its corporate partners. From The First Shift to the National Coach Certification Program, Officiating Program of Excellence, and skills camps hosted from coast to coast to coast, Hockey Canada has proved itself a world leader in the game.

Hockey Canada believes in

- a positive hockey experience for all participants, in a safe, sportsmanlike environment;
- the development of life skills that will benefit participants throughout their lives;
- the values of fair play and sportsmanship, including the development of respect for all people by all participants;
- hockey opportunities for all people regardless of age, gender, colour, race,

ethnic origin, religion, sexual orientation, or socio-economic status, and in both official languages;

- the importance for participants to develop dignity and self-esteem;
- the ability to instill the values of honesty and integrity in participants at all times;
- the promotion of teamwork and the belief that what groups and society can achieve as a whole is greater than what can be achieved by individuals;
- the country of Canada, its tradition in the game of hockey, and the proud and successful representation of this tradition around the world;
- the value of hard work, determination, the pursuit of excellence, and success in all activities; and
- the benefits of personal and physical well-being.

Get Involved

Whether you want to be a player, coach, or official, or you want to volunteer your time to be a part of Canada's game, contact your minor hockey association or provincial member to get more information on how to get started. Visit Hockey Canada on the web at www.Hockey-Canada.ca, Facebook at www.facebook.com/HockeyCanada, Twitter at @HockeyCanada, and Instagram at www.Instagram.com/Hockey-Canada.

©Hockey Canada

Reviewing Concepts and Vocabulary

Complete the following in order to show your growing understanding of fitness, health, and wellness. Answer items 1 through 5 by correctly completing each sentence with a word or phrase.

1. The muscles that support your spine and keep your rib cage and spine stable are referred to as your _____ muscles.
2. About _____ percent of adults experience back pain at some point.
3. _____ are exercises that use all or part of your body weight to provide resistance.
4. _____ is the real name of the supplement sometimes called andro.
5. The full name for the substance called HGH is _____.

For items 6 through 10, match each term in column 1 with the appropriate phrase in column 2.

6. rhabdomyolysis   a. swayback
7. periodization   b. rounded shoulders
8. lordosis   c. breakdown of muscle fibre
9. kyphosis   d. varying your program schedule for muscle fitness
10. ptosis   e. protruding abdomen

For items 11 through 15, respond to each statement or question.

11. What are some of the best exercises for building your core muscles?
12. Describe three guidelines for properly lifting, carrying, and moving objects.
13. What self-assessments can you do to determine whether you are at risk for back pain?
14. What are some harmful effects of steroids?
15. What are some good strategies for preventing relapse?

Thinking Critically

Write a paragraph to answer the following question.

A friend of yours is excited about an advertisement in a muscle magazine. The ad describes a pill that is "guaranteed to add size to your muscles in two weeks without exercise." What advice would you give your friend? Justify or support your advice with sound reasoning.

Project

Assume that you've been hired as a reporter for a local newspaper. Write an article about preventing back pain or injury. Interview relevant people, such as a physical therapist, a physical education teacher, an athletic trainer, and a person who has experienced back pain or injury. Present your article in class or submit it to a newspaper for publication.

12

Developing Flexibility

(www) **Student Web Resources**
www.fitnessforlife.org/student

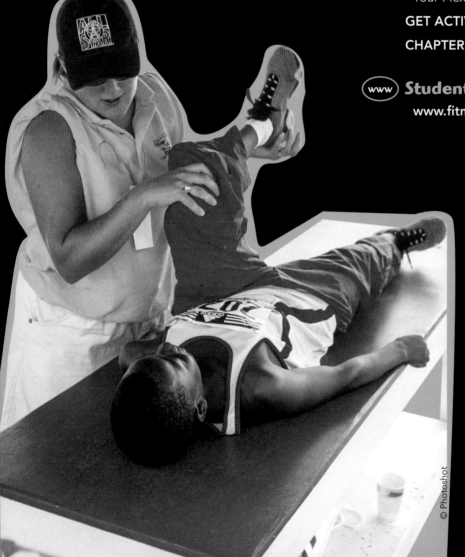

© Photoshot

Lesson 12.1

Flexibility Facts

Lesson Objectives

After participating in this lesson, you should be able to

1. explain the difference between a warm-up and a flexibility workout,
2. describe flexibility and some of the factors that influence it,
3. explain the benefits of good flexibility,
4. describe types of flexibility exercise and the FIT formula for each, and
5. explain why it is important to balance strength and flexibility exercise.

Lesson Vocabulary

active stretch, antagonist, ballistic stretching, CRAC, dynamic movement exercise, dynamic stretching, hypermobility, muscle–tendon unit (MTU), passive stretch, PNF stretching, range of motion (ROM), range-of-motion (ROM) exercise, static stretch

Do you have good flexibility? Do you do any regular stretching to improve your flexibility? In this lesson, you'll learn about the importance of being flexible and how to improve your flexibility by applying fitness principles. You'll also learn to evaluate your flexibility.

Sometimes people confuse a warm-up with a flexibility workout, but these are two different things. A warm-up is a group of exercises done to get ready for a specific workout or competition. A flexibility workout is a group of exercises done to build flexibility. Stretching exercises are now used less frequently in warm-ups than in the past, especially when preparing for certain types of activity, such as those involving strength, speed, and power. But this does not mean that flexibility exercises, including stretching, are not important. Flexibility is a key component of health-related physical fitness.

What Is Flexibility?

Flexibility is the ability to move your joints through a full **range of motion (ROM)**. A joint is a place in your body where bones come together. The best-known joints include the knees, ankles, elbows, wrists, knuckles, shoulders, hips, and the joints between the vertebrae in the spine. Some joints, such as your knees and elbows, work like a hinge, permitting movement in only two directions. Other

joints, such as your hips and shoulders, work like a ball and socket, allowing movement in all directions. Range of motion is the amount of movement you can make in a joint (figure 12.1).

Your bones are connected at your joints by non-elastic bands called ligaments; as you'll see later, they should not be stretched. Your bones are connected to your muscles by tendons. When your muscles contract, they pull on your tendons to cause your bones to move. Unlike ligaments, muscles and tendons need to be stretched in order to maintain a healthy length. Together, muscles and tendons are called a **muscle–tendon unit (MTU)** (figure 12.1). Both parts of the MTU are stretched when performing flexibility exercises, but we frequently refer only to "stretching the muscle" for simplicity. If your muscles and tendons are too short, they restrict a joint's ROM.

Benefits of Good Flexibility

Flexibility is sometimes referred to as the forgotten part of health-related fitness because many people focus exclusively on the other parts. We know, however, that good flexibility provides many benefits, including health benefits, especially when you grow older.

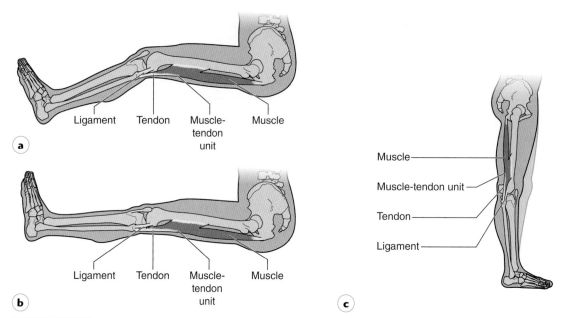

FIGURE 12.1 *(a)* Poor joint range of motion—knee does not fully extend because of short hamstring muscles; *(b)* good range of motion—knee fully extends because of long hamstrings; *(c)* too much range of motion—knee bends backward.

Improved Function

Everyone needs at least some flexibility in order to maintain health and mobility. The exact amount of flexibility needed for normal daily function depends on the demands of the activities that you perform. For example, plumbers, painters, and dentists often need to bend and stretch, and some musicians need very flexible fingers and wrists. As people grow older, their flexibility tends to decrease, which can limit simple movements such as looking over the shoulder while driving. Therefore, it's especially important for older people to do exercises that build and maintain a full ROM.

Flexibility is also important to many athletes, especially in certain sports. Dancers and gymnasts must be very flexible to perform their routines. Swimmers need good flexibility to get maximum performance, as do kickers in football. Good flexibility also allows a longer backswing—and therefore a faster forward swing—in the throwing and striking movements that are crucial in golf, tennis, and baseball pitching. While some research has questioned the value of stretching right before a competition or performance, muscles of adequate length can be beneficial even in such activities as weightlifting and the shot put.

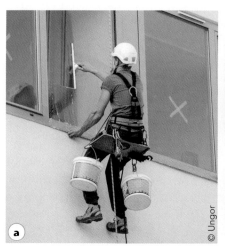
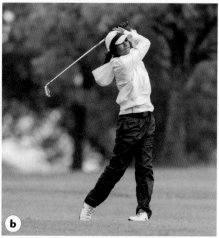

Good flexibility is needed *(a)* for some jobs and *(b)* by most athletes.

Improved Health and Wellness

Good flexibility is important for your back health and your posture. For example, back pain and poor posture are associated with short hamstring and hip flexor muscles. More generally, very short muscles are at risk of being overstretched and injured. Stretching exercises also have a beneficial effect on a number of conditions. Flexible musicians are less likely to have pain in their joints. Stretching exercises can often alleviate menstrual cramps in women. They can prevent or provide relief from leg cramps and shinsplints (pain in the front of the shins caused by overuse). Stretching a muscle can also help it relax, and some forms of stretching can help you manage stress.

Rehabilitation From Injury and Medical Problems

Flexibility exercises are used for rehabilitation from a variety of injuries and medical problems. Both physiotherapists (PTs) and athletic trainers (ATs) use a variety of techniques, including stretching and muscle fitness exercises, in their work. Physiotherapists treat patients after surgery and patients with medical conditions such as arthritis, back pain, stroke, and osteoporosis. Athletic trainers help athletes train to prevent injury and help them recover when injury does occur.

FIT FACT

Physiotherapists are health care professionals who treat patients with medical problems or those who have had surgery. They help patients manage pain and improve their mobility. They also help people perform regular exercises to prevent muscle-related problems and to maintain or regain their ability to function normally. Physiotherapists have many years of advanced education and, in Canada, must be licensed in the province in which they practice. They work in many settings, including private practices, hospitals, nursing homes, outpatient clinics, schools, and sport and fitness facilities. More than 12,000 PTs and PT students belong to the Canadian Physical Therapy Association, a professional group whose goal is to help people improve their health and quality of life.

" I want to get old gracefully. I want to have good posture, I want to be healthy and be an example to my children. "

—Sting, musician

Factors Influencing Flexibility

You already know that short muscles and tendons reduce flexibility and that they can be stretched to improve flexibility. Your flexibility is also influenced by the following factors.

Heredity

Inherited anatomical differences in our bodies help determine what we can and cannot do. Some people inherit joints that do not favour a large ROM. These people have to exercise regularly in order to develop a healthy ROM. Other people have an unusually large ROM in certain joints—a condition sometimes referred to as being double jointed but officially called **hypermobility**. People with hypermobility score better on flexibility tests and can extend the knee, elbow, thumb, or wrist joint past a straight line, as if the joint could bend backward. Some people who have hypermobile joints are prone to joint injury and may be more likely to develop arthritis, a disease in which the joints become inflamed. For the most part, however, those with hypermobile joints do not have problems other than a slight disadvantage in some sports. For example, when doing push-ups, the elbows of a hypermobile person might lock when the arms straighten, making it difficult to unlock the elbows to begin the downward movement.

Body Build

Can short people touch their toes more easily than tall people? In most cases, this is not true, because a shorter person tends to have not only shorter legs and trunk but also shorter arms (though there are exceptions). In contrast, a taller person tends to have longer legs and trunk and longer arms. Some people do have exceptionally long arms or legs, and these characteristics may make it easier or harder for them to score well on flexibility tests, but this is the exception rather than the rule.

Sex and Age

Generally, females tend to be more flexible than males. About twice as many females as males are hypermobile, and at most ages more females than males meet minimum fitness standards for flexibility. Similarly, younger people tend to be more flexible than older people. As people grow older, their muscles typically grow shorter because they are used less, and their joints tend to allow less movement due to conditions such as arthritis. With this in mind, one important reason for doing regular flexibility exercises when you're young is to reduce your risk of joint problems when you're older. Good flexibility also enhances performance in a variety of tasks for people of all ages.

Different Types of Flexibility Exercise

 The following discussion presents methods of building and maintaining flexibility. For best results, perform exercises especially designed to improve your flexibility (step 5 of the Physical Activity Pyramid; figure 12.2). The four major types of exercise for building flexibility are ROM exercise, static stretching, ballistic stretching, and dynamic stretching.

Range-of-Motion Exercise

Technically, all flexibility exercises are ROM exercises because they are all designed to help allow a healthy ROM in the joints. More specifically, the term **range-of-motion (ROM) exercise** refers to exercise that requires a joint to move through a full ROM, powered either by the body's own muscles or by assistance from a partner or therapist. Such exercises are commonly used in physical therapy for people who have lost ROM or who want to avoid loss of ROM associated with an injury or medical problem. The exercise movement is typically continuous and performed at a slow to moderate pace.

Each joint has its own normal or healthy range of movement, so exercises are designed specifically for each joint. Examples include shoulder rotation exercises for people with shoulder injuries (for example, baseball pitchers) and knee flexion and extension of the fingers for people with arthritis. The weight of the body part and the momentum of the movement do cause some stretch in the muscles and connective

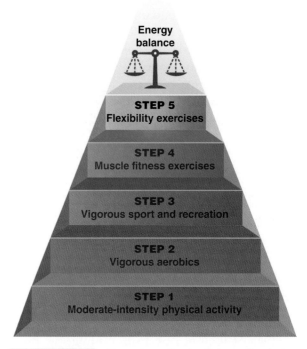

FIGURE 12.2 Exercises for building flexibility are represented by step 5 of the Physical Activity Pyramid.

Adapted from *Physical Activity Pyramid for Teens*, source: C.B. Corbin.

tissues, but these exercises typically do not use the same intensity of stretch as those described in the next section; therefore, ROM exercises are not as good as stretching exercises for improving flexibility.

Muscles often work as **antagonists**—meaning that they perform opposite functions—to allow multiple movements and full ROM. For example, if you're sitting in a chair and contract the quadriceps muscles on the front of your thigh, they lift your lower leg and foot off the floor; at the same time, the muscles on the back of your thigh, which are the antagonists, relax to allow the quadriceps to lift your leg.

Static Stretching

A **static stretch** involves stretching slowly as far as you can without pain, until you feel a sense of pulling or tension. For best results, static stretches are held for 10 to 30 seconds. The FIT formula for static stretching is outlined in table 12.1. Done correctly, static stretching increases your flexibility and can help you relax. Some experts think that static stretching exercises are safer than ballistic stretching

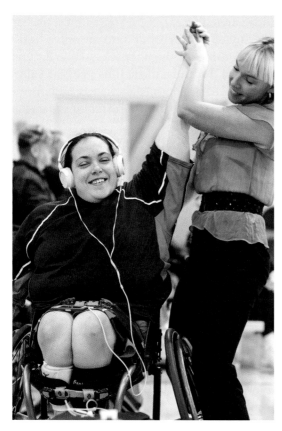

Range-of-motion exercises are commonly used in physical therapy for people who have lost ROM associated with an injury or medical condition.

exercises because you're less likely to stretch too far and injure yourself.

Static stretching can be performed using either **active stretch** or **passive stretch**. A static stretch requires an assist from an external source, such as gravity, a partner, or some other source. Active static stretch is caused by contracting your own antagonist muscles—for example, contracting your shin muscle to move your toes upward, thus causing a stretch in your calf muscles (figure 12.3*a*). Passive static stretch is achieved without use of an antagonist muscle. The calf stretch, for example, can be done by having a partner push gently on your foot or by using your own arms to pull your foot upward (figure 12.3*b*).

Some experts consider active static stretch to be safer than other types of stretch because you don't have to worry about the external force overstretching your muscle (for example, if a partner pushes too hard). The advantage of passive static stretch is that it is easier to create adequate stretch in order to improve the length of the muscle.

PNF Stretching

PNF stretching (PNF stands for proprioceptive neuromuscular facilitation) is a stretching technique originally used by PTs and occupational therapists (OTs) to help soldiers who had been injured. It is now widely used by many people interested in improving their flexibility, including athletes. PNF stretching is a variation of static stretching. Some experts believe that it is the most effective type of exercise for improving flexibility, though it may cause more soreness than static stretching. PNF involves contracting the muscle before you stretch it to help the muscle relax so that it can be more easily stretched. Active stretch is sometimes called "active isolated stretch" because the contraction before the stretch isolates, or identifies, the muscle to be stretched. One popular form of PNF is called **CRAC** (contract-relax-antagonist-contract). After you contract a muscle that you want to stretch,

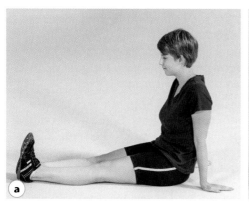
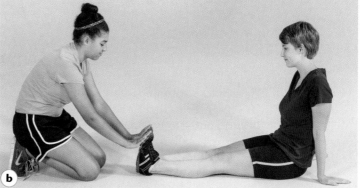

FIGURE 12.3 Stretching the calf: *(a)* active stretch; *(b)* passive stretch (with a partner assisting).

the muscle automatically relaxes. Contracting the opposing (antagonist) muscles during the stretch also makes the muscle you're stretching relax. CRAC does both of these actions.

The static stretch exercise shown in figure 12.3*b* can be made into a CRAC form of PNF exercise by contracting the calf muscles by pushing the toes against the partner's hands before doing the stretch.

The FIT formula for PNF stretch is described in table 12.1.

Ballistic Stretching

Ballistic stretching involves a series of gentle bouncing or bobbing motions that are not held for a long time. The FIT formula for ballistic stretch is outlined in table 12.1. Like static stretching and PNF, ballistic stretching exercises are designed to use the joints through a full range of movement and cause the muscles and tendons to stretch beyond their normal length. Most of the static stretching exercises shown in this chapter can be made into

ballistic stretching exercises. For example, the hamstring stretch can be made into an active ballistic stretch by using the thigh muscles to bob the upper leg forward. It can be made into a passive ballistic stretch by having a partner alternately push forward and pull backward to produce a bobbing movement of the upper leg.

Sport movement stretching uses movements that closely mimic those of a specific sport. Examples include baseball batters who swing with a weighted bat and golfers who swing the club several times before beginning a round of golf. This type of warm-up has also been referred to as sport-specific ballistic stretching. Regardless of the name preferred, it involves using the muscles to initiate a sport-specific movement that causes the muscles to be used beyond their normal ROM. Consult with your instructor or coach to find out about recommended exercises for a given sport.

Some teachers and coaches have concerns about ballistic stretching because of the possibility of overstretching and injuring muscles if it is not done

TABLE 12.1 FIT Formula and Fitness Target Zones for Stretching Exercise

	Static and PNF	Ballistic
Frequency	**Threshold of training:** Stretch each muscle group on 2 or 3 days each week. **Target zone:** Stretch each muscle group on 2-7 days each week.	**Threshold of training:** Stretch each muscle group on 2 or 3 days each week. **Target zone:** Stretch each muscle group on 2-7 days each week.
Intensity	**Threshold of training:** Stretch the muscle beyond its normal length until you feel tension, then hold. **Target zone:** Stretch the muscle beyond its normal length, from first point of tension to point of mild discomfort (not pain). Hold.	**Threshold of training:** Stretch the muscle beyond its normal length until you feel tension. Use slow, gentle bounces or bobs. Use the motion of your body part to stretch the specific muscle. **Target zone:** Stretch the muscle beyond its normal length, from first point of tension to point of mild discomfort (not pain). Use the same gentle bouncing stretch as for threshold. *Caution: No stretch should cause pain, especially sharp pain. Be especially careful when doing ballistic stretching.*
Time	**Threshold of training:** Do 2 stretches of 10-30 sec for each muscle group. **Target zone:** Do 2-4 stretches with a goal of 60 sec (total) of stretching for each muscle group (6 × 10, 4 × 15, or 2 × 30 sec). Rest for 15 sec between stretches.	**Threshold of training:** For each muscle group, perform 2 sets. Bounce against the muscle slowly and gently. Perform 15 reps. Rest for 10 sec between sets. **Target zone:** For each muscle group, perform 2-4 sets of 15 reps. Rest for 10 sec between sets. Start with 2 sets and progress to 4.

❤ FITNESS TECHNOLOGY: Goniometers

When you perform flexibility self-assessments, you use low-tech aids such as a yardstick or ruler. In some cases, you may use a flexibility box that includes a built-in measuring stick. When experts do research on flexibility, they use more sophisticated instruments, such as a goniometer, which measures joint angles. Some goniometers are electronic. Your school may have an inexpensive goniometer, such as the one shown, that you can use when assessing the ROM in your joints.

Using Technology

Do some investigation to learn more about goniometers and other devices for measuring flexibility.

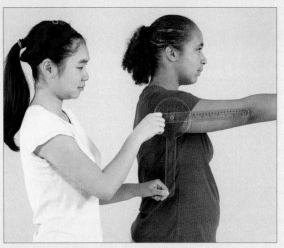

A goniometer can be used to assess range of motion and flexibility.

FIT FACT

The Canadian Society of Exercise Physiology (CSEP) refers to dynamic stretching exercises as an additional way to build flexibility. They are similar to static stretching exercises, but the stretch is slow, gradual, and continuous until the muscle is fully stretched. Developmental stretching is another type of flexibility exercise recommended by some experts. It is performed slowly like dynamic stretching, and the stretch is held for 10 to 30 seconds (the same as for static stretching). The difference is that in developmental stretching you stretch until you feel slight tension and then reduce the stretch for three to five seconds. The stretch is then increased slightly beyond the previous stretch. You repeat these steps (stretch, reduce stretch, stretch) until you reach a full stretch as outlined in table 12.1. Both dynamic and developmental stretching exercises are good alternatives for people who have been injured or who are just beginning a stretching program.

carefully. However, studies show that, if performed properly, ballistic stretching can be safe and does not cause as much muscular soreness as static stretching. Therapists do caution against ballistic stretching after a muscle or tendon injury, and they recommend consulting an expert to determine the best method of stretch for rehabilitation.

Balancing Muscle Fitness and Flexibility

You should do muscle fitness and flexibility exercises together. We now know that muscle fitness exercises, when properly performed, need not limit flexibility. In fact, when done through a full ROM, they can even help you build flexibility. But muscle fitness exercises are best for building muscle fitness, and flexibility exercises are best for building flexibility.

Therefore, a balanced exercise program includes both muscle fitness and flexibility exercises for all of your muscles so that they can apply equal force on all sides of a joint. People commonly use the arm flexors (muscles on the front of the body) a great deal because many daily activities emphasize the use of those muscles. For example, the majority of people have strong biceps muscles (on the front of the arms) and pectoral muscles (on the front of

⚛ SCIENCE IN ACTION: Dynamic Movement Exercise

Dynamic movement exercises include jumping, skipping, and other calisthenics (such as lunges and squats) used in a warm-up. This type of exercise is also referred to as dynamic calisthenics, because the only resistance encountered is the person's body weight. Dynamic movement exercises move the joints beyond normal resting ROM and cause the muscles and tendons to stretch. The stretch caused by dynamic movement exercise is followed by a contraction of the stretched muscle. For example, jumping stretches the calf muscle; after the stretch caused by landing from a jump, the muscle contracts again to provide the force for the next jump. Dynamic movement exercises should not be confused with dynamic stretching exercises (see the Fit Fact on dynamic stretching).

Experts who pioneered the use of dynamic movement exercises point out that they are not the same as ballistic stretching exercises because they do not involve bobbing or bouncing against the muscle. Dynamic movement exercise routines use many kinds of movement, including muscle fitness calisthenics (such as push-ups, lunges, and half squats) and several types of sport- and activity-specific movements that prepare an athlete for activity.

Whereas dynamic *stretching* exercises are done primarily to build flexibility, that is not the primary intent of dynamic *movement* exercises (calisthenics). For this reason, a specific FIT formula is not provided for this type of exercise. However, it is often included in a warm-up and as

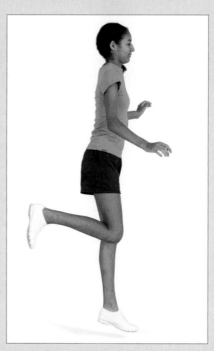

Dynamic movement exercises, such as the backward hop, stretch muscles and tendons.

part of other exercise circuits, and it does provide flexibility benefits and improve muscle fitness and power. Typically, when dynamic movement exercises are included in a warm-up, exercises are chosen for different muscle groups, and the total time for the exercise is 5 to 10 minutes.

Student Activity

Prepare a blog explaining dynamic movement exercise and the reasons for doing it.

---

the chest). In addition, most people have strong quadriceps muscles (on the front of the thighs) and tight hip flexors (also on the front of the body). The pull of these strong muscles results in the body hunching forward. To avoid becoming permanently hunched over, you need to make certain that these strong, short muscles on the front of your body get stretched. At the same time, you must strengthen the weak, relatively unused muscles on the back of your body. Table 12.2 lists the muscles for which most people need the most flexibility exercise.

Specificity of Stretching

Are there any muscles that do not need stretching? For many people, the answer is yes. For example, some people eventually begin to develop a hunched-over posture often called humpback at some point in life. Because the upper back muscles become overstretched in people with this postural problem, they should avoid further stretching of those muscles. The abdominal muscles are another example. You do need to keep your abdominal muscles strong, but

TABLE 12.2 Muscles That Need the Most Stretching

Muscle(s)	Reason for stretching
Chest	Prevent poor posture
Front of shoulders	Prevent poor posture
Front of hip joints	Prevent swayback posture, backache, pulled muscle
Back of thighs (hamstring)	Prevent swayback posture, backache, pulled muscle
Inside of thighs	Prevent back, leg, and foot strain
Calf	Avoid soreness and Achilles tendon injury (may result from running and jumping)
Lower back	Prevent soreness, pain, back injury

most people don't need to stretch them. In fact, if they're stretched, they begin to sag, and the abdomen protrudes, leading to poor posture.

Each person must evaluate his or her own needs to avoid stretching already overstretched muscles and avoid strengthening muscles that are already so strong that they are out of balance with their opposing muscles. Keeping muscles on opposites sides of a joint in balance helps them pull with equal force in all directions. This balance helps align your body parts properly, ensuring good posture.

Lesson Review

1. How does a stretching warm-up differ from a flexibility (stretching) workout?
2. What is flexibility, and what factors influence it?
3. What are the benefits of good flexibility?
4. What are the types of flexibility exercise, and what is the FIT formula for each?
5. Why is it important to balance strength and flexibility exercise?

In this self-assessment, you'll evaluate the flexibility in several areas of your body. Use these general directions for the tests that follow. Then score yourself using table 12.3.

- Perform each exercise as described and illustrated here.
- Stretch and hold the position for two seconds while a partner checks your performance.
- Score 1 point for each test for which you meet the standard. Total your score for all tests.
- Determine your rating using table 12.3. Record your results.

You are expected to do these tests in class only once, unless your instructor tells you otherwise. However, you may want to retest yourself periodically. A retest helps you to see progress and can also be used to help set new goals. If you're working with a partner, remember that self-assessment information is personal and considered confidential. It shouldn't be shared with others without the permission of the person being tested.

Safety tip: Before taking a flexibility test, do a general warm-up and try each movement two or three times.

TABLE 12.3   Rating Chart: Flexibility

Fitness rating	Score (items passed)
Good	8–11
Marginal	5–7
Low	0–4

Arm Lift

1. Lie facedown. Hold a ruler or stick in both hands. Keep your fists tight and your palms facing down.
2. Raise your arms and the stick as high as possible. Keep your forehead on the floor and your arms and wrists straight.
3. Hold this position while your partner uses a ruler to check the distance of the stick from the floor.
4. Record 1 point if you meet the standard: 25 centimetres (10 inches) or more.

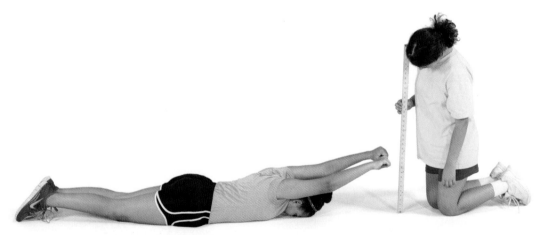

This test evaluates your chest and shoulder flexibility.

Zipper

1. Reach your left arm and hand over your left shoulder and down your spine, as if you were going to pull up a zipper.

2. Hold this position while you reach your right arm and hand behind your back and up your spine to try to touch or overlap the fingers of your left hand.

3. Hold the position while your partner checks it.

4. Repeat, this time reaching your right arm and hand over your right shoulder and your left arm and hand up your spine.

5. Record 1 point for each side on which you meet the standard: touching or overlapping fingers.

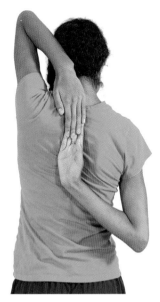

This test evaluates your shoulder, arm, and chest flexibility.

Trunk Rotation

1. Stand with your toes on the designated line. Your left shoulder should be an arm's length (with fist closed) from the wall and directly on a line with the target spot located on the wall.

2. Drop your left arm and extend your right arm to your side at shoulder height. Make a fist with your palm down.

3. Without moving your feet, rotate your trunk to the right as far as possible. Your knees may bend slightly to permit more turn, but don't move your feet. Try to touch the target spot or beyond with a palm-down fist.

4. Hold the position while your partner checks it.

5. Repeat, rotating to the left.

6. Record 1 point for each side on which you meet the standard: touch the centre of the target or beyond.

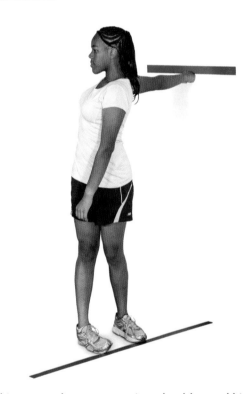

This test evaluates your spine, shoulder, and hip flexibility.

Wrap-Around

1. Raise your right arm and reach behind your head. Try to touch the left corner of your mouth. You may turn your head and neck to the left.
2. Hold the position while your partner checks it.
3. Repeat with your left arm.
4. Record 1 point for each side on which you meet the standard: touching the corner of the mouth.

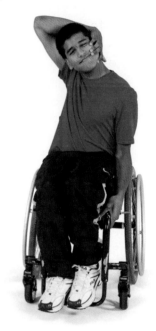

This test evaluates your shoulder and neck flexibility.

Knee to Chest

1. Lie on your back and extend your right leg. Place your hands on the back of your left thigh and pull toward you to draw the knee closer to the chest. Do not place your hands on top of the knee.
2. Keep your right leg straight and on the floor if possible. Keep your lower back flat on the floor.

3. Hold the position. Have your partner check to see if your upper left thigh and knee are against your chest and your right leg is straight and on the floor.
4. Repeat with the opposite leg.
5. Record 1 point for each side on which you meet the standard: thigh and knee against the chest and calf on the floor.

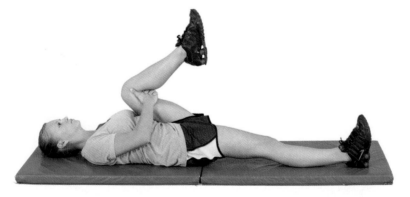

This test evaluates the flexibility of your hamstrings, your lower back, and the hip flexor muscles.

Ankle Flex

1. Sit erect on the floor with your legs straight and together. You may lean backward slightly on your hands if necessary.

2. Start with the soles of your shoes at 90 degrees (perpendicular) to the floor.

3. Flex your ankles by pulling your toes toward your shins as far as possible. Hold this position while your partner checks whether the angle that the sole of each foot makes with the floor is 75 degrees. (You can use a protractor to make a 75-degree angle on a sheet of paper.).

4. Record 1 point for each ankle for which you meet the standard: soles angled 75 degrees or more.

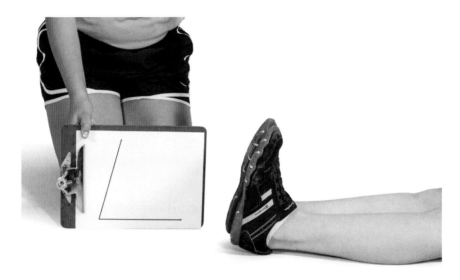

This test evaluates the flexibility of your calf muscles and your range of ankle movement.

Lesson 12.2
Preparing a Flexibility Program

Lesson Objectives

After participating in this lesson, you should be able to

1. describe several basic flexibility (stretching) exercises,
2. describe other forms of activity that build flexibility,
3. describe and explain how to apply basic guidelines for stretching, and
4. select flexibility exercises and prepare a written flexibility exercise plan.

 Lesson Vocabulary

tai chi, yoga

Do you know which specific exercises are best for developing flexibility using the different types of stretching? Have you ever considered safety issues when performing flexibility exercise? In the previous lesson, you learned about several types of flexibility exercise. In this lesson, you'll learn some of the most common exercises used to build flexibility; you'll also learn how to plan a personal flexibility exercise program.

Exercise Choices for Building Flexibility

The type of exercises that you choose for building flexibility depends on your personal goals. The following sections describe some of the most popular flexibility exercises.

Basic Flexibility Exercises

The Canadian Society for Exercise Physiology (CSEP) recommends that you perform exercises to stretch all of your major muscle groups. The 12 exercises described at the end of this lesson allow you to do so by choosing 8 to 10 exercises. As you'll see, all of these exercises can be done using static stretching, and some can also be done using PNF or ballistic stretching. The following guidelines will help you perform these exercises effectively.

- Consider the FIT formula information in table 12.1. Also consider the recommendations for the appropriate number of reps, sets, and time that accompany each of the exercises described in this lesson.

- The exercises labelled PNF include a contraction of the muscle before stretching. To perform them as static stretches, omit the contraction phase.

- The exercises labelled ballistic can be made ballistic by using a gentle bobbing movement rather than a static stretch.

Range-of-Motion Exercises

As noted in this chapter's first lesson, ROM exercises are commonly used in physical therapy and can be performed daily to help retain a healthy ROM. Dynamic and developmental stretching exercises can also be used by people recovering from injury and by beginners. Specific details for these types of exercises are not provided here because the static, PNF, and ballistic exercises are better choices for healthy teens. However, most of the basic exercises listed here can be done using dynamic or developmental stretching.

Yoga, Tai Chi, and Pilates

In addition to the static, PNF, and ballistic stretching exercises described in this chapter, there are other popular activities that can be good for building flexibility. The American College of Sports Medicine (ACSM) refers to these types of activities as functional fitness training because they help people (especially older people) perform tasks of daily living effectively. They also have health benefits (see Fit Fact). Tai chi and yoga are sometimes called neuromotor exercises because they build components of skill-related fitness such as agility and balance that require the nerves *(neuro)* and muscles to work together.

Tai chi is an ancient form of exercise that originated in China. It is considered to be a martial art and has many different forms. Tai chi is now practiced worldwide as a form of exercise rather than a martial art, and its basic movements have been shown to increase flexibility and reduce symptoms of arthritis in some people. When practiced regularly, it can help in developing muscle fitness, preventing back pain, and improving posture and balance.

FIT FACT

Research studies show that tai chi provides a variety of benefits, including improved bone health; improved functional fitness; better quality of life; and, among older people, reduced risk of falls.

Yoga was introduced centuries ago in India. Traditional forms include meditation as well as the exercises and breathing techniques that are common in modern forms. Yoga poses, called *asanas,* are similar to many flexibility exercises and can contribute to improved flexibility and provide other health benefits similar to those for tai chi. Yoga is practiced by millions of young adults as a method of relaxing and training, and many schools now have yoga clubs. However, yoga should be undertaken with care. Physical therapists and other health experts caution against performing certain yoga poses because they are considered to be risky exercises. In addition, beginners are cautioned to progress gradually; it can be more harmful than helpful to try advanced poses without weeks or even months of practice.

Pilates was originally developed as a form of therapy but is now practiced as a method of building muscle fitness and flexibility. It focuses on core muscle fitness but also includes exercises for building flexibility. When practiced properly, it helps prevent back pain, improves posture, and aids functional capacity in daily life.

If you're considering tai chi, yoga, or Pilates, you should seek qualified instruction and follow the guidelines outlined in this chapter for building flexibility.

Guidelines for Flexibility Exercise

To get the most benefit and enjoyment from your exercise program, perform the exercises correctly and use caution to avoid injury. Before you begin stretching, follow these guidelines and cautions to help you safely achieve and maintain flexibility.

- **Before stretching, do a general warm-up.** Warm muscles respond better than cold ones, and the CSEP recommends doing a general warm-up of 5 to 10 minutes before performing stretching exercise.
- **Make flexibility exercises part of your workout.** Don't rely on warm-up exercises to build flexibility. Select an appropriate type of exercise and follow the FIT formula for that type.
- **Choose exercises for all major muscle groups.** Twelve different exercises for the various muscle groups are described later in this lesson.

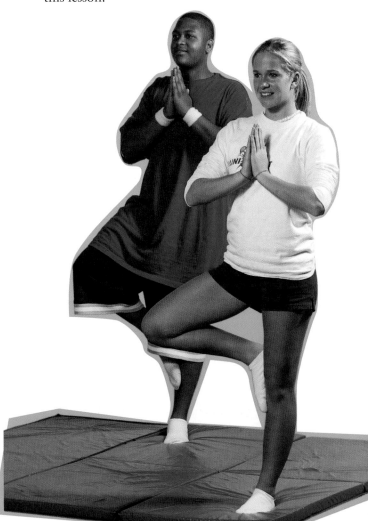

- **When beginning (or for general health), use static stretching or PNF.** Consider ballistic stretching after achieving the good fitness zone. Dynamic and developmental stretching may also be beneficial.

- **Progress gradually.** Regardless of the type of flexibility exercise you choose, progress gradually. Some flexibility exercises may seem easy, but, as with muscular endurance exercise, it does not take much to make your muscles sore. Gradually increase the time and number of repetitions and sets.

- **Avoid risky exercises.** Exercises that hyperflex or hyperextend a joint should be avoided, as should exercises that cause joint twisting and compression.

- **Do not stretch joints that are hypermobile, unstable, swollen, or infected.** People with these conditions or symptoms are at risk of injury from overstretching.

- **Do not stretch to the point of feeling pain.** The old saying "no pain, no gain" is wrong. Stretch only until your muscle feels tight and a little uncomfortable.

- **Avoid stretching muscles that are already overstretched from poor posture.** The abdominal muscles, for example, typically do not need to be stretched.

- **Avoid stretches that last 30 seconds or more before performing strength and power activities.** Research suggests that stretches lasting longer than 30 seconds may have a negative effect on performances of strength and power in sport and other activities. As a result, some experts recommend doing dynamic movement exercises rather than stretching before strength and power performances.

> " I never struggled with injury problems because of my preparation—in particular my stretching. "
>
> —Edwin Moses, U.S. Olympic gold medalist

FIT FACT

Once you've reached an acceptable level of muscle flexibility, you must continue to move all of your joints and muscles through this new and improved ROM on a regular basis. If you don't, your muscles will begin to shorten again, and you'll lose that flexibility. All types of exercise described in this lesson help maintain flexibility.

Planning a Flexibility Exercise Program

Elijah is a 16-year-old who used the five steps of program planning to prepare a flexibility exercise program. His program is described here.

Step 1: Determine Your Personal Needs

To get started, Elijah prepared a table summarizing his flexibility activity (or lack thereof) over the past two weeks and his flexibility scores. (He wrote his plan during the summer when he was not in school.) As you can see in figure 12.4, he did no flexibility exercise during that two-week period. He also had

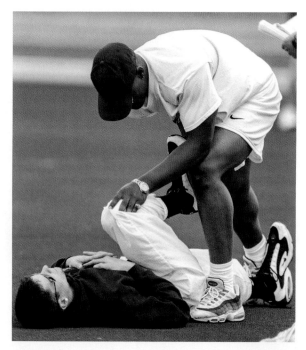

Stretching works best after a 5- to 10-minute general warm-up.

Day	Flexibility exercises	Amount
Mon.	None	None
Tues.	None	None
Wed.	None	None
Thurs.	None	None
Fri.	None	None
Sat.	None	None
Sun.	None	None

Fitness self-assessments	Score	Rating
Arm lift	20 cm (8 in.)	Need improvement
Zipper Right Left	Fingers touch Fingers do not touch	Met standard Need improvement
Trunk rotation Right Left	Reached target Did not reach target	Met standard Need improvement
Wrap-around Right Left	Touched mouth Touched mouth	Met standard Met standard
Knee to chest Right Left	Calf lifted >2.5 cm (1 in.) Calf lifted >2.5 cm (1 in.)	Need improvement Need improvement
Ankle flex Right Left	75° 80°	Met standard Need improvement
Total score	6 items passed	Marginal fitness
Back-saver sit and reach	13 cm (5 in.)	Low fitness

FIGURE 12.4 Elijah's flexibility exercise (physical activity) and fitness profiles.

not done any recent flexibility tests, but he did have scores from tests he had done in school during the previous semester.

Elijah obviously did not meet the CSEP recommendation of performing flexibility exercise for the major muscle groups on at least two days a week. Even so, he had passed several of his recent flexibility tests (and he had been doing some flexibility exercises at that time).

Step 2: Consider Your Program Options

Elijah listed seven types of flexibility exercise that he wanted to consider. He reviewed many types of exercises before preparing a list of exercises that he thought would be good for him and that he would be most likely to perform.

- Static stretching exercises
- PNF exercises
- Ballistic stretching exercises
- Yoga
- Tai chi
- Pilates
- Dynamic movement exercises (for warm-up)

Step 3: Set Goals

For his flexibility exercise plan (see figure 12.5), Elijah chose a time period of two weeks. This was too short a time for setting long-term goals, so he developed only short-term physical activity goals for this plan. Later, he'll develop long-term goals, including some flexibility improvement goals, when he prepares a longer plan. For now, he just wanted

Day	Exercise type	✔	Time, sets, reps
Mon.	**Static stretch** Back-saver sit and reach Knee to chest Side stretch Sitting stretch Zipper Hip stretch Chest stretch Calf stretch		3:00 p.m. after daily jog 1 set of 2 repetitions for each exercise Hold each exercise 15 sec
Tues.	**Dynamic movement exercise warm-up** High-knee march Standing flutter Quarter-turn cha-cha Shutter Grapevine Frankenstein Knee-high skip Jump and tuck Slow jog, fast sprint		1:00 p.m. before soccer Approximately 10 min. Perform each exercise five times, then continue on to the next exercise. Exercises followed by a slow jog for 30 sec and a fast sprint for 10 sec repeated three times.
Wed.	**Static stretch** Back-saver sit and reach Knee to chest Side stretch Sitting stretch Zipper Hip stretch Chest stretch Calf stretch		3:00 p.m. after daily jog 1 set of 2 repetitions for each exercise Hold each exercise 15 sec
Thurs.	**Dynamic movement exercise warm-up** High-knee march Standing flutter Quarter-turn cha-cha Shutter Grapevine Frankenstein Knee-high skip Jump and tuck Slow jog, fast sprint		1:00 p.m. before soccer Approximately 10 min. Perform each exercise five times, then continue on to the next exercise. Exercises followed by a slow jog for 30 sec and a fast sprint for 10 sec repeated three times.
Fri.	**Static stretch** Back-saver sit and reach Knee to chest Side stretch Sitting stretch Zipper Hip stretch Chest stretch Calf stretch		3:00 p.m. after daily jog 1 set of 2 repetitions for each exercise Hold each exercise 15 sec
Sat.	Yoga class		10:00–10:30 a.m. with sister
Sun.	None		None

FIGURE 12.5 Elijah's written flexibility exercise plan.

to get started by trying some new exercises. Besides, it was summer, and he didn't have access to school facilities, nor was he a member of a fitness club. So he chose SMART goals for his specific situation and wrote them down.

1. Perform one set of eight static stretching exercises on three days a week, including back-saver sit and reach, knee to chest, side stretch, sitting stretch, zipper, hip stretch, chest stretch, and calf stretch.
2. Perform a dynamic movement exercise warm-up for 10 minutes including nine basic exercises before playing sports.
3. Perform yoga for 30 minutes on one day a week.

Step 4: Structure Your Program and Write It Down

Elijah's next step was to write down his two-week flexibility exercise plan (see figure 12.5). He chose

static stretching that he could do at home three days a week. Because he played soccer two days a week, he also decided to do a dynamic movement exercise warm-up prior to his matches. He didn't expect the warm-up to be his main source of flexibility development, but he thought it would supplement his other flexibility exercise. He also agreed to go to yoga class with his sister Nicole, who was allowed to bring a guest for two free sessions.

Step 5: Keep a Log and Evaluate Your Program

Over the next two weeks, Elijah will self-monitor his activities and place a checkmark beside each activity he actually performs. At the end of the two weeks, Elijah will evaluate his activity to see whether he met his goals. He can then use the evaluation to help him write a future activity plan.

Lesson Review
1. Describe several basic flexibility (stretching) exercises.
2. What are some other forms of activity that build flexibility?
3. What are the basic guidelines for stretching?
4. What flexibility exercises should you include in your written flexibility exercise plan? Why?

BACK-SAVER SIT AND REACH (PNF OR STATIC)

1. Assume the back-saver sit-and-reach position with your right knee bent and your left leg straight.

2. Bend your left knee slightly and push your heel into the floor as you contract your hamstrings hard for three seconds. Relax.

    Note: For a static stretch, omit step 2.

3. Immediately grasp your ankle with both hands and gently pull your chest toward your knee. Hold the position for 15 seconds.

4. Repeat the exercise on the other leg.

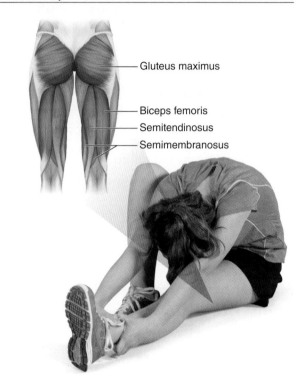

Gluteus maximus

Biceps femoris

Semitendinosus

Semimembranosus

This exercise stretches your hamstrings and lower back muscles.

KNEE TO CHEST

1. Lie on your back and extend your right leg. Place your hands on the back of your left thigh and pull toward you to draw the knee closer to the chest. Do not place your hands on top of the knee.

2. Keep your right leg straight and on the floor if possible. Keep your lower back flat on the floor.

3. Hold the position for 15 seconds.

4. Repeat with the opposite leg.

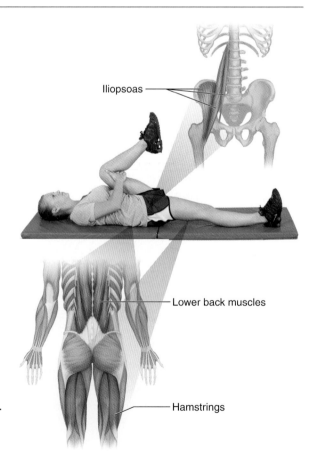

Iliopsoas

Lower back muscles

Hamstrings

This exercise stretches your hamstrings, your lower back, and the hip flexor muscles.

BACK AND HIP STRETCH (PNF OR STATIC)

1. Lie on your back with your knees bent and your arms at your sides.

2. Lift your hips until there is no bend at the hip joint. Squeeze the buttocks muscles hard for three seconds. Relax by lowering your hips to the floor.

    Note: For a static stretch, omit step 2.

3. Immediately place your hands under your knees and gently pull your knees to your chest. Hold the position for 15 seconds or more.

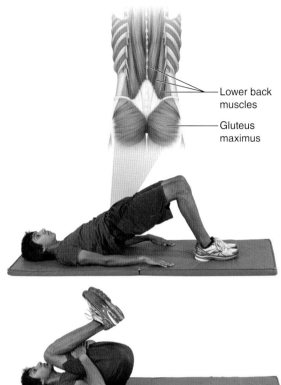

Lower back muscles

Gluteus maximus

This exercise stretches your lower back and gluteal muscles.

SIDE STRETCH (STATIC OR BALLISTIC)

1. Stand with your feet slightly wider than shoulder-width apart.

2. Lean to your left.

3. Reach down to your left foot with your left hand. Reach over your head with your right arm. Hold for a count of 10 to 30 seconds.

    Caution: Do not twist or lean your body forward.

4. Repeat the exercise on your right side.

Note: For a ballistic stretch, do a gentle bouncing stretch.

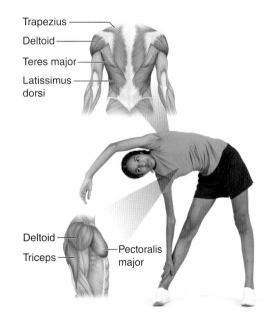

Trapezius

Deltoid

Teres major

Latissimus dorsi

Deltoid

Triceps

Pectoralis major

This exercise stretches the muscles of your arms and shoulders and the sides of your body.

TRUNK AND HIP STRETCH (STATIC)

1. Lie on your back with your knees bent and your arms extended at shoulder level.
2. Cross your left leg over your right leg.
3. Keep your shoulders and arms on the floor as you rotate your lower body to the left and touch your right knee to the floor. Stretch and hold the position for 10 to 30 seconds.
4. At the end of the stretch, reverse the position of your legs (cross your right leg over your left), then rotate to the right and hold the position.

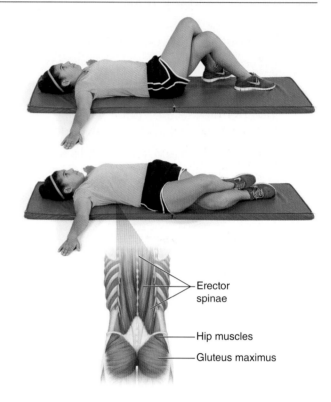

Erector spinae

Hip muscles

Gluteus maximus

This exercise stretches the muscles of your hips and lower back.

SITTING STRETCH (PNF OR STATIC)

1. Sit with the soles of your feet together and your elbows or hands resting on your knees.
2. Contract the muscles on the inside of your thighs, pulling up as you resist with your arms pushing down. Hold the position for three seconds. Relax your legs.
   Note: For a static stretch, omit step 2.
3. Immediately lean your trunk forward and push down on your knees with your arms to stretch your thighs. Hold the position for 10 to 30 seconds.

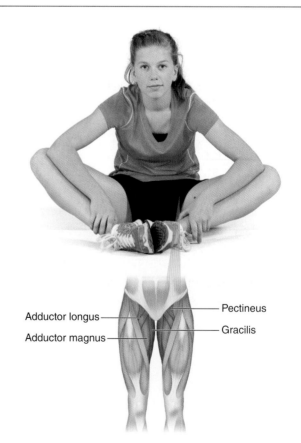

Adductor longus

Adductor magnus

Pectineus

Gracilis

This exercise stretches the muscles of the inside of your thighs.

ZIPPER (PNF OR STATIC)

1. Stand or sit. Lift your right arm over your right shoulder and reach down your spine.

2. With your left hand, press down on your right elbow. Resist the pressure by trying to raise that elbow, contracting the opposing muscles. Hold the position for three seconds. Relax.

    Note: For a static stretch, omit step 2.

3. Immediately stretch by reaching down your spine with your right arm as your left arm assists by pressing on your elbow. Hold the position for 10 to 30 seconds.

4. Repeat the exercise with your other arm.

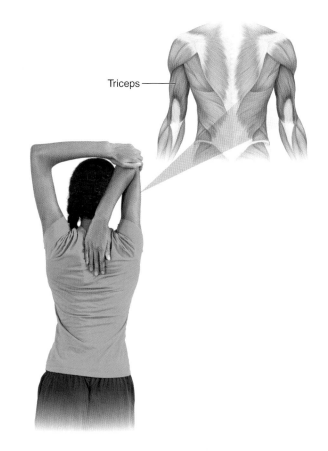

Triceps

This exercise stretches your triceps and latissimus muscles.

ARM PRETZEL (STATIC OR BALLISTIC)

1. Stand or sit. Bend your elbows and hold both hands as if shaking hands. Cross your right hand over your left so that the backs of the two hands are facing each other about 5 centimetres (2 inches) apart. Turn your right palm upward and point your thumb down over the left hand.

2. Grasp your right thumb with your left hand and pull down gently. Stretch and hold the position for 10 to 30 seconds.

3. Reverse arm positions and stretch your left shoulder.

Note: For a ballistic stretch, do a gentle bouncing stretch.

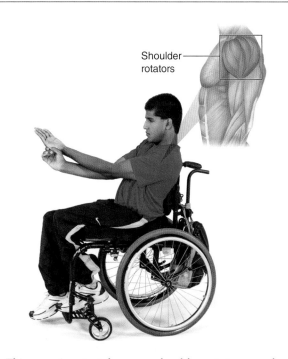

Shoulder rotators

This exercise stretches your shoulder rotator muscles.

HIP STRETCH (STATIC OR BALLISTIC)

1. Take a long step forward on your right foot and kneel on your left knee. Your right knee should be directly over your ankle and bent at a right angle.

2. You should feel a stretch across the front of your left hip joint and in the front of your thigh muscles.

3. Place your hands on your right knee for balance. Stretch by shifting your weight forward as you tilt your pelvis and trunk backward slightly. Keep your back knee in the same spot to stretch your hip and thigh muscles. Hold the position for 10 to 30 seconds.

4. Repeat the exercise with your other leg.

Note: For a ballistic stretch, do a gentle bouncing motion forward as you tilt your pelvis back.

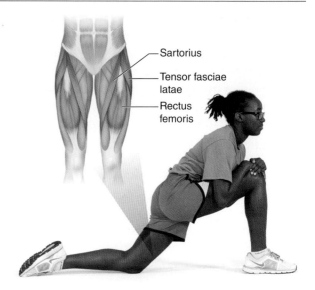

This exercise stretches the quadriceps muscles on the front of your thighs and the muscles on the front of your hips.

ARM STRETCH (STATIC)

1. Sit or stand and cross your right arm over your left (just above your head) with your palms facing each other. Lace your fingers together.

2. Straighten your elbows to raise your arms overhead as high as possible (your upper arms should touch your ears). Hold the position 10 to 30 seconds.

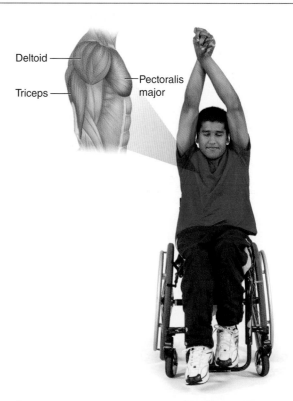

This exercise stretches the muscles of your shoulders, arms, and chest.

CHEST STRETCH (PNF, STATIC, OR BALLISTIC)

1. Stand in a forward-stride position in a doorway. Raise your arms slightly above shoulder height. Place your hands on either side of the doorway.

2. Lean your body into the doorway. Resist by contracting your arm and chest muscles. Hold the position for three seconds. Relax.

3. Immediately lean farther forward, letting your body weight stretch your muscles. Hold the position for 10 to 30 seconds.

4. For a ballistic stretch, gently bounce your body forward.

Note: For a static stretch, omit steps 2 and 4.

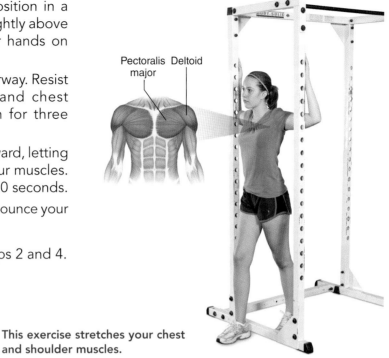

This exercise stretches your chest and shoulder muscles.

CALF STRETCH (STATIC OR BALLISTIC)

1. Step forward with your right leg in a lunge position. Keep both feet pointed straight ahead and your front knee directly over your front foot. Place your hands on your right leg for balance.

2. Keep your left leg straight and the heel on the floor. Adjust the length of your lunge until you feel a good stretch in your left calf and Achilles tendon. Hold the position for 10 to 30 seconds.

3. Repeat the exercise with your other leg.

Note: For a ballistic stretch, gently bounce your heel toward the floor.

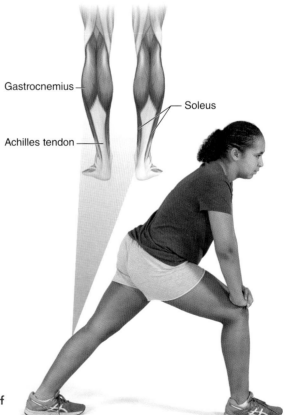

This exercise stretches your calf muscles and Achilles tendons.

TAKING CHARGE: Building Positive Attitudes

Allen and Matt are friends who often do things together, including sport activities. Sometimes they play tennis together on the weekend. Lately, Allen has been winning most of their matches.

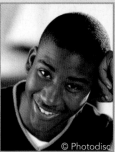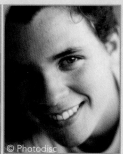

© Photodisc © Photodisc

"You ready to hit the court?" Allen asked Matt as he grabbed his tennis racket.

"I don't feel like playing today," Matt said. "Anyway, there's a good show on TV." He walked into the family room and sat on the couch.

Allen followed him. "I think you just don't want to lose again."

"You're right," Matt admitted. "I hate losing."

"You win sometimes, Matt. The competition is what makes tennis fun."

"Not when I lose," Matt replied.

Allen thought for a minute. "How about taking a jog around the block?" he asked. "There'll be no winner or loser that way."

"I don't want to get all sweaty," Matt replied. "I'd rather relax watching TV."

"Oh, come on, Matt. Jogging will help you relax. We need to stay in shape."

Matt looked at Allen and said, "I'm thinking about it."

For Discussion

What does Allen like about being physically active? What does Matt like—and not like—about physical activity? How could Matt change his negative attitudes and become more active? What are some other negative attitudes that keep people from being active, and how can they be changed? What are some positive attitudes that help people stay active? Consider the information in the Self-Management feature when answering the discussion questions.

SELF-MANAGEMENT: Skills for Building Positive Attitudes

Most of us have had both positive and negative attitudes about physical activity at one time or another. Experts have shown that people with more positive attitudes toward physical activity than negative ones are likely to be active. Here are some examples of positive and negative attitudes toward physical activity:

Positive attitudes:

- **"Physical activities are a great way to meet people."** Many activities provide opportunities to meet people and strengthen friendships. For example, aerobic dance and team sports are good social activities.

- **"I enjoy the challenge."** When the famous mountain climber George Mallory was asked why he climbed Mount Everest, he replied, "Because it's there." Helen Keller was deaf and blind but became a famous author. She said in one of her books that "life is either a daring adventure or nothing at all." Some people just enjoy a challenge. Are you one of them?

- **"Physical activity just makes me feel good."** Many people just feel better when they exercise, and many have a sense of loss or discomfort when they don't exercise.

Negative attitudes:

- **"I don't have the time."** You can make this attitude more positive by saying, "I will plan a time for physical activity." If you planned time for physical activity, you would feel better, function more efficiently, and therefore have more time to do other things that you want to do.

- **"People might laugh at me."** You can make this attitude more positive by saying, "When they see how fit I get, they'll wish they were exercising too." Find friends who are interested in getting fit. Anyone who does laugh may simply be jealous of your efforts and results.

- **"None of my friends work out, so neither do I."** You can make this attitude more positive by saying, "I'll ask my friends to join me, and maybe we'll work out together." Talk with your friends. Some of them may be interested in working out or doing lifestyle activities together.

Use the following guidelines to build positive attitudes and get rid of negative ones.

- **Assess your attitudes.** Make a list of your positive and negative attitudes toward physical activity.

- **Identify your reasons for any negative attitudes.** Your self-assessment will help you identify any negative attitudes you hold. Ask yourself why you feel negative about physical activity. If you can find the reason, it may help you change. For example, you may not have liked playing a sport when you were young because you didn't like a particular coach or player. Maybe you can now find a situation that will make an activity more fun. Consider the alternatives to negative attitudes described earlier.

- **Find activities that bring out fewer negative attitudes.** People have different attitudes and feelings about different activities. For example, maybe you don't like team sports but you do enjoy recreational activities. List your negative attitudes, then ask yourself whether there are activities you don't dislike. If so, consider trying them.

- **Choose activities that accentuate the positive.** If you really like certain activities and feel good about them, focus on these activities rather than ones you don't like as much.

- **Change the situation.** You may feel negatively about an activity because of things unrelated to the activity. For example, if you hated playing basketball because you had too little time to get dressed and groomed after participating, maybe you can find a situation in which you can do the activity and also have more time to shower and dress.

- **Be active with friends.** Activities are often more fun when you do them with friends. Sometimes participating with other people you like is enough to change your feelings about an activity.

- **Discuss your attitudes.** Just talking about your attitudes can sometimes help. People sometimes think they're the only ones who have problems in certain situations. Talking about it with others can help you change the situation to make it more fun for everyone concerned.

- **Help others build positive attitudes.** The ways in which others react can affect a person's feelings about physical activity. Your positive reactions can help others change negative feelings about physical activity. Consider the following suggestions when you interact with others in physical activity.

  - **Instead of laughing, provide encouragement.** Do you remember how difficult it is to start something new or different? You can encourage others by saying things such as "Good to see you exercising. Way to go!"

  - **Try to make new friends through participation in physical activities.** Introduce yourself to others and offer to help others when appropriate.

  - **Don't hesitate to ask for help from others.** Start or join a sport or exercise club at school. An activity club can be a great way for you and your friends to combine socializing with physical activity. If you're thinking about starting a club, check with your school's activity coordinator first.

  - **Be sensitive to people with special needs.** Some people need certain accommodations or modifications when performing physical activity. People with no special needs can help by participating with those who do have special challenges and by being sensitive to their needs.

  - **Be considerate of differences.** The popularity of physical activities varies from culture to culture. What is popular in one culture is not necessarily popular in another. For example, orienteering and men's field hockey are not popular in Canada but are very popular in other countries. Similarly, what one person enjoys may not be so enjoyable to another. Learning to accept cultural and personal differences helps all people enjoy activity and contributes to better interpersonal understanding.

Prepare a two-week muscle fitness flexibility exercise plan. Prepare tables similar to those used by Elijah and use the five steps of program planning. Try out your program and see if you can meet your goals. The goal is to perform flexibility exercises three days a week. Carry out it over a two-week period. Your teacher may give you time in class to do some of the activities in your plan. Consider the following suggestions for taking action.

- Before performing stretching exercises, do a general warm-up.
- Consider the guidelines for flexibility exercise presented in lesson 2 of this chapter.
- If you're already participating in organized sport or physical activity, consider doing your flexibility exercise during the cool-down portion of your workout.

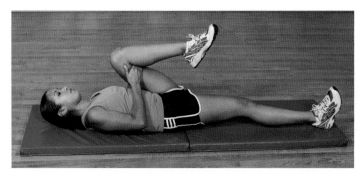

Take action by performing your flexibility exercise plan.

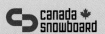 GET ACTIVE WITH CANADA SNOWBOARD

©Canada Snowboard

Who We Are

Canada Snowboard is the national sport organization dedicated to making Canada a leading snowboarding nation. From park to podium, we hope to inspire young athletes, encourage self-expression and promote the sport of snowboarding.

What We Do

In partnership with our provincial and territorial associations, Canada Snowboard ensures Canadian athletes have the opportunity to compete at any level, from grassroots to the international stage, and help inspire a nation. Whether competing in a slopestyle contest or in a snowboardcross race, our athletes are provided with the best possible chance of success through numerous camps, programs and initiatives. Through our Riders program, aimed at getting young boarders into snowboarding, all the way up to our national team jump camps, we are there every step of the way to provide the coaching and tools necessary for our athletes to perform at their absolute best.

Get Involved

From PEI to BC, there are snowboard clubs and associations to sign up with throughout the country. If freestyle is your thing, dozens of contests are held throughout the country where you can showcase your skills in slopestyle, big air and halfpipe contests. In speed disciplines such as Alpine or snowboardcross, speed and strategy come into play. One of the best ways to get involved is to find a local club or event, grab a couple of friends and head to your local mountain. No matter your level of riding, there are countless ways to get involved. Check out our website (www.canadasnowboard.ca) and social media pages where you'll find videos, articles and links to our provincial associations to help you get the most out of your riding.

©Canada Snowboard

Reviewing Concepts and Vocabulary

Complete the following in order to show your growing understanding of fitness, health, and wellness. Answer items 1 through 5 by correctly completing each sentence with a word or phrase.

1. The amount of movement you can make in a joint is called your _____.
2. Exercises including jumping, skipping, and calisthenics (such as those used in a warm-up) are called _____ exercises.
3. Being able to move beyond a typical healthy range of motion is called _____.
4. _____ is an ancient form of exercise that originated in China.
5. Gentle bouncing motions are part of _____.

For items 6 through 10, match each term in column 1 with the appropriate phrase in column 2.

6. zipper
7. passive stretch
8. active stretch
9. PNF
10. yoga

a. stretch created by gravity or an outside force
b. form of exercise from India
c. stretch created by an antagonist muscle
d. stretch after muscle contraction
e. arm stretching exercise

For items 11 through 15, respond to each statement or question.

11. What are some benefits of good flexibility?
12. What are some factors that influence flexibility other than stretching?
13. What are some good tests of flexibility described in this chapter?
14. What are some good basic flexibility (static stretching) exercises for the major muscle groups?
15. What are some guidelines for building positive attitudes toward physical activity?

Thinking Critically

Write a paragraph to answer the following question.

André's father went to a physical therapist to get treatment after a hip injury. The therapist recommended static stretching with a passive assist. André's dad asked him to help with the exercises. What safety concerns should André have in helping his father?

Project

Young people typically have better flexibility than older people. For this reason, parents and grandparents are likely to be less flexible than their children or grandchildren. Interview a parent or grandparent. Prepare a list of five questions related to current flexibility, past flexibility (at an earlier age), steps taken to maintain flexibility, and future plans for flexibility exercise. Prepare a report presenting your findings.

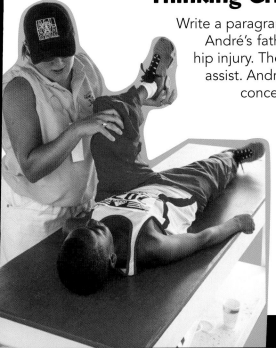

UNIT V

Making Healthy Food and Fitness Choices

• • • • • • • • • • • • • • • • •

Self-Assessment Features in This Unit
- Body Measurements
- Energy Balance
- Your Personal Fitness Test Battery

Taking Charge Features in This Unit
- Improving Physical Self-Perception
- Saying No
- Learning to Think Critically

Self-Management Features in This Unit
- Skills for Self-Perception
- Skills for Saying No
- Skills for Thinking Critically

Taking Action Features in This Unit
- Elastic Band Workout
- Burn It Up Workout
- My Health and Fitness Club

Canadian Sport and Health Organization Features in This Unit
- Get Active With Swimming Canada
- Get Active With Dietitians of Canada
- Get Active With the YMCA

13

Maintaining a Healthy Body Composition

In This Chapter

www. **Student Web Resources**
www.fitnessforlife.org/student

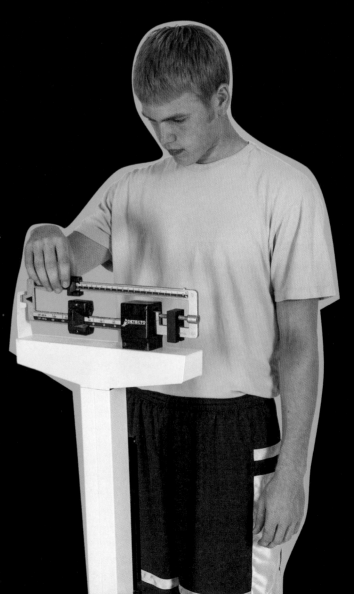

Lesson 13.1
Body Composition Facts

Lesson Objectives

After participating in this lesson, you should be able to

1. define *body composition, overweight,* and *obesity;*
2. describe some factors that influence body composition;
3. define *anorexia nervosa, bulimia,* and *anorexia athletica;*
4. explain how excess body fat levels can affect health; and
5. describe several laboratory and nonlaboratory tests for measuring body composition.

Lesson Vocabulary

anorexia athletica, anorexia nervosa, basal metabolism, body composition, body fat level, bulimia, essential body fat, lean body tissue, metabolic syndrome, obesity, overweight, skinfold, underweight

---

Body composition is a part of health-related physical fitness. It refers to all the tissues that make up your body. In this lesson, you'll learn about the types of tissue that make up your body and about key terms related to **body composition**. You'll also learn how to assess your current body composition and determine whether it is optimal for good health.

Body Composition Definitions

Your body is made up of two major types of tissue. In a healthy person, the great majority of the body consists of **lean body tissue**, including muscle, bone, skin, and body organs such as the heart, liver, kidneys, and lungs. All of the types of physical activity included in the Physical Activity Pyramid build lean body tissue, but muscle fitness exercises are especially good because they both build muscle and enhance bone development.

The other major type of body tissue is fat. Your **body fat level** refers to the percentage of your body that is fat tissue. A fit person has a healthy amount of body fat—neither too much nor too little.

About half of your body fat is located deep within your body. The remaining fat is located between your skin and your muscles. People who do regular physical activity typically have a larger percentage of lean body weight (especially from muscle and bone) and less body fat than people who do not do such activity. It's good if fat accounts for a relatively low percentage of your total body weight. However, for good health, you do need some body fat. Determining your body fatness requires special equipment and expertise. Later, you'll learn how to measure the fat between your skin and muscles to estimate your total body fatness.

The terms **underweight** and **overweight** are commonly used to refer to a body weight that is outside the healthy weight range—either below the range or above it. These terms have limitations because weight, or the combination of weight and height, does not always accurately reflect the amount of fat and lean tissue in the body. You'll learn more about underweight and overweight later in this chapter. The term **obesity** refers to the condition of being especially overweight or high in body fat.

FIT FACT

About two-thirds of all Canadian adults are considered overweight or obese. Since obesity has been linked with many chronic diseases, including hypertension, type 2 diabetes, cardiovascular disease, osteoarthritis, and certain types of cancer, this is cause for concern for the health and wellness of Canadians.

Factors Influencing Body Fatness

Many factors influence a person's level of body fat. Some are discussed in the following sections.

Heredity

You inherit your body type from your parents. Some people are born with a tendency to be lean, or muscular, or heavy. Inherited tendencies make it easier for some people and harder for others to keep their body fat level in the good fitness zone. You can't control your heredity, but you can be aware of tendencies in your family.

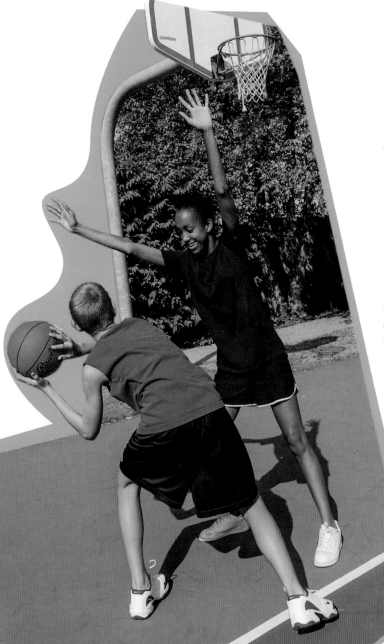

Metabolism

Your **basal metabolism** is the amount of energy (calories) your body uses just to keep you living. Your basal metabolism does not include the calories you burn while working, enjoying recreation, studying, or even sitting and watching television. Some people have a higher basal metabolism than others. This means that their bodies, at complete rest, burn more calories than the bodies of people with a lower metabolism. People with more muscle mass have a higher metabolism than people with less muscle mass. People with a higher metabolism can consume more calories than others can without increasing their level of body fat.

Your metabolism is affected by your heredity, age, and maturation. Most young people have a high metabolism because their bodies are growing and building muscle. As you grow older and lose muscle mass, your metabolism typically slows, which means that most people need to reduce the number of calories in their diet in order to avoid gaining fat.

Maturation

As you grow older and your hormone levels begin to change, your level of body fat also changes. During the teen years, female hormones cause girls to develop more body fat than boys, which is absolutely normal and healthy. Because of male hormones, teenage boys experience greater muscle development.

Body Fat Levels Early in Life

Children who have excessive amounts of fat have developed extra fat cells that make it more difficult to control their fat level later in life. Therefore, keeping your body fat level within the good fitness zone during your childhood and teen years will help you keep it in check throughout life.

Diet

The amount of energy contained in foods is measured in calories. Teens typically need more calories than adults. A typical teen male needs to consume about 2,500 to 3,000 calories a day to maintain an ideal level of body fat. A typical teenage female needs about 2,000 to 2,500 calories a day. Most males need more calories than most females because they are larger and have more muscle mass.

Physical Activity

Your body burns calories for energy. Therefore, the more vigorous activity you do (the more energy your body uses), the more calories you need. An inactive person uses less energy each day than an active person and thus needs to consume fewer calories. Teens who participate in vigorous activities such as sports need to consume more calories than less active teens. The key is to balance energy expenditure with calorie consumption.

Body Fatness, Health, and Wellness

Having too much fat can be unhealthy. Scientists report that people who are high in body fat have a higher risk of heart disease, high blood pressure, diabetes, cancer, and other diseases. Until recently, type 2 diabetes was considered to be an adult disease, but it has become more common among youth primarily because of increases in body fat levels among youth. High levels of body fat are also associated with a condition called **metabolic syndrome**. This syndrome occurs when a person has a high level of body fat, large waist girth, and other health risks, such as high blood pressure, high blood fat, and high blood sugar.

In addition, health costs for obese people total thousands of dollars a year more than for people with healthy levels of body fat, and being high in body fat reduces a person's chances of successful surgery. A person with too much body fat also tires more quickly and easily than a lean person and

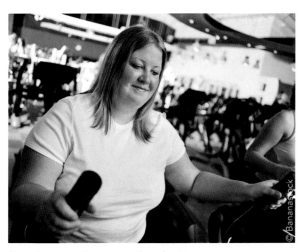

Regular exercise expends calories.

FIT FACT

Fewer children and teens are considered overweight or obese compared to adults, and the percentage varies by age, sex, and province. Obesity is highest among those living in the Atlantic provinces (Newfoundland and Labrador, Prince Edward Island, Nova Scotia, and New Brunswick) as well as Saskatchewan and the Northwest Territories. Quebec and British Columbia have the lowest rates of obesity. Obesity rates continue to rise across Canada.

therefore may be less efficient in both work and recreation. Many experts believe that the reason so many adults have too much body fat is that they try to achieve an unrealistic weight or fat level. For example, many people try to be as lean as a movie star or an athlete shown in a commercial. When they cannot attain or maintain such an exceptionally low level of body fat, they give up and gain body fat. Instead, experts recommend setting less extreme goals that are achievable, which helps people maintain a healthy level of body fat throughout life.

 We have to make sure that our kids still feel good about themselves no matter what their weight, no matter how they feel. We need to make sure that our kids know that we love them no matter who they are, what they look like.

—Michelle Obama, former First Lady of the United States

Too Little Body Fat

Having too little body fat is also a health risk. Eating disorders such as **anorexia nervosa**, **anorexia athletica**, and **bulimia** have many negative health consequences and can even be fatal. It is extremely important to identify the symptoms of an eating disorder as early as possible. An excessive desire to lose fat or maintain a very low fat level can lead to serious health problems.

The minimum amount of body fat required for healthy body functioning is called **essential body**

fat. Having too little body fat can cause abnormal functioning of various organs. In fact, exceptionally low body fat can result in serious health problems, particularly among teenagers. Females with especially low body fat experience health problems related to their reproductive system and risk losing bone density. The following list summarizes several reasons your body needs some fat.

The Importance of Body Fat

- Fat is an insulator; it helps your body adapt to heat and cold.

- Fat acts as a shock absorber; it can help protect your organs and bones from injury.

- Fat helps your body use vitamins effectively.

- Fat is stored energy that is available when your body needs it.

- In reasonable amounts, fat helps you look your best, thus increasing your feelings of well-being.

Anorexia Nervosa

Anorexia nervosa is a serious eating disorder. A person who has this disorder severely restricts the amount of food that he or she eats in an attempt to have an exceptionally low level of body fat. In addition, many people with anorexia do extensive physical activity, thus further lowering their body fat to extremely dangerous levels.

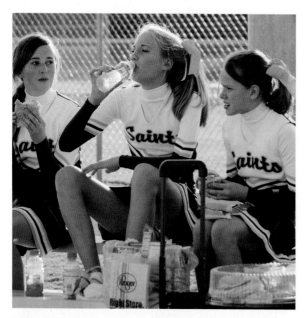

Even if you're in a sport where low body weight is desirable, it's still important to eat healthfully.

Anorexia is most common among teenage girls, but it is becoming increasingly common among teenage boys. People with this disorder are usually very hard workers and high achievers. They have a distorted view of their body and see themselves as being too fat even when they are extremely thin. Persons with this disorder often fear maturity and the weight gain associated with adulthood. They often try to hide their condition by wearing baggy clothing, pretending to eat, and exercising in private. Anorexia is a life-threatening condition, and people who have it need immediate professional help.

Anorexia Athletica

Anorexia athletica has many symptoms similar to those of anorexia nervosa. It is most common among athletes involved in sports—such as gymnastics, wrestling, and cheerleading—in which low body weight is desirable. This disorder can lead to anorexia nervosa. It is thought to be related to the pressure to maintain low weight and an excessive preoccupation with dieting and exercising for weight loss.

Bulimia

Bulimia is an eating disorder in which a person engages in binge eating—eating a very large amount of food in a short time. Bingeing is followed by purging, perhaps by vomiting or by the use of laxatives to rid the body of food and prevent its digestion. Bulimia can result in severe digestive problems and other health problems such as tooth loss and gum disease.

FIT FACT

Studies show that the number of teens who think they are overweight is four to five times the number who really are. At the same time, interviews with teens who actually are overweight show that 44 percent either have been or currently are teased about their body weight. Getting teased for being overweight—or just feeling as though one is overweight—can result in low physical self-perceptions. Teens can help other teens improve their self-perceptions by being supportive rather than critical.

⚛ SCIENCE IN ACTION: Media Misrepresentation

Over the years, both exercise psychologists and nutrition scientists have conducted research about physical self-perceptions. They have found that people of all ages are self-conscious about the way they look. In fact, most people are far more critical of their own body than other people are. One reason is that we often compare ourselves with movie stars and other celebrities. Experts point out that the pictures we see of these people have been designed specifically to make them look as glamorous as possible and are touched up to enhance appearance. For example, computer programs can be used to make a female movie star's waist smaller and a male star's muscles larger. Some magazines have promised to limit changes in photos, but there are no regulations, and each magazine can do as it pleases.

Websites also use fake or altered pictures. Advertisements frequently show supposed before-and-after pictures to promote a product. The "before" photos often are taken with bad lighting and in unflattering conditions. The "after" photos are taken with better lighting and are sometimes altered. Video games also present unrealistic images of the human body. For example, body proportions for some male and female video game figures are literally impossible for real-life people.

Many experts believe that the misrepresentation of the human body in the media results in an obsession with leanness. Statistics indicate that many teens, especially girls, set unrealistic standards in judging their body composition. Many feel that they have more fat than they really do, and they try to lose weight unnecessarily. Because we are all a bit self-conscious, it is easy

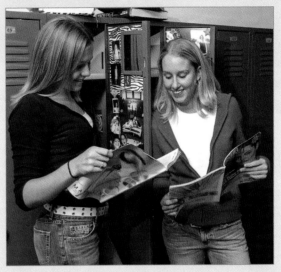

Magazines and websites often alter photos of models and celebrities to make their bodies look unrealistically thin.

to overreact when others make comments about the way we look. For this reason, experts point out the importance of not making critical comments about others. It is also important to keep personal information, such as self-assessment results, confidential. You'll learn more about self-perceptions in the Taking Charge feature in the next lesson of this chapter.

Student Activity

Explore a variety of media sources to find examples of misrepresentation of the human body. Look for websites that provide pictures and explanations of how photos of stars and models in advertisements are altered.

Laboratory Measurements for Assessing Body Composition

The most accurate methods for measuring body composition require special equipment and trained people. They are typically done in a laboratory. Three of the best methods are DXA, underwater weighing, and the Bod Pod (figure 13.1). All three

are useful in determining how much of the body weight is fat and how much is lean tissue.

Dual-Energy X-Ray Absorptiometry

Dual-energy X-ray absorptiometry (DXA) is now considered the best method of assessing body composition (figure 13.1*a*) because it can accurately detect body fat, bone, muscle, and other body

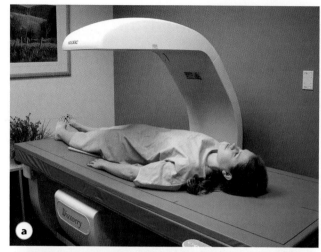
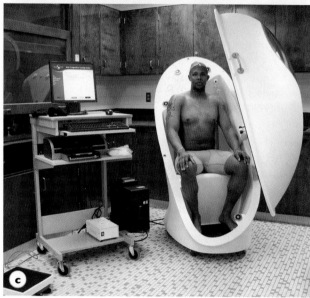
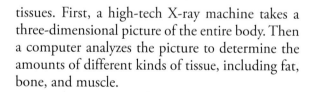
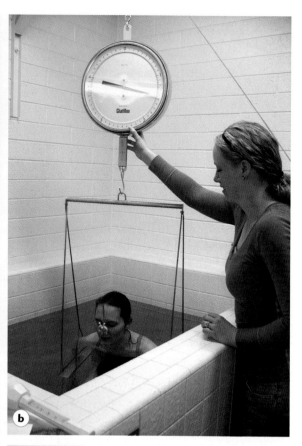

FIGURE 13.1 Laboratory methods for assessing body composition: *(a)* DXA; *(b)* underwater weighing; *(c)* Bod Pod.

Photos courtesy of Dale Wagner.

tissues. First, a high-tech X-ray machine takes a three-dimensional picture of the entire body. Then a computer analyzes the picture to determine the amounts of different kinds of tissue, including fat, bone, and muscle.

Underwater Weighing

Until recently, underwater weighing was considered the best way to assess body fat level, and it is still a very good laboratory method. With this technique, you are weighed on land, then immersed in a tank of water and weighed again (figure 13.1*b*). Measurements of your lung capacity are also taken because the amount of air in your lungs influences your weight in water. A formula is then applied to determine your body fat level based on your land weight, your underwater weight, and your lung capacity.

Bod Pod

A third type of laboratory assessment of body composition uses a machine called the Bod Pod. In this method, the person being tested sits in an egg-shaped chamber or pod (figure 13.1*c*). The person's body, of course, takes up space in the pod, thus causing air to be moved from the pod. Information gained from changes in the pod's air is then plugged into a special formula to determine the person's body fatness.

Nonlaboratory Measures

Because laboratory measures require special equipment and special training, they are rarely used in schools. For school and home use, nonlaboratory measures are available. Several practical methods of assessment are described here. However, not all of these measures accurately predict the amount of fat and lean body tissue; for this reason, they are typically referred to as body measurements. Body measurements are easier to use than laboratory measures and can be performed at school and often at home. Because you will probably encounter all of these measures at some time in your life, you should try each one of them.

Skinfold Measurements

Your body fat level can also be estimated by measurement of **skinfold** thickness (the amount of fat under your skin). Skinfold thickness is measured by means of a special instrument called a calliper (see figure 13.2). Skinfold measurements can be used to provide an estimate of the total amount of fat in the body. As noted earlier, a high level of body fat is associated with a variety of health problems, including diabetes, heart disease, and other chronic diseases. You'll learn to do skinfold measurements in this chapter's Self-Assessment feature.

Height–Weight and BMI

Height and weight are commonly used in two ways. One method uses height–weight tables that show "normal" weight ranges for people according to age, height, and sex. These tables indicate what the average person of a given sex weighs at a given height. However, because about two-thirds of adults in Canada are overweight or obese, many people who are classified as "normal" or "average" are still overweight or obese. For this reason, height–weight tables are considered less useful than some other methods presented in this chapter. You'll get a chance to use height–weight charts in the self-assessment that follows this lesson.

Height and weight are also used to calculate a person's body mass index (BMI). This index is considered to be a better measure than height and weight alone, but it still does not give as accurate an assessment of body fatness as DXA, underwater weighing, Bod Pod analysis, or skinfold measurement. Both the BMI and the height–weight charts can provide inaccurate measurements for people who have a lot of muscle (athletes, for example) because muscle weighs a lot more than fat. As a result, a very muscular person could be high in weight but not too fat. Similarly, a person who appears normal according to height–weight and BMI charts could actually have an unhealthy level of body fat. This is why skinfolds and laboratory techniques are often considered to be better measures.

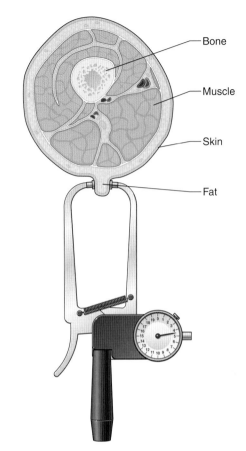

Bone

Muscle

Skin

Fat

FIGURE 13.2 A calliper measures skinfolds.

In spite of the limitations of BMI, high BMI has been associated with a variety of health problems among both teens and adults. In addition, BMI is often used because it's easy to measure, especially in large groups.

Waist-to-Hip Ratio

The waist-to-hip ratio is used not to determine body fatness but to assess health risk. Scientists now know that people who carry more weight in the middle of the body have a higher risk of disease than people who carry more weight in the lower body (legs and hips). People who carry too much weight in their midsection are said to have an apple body type, whereas people who carry more weight in their hips are said to have a pear body type. In general, women are more likely to be the pear type, and men are more likely to be the apple type.

The waist-to-hip ratio is a simple method for assessing the risk associated with body type. As you'll see when you do the self-assessment for this chapter,

FITNESS TECHNOLOGY: Bioelectrical Impedance Analysis

Computers and other machines have been developed to test body fat levels. For example, bioelectrical impedance analysis (BIA) requires a special machine and expertise to administer the test. However, in recent years BIA machines have become more common in schools because of lower prices and improved ease of use. Used properly, they can provide reliable and accurate estimates of body fatness. One limitation is that different machines can give different results, so it is important to use the same machine and to be sure that the machine is properly calibrated (tested for accuracy). In addition, testing should be done under similar conditions each time you are tested—for example, at the same time of day and not at times when you might be dehydrated. Some health and fitness clubs and doctors' offices now have BIA machines. Results of a BIA test can help determine the accuracy of measurements made using other techniques described in this chapter.

> **Using Technology**
>
> If possible, arrange to have a BIA test done. Compare your BIA results with the results of other self-assessments presented in this chapter. If a BIA test is not available, do some research about BIA testing and report your findings.

you determine this ratio by using a tape to measure your waist circumference and your hip circumference. It is desirable to have a waist circumference smaller than your hip circumference.

Waist Girth (Circumference)

Waist girth (also called waist circumference) can be used by itself as an indicator of health risk. Evidence indicates that people with a very large waist are at risk for health problems. As people grow older, their waist size often increases, thus exposing them to greater health risk. Thus waist girth is a useful health risk indicator that you can use throughout your life.

What Is My Ideal Body Weight?

Even after learning about the various forms of assessment, many people wonder what their ideal body weight is. Experts agree that there is no such thing as one ideal body weight for all people; that is, there is no single table or test that provides a best number for everyone. The best advice is to set a long-term goal of achieving a body fat level in the good fitness zone. Once you have achieved a body fat level that you are comfortable with and that puts you in the good fitness zone, weigh yourself and maintain that weight (this is sometimes referred to as target weight). It's a desirable lifetime goal to maintain this weight and a fat level in the good fitness zone.

If you're in the marginal or low fitness zone, develop a plan that will gradually move you to the next zone. Trying to achieve the good fitness zone when you're too far from it is unrealistic. Instead, people in the low fitness zone should try to move to the marginal zone. Those in the marginal zone should try to move to the good fitness zone. If you're already in the good fitness zone, a reasonable goal for you is simply to stay there.

Some athletes and people in careers that require high levels of fitness may be in the very lean zone, and some people can be very lean because of hereditary factors. While it is possible to be fit and healthy and be in the very lean zone, exceptional leanness is not necessarily a sign of good health and may not be a realistic goal for all people. As noted earlier in this chapter, your body needs a certain amount of body fat (essential body fat), and having too little can cause health problems. Too little body fat can also indicate an eating disorder. If you already have too little fat, increase your weight by gaining body fat. People with eating disorders often try to reduce body fat even when they already have too little for good health. It is important for all people to eat well in order to increase fitness, health, and wellness while also reducing disease. Athletes and those who perform jobs that require high levels of fitness have to eat well in order to be healthy and well, but also in order to reach their peak performance.

As part of a lifelong self-assessment plan, you may choose to monitor your waist-to-hip ratio and your waist girth, especially if you find it difficult to get a good assessment of your body fat level. These measurements are good indicators of health risk. You may also choose to track your BMI over time because physicians often use this measure. High scores are associated with health risks, but because BMI does not estimate body fat levels or lean body mass, it may misclassify some people as overweight or obese when they are not. Similarly BMI may classify a person as "normal" in weight when the person has a higher than healthy level of body fat. The same is true for height–weight charts.

Assessment Confidentiality

Self-assessments are done to gain information that will help the person build an accurate personal profile and plan for healthy active living. The results of self-assessments are personal information. In many assessments, you'll work with a partner, and you and your partner must agree to keep test results private. Information may be submitted to an instructor or a parent or guardian but always with the expectation that the information is private. Assessment-related information should not be shared with others without permission from the person being tested.

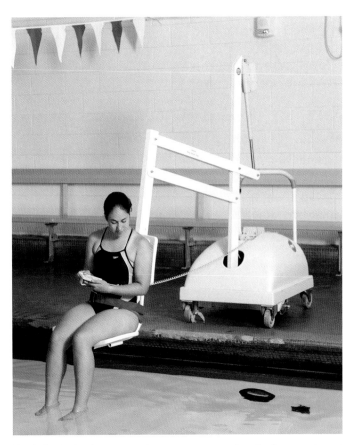

Body fat helps buoyancy in water, so people who have reduced or limited movement abilities can do exercises in water that they can't do on land.

Lesson Review

1. What do the terms *body composition*, *overweight*, and *obesity* mean?
2. What are some factors that influence body composition? How do they influence body composition?
3. What do the terms *anorexia nervosa*, *bulimia*, and *anorexia athletica* mean?
4. How do excess body fat levels affect health?
5. What are some laboratory and nonlaboratory tests for measuring body composition?

Earlier in this chapter, you learned about ways to determine body composition. Laboratory measures are the most accurate, but they typically require expensive equipment and people who know how to use the equipment correctly. Height and weight are the most commonly used nonlaboratory measures because they can be determined easily and do not require a lot of equipment.

In addition, body circumferences (such as waist-to-hip ratio and waist girth) can be used to determine health risks, and skinfold measurements can be used both to estimate body fat and to assess health risk. Your fitness scores are your personal information and should be kept confidential. You should also be sensitive to the feelings of others when body fat measurements are being taken; it may be appropriate to take measurements privately and to record and store them privately.

Height–Weight Charts

1. Locate the appropriate part of table 13.1 for your sex. Next, find your height (to the nearest centimetre) at the left and your age at the top of the table. The "normal" weight range for your sex, height, and age is shown in the box where your height row and your age column intersect.

2. Record the weight range for your sex, age, and height.

TABLE 13.1 Normal Weight Ranges in Kilograms

Male Height cm	13 or 14	15 or 16	17–20	Female Height cm	13 or 14	15 or 16	17–20
137	31–33			137	33–34		
140	33–34			140	34–36		
142	35–37			142	36–37		
145	37–39	37–39		145	39–40	41–43	
147	39–41	39–41		147	41–43	44–46	45–46
150	40–41	40–41		150	44–45	46–48	47–49
152	40–42	44–45	46–47	152	47–49	48–49	49–51
155	44–45	46–47	48–49	155	48–49	49–51	51–52
157	45–47	48–49	52–53	157	48–49	51–52	52–54
160	48–49	50–52	55–56	160	50–51	52–54	54–56
163	51–53	52–54	56–58	163	52–54	54–56	57–58
165	53–54	54–56	59–60	165	54–55	56–58	59–60
168	54–56	57–59	61–62	168	57–59	58–59	61–62
170	57–59	60–61	62–64	170	58–59	59–61	62–64
173	59–60	61–63	64–65	173	58–59	61–63	65–66
175	61–63	63–64	67–68	175	59–60	62–64	67–68
178	64–65	64–66	68–69	178	59–60	63–64	69–71
180	66–68	68–69	69–70	180		64–66	72–73
183	68–70	69–70	71–72	183		66–68	74–75
185		72–73	73–75				
188		73–74	76–77				
191			80–82				

To convert centimetres to inches, multiply centimetres by 0.39. To convert kilograms to pounds, multiply kilograms by 2.2. Alternatively, you can use the Internet to find a calculator that converts centimetres to inches and kilograms to pounds. Values have been rounded off to the nearest whole number.

Waist-to-Hip Ratio (Male and Female)

1. Measure your hips at the largest point (the largest circumference of your buttocks). Make sure that the tape is at the same level (horizontal to ground) in the front, in the back, and on your sides. The tape should be snug but not so tight as to cause indentations in your skin (do not use an elastic tape). Stand with your feet together when making the measurement.

2. Measure your waist at the smallest circumference (called the natural waist). If there is no natural waist, measure at the level of the umbilicus (belly button). Measure at the end of a normal inspiration (just after a normal in-breath). Do not suck in to make your waist smaller. This measurement is slightly different from the one used to measure waist girth by itself.

3. To calculate your waist-to-hip ratio, divide your waist girth by your hip girth.

4. Find your ratio in table 13.2 to determine your rating.

5. Record your hip and waist measurements and rating.

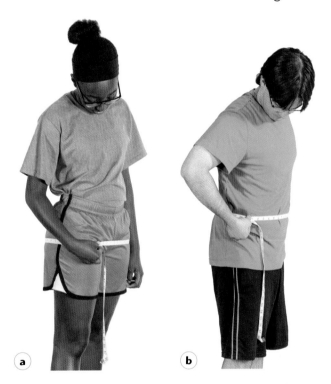

To determine your waist-to-hip ratio, measure (a) your hips and (b) your waist.

TABLE 13.2 Rating Chart: Waist-to-Hip Ratio

	Male	Female
Good fitness zone	≤0.90	≤0.79
Marginal	0.91–1.0	0.80–0.85
Low fitness zone	≥1.1	≥0.86

Waist Girth (Circumference)

1. Measure your waist at a level just above the top of your hipbones. Mark the top of your hipbone on each side and hold the tape just above the marks.

2. Measure after a normal inspiration (at the end of a normal in-breath). Do not suck in to make your waist smaller. Keep the tape horizontal to the ground when making the measurement.

3. Use table 13.3 to determine your rating.

4. Record your waist girth and rating.

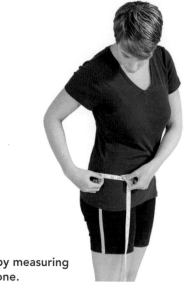

Waist girth is determined by measuring your waist above the hipbone.

TABLE 13.3 Rating Chart: Waist Girth in Centimetres

Age (years)	12	13	14	15	16	17	≥18
Male							
Good fitness zone	≤73.4	≤75.9	≤78.5	≤81.0	≤83.6	≤86.1	≤88.6
Marginal	73.5–85.0	76.0–87.4	78.6–91.2	81.1–94.9	83.7–97.5	86.2–101.3	88.7–105.2
Low fitness zone	≥85.1	≥87.5	≥91.3	≥95.0	≥97.6	≥101.4	≥105.3
Female							
Good fitness zone	≤73.6	≤75.9	≤78.5	≤81.0	≤82.3	≤84.8	≤87.4
Marginal	73.7–82.3	76.0–86.1	78.6–88.8	81.1–91.2	82.4–97.5	84.9–97.5	87.5–101.3
Low fitness zone	≥82.4	≥86.3	≥88.9	≥91.3	≥97.6	≥97.6	≥101.4

To convert centimetres to inches, multiply centimetres by 0.39. Alternatively, you can use the Internet to find a calculator that converts centimetres to inches.

Skinfold Measurements

Skinfold measurements require a special calliper, and using the calliper requires special training. But when done properly by a trained expert, skinfold measurements can provide a good estimate of body fatness. For best results, an expensive calliper is used, but research has shown that inexpensive plastic callipers, such as those shown in the photos here, can be quite accurate if used properly by a trained person who practices the measurement technique. Various measurements can be used; in this book, the calf and triceps are used because of their ease of measurement.

Use the following procedures to complete the various measurements and determine your ratings for each assessment. You can use skinfold measurements to estimate your body fat percentage and determine your target weight. For teenagers, upper arm (triceps) and calf measurements provide a good estimate of body fat percentage. If possible, have the measurements done by an expert. If not, work with a partner to take each other's measurements. With practice, you and your partner will improve your measurement skills. Comparing your measurements to those done by an expert will help you determine the accuracy of the measurements. If you're working with a partner, remember that self-assessment information is personal and considered confidential. It shouldn't be shared with others without the permission of the person being assessed.

For the triceps skinfold, pick up a skinfold on the middle of the back of the right arm, halfway between the elbow and the shoulder. The arm should hang loose and relaxed at the side.

For the calf skinfold, the person being tested should stand and place his or her right foot on a chair. Pick up a skinfold on the inside of the right calf, halfway between the shin and the back of the calf where the calf is largest.

1. Use your left thumb and index finger to pick up the skinfold. Do not pinch or squeeze the skinfold.

2. Hold the skinfold with your left hand while you pick up and use the calliper with your right hand to get a reading.

3. Place the calliper over the skinfold about 1.3 centimetres (0.5 inches) below your finger and thumb. Hold the calliper on the skinfold for three seconds, then note the measurement. If possible, read the calliper measurement to the nearest half-millimetre.

4. Make three measurements each for the triceps and the calf skinfolds. Allow at least 10 seconds between measurements. Use the middle of the three measures as the score. For example, an 8, 9, and 10 give a score of 9. If your three measurements differ by more than 2 millimetres, take a second, or even a third, set of three measurements.

5. Now determine your percent body fat and your body fatness rating. Add your triceps and calf scores to get your sum in millimetres; then use table 13.4 to estimate your body fat percentage based on your sum. Use the appropriate table for your sex and find your skinfold sum. Your percent body fat is the number just to the right. For example, if you're male and your skinfold sum is 26, your percent body fat is 21.

6. Once you have determined your percent body fat, use table 13.5 to determine your body fatness rating.

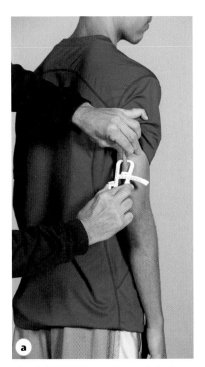 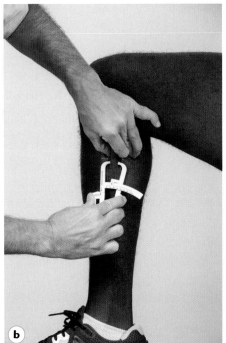

Skinfold measurements: *(a)* triceps; *(b)* calf.

TABLE 13.4 Percent Body Fat From Skinfolds

Sum (mm)	% fat	Sum (mm)	% fat	Sum (mm)	% fat	Sum (mm)	% fat	Sum (mm)	% fat	Sum (mm)	% fat
					Male						
5	6	15	13	25	20	35	28	45	35	55	42
6	7	16	14	26	21	36	28.5	46	36	56	43
7	7.5	17	14.5	27	21.5	37	29	47	36.5	57	43.5
8	8	18	15	28	22	38	30	48	37	58	44
9	9	19	16	29	23	39	30.5	49	37.5	59	44.5
10	10	20	17	30	24	40	31	50	38	60	45
11	10.5	21	17.5	31	25	41	32	51	39		
12	11	22	18	32	26	42	33	52	39.5		
13	11.5	23	18.5	33	26.5	43	33.5	53	40		
14	12	24	19	34	27	44	34	54	41		
					Female						
5	7	15	14	25	21	35	29	45	36	55	43
6	8	16	15	26	22	36	29.5	46	37	56	44
7	8.5	17	15.5	27	22.5	37	30	47	37.5	57	44.5
8	9	18	16	28	23	38	30.5	48	38	58	45
9	10	19	17	29	24	39	31	49	38.5	59	45.5
10	11	20	18	30	24.5	40	32	50	39	60	46
11	12	21	18.5	31	25	41	33	51	40		
12	12.5	22	19	32	26	42	34	52	40.5		
13	13	23	19.5	33	27	43	34.5	53	41		
14	13.5	24	20	34	28	44	35	54	42		

Adapted from "Triceps Plus Calf Skinfolds: Males" and "Triceps Plus Calf Skinfolds: Female"; reprinted by permission of Dr. Tim G. Lohman, Department of Exercise and Sport Sciences, University of Arizona.

TABLE 13.5 Rating Chart: Body Fatness

	Age (years)					
Rating	13	14	15	16	17	18 or older
			Male			
Very lean	≤7.7	≤7.0	≤6.5	≤6.4	≤6.6	≤6.9
Good fitness	7.8–22.8	7.1–21.3	6.6–20.1	6.5–20.1	6.7–20.9	7.0–22.2
Marginal	22.9–34.9	21.4–33.1	20.2–31.4	20.2–31.5	21.0–32.9	22.3–35.0
Low fitness	≥35.0	≥33.2	≥31.5	≥31.6	≥33.0	≥35.1
			Female			
Very lean	≤13.3	≤13.9	≤14.5	≤15.2	≤15.8	≤16.5
Good fitness	13.4–27.7	14.0–28.5	14.6–29.1	15.3–29.7	15.9–30.4	16.6–31.3
Marginal	27.8–36.2	28.6–36.7	29.2–37.0	29.8–37.3	30.5–37.8	31.4–38.5
Low fitness	≥36.3	≥36.8	≥37.1	≥37.4	≥37.9	≥38.6

Lesson 13.2

Energy Balance

Lesson Objectives

After participating in this lesson, you should be able to
1. explain how to use the FIT formula for fat control,
2. explain how many calories are expended in doing various physical activities,
3. explain how physical activity helps a person maintain a healthy body fat level, and
4. name some common myths about fat control.

Lesson Vocabulary

calorie, calorie expenditure, calorie intake, energy balance

Do you know how many **calories** you expend in a typical day? Do you know how many calories you consume in a typical day? One major health goal is to achieve and maintain an acceptable level of body fat throughout your life. To do this, you must balance the calories you consume and the calories you expend. In this lesson, you'll learn the FIT formula for fat control and appropriate activities for gaining weight and losing body fat.

Balancing Calories

The term *calorie* is commonly used to refer to the amount of energy in a food. The true term is *kilocalorie* (a unit of energy or heat), but when we are talking about diet and nutrition, *calorie* is typically used. **Energy balance** refers to balancing **calorie**

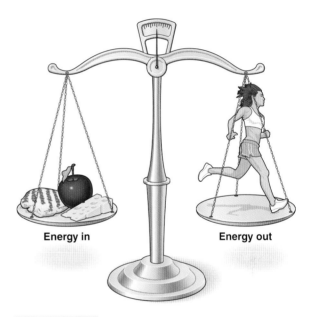

Energy in   Energy out

FIGURE 13.3 Balancing energy (calorie) intake with energy (calorie) output is essential for healthy weight maintenance.

FIT FACT

One pound of fat (0.45 kilograms) contains 3,500 calories. Therefore, you can lose 0.45 kilograms of fat by eating 3,500 calories fewer than you normally eat in a given time or by burning 3,500 calories more than normal in physical activity. Eating food that provides more calories than your body uses will cause you to gain weight. Therefore, you can gain 0.45 kilograms of fat by eating 3,500 calories more than you usually eat within a given time or by expending 3,500 calories fewer than usual in physical activity within a given time.

intake and **calorie expenditure** (figure 13.3; also see figure 13.4 and notice the energy balance scale at the top of the Physical Activity Pyramid). Calorie intake is the number of calories or total energy in the foods you eat. Calorie expenditure is the number of calories (energy) you expend in physical activity. If you take in (eat) more calories than you expend (in activity), you will gain weight because extra energy is stored in the body as fat. If you expend more calories than you take in, you will lose weight. If you balance the calories you consume and expend, you will maintain your current weight.

The FIT Formula

Both diet and physical activity are important for fat control. For this reason, each has a target zone, as shown in table 13.6.

Gaining Weight

Combining proper physical activity and diet is the best way to gain weight. In terms of activity, strength and muscular endurance exercises can help you gain weight. Resistance exercises that help build muscle are especially effective because muscle weighs more than fat.

Remember that every physical activity burns calories. Therefore, when you're active, you need to increase your intake of calories in order to gain weight. You do not, however, need to eat a special diet or take protein supplements; you need only eat a well-balanced diet that contains more calories. Ideally, the extra calories come from foods that contain a lot of nutrients like green vegetables, lean meats (e.g., chicken and fish), and colourful fruits.

Physical Activity and Calories

You might wonder how many calories are burned by different activities. Table 13.7 shows the approxi-

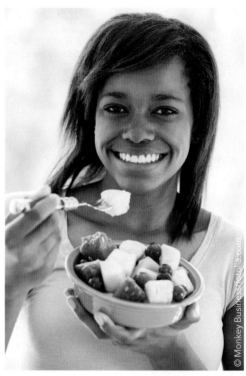

Eating a healthy diet is an essential component of maintaining a healthy weight.

mate number of calories burned each hour during selected vigorous recreational activities. To use the table, find the weight value nearest to your own weight. If you weigh more than the nearest weight,

TABLE 13.6   FIT Formula for Fat Control

	Diet*	Physical activity**
Frequency	Eat three regular meals or four or five small meals daily. Regular, controlled eating is best for losing fat. Skipping meals and snacking is usually not effective.	Participate in physical activity daily. Regular physical activity is best for losing fat.*** Short or irregular physical activity does little to control body fat.
Intensity	To lose 1 lb (about 0.5 kg) of fat, you must eat 3,500 fewer calories than normal over a given span of time. To gain 1 lb (0.5 kg) of fat, you must eat 3,500 more calories than normal over a given span of time. To maintain your weight, you must keep eating the same number of calories over a given span of time.	To lose 1 lb (0.5 kg) of fat, you must use 3,500 more calories than normal over a given span of time. To gain 1 lb (0.5 kg) of fat, you must use 3,500 fewer calories than normal over a given span of time. To maintain your weight, you must keep your level of physical activity the same over a given span of time.
Time	Neither dietary change nor physical activity results in quick fat loss. Medical experts recommend that a person lose no more than 2 lb (1 kg) per week without medical supervision.	Together, diet and physical activity can be used to safely lose 1 or 2 lb (0.5–1.0 kg) per week.

*Assumes that physical activity is constant.
**Assumes that diet is constant.
***Weight maintenance is only one reason to exercise or be physically active. Physical activity increases fitness, health, and wellness. Physical activity improves mood, mental functioning, and quality of life. Physical activity also reduces your risk of several diseases (e.g., heart disease, diabetes, and hypertension).

TABLE 13.7 Energy Expenditure

	Calories used per hour based on weight				
	45 kg (100 lb)	54 kg (120 lb)	68 kg (150 lb)	82 kg (180 lb)	91 kg (200 lb)
Backpacking/Hiking	307	348	410	472	513
Badminton	255	289	340	391	425
Baseball	210	238	280	322	350
Basketball (half-court)	225	240	300	345	375
Bicycling (normal speed)	157	178	210	242	263
Bowling	155	176	208	240	261
Canoeing (6.5 kph [4 mph])	276	344	414	504	558
Circuit training	247	280	330	380	413
Curling	181	218	272	327	363
Dance (aerobic)	300	360	450	540	600
Dance (ballet/modern)	240	300	360	432	480
Dance (social)	174	222	264	318	348
Fitness calisthenics	232	263	310	357	388
Football	225	255	300	345	375
Golf (walking)	187	212	250	288	313
Gymnastics	232	263	310	357	388
Ice hockey	363	435	544	653	726
Interval training	487	552	650	748	833
Jogging (9 kph [5.5 mph])	487	552	650	748	833
Judo/Karate	232	263	310	357	388
Lacrosse	363	435	544	653	726
Racquetball/Handball	450	510	600	690	750
Rope jumping (continuous)	525	595	700	805	875
Running (16 kph [10 mph])	625	765	900	1,035	1,125
Skating (ice or roller)	262	297	350	403	438
Skiing (cross-country)	525	595	700	805	875
Skiing (downhill)	450	510	600	690	750
Snowboarding	281	337	422	506	526
Snowshoeing	363	435	544	653	726
Soccer	405	459	540	575	621
Softball (fast pitch)	210	238	280	322	350
Swimming (slow laps)	240	272	320	368	400
Swimming (fast laps)	420	530	630	768	846
Tennis	315	357	420	483	525
Ultimate	363	435	544	653	726
Volleyball	262	297	350	403	483
Walking	204	258	318	372	426
Weight training	352	399	470	541	558

add 5 percent to the number of calories for each 4.5 kilograms (10 pounds) you weigh above the listed weight value. If you weigh less than the nearest weight, subtract 5 percent from the number of calories for each 4.5 kilograms you weigh below the listed weight value. Use this table to determine which physical activities are best for burning calories, then see which activities appeal to you.

> " Choice, not chance, determines your destiny. "
>
> —Aristotle, Greek philosopher

Physical Activity and Fat Loss

The best way to lose fat is to combine regular physical activity with a healthy diet. Research shows that a person who reduces calorie intake without increasing activity will lose both fat and muscle tissue, whereas a person who increases physical activity and reduces calorie consumption loses mostly body fat. Notice that physical activities from all steps of the Physical Activity Pyramid (figure 13.4) are

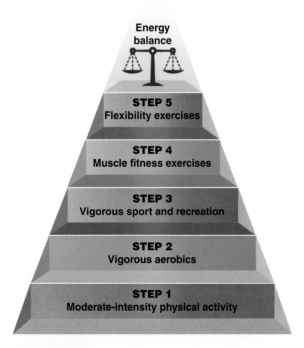

FIGURE 13.4 All activities in the Physical Activity Pyramid result in calorie expenditure and aid in energy balance.

Adapted from Physical Activity Pyramid for Teens, source: C.B. Corbin.

appropriate for helping to control body fat level and provide energy balance.

Moderate-Intensity Physical Activity

Moderate-intensity physical activity is especially effective in long-term fat control. In fact, studies indicate that moderate-intensity activity is just as effective as organized sports and games for losing fat—and more effective for permanent fat loss. You can do moderate-intensity activities for relatively long periods of time, thus burning many calories.

Vigorous Aerobics

Because vigorous aerobic activity is more intense than moderate-intensity physical activity, you can burn more calories in a shorter time with this type of activity. It is most often continuous, thus allowing you to expend calories for the full duration of the activity. Vigorous aerobic activities can be sustained for a relatively long time and therefore have potential for considerable calorie expenditure.

Vigorous Sport and Recreation

Like vigorous aerobics, vigorous sport and recreational activities are more intense than moderate-intensity physical activities. Therefore more calories are expended per unit of time than in moderate-intensity activities. The way you perform these activities makes a difference in the number of calories you expend. For example, shooting baskets typically expends fewer calories than playing a game of full-court basketball. The greater the intensity of the activity, the greater the number of calories expended over a similar length of time.

Muscle Fitness Exercises

Muscle fitness exercise expends considerable calories and is therefore beneficial in maintaining a healthy level of body fat. In addition, the extra muscle tissue you build with these exercises provides a second benefit by helping you expend more calories even when you're resting.

Flexibility Exercises

Flexibility exercises do not expend as many calories as the other four types of activity represented in the Physical Activity Pyramid. They do, however, expend more calories than resting, and any calories expended above normal can help you control body fatness.

Calculating Your Daily Calorie Expenditure

If you keep a record of all the activities you perform in a day, you can determine the total calories you expended. As directed by your teacher, keep a daily record. After recording your activities for a full day, you can calculate your daily calorie expenditure and compare it with your daily calorie intake. To maintain weight, you must expend as much energy as you take in. To lose weight, you must expend more energy than you take in. To gain weight, you must take in more calories than you expend.

Myths About Fat Loss

Some people hold incorrect ideas about physical activity and fat loss. Read table 13.8 to identify

FIT FACT

If you maintain your normal calorie intake and increase your activity by playing 30 minutes of tennis daily, you will lose 7 kilograms (16 pounds) in a year. If you walk briskly for 15 minutes a day instead of watching TV, you will lose 2.5 kilograms (about 6 pounds) in a year. On the other hand, if you sit for 15 minutes instead of taking a regular 15-minute walk each day, you will gain 2.5 kilograms (about 6 pounds) in a year.

some mistaken ideas and learn some facts about losing body fat. No matter what your body is like now, regular physical activity and proper diet will help you control body fatness. When you're fit, you look better, feel better, and have fewer health problems than people who have a high level of body fat and are unfit.

TABLE 13.8 Myths and Facts About Fat Loss

Myth	Fact
Exercise cannot be effective for fat loss because it takes many hours of exercise to lose even 1 lb (0.5 kg) of fat.	You can lose body fat over time with regular physical activity if your calorie intake remains the same. Fat lost through physical activity tends to stay off longer than fat lost through dieting alone.
Exercise does not help you lose fat because it increases your hunger and encourages you to overeat.	If you are moderately active instead of inactive, your hunger should not increase. Even moderate to vigorous activity will not cause hunger to increase so much that you overeat. People who overeat usually do so for other reasons (habit, anxiousness, presence of empty calories, large portion sizes, and so on).
Most people with too much body fat have glandular problems.	While some people do have glandular problems, most people who are high in body fat eat too much, do too little physical activity, or both.
You can spot-reduce by exercising a specific body part to lose fat in that area.	Any exercise that burns calories will cause the body's general fat deposits to decrease. A given exercise does not cause one area of fat to decrease more than another.

Lesson Review

1. How can you use the FIT formula to control your body fat level?
2. How many calories are expended in the five most common physical activities that you perform?
3. How can physical activity help you maintain a healthy body fat level?
4. What are some common myths and facts about fat control?

TAKING CHARGE: Improving Physical Self-Perception

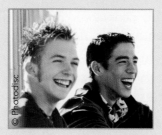

Each person has a mental picture of himself or herself. If you think you do well in a certain activity, you'll probably take part in that type of activity. If you feel embarrassed about your appearance or ability level while doing an activity, you'll probably avoid that activity. Here are two very different examples of physical self-perception.

Michal was not sure that he wanted to go back to school after the summer break. It seemed as if all of his friends had grown taller in the last few months, but he had stayed the same height. Michal felt embarrassed and a little jealous, even though none of his friends seemed to notice. His height certainly did not alter his ability to play tennis. In fact, his friends still called him "King of the Court" because he usually won.

Raul was one of the shortest people in his class, but his height did not stop him from being involved in activities. He realized that he had never been a great basketball player, but he still liked to play with his friends from school. He also discovered that height had nothing to do with his ability to go hiking, nor did it prevent him from being a good wrestler.

For Discussion

Michal had a negative self-perception because of his height. What can he do to change his negative perception? How does Raul keep a positive self-perception? What else can a person do to develop a positive self-perception? Consider the guidelines presented in the Self-Management feature as you answer the discussion questions.

SELF-MANAGEMENT: Skills for Self-Perception

A self-perception is an idea you have about your own thoughts, actions, or appearance. It is influenced by how you think other people view you. Some of the many kinds of self-perception are academic, social, and artistic. In this book, the focus is on physical self-perceptions—the way you view your physical self.

Four aspects of physical self-perception are strength, fitness, skill, and physical attractiveness. People with good physical self-perceptions are happy with their current strength and fitness levels; they also feel that their skills are adequate to meet their needs, and they like the way they look. We know that people who have positive physical self-perceptions are more likely to be physically active than those who do not. The following list provides guidelines you can use to maintain or improve your physical self-perceptions.

- **Assess your physical self-perceptions.** You may use the worksheet provided by your instructor.

- **Consider your self-assessment results.** Use the self-assessment worksheet to determine whether you have any areas in which your physical self-perceptions are especially low (strength, fitness, skill, or physical attractiveness).

- **Perform regular physical activity to improve your physical fitness or practice regularly to improve your physical skills.** Regular physical activity can help you look your best, and learning skills can help you perform your best.

- **Consider a new way of thinking about yourself.** People often set unrealistic standards for themselves, such as looking like someone they see on television or in the movies. Understand that in real life these people do not look the way they look on the screen. In fact, their appearance is often enhanced by special cameras and computer programs. You also do not know whether a movie star has an eating disorder or practices healthy habits. Consider your heredity and set realistic standards for yourself.

- **Think positively.** Almost all people have a physical characteristic that they would like to change. But studies show that the things people don't like about themselves are rarely seen as problems by other people. You're often your own worst critic, and thinking positively can help you present yourself in a positive way.

- **Do not let the actions of a few insensitive people cause you to feel negatively about yourself.** There will always be some people who are insensitive to others' feelings. These people often have low self-perceptions and try to build themselves up by tearing other people down. Recognize that criticism from these people is their problem, not yours.

- **Consider how your behaviour and actions influence the way other people view you.** Acting cheerful and friendly has as much to do with how others perceive you as your physical characteristics.

- **Realize that all people have some imperfections.** Try to build on your strengths and improve your areas of weakness.

- **Find a realistic role model and be a role model for others.** Instead of trying to be like someone who is totally unlike you, find someone you admire who has characteristics you can realistically achieve. And, just as you look to others for models, remember that others may look to you as a model. Providing a positive model for others can help you think positively about yourself.

Muscle fitness exercises provide a triple benefit in helping you maintain a healthy body composition. First, they build muscles that help you look your best. Second, they expend energy, thus helping you to achieve a good energy balance. Finally, the extra muscle that you build through resistance exercise causes you to burn extra calories even at rest.

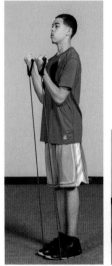

You can take action by completing an elastic band resistance circuit. Elastic bands are beneficial because they are affordable, travel well, and allow you to easily exercise many muscles. They are appropriate for people of all fitness levels, and they will help you improve your overall coordination and your muscular fitness. Consider the following guidelines for performing resistance band (elastic band) exercises.

- When choosing bands, make sure they are the right length for you and that they do not have cracks or other signs of wear.
- Choose a band that provides the proper resistance, allowing you to perform the recommended number of sets and reps.
- You can also do resistance exercises that use your body weight to add variation and create a good workout circuit.

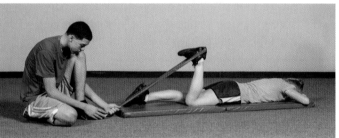

Take action by performing elastic band exercises.

 ## GET ACTIVE WITH SWIMMING CANADA

©Swimming Canada

Who We Are

Swimming Canada is responsible for the sport of competitive swimming in Canada. Our core business is governing and developing the sport through 430 swim clubs across Canada as well as four high-performance centres. Ultimately we are judged every four years by our team's performance at the Olympic and Paralympic Games.

What We Do

Swimming Canada doesn't just produce Olympic and Paralympic athletes to represent Canada. We work with aquatic partners such as the Canadian Red Cross, Lifesaving Society Canada, and YMCA Canada to teach every Canadian child how to swim. We believe that every Canadian should know how to swim because it's the only sport that can both get you fit and save your life!

Get Involved

Swimming is a gateway sport to virtually any sport that happens in or on the water. Learning to swim not only helps keep you safe but also opens up a world of recreational opportunities for a lifetime of fitness and health. Anyone can swim. It doesn't matter how big, flexible, strong, or coordinated you are. When you're with or without disability, swimming is a safe, nonimpact sport that is good for your heart, muscles, and joints. Swimming gives you a full-body workout you can do alone or with a group.

Swimming is also inexpensive. Take your swimsuit and a pair of goggles to the local pool and you're all set. Use some of the pool's training aids such as flippers, kickboards, or even lifejackets to give your workout variety. Track your distance in each workout and try to go just one length further or faster each time out. Learn more by visiting us at www.swimming.ca/en.

Reprinted, by permission, from Swimming Canada.

Reviewing Concepts and Vocabulary

Complete the following in order for you to determine your growing understanding of fitness, health, and wellness. Answer items 1 through 5 by correctly completing each sentence with a word or phrase.

1. A term used to describe a person who has a high body fat level is _____.
2. An eating disorder characterized by bingeing and purging is called _____.
3. The minimum amount of body fat needed for good health is _____.
4. People with _____ see themselves as too fat even when they are extremely thin.
5. Keeping your calories consumed equal to your calories expended is called _____.

For items 6 through 10, match each term in column 1 with the appropriate phrase in column 2.

6. metabolic syndrome
7. calliper
8. DXA
9. anorexia athletica
10. basal metabolism

a. best measure of body composition
b. used to measure skinfolds
c. condition associated with health risk factors
d. energy your body uses just to keep you living
e. eating disorder most common among athletes

For items 11 through 15, respond to each statement or question.

11. Discuss why 3,500 calories is an important number for maintaining a healthy body composition.
12. Why is confidentiality so important when making body composition assessments?
13. Why is it important to maintain essential body fat?
14. Name one myth about fat loss and explain how it is incorrect or misleading.
15. What are some guidelines for improving physical self-perceptions?

Thinking Critically

Each year, people spend billions of dollars on weight loss and muscle-building products that do not work. Look at a newspaper, popular magazine, or website and find an advertisement for a weight loss product. Read the ad and make a list of its claims. Place a checkmark by the claims that are consistent with the information presented in this chapter. Place an "X" by those that appear to be false or questionable. Write a paragraph evaluating the advertisement.

Project

Canada releases statistics about obesity and being overweight. Data include the national average as well as provincial percentages for multiple age groups. Prepare an index card showing information on overweight and obesity statistics for your assigned province as well as the national average. Each group will then add their index card to the map of Canada so that we can examine this issue from a national perspective. On the back of the index card, list our province's statistics and five factors that you think may cause our province to rank as it does.

14

Choosing Nutritious Food

 Student Web Resources
www.fitnessforlife.org/student

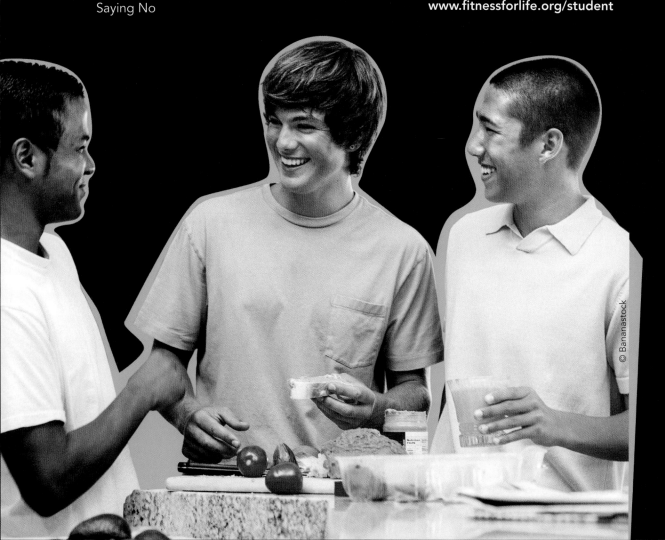

© Bananastock

Lesson 14.1
A Healthy Diet

Lesson Objectives

After participating in this lesson, you should be able to

1. list the three types of nutrients that provide energy, and list the recommended percentage of calories from each that is needed for good health;
2. explain why vitamins, minerals, and water are necessary for good health;
3. describe the four food groups and explain how knowledge of these groups can help you plan for healthy eating;
4. explain how to create a balanced diet using the Eat Well Plate; and
5. list three general guidelines for healthy eating.

Lesson Vocabulary

Adequate Intake (AI), amino acid, basal metabolism, carbohydrate, complete protein, creeping obesity, Dietary Reference Intake (DRI), dietician, empty calories, fat, fibre, incomplete protein, macronutrient, micronutrient, protein, Recommended Dietary Allowance (RDA), resting metabolism, saturated fat, Tolerable Upper Intake Level (UL), trans-fatty acid, unsaturated fat

What kinds of food are important to your health? How much food do you need to eat? In this lesson, you'll learn about healthful foods and learn how to select foods for a balanced diet.

Nutrients Your Body Needs

Scientists have identified 45 to 50 nutrients—food substances required for the growth and maintenance of your cells. These nutrients have been divided into six groups—carbohydrate, protein, fat, vitamin, mineral, and water. Each of these is discussed in this chapter.

Nutrients That Provide Energy

Three types of nutrient supply the energy that your body needs in order to perform its daily tasks: **fat**, **carbohydrate**, and **protein**. They are referred to as **macronutrients**. Fat contains more calories than protein or carbohydrate per unit of weight. One gram of fat contains 9 calories, whereas one gram of carbohydrate or protein contains 4 calories. Health Canada recommends that most of the calories in your diet come from carbohydrate. Fewer of your calories typically come from fat and protein.

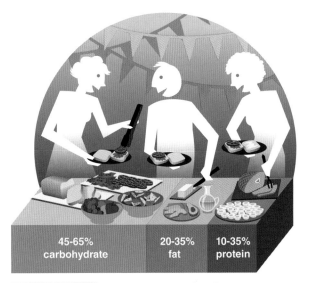

FIGURE 14.1 Percentage of calories recommended by Health Canada for carbohydrate, protein, and fat.

Figure 14.1 shows the recommended percentage of calories from each of the three types of energy-providing nutrient.

Carbohydrate

Carbohydrate is your main source of energy, and it comes in two types: simple and complex. Simple carbohydrate includes sugars such as table sugar, fructose, and sucrose. Fructose and sucrose are

Choosing Nutritious Food **331**

commonly found in soft drinks and other sweetened foods. Simple carbohydrate provides a quick source of energy but contains few nutrients (figure 14.2a). Most of your carbohydrate calories should come from complex carbohydrate. Complex carbohydrate has a more complex chemical structure, so it takes longer to digest (figure 14.2b). It contains more nutrients than simple carbohydrate and is often rich in **fibre**. Fibre is found in foods such as whole grains and vegetables. You should minimize your intake of simple carbohydrate, although some simple carbohydrate sources are better than others. For example, bananas and oranges contain simple carbohydrate but also contain essential nutrients such as vitamins, minerals, and fibre. Foods containing simple carbohydrate—such as candy, pastry, and sugared soft drinks—contain **empty calories**, which provide energy but few if any other nutrients such as vitamins and minerals.

Fibre is a type of complex carbohydrate that your body cannot digest. It supplies no energy. Fibre sources include the leaves, stems, roots, and seed coverings of fruits, vegetables, and grains (figure 14.2c). Examples of foods high in fibre include whole-grain bread and cereal, the skin of fresh fruits, raw vegetables, nuts, and seeds. Fibre helps you avoid intestinal problems and might reduce your chances of developing some forms of cancer.

> " I was eating bad stuff. Lots of sugar and carbs, junk food all the time. It makes you very irritated. "
>
> —Avril Lavigne, singer/songwriter and actress

Protein

Protein is the group of nutrients that builds, repairs, and maintains body cells; they are the building blocks of your body. Protein is contained in animal products (such as animal milk, eggs, meat, and fish) and in some plants (such as beans and grains). Protein provides energy but not as many calories as fat. If you consume more protein than is needed to build your body tissue, the additional calories will either be used to produce energy for daily activity or be stored as body fat.

During digestion, your body breaks protein down into simpler substances called **amino acids**, which your small intestine can absorb. Your body can manufacture 11 of the 20 known amino acids; you need to get the other 9—known as the essential amino acids—from food.

Foods containing all nine essential amino acids are said to provide **complete protein**. Animal sources such as meat, milk products, and fish provide complete protein. A grain called quinoa (pronounced keen' wah) and some forms of soy contain all nine essential amino acids. Quinoa can be served hot, like rice, or cold in a salad.

Foods that contain some, but not all, essential amino acids are said to contain **incomplete protein**. Examples include beans, nuts, rice, and certain other plants. You can usually get enough essential amino acids from a daily diet that includes some foods with complete protein and some with incomplete protein. People who do not eat meat need to eat a variety of foods that contain incomplete protein and, taken together, provide all the essential amino acids.

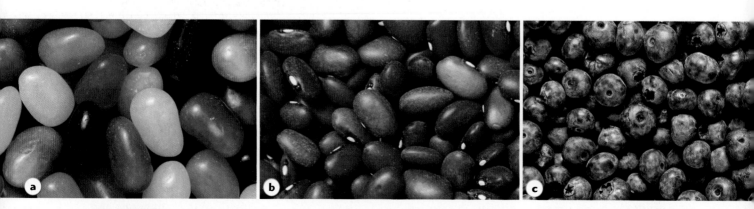

FIGURE 14.2 Types of carbohydrate: (a) Simple carbohydrate (such as in candy) contains empty calories, but (b and c) complex carbohydrate (such as in vegetables and fruit) contains more nutrients and fibre.
© 1999 PhotoDisc, Inc.

Fat

Fat is contained in animal products and some plant products, such as nuts and vegetable oils. Fat is necessary to grow and repair your cells; it dissolves certain vitamins and carries them to your cells. In addition, fat enhances the flavour and texture of many foods. Fat is classified as either saturated or unsaturated. In general, **saturated fat** is solid at room temperature, and **unsaturated fat** is liquid. Saturated fat comes mostly from animal products, such as lard, butter, milk, and meat fat. Unsaturated fat comes mostly from plants, such as sunflower, corn, soybean, olive, almond, and peanut. In addition, fish produce unsaturated fat in their cells.

At most, fewer than 35 percent of the total calories you consume should come from fat, and many experts recommend a level closer to 20 percent. The bulk of the fat in your diet should come from unsaturated fats, including fish oils. You should minimize your intake of calories from saturated fat. **Trans-fatty acids** (also called trans fat) should not be included in the diet. Trans fat is created through a process that makes unsaturated fat solid at room temperature—as, for example, in solid margarine. In 2007, Health Canada adopted the two recommendations of the Trans Fat Task Force, which were to limit the trans fat content in oils and spreadable margarines, as well as the trans fat content in all other foods. The U.S. Food and Drug Administration (FDA) indicates that trans fats are not "recognized as safe," so they can no longer be included in foods. The FDA has given U.S. companies until 2018 to phase out all artificial trans fats from foods. Hopefully Canada will follow the FDA's lead.

FIT FACT

Canada was the very first country requiring trans fat amounts to appear on packaged foods. Health Canada also has the Trans Fat Task Force, which monitors the amount of trans fats included in foods in restaurants, fast food chains, quick service restaurants, cafeterias located in institutions, and establishments serving various ethnic cuisines, as well as in prepackaged foods. In addition, Canada's Food Guide contains explicit recommendations to limit trans fat and saturated fat in your diet.

Cholesterol is a waxy, fatlike substance found in the saturated fat of animal cells, including those of humans. You consume cholesterol in foods that are high in saturated fat, such as meat. Because you are an animal, you also produce your own cholesterol. People who eat a lot of saturated fat produce more cholesterol than those who limit their consumption of saturated fat. A high level of blood cholesterol can contribute to atherosclerosis (clogged arteries) and other heart diseases. Medical experts recommend eating foods that are low in cholesterol and saturated fat. Trans-fatty acids also affect cholesterol, which was the primary reason they were banned in foods. Some kinds of fat, such as fish oil, are considered to be healthier than others.

Nutrients That Do Not Provide Energy

Minerals, vitamins, and water have no calories and provide no energy, but they all play a vital role in your staying fit and healthy. Minerals and vitamins are called **micronutrients** because the body needs them in relatively small amounts as compared with carbohydrate, protein, and fat.

The **Dietary Reference Intake (DRI)** is a system used by Health Canada to specify recommended amounts of each micronutrient. Three types of DRI help you know how much of each vitamin or mineral you should consume. The first, **Recommended Dietary Allowance (RDA)**, is the minimum amount of a nutrient necessary to meet the health needs of most people. The second, **Adequate Intake (AI)**, is used when there is not sufficient evidence to establish an RDA for a given micronutrient. And the third, the **Tolerable Upper Intake Level (UL)**, refers to the maximum amount of a vitamin or mineral that can be consumed without posing a health risk.

Minerals

Minerals are essential nutrients that help regulate the activity of your cells. They come from elements in the earth's crust and are present in all plants and animals. You need 25 minerals in varying amounts. Table 14.1 shows major functions and food sources of the most important minerals.

Some minerals are especially important for young people—for example, calcium, which builds and maintains bones. During your teen years, your body needs calcium to build your bones. During young adulthood, your bones become less efficient in getting calcium from food and begin to lose calcium. Later, typically around age 55, women experience a change in hormones that leads them to experience much more bone loss than men do. In fact, a large percentage of older women develop osteoporosis, a condition in which their bones become porous and break easily. Men can also have this disease, but they get it less often and much later in life. You can reduce your risk for osteoporosis by getting enough calcium and doing weight-bearing exercise (such as walking and jogging) and resistance exercise throughout your life.

Another important mineral is iron, which is needed for proper formation and functioning of your red blood cells. These cells carry oxygen to your muscles and other body tissues. Iron deficiency is especially common among girls and women. If your body has insufficient iron, you have a condition called iron-deficiency anaemia, which causes you to feel tired all the time. Iron from animal foods is more easily absorbed than iron from plants. The best sources of iron are meat (especially red meat), poultry, and fish. You can also help your body absorb iron by getting an adequate amount of vitamin C.

Sodium is a mineral that helps your body cells function properly. It's present in many foods and is especially high in certain foods, such as snack foods, processed foods, fast foods, and cured meats (for example, ham). For many people, dietary sodium comes primarily from table salt (sodium chloride). Most people eat more sodium than they need. Canadians eat more than double the amount of salt needed, about 3,400 milligrams. People with high blood pressure, or hypertension, need to be especially careful to limit sodium because it can cause their body to retain water, thus contributing to keeping their blood pressure high.

Vitamins

You need vitamins for the growth and repair of your body cells. Vitamin C and the B vitamins are water soluble, so they dissolve in your blood and are carried to cells throughout your body. Because your body cannot store excess B and C vitamins, you need to eat foods containing these vitamins every day. In contrast, vitamins A, D, E, and K dissolve in fat, and excess amounts of these vitamins are stored in fat cells in your liver and other body parts. Folacin, or folic acid, is especially important for girls and young women. Research shows that children born to women low in folacin are at risk of birth defects. Table 14.2 gives you more information about specific vitamins.

Water

Dieticians usually say that water is the single most important nutrient. It carries the other nutrients to your cells, carries away waste, and helps regulate

TABLE 14.1   Functions and Sources of Minerals

Mineral	Function in the body	Food sources
Calcium	Builds and maintains teeth and bones; helps blood clot; helps nerves and muscles function	Cheese, milk, dark green vegetables, sardines, legumes
Iron	Helps transfer oxygen in red blood cells and other cells	Liver, red meat, dark green vegetables, shellfish, whole-grain cereals
Magnesium	Aids breakdown of glucose and proteins; regulates body fluids	Green vegetables, grains, nuts, beans, yeast
Phosphorus	Builds and maintains teeth and bones; helps release energy from nutrients	Meat, poultry, fish, eggs, legumes, milk products
Potassium	Regulates fluid balance in cells; helps nerves function	Oranges, bananas, meat, bran, potatoes, dried beans
Sodium	Regulates internal water balance; helps nerves function	Most foods, table salt
Zinc	Aids transport of carbon dioxide; aids healing of wounds	Meat, shellfish, whole grains, milk, legumes

your body temperature. Most foods contain water. In fact, 50 to 60 percent of your own body weight comes from water. Your body loses 1.9 to 2.8 litres of water a day through breathing, perspiring, and elimination of waste from your bowels and bladder. You lose even more water than usual in very

TABLE 14.2   Functions and Sources of Vitamins

Vitamin	Function in the body	Food sources
A (retinol)	Helps produce normal mucus; part of the chemical necessary for vision	Butter, margarine, liver, eggs, green or yellow vegetables
B_1 (thiamin)	Helps release energy from carbohydrate	Pork, organ meat, legumes, greens
B_2 (riboflavin)	Helps break down carbohydrate and protein	Meat, milk products, eggs, green and yellow vegetables
B_6 (pyridoxine)	Helps break down protein and glucose	Yeast, nuts, beans, liver, fish, rice
B_{12} (cobalamin)	Aids formation of nucleic and amino acids	Meat, milk products, eggs, fish
Biotin	Aids formation of amino, nucleic, and fatty acids and glycogen	Eggs, liver, yeast
C (ascorbic acid)	Aids formation of hormones, bone tissue, and collagen	Fruits, tomatoes, potatoes, green leafy vegetables
D	Aids absorption of calcium and phosphorus	Liver, fortified milk, fatty fish
E (tocopherol)	Prevents damage to cell membranes	Vegetable oils
Folacin	Helps build DNA and protein	Yeast, wheat germ, liver, greens
K	Aids blood clotting	Leafy vegetables
Niacin	Helps release energy from carbohydrate and protein	Milk, meat, whole-grain or enriched cereals, legumes
Pantothenic acid	Necessary for converting food to fuel for producing energy and helps nervous system function properly	Most unprocessed foods

 ## SCIENCE IN ACTION: Vitamin and Mineral Supplements

Scientists who study nutrition and medicine have researched the value of vitamin and mineral supplements. The most common type of supplement is taken daily and contains the amounts of vitamins and minerals recommended for daily intake. If you eat a balanced diet, however, you will most likely get the proper amounts without a supplement. **Dieticians** worry that people might think a supplement can take the place of eating well. Some medical and nutrition experts, however, recommend a multivitamin for people who do not eat regular meals and thus may not get the vitamins and minerals they need. Other experts, including scientists from the Dietitians of Canada, say there is not enough evidence to indicate that a daily supplement is beneficial for most people.

With all this in mind, the decision to take a vitamin or mineral supplement should be done only with the advice of a nutrition or medical expert based on your medical history and personal nutrition habits. Unless an expert advises otherwise, a supplement should contain no more than the RDA or AI value for each mineral and vitamin. Excessive amounts can lead to health problems.

Student Activity

Investigate a multivitamin supplement. Determine whether it contains more than 100 percent of the recommended amount of each vitamin.

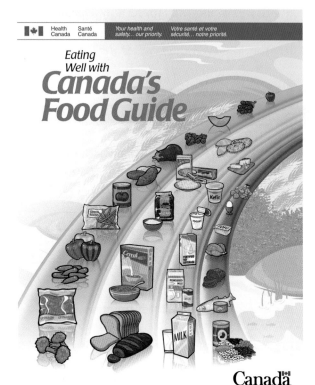
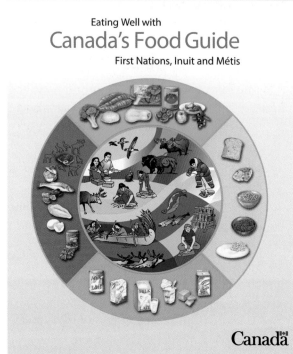

FIGURE 14.3 Canada's Food Guide to healthy eating shows the four basic food groups and how much is required daily to make up a healthy diet.

hot weather and when you exercise vigorously. As a result, you need to drink plenty of extra fluid.

The best beverages for this purpose are water, fruit juice, and milk. The type of juice or milk makes a difference. Pure fruit juices contain vitamins and minerals, and some contain fibre (for example, orange juice pulp). Some juice drinks contain small amounts of real juice and are supplemented with simple sugar. Skim milk provides the same basic nutrients as whole milk but without the fat.

Soft drinks that contain caffeine are not as effective as water. Sport drinks usually contain sodium and other ingredients that you don't need unless you engage in moderate-intensity exercise for several hours or vigorous-intensity exercise for more than 1.5 hours.

Food Groups

Health Canada's guide to healthy eating illustrates the four basic food groups (see figure 14.3). Each coloured area represents the four basic types of food—grain products, vegetables and fruits, meat

FIT FACT

Health Canada updates Canada's Food Guide periodically in order to continue to provide current and relevant easy-to-use information about eating for good health. One such update has been the addition of the Guide for First Nations, Inuit and Métis. There is also an opportunity to create your own food guide on Health Canada's website. Guides are available in over 15 languages. All guides can either be ordered online at no cost or be downloaded.

and alternatives, and milk and alternatives—that make up part of a healthy diet. Canada's Food Guide describes healthy eating for Canadians two years of age or older. Choosing the amount and type of food recommended in Canada's Food Guide will help children and teens grow and thrive; meet your needs for vitamins, minerals, and other nutrients; and lower your risk of obesity, type 2 diabetes, heart disease, certain types of cancer, and osteoporosis (weak and brittle bones).

Foods from each of the groups contain macro-nutrients (carbohydrate, protein, and fat), micro-nutrients (vitamins and minerals), and water. Some foods are richer in nutrients than others. The goal is to eat more foods that are high in nutritional value and fewer foods containing empty calories. Foods with empty calories are typically high in fat, simple sugar, or both.

The yellow area on the guide represents grain products; it is relatively large because grains make up a large part of a healthy diet. At least half of your grain choices should be whole grain. Look for the whole-grain label on bread, cereal, and other grain products. Also look for products low in fat, sugar, or salt. Try a variety of grain products such as barley, brown rice, oats, quinoa, and wild rice. The green area represents vegetables and fruit; the blue area represents milk and alternatives; and the red area represents meat and alternatives. Together, vegetables and fruits should constitute approximately half of your total diet. Fruits and vegetables contain fibre, vitamins, minerals, carbohydrate, some protein, and very little fat. They are considered nutrient-dense foods and often have few calories. This is directly opposite to the situation with many processed snack foods, candy, and sugary drinks (e.g., fruit juices, pop), often called empty calories; they have few nutrients (i.e., vitamins and minerals) and lots of calories. The guidelines suggest eating at least one dark green and one orange vegetable each day. Furthermore, enjoying vegetables and fruit prepared with little or no added fat, sugar, or salt is recommended. Eating vegetables and fruits more often than fruit juice is suggested because much juice has high simple sugar (i.e., simple carbohydrate) content. In fact, at the time this textbook was being written, Health Canada was reviewing whether fruit juice should be removed from Canada's Food Guide to healthy eating.

> " An apple a day keeps the doctor away. "
>
> —Anonymous proverb

The red area represents meats and alternatives. You don't need to eat as much of these foods as other foods (indicated by the smaller suggested servings), but they are essential to good health. This group includes meats (such as beef, poultry, and pork), meat alternatives (veggie burgers), tofu, seafood (fresh and canned), beans and peas, and nuts and seeds. You should limit your intake of processed meats such as hot dogs and some lunch meats, which contain very high levels of salt. Recommended foods in the protein group include lean meat cuts, poultry (without skin), and fish high in omega-3 fatty acids (such as salmon and trout). You should also use cooking methods that do not add fat to your food. For example, broiling lets fat drip away, whereas frying, especially deep-fat frying, adds many extra calories and extra fat, even to vegetables (as in French fries).

Some foods—beans, peas, nuts, and seeds—are included in the protein group and the vegetable group because they are vegetables that are high in protein. These foods are especially important for vegetarians or people who do not eat a lot of meat.

The blue area represents the milk and alternatives group. This group includes milk, fortified soy beverages, non-dairy beverages (rice, almond, coconut, cashew milk—preferably unsweetened), cheese, milk-based desserts, and yogurt. These foods are good sources of calcium. When choosing foods from this group, consider low-fat, fat-free, and unsweetened options.

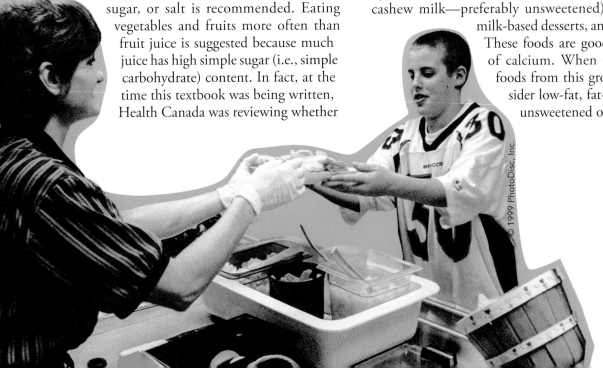

© 1999 PhotoDisc, Inc.

337

The Ideal Diet?

Dietary guidelines emphasize that no single diet is best for all people. The exact amount of food that should be consumed from each food group depends on factors such as age, sex, and activity level. Canada's Food Guide does provide serving suggestions for children, teens, and adults. Additional information on how to use Canada's Food Guide has been developed by the Canadian Heart and Stroke Foundation for people with heart problems and those who wish to reduce their risk of heart problems.

Here are some general guidelines for healthy eating from Health Canada and the Dietitians of Canada.

- Make half of your plate fruits and vegetables.
- Increase dietary complex carbohydrate.
- Make at least half your grains whole.
- Reduce consumption of calories from added sugar.
- Drink water instead of sugary drinks.
- Switch to skim or 1 percent milk.
- Reduce dietary fat, especially saturated fat.
- Reduce daily salt (sodium) intake.
- Consume adequate dietary calcium.
- Avoid oversized portions.

Some of the guidelines described previously deserve elaboration because of their importance to a healthy diet. Consider the following strategies.

Avoid Empty Calories

Minimize your consumption of foods high in empty calories. Examples include cake, candy, donuts, drinks with added sugar (including soft drinks and many energy and sport drinks), processed meats (such as hot dogs, bacon, and sausage), ice cream made with real cream and added sugar, and condiments (such as ketchup and mayonnaise). Nutrition scientists have shown that from age 20 through age 40, the average North American gains a pound (about 0.5 kilograms) a year; this increase is sometimes referred to as **creeping obesity** because the weight gain is gradual—it creeps up on you. Consumption of empty calories is a principal reason for gradual weight gain in early adulthood.

FIT FACT

Revisions to Canada's Food Guide are planned for 2017 and 2018. In 2017, key nutritional messages and resources for Canadians will be released. In 2018, new guidelines for healthy eating patterns (i.e., recommended amounts and types of food) will be released.

Choose Oils Carefully

Oil is fat that is liquid at room temperature. Oils do not constitute a separate food group, but they do provide important nutrients. Because oil is fat, you should limit consumption, but some oils are better than others. For example, fish oils containing omega-3 fatty acids are considered to be a healthy part of your diet. When considering other oils, choose monounsaturated oils (such as canola oil). Polyunsaturated oils (such as corn oil) are preferred over the saturated fat in butter, lard, and margarine. Even some oils made from plants (for example, coconut and palm) contain saturated fat and therefore are not healthy diet options.

Watch Servings and Serving Sizes

You now know that you need to eat appropriate amounts of macro- and micronutrients from the four food groups. But how much do you need from each group? Table 14.3 shows the recommended number of servings from each food group, as well as the appropriate serving size. The recommended number of servings from a given food group depends on your daily calorie intake. In general, boys require more servings than girls because they are larger and have more muscle mass. Most teen girls need about 1,700 to 2,400 calories per day, whereas teen boys typically need 1,900 to 3,300. The lower calorie amounts are appropriate for more sedentary teens, and the higher amounts are appropriate for active teens. Sedentary adults need fewer calories (2,000 or below).

Be Active to Balance Calories

To maintain a healthy body composition throughout your life, you must balance the calories you

TABLE 14.3   Recommended Number and Size of Servings

	Children 9–13 years (males and females)	Teens 14–18 years		Adults 19–50 years		Adults 51+ years		Serving size examples
		Females	Males	Females	Males	Females	Males	
Vegetables and fruit	6	7	8	7–8	8–10	7	7	250 mL (1 cup) raw leafy vegetables or salad; 125 mL (1/2 cup) cooked vegetables; 1 piece of fruit
Grain products	6	6	7	6–7	8	6	7	1 slice bread; 1/2 a pita or tortilla; 125 mL (1/2 cup) cooked rice, pasta, or couscous; 175 mL (3/4 cup) hot cereal
Milk and alternatives	3–4	3–4	3–4	2	2	3	3	250 mL (1 cup) milk or fortified soy beverage; 175 g (3/4 cup) yogurt; 50 g (1 1/2 oz) cheese
Meat and alternatives	1–2	2	3	2	3	2	3	5 g (1/2 cup) cooked fish, shellfish, poultry, or lean meat; 175 mL (3/4 cup) cooked beans; 2 eggs; 30 mL (2 Tbsp) peanut butter

More information about servings of specific foods is available in the student section of the Fitness for Life Canada website.

take in with the calories you expend. Nutrition guidelines now acknowledge that both physical activity and healthy eating are important. Studies show, however, that most people overestimate their activity and underestimate how many calories they eat each day. Over time, this misperception can lead to unnecessary weight gain. The self-assessment in this chapter helps you determine how many calories you consume and how many you expend each day.

Lesson Review

1. How much dietary carbohydrate, protein, and fat are desirable for good health?
2. Why are vitamins, minerals, and water necessary for good health?
3. Describe the four basic food groups and explain why each is important.
4. How can the Eat Well Plate help you create a balanced diet?
5. What are three general guidelines for healthy eating?

This self-assessment helps determine how many calories you take in (your calorie intake) and how many calories you expend each day. As directed, record the required information on worksheets provided by your instructor.

Remember that self-assessment information is personal and considered confidential. It shouldn't be shared with others without the permission of the person self-assessing.

Step 1: Determine Your Calorie Intake

Prepare a chart indicating food types, foods, and food amounts for your consumption on one day. Figure 14.4 shows a sample food log prepared by Sandy, a 15-year-old boy in the ninth grade. Sandy kept a food log for one day to see how many calories he consumed and how many servings he ate from each food group. He recorded the number of servings for each food and made a checkmark by the food group it came from to help him see if he was eating from each group. To help him determine serving sizes, he used table 14.3. Then he used a food calculator to determine the number of calories in each food. Finally, he added the calories and the number of servings of each food to determine his total calorie intake and see if he had met the recommended guide-

lines for each food group. Sandy's total calorie intake for Wednesday was 2,551, which falls in the recommended range for a male teen.

Prepare a one-day food log similar to Sandy's for your own consumption. Check to see if all food groups were represented. Use a free food calculator app or search the web for a free food calculator to determine the number of calories in the foods you ate. Sandy used the free Eat Well Plate from the Healthy Canadians website and a My Food Guide mobile app. Dietitians of Canada also provide a free website and app (eaTracker) to help you reach your goals by supporting you in planning your meals, analyzing your food, and tracking your activity. The United States Department of Agriculture also has a free FoodTracker on the MyPlate website.

Step 2: Estimate Your Calorie Expenditure

First, determine your **resting metabolism**—the number of calories expended by your body for its basic functions and the typical light activities done during the day. In other words, resting metabolism includes your **basal metabolism** (the calories required for sleeping, digesting food, and other nonactive behaviour) plus the calories you use for light daily activities such as tooth brushing, eating, reading, and typing. Sandy used table 14.4 to determine his resting metabolism based on his sex, age (15 years), weight (68 kilograms, or 150 pounds), and height (1.8 metres, or 71 inches). The chart indicated a resting metabolism of 1,800 calories each day. Sandy recorded this figure in his activity log.

Determine your resting metabolism using the appropriate table. For boys, use table 14.4 (ages 12 through 15) or table 14.5 (age 16 or older). For girls, use table 14.6 (ages 12 through 15) or table 14.7 (ages 16 or older). Record your resting metabolism.

Next, prepare a log of your physical activity for one day. Like Sandy, record each activity you performed and its length. Here are Sandy's calculations.

Sandy looked at a physical activity compendium (see the student section of the Fitness for Life Canada website) and found that a person weighing 68 kilograms (150 pounds) expends 318 calories in one hour of walking. For each minute of walking, then, Sandy expends 5.3 calories (318 calories ÷ 60 minutes = 5.3 calories per minute). Therefore, he expends 53 calories in a 10-minute walk (5.3 × 10 = 53).

Sandy also did 30 minutes of the Burn It Up workout in physical education class. This activity causes a 68-kilogram (150-pound) person to expend 340 calories per hour, or 5.67 calories per minute (340 ÷ 60 = 5.67). Therefore, in 30 minutes, Sandy expended about 170 calories (5.67 × 30 = 170).

Mowing the lawn expends 314 calories per hour for a person of Sandy's size, or about 5.25

Food	Servings	Calories	Grain products	Vegetables and fruit	Meat and alternatives	Milk and alternatives	Other
Breakfast							
Scrambled egg	1	104			✔		
Fried ham slice	1	82			✔		
Whole wheat toast slice	2	138 (69 × 2)	✔				
~0.2 L (8-oz) glass of orange juice	1	112		✔			
Breakfast total		436					
Lunch							
Cheese pizza slice	3	693 (231 × 3)	✔		✔	✔	
Small salad	1	33		✔			
Salad dressing	1	71					✔
~0.4 L (12-oz) soda	1	150					✔
Lunch total		947					
Dinner							
Green beans	2	88 (44 × 2)		✔			
Baked potato	2	242 (121 × 2)		✔			
Sour cream for potato	1	62				✔	
Broiled chicken breast	2	282 (141 × 2)			✔		
~0.5 L (16-oz) glass of fat-free milk (two 0.25 L servings)	2	166 (83 × 2)				✔	
Salad	1	33		✔			
Salad dressing	1	71					✔
Dinner total		944					
Snack							
Bag of chips	1	152		✔			✔
Apple	1	72		✔			
Snack total		224					
Daily total		2,551					

Figure 14.4   Sandy's food log for Wednesday.

TABLE 14.4   Resting Metabolism (Calories) for Males Aged 12 to 15

Height m (in.)	Weight kg (lb)					
	45 (100)	54 (120)	68 (150)	81 (180)	90 (200)	≥99 (≥220)
1.52–1.63 (60–64)	1,380	1,500	1,700	1,900	2,000	2,100
1.65–1.73 (65–68)	1,430	1,550	1,750	1,950	2,050	2,200
1.76–1.83 (69–72)	1,480	1,600	1,800	2,000	2,100	2,230
≥1.85 (≥73)	1,500	1,630	1,820	2,010	2,130	2,240

TABLE 14.5   Resting Metabolism (Calories) for Males Aged 16 or Older

Height m (in.)	Weight kg (lb)					
	45 (100)	54 (120)	68 (150)	81 (180)	90 (200)	≥99 (≥220)
1.52–1.63 (60–64)	1,360	1,480	1,670	1,860	1,980	2,110
1.65–1.73 (65–68)	1,410	1,540	1,720	1,910	2,035	2,140
1.76–1.83 (69–72)	1,460	1,590	1,770	1,960	2,085	2,210
≥1.85 (≥73)	1,490	1,610	1,800	1,985	2,110	2,235

TABLE 14.6 Resting Metabolism (Calories) for Females Aged 12 to 15

Height m (in.)	Weight kg (lb)					
	41 (90)	45 (100)	54 (120)	68 (150)	81 (180)	≥90 (≥200)
1.52–1.63 (60–64)	1,275	1,320	1,410	1,540	1,670	1,755
1.65–1.73 (65–68)	1,295	1,340	1,425	1,560	1,690	1,775
1.76–1.83 (69–72)	1,315	1,360	1,445	1,575	1,705	1,795
≥1.85 (≥73)	1,325	1,370	1,455	1,585	1,715	1,800

TABLE 14.7   Resting Metabolism (Calories) for Females Aged 16 or Older

Height m (in.)	Weight kg (lb)					
	41 (90)	45 (100)	54 (120)	68 (150)	81 (180)	≥90 (≥200)
1.52–1.63 (60–64)	1,260	1,300	1,390	1,520	1,650	1,740
1.65–1.73 (65–68)	1,275	1,320	1,405	1,540	1,670	1,755
1.76–1.83 (69–72)	1,295	1,340	1,425	1,555	1,685	1,775
≥1.85 (≥73)	1,305	1,350	1,440	1,565	1,700	1,785

calories per minute (314 ÷ 60 = about 5.25). Thus in mowing the lawn for 15 minutes, he expended about 79 calories (5.25 × 15 = 79).

Sandy recorded his calories expended in his activity log (see figure 14.5). His calories expended in physical activity totalled 355. He added this number to his resting metabolism of 1,800 to determine that his total energy expenditure for the day was 2,155 calories (355 + 1,800 = 2,155).

Prepare an activity log similar to the one that Sandy prepared. Record each activity you performed on the day of your log. Use the compendium for physical activity or a physical activity calculator to determine the number of calories you expended in each activity that you performed. Total the calories expended in these activities. Then add this calorie total to your resting metabolism calories to determine your total calories expended for the day.

Activity	Minutes	Calories per hour	Calories
Morning			
Physical education: Burn It Up workout	30	340	170
Walk to and from classes	10	318	53
Afternoon			
Walk to and from classes	10	318	53
Evening			
Mow lawn	15	314	79
Daily activity total	65		355
Resting metabolism			1,800
Total daily calories expended			2,155

Figure 14.5 Sandy's activities for Wednesday.

Step 3: Evaluate Your Calorie Balance

Compare your calorie expenditure to your calorie intake to see if your calories balance for the day. Sandy expended 2,155 calories for the day but consumed 2,551, so he consumed 396 calories more than he expended (2,551 – 2,155 = 396). It's not unusual to consume more calories than expended on one day, then consume less than expended on another. However, if Sandy regularly consumed 396 calories a day more than he expended, he would gain body fat over time.

Determine if you have energy balance (calorie intake equals calorie expenditure) or if you have imbalance. Subtract the smaller number (whether calorie intake or calorie expenditure) from the larger number.

Lesson 14.2
Making Healthy Food Choices

Lesson Objectives

After participating in this lesson, you should be able to

1. describe the FIT formula for meeting nutritional needs,
2. identify several important elements of food labels and describe the information they provide,
3. identify some nutrients that should be limited in your diet, and
4. name some common myths about nutrition and explain why they are not true.

 Lesson Vocabulary

calorimeter, food label, natural health product (NHP)

Do you know how to read a nutrition label? Have you ever wondered if your portion sizes are the same as the serving size listed on a nutrition label? In the previous lesson, you learned how to choose foods from different food groups in order to build a nutritious diet. You also learned how following dietary guidelines can help you attain and maintain good health. In this lesson, you'll learn more about choosing healthy foods for a balanced diet.

The FIT Formula and Nutrition

Table 14.8 shows how you can use the FIT formula as a guideline for nutritional fitness. Too often, teens in particular violate the FIT formula. For example, some skip breakfast or lunch, which often leads them to overeat later in the day. Skipping meals can make you feel tired during the day and can make it difficult to concentrate, thus contributing to poor school performance. If you play on a sport team, skipping meals can negatively affect your performance.

In addition, many people don't know how many calories they should consume each day. This number, however, is easy to determine (see this chapter's self-assessment). As you learned earlier, a person's nutrient needs vary according to age, sex, height, weight, and daily physical activity. Young people who are going through puberty or are still growing have special nutritional needs; specifically, they need to eat foods high in minerals (potassium, calcium, iron) that aid in the development of bones and blood. If you eat the recommended number of servings from each of the food groups, you're well on your way to consuming a diet that meets your nutritional needs.

Servings and Portions

A serving of food and a portion of food are not necessarily the same thing. As seen in table 14.3, a serving is a recommended amount. A portion, on the other hand, is the amount of food you put on your plate (or, at a restaurant, the amount put there for you). Therefore, a portion can be large or small. A large portion can contain much more than

TABLE 14.8 Fitness Target Zones and Nutrition

	Nutrition target zone
Frequency	Eat three meals a day. Healthy planned snacks can be part of a healthy diet.
Intensity	The number of calories you consume daily should fall within the range determined by factors described in this chapter's self-assessment. Calories should come from recommended servings for each food group (see table 14.3).
Time	Eat meals at regular intervals, such as morning, noon, and evening.

a recommended serving, and a small portion can contain less than a recommended serving. Use the following strategies to control your portion sizes so that you eat an appropriate amount of food.

- Know the size of a recommended serving (see table 14.3).
- Choose portions equal to recommended servings.
- Eat only part of large portions; save extra food for another meal.
- Read food labels carefully. Calorie totals listed on food labels (see figure 14.6) typically show the number of calories in one serving, but a package often contains several servings. To consume the number of calories on the label, choose only an amount from the package that is equal to a recommended serving.

FIT FACT

One reason for Canadians' increase in portion sizes in recent years is the marketing of larger meals sometimes referred to as "super-sized." For example, the original size of most French fry orders contained 450 calories, but the size of a large order currently promoted by many fast food outlets contains more than 600 calories. Another example is the all-you-can-eat buffet offered at a set price, which can motivate people to eat large portions in order to get their money's worth. Use the information presented in table 14.3 in the previous lesson to help you determine how much you eat. You may find that one portion is equal to several servings.

You can also get an idea of appropriate serving sizes by referring to certain common objects typically found around the house. The following list provides some examples of approximate sizes of single servings.

- Baked potato: computer mouse
- Bagel: can of tuna
- Apple: baseball
- Hard cheese: three game dice
- Lean beef: deck of cards

Food Labels

Many teenagers do not shop for groceries, plan meals, or cook for a family. But it's important for you to start learning how to do these things now because you'll need these skills at some point in your life. Reading and understanding **food labels** can help you plan your diet and shop for healthy foods. By law, manufacturers must now use a standard format for food labels. In 2015, Health Canada made changes to the food label based on feedback from more than 10,000 Canadians. Food manufacturers have until 2020 to institute the proposed changes to the food labels. The changes proposed by Health Canada will appear in the following sections. Be aware that the food labels required by the government are not the same as the food labels sometimes provided by manufacturers on the front of food packages (for example, cereal boxes). Front-of-box labels are not regulated and may not be accurate. In fact, nutrition experts criticize these labels because they are often deceptive and are really part of a strategy to sell the food rather than provide nutrition information. Experts worry that consumers will look at the front-of-box label rather

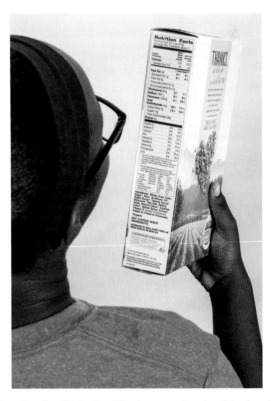

Reading food labels will help you select healthy foods.

than the regulated side-of-box label that provides scientifically sound information.

You've probably already used side-of-box nutrition labels at one time or another, but you may not know how to use them most effectively. When reading a food label, start at the top and use the following six steps, which refer to the sample label from a package of food presented in figure 14.6. (Food labels are typically all white on food containers, but colours are used in this example to help you easily find each area on the label.)

Step 1: Servings

The number of servings in the container is shown in the green area. In this case, two servings are listed, and the size of each serving is 1 cup, thus making a total of 2 cups in the package. By 2020, food manufacturers in Canada will have to present serving sizes that reflect portions people typically eat. For example, many bread products present a serving size as one slice and provide nutrition information

based on that serving, but if you eat a sandwich you typically have two slices.

Step 2: Calories

The white area shows the number of calories per serving—in this case, 130 calories. Therefore, the total calorie content of the food package is 260 (130 calories × 2 servings = 260 calories). Some food labels include both total calories in the package and calories per serving. However, many labels include only calories per serving, which may lead people to think that the calorie number listed (130) is the amount in the total package. The real calorie content is 260 (2 servings × 130 = 260 calories).

Step 3: Nutrients That Should Be Limited

The yellow area presents information about some nutrients that should be limited in your diet, such as fat, salt, and cholesterol. The number beside

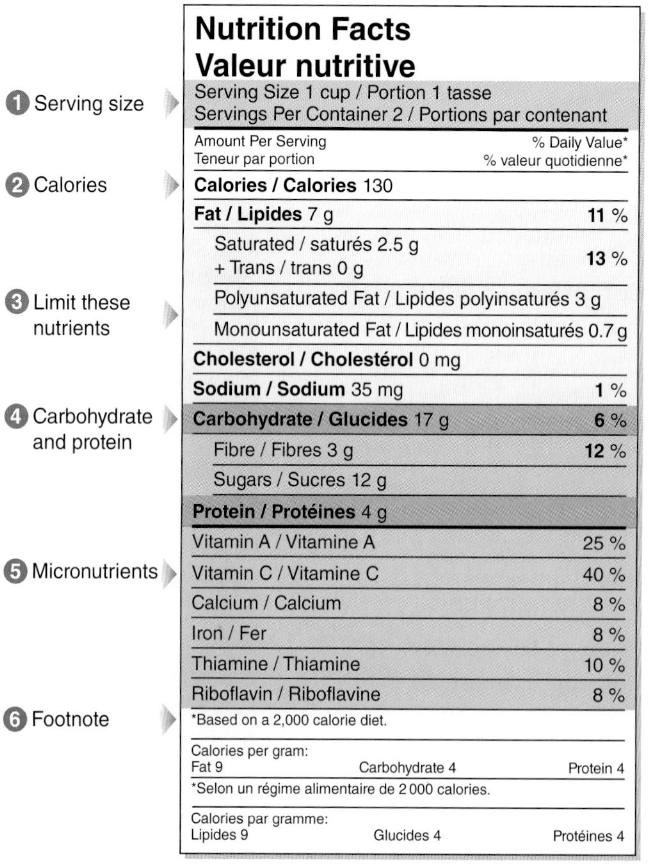

FIGURE 14.6 Sample food label.
From Canadian Food Inspection Agency.

each nutrient indicates the amount in grams (g) or milligrams (mg) and the percentage of that nutrient's daily amount provided by one serving. In this case, one serving of the food provides 11 percent of the total fat and 1 percent of the salt you should consume each day. If you eat two servings, you need to double the listed numbers to know how much fat and salt you're consuming. Trans fat amounts are shown in figure 14.6 even though they could be excluded from foods in the future. In addition, amounts of healthy fats such as mono- and polyunsaturated fats are provided on some labels.

Step 4: Carbohydrate and Protein

Carbohydrate and protein are two of the three macronutrients that provide your body with energy. Two types of carbohydrate are listed on the label (in blue): dietary fibre and sugars. As shown in pink, 6 percent of the daily requirement of carbohydrate

is provided by one serving. Dietary fibre, a type of carbohydrate, is desirable in the diet, and the label helps you determine if you eat enough of it. Sugars should be limited in the diet like fat and sodium. One of the main changes Health Canada will require of food manufacturers by 2020 is to provide more detailed information about added sugars in the ingredients list. Specifically, products that have sugar added (like granola bars, cereal, and fruit bars) will be required to group the different types of added sugars into a category called "sugars." For example, if a product adds brown sugar, fancy molasses, and sugar, the ingredients list would group them as "sugars (brown sugar, fancy molasses, and sugar)." In addition, the ingredients list on products with added sugars must list the ingredients by weight, beginning with the ingredients that contribute the most weight to the product. What this means for many products is that sugars will now appear as the first ingredient (indicating that it is the number-one

 FITNESS TECHNOLOGY: What's in Your Food?

A **calorimeter** is an apparatus designed to determine the amount of heat generated by a chemical reaction. In Latin, *calor* means heat and *metron* means measure; thus a calorimeter measures heat. A special type of calorimeter is used to determine the amount of heat created when different types of food are burned. In this way, nutrition scientists have determined the calorie counts of various foods. The Dietitians of Canada provides a free website and app (eaTracker) that allows you to determine the calorie counts of many foods. The eaTracker is also a useful tool that can support you in reaching your goals with meal planning, food analysis, and physical activity. The U.S. Department of Agriculture's Food Tracker, a

part of the SuperTracker found at the MyPlate website, will also help you determine the calorie counts of various foods. As part of their Healthy Canadians website, the Government of Canada has created a Healthy Eating resource that allows you to gather information about nutrients in foods, healthy eating recommendations, and nutrition programs that support Canadians.

The web has also made it relatively easy for you to find other information about food content. For example, some nutrition websites list the specific nutrient content (carbohydrate, protein, fat, vitamins, and minerals) of various foods. Some address foods of all kinds, and others provide information specifically about fast food.

Using Technology

Find the Dietitians of Canada eaTracker website (www.eatracker.ca). Notice that it includes online tools for meal planning, meal analysis, physical activity tracking, and goal setting. You could also try the SuperTracker at the MyPlate website (www.ChooseMyPlate.gov). Notice that it includes six different online tracking tools, including FoodTracker and Physical Activity Tracker. Alternatively, you could use a free web tool such as Food-O-Meter at webMD.com or MyFitnessPal at MyFitnessPal.com. Try one of the tools and write an evaluation of it that is several paragraphs long. Explain how the tool would or would not be useful.

ingredient by weight). The number of grams of protein is shown on the label in pink. Health Canada recommends 0.8 grams of protein per kilogram of body weight each day (54.5 grams for a person weighing 68 kilograms [150 pounds]).

Step 5: Micronutrients

Micronutrients, such as vitamins and minerals, are especially important to your diet. You need to get 100 percent of these each day. Six types of micronutrients, four vitamins and two minerals, are highlighted in blue on the label. As you can see from the label in figure 14.6, one serving of the food

FIT FACT

Calories from soft drinks add up fast. Most soft drinks contain about 150 calories in a 12-ounce (about 0.4-litre) can—that's 450 calories in three cans—and many teens drink multiple cans per day. A 64-ounce (about 2-litre) drink, such as those sold at many fast food and convenience stores, contains almost 800 calories. Not surprisingly, studies show that excessive consumption of soft drinks may be one reason for the high incidence of overweight in developed countries. In fact, if all other aspects of your diet stayed the same, adding one soft drink a day would cause you to gain about 7 kilograms (~15 pounds) of fat in a year. The solution? Water quenches your thirst and contains zero calories.

provides 8 percent of daily calcium and iron, and between 8 and 40 percent of the vitamins.

Step 6: Footnote

Use the information in the white area at the bottom of the label to make adjustments for the total number of calories you consume. The total number of calories needed each day varies from person to person depending on age and body size. People who require more calories need to adjust the nutrient amounts, and the information presented at the bottom of the label helps you make these adjustments. For example, a person requiring 2,200 calories per day is allowed more fat, and needs more fibre, than a person requiring 2,000 calories per day.

Other Food Labels

You've learned that side-of-box labels provide useful information and that front-of-box labels can be deceiving. But there are also other food labels you should know about. One type of label refers to a food's fat content. In Canada, labels such as "fat free" can be displayed on food containers only if the food meets legal standards set by the government's Food Inspection Agency. The terms presented in table 14.9 were developed to prevent false advertising. Even with these standardized terms, however, you can still be fooled by advertisements relating to a food's fat content. Some foods, such as milk and packaged meats, are advertised as 2 percent fat—that is, 98 percent fat free. This is true if fat is measured by the product's weight, but it is not true if fat is measured by the total number of calories in the food. For example, only 2 percent of the weight

TABLE 14.9 Key Words on Food Labels and What They Mean

Key words	What they mean
Fat free	Less than 0.5 g of fat per 100 g serving
Low fat	3 g or less of fat per serving
Lean	Contains 10% or less fat
Extra lean	Contains 7.5% or less fat
Free (no, zero, without)	Less than 2 mg of cholesterol, less than 200 mg of saturated fatty acids, and less than 200 mg of trans fatty acids combined
Reduced (less, lower, lower in, fewer, light)	At least 25% less calories, fat, cholesterol, sodium, or sugars than the food to which it is compared

of a glass of 2 percent milk is fat, but more than 30 percent of the calories come from fat.

You can calculate the true percentage of fat calories in food for yourself. Simply divide the calorie total per serving into the calorie total for fat per serving. For the food label shown in figure 14.6, the calorie total per serving is 130 and the calorie total for fat per serving is 63 (7 g × 9 cal/g), so the percentage of fat calories in this food is 48 percent (63 calories ÷ 130 calories = 0.48).

You also might see health claims such as "good for heart health" on food labels. Manufacturers must comply with government regulations regarding such labelling. For example, if it is advertised that a product's fat content is good for your heart, the product must be low in fat, saturated fat, and cholesterol. Fruits, vegetables, and grain products for which such claims are made must not only be low in fat, saturated fat, and cholesterol but also contain at least the minimum amount of fibre per serving. Foods that display health claims related to blood pressure must be low in sodium.

Common Food Myths

You may have heard a number of incorrect or misleading statements about nutrition. Some common nutrition myths are exposed in the following list.

Myth: Skipping meals is a good way to lose weight.

Fact: Studies show that people who skip meals typically eat more than those who eat regular meals. Skipping meals stimulates the appetite, so eating fewer meals can lead to eating more food at each meal, whereas eating more meals usually means eating less at each meal. Skipping breakfast or lunch is common but is ineffective in weight loss and results in lower work and school performance.

Myth: A **natural health product (NHP)** is tested to ensure that it is safe and that it meets the claims advertised by the seller.

Fact: The Natural and Non-prescription Health Products Directorate (NNHPD) regulates food supplements in Canada. This agency tries to provide consumers with quality assurance. Unfortunately, the Canadian government has

not been able to keep up with the ever-growing number of commercial NHPs; thousands of NHPs on the market have not been reviewed for safety or efficacy. So beware of food supplements with claims that are too good to be true.

Myth: A high-protein diet is best for losing weight, building muscle, and maintaining good health.

Fact: A review of a large number of studies shows that a balanced diet—based on the nutrient percentages listed in this chapter's first lesson—is most effective in both fat loss and weight maintenance. Popular high-protein diets cause quick loss of body water, but a diet is effective for fat loss only if it results in consumption of fewer calories. Because these diets are high in fat, experts fear that they can result in increased health problems if used for a long time. Active people need more protein than inactive people, but because active people consume more calories they also get the protein they need through a balanced diet.

Myth: If you limit the amount of fat in your food, you do not need to be concerned with how many calories a food contains.

Fact: It's the total number of calories you consume that makes a difference in weight maintenance. Fat does contain more calories per gram than carbohydrate and protein, but many foods advertised as low in fat actually contain more calories than foods higher in fat.

Myth: Diets very low in calories are effective for weight loss.

Fact: Your body needs calories in order to function. Eating too few calories in a day (800 or less) causes the body to conserve calories to keep the body functioning, which means your body uses fewer calories than it normally would. Therefore, eating too few calories is not an effective way to reduce body fat. In fact, it can be dangerous because very low calorie diets typically do not provide the basic nutrients (such as vitamins and minerals) that your body needs.

"You are what you eat."

—Ludwig Feuerbach, philosopher

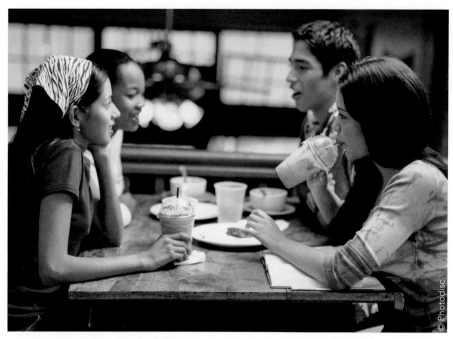

Snacks with friends can be all right if they are low in empty calories and included as part of a total dietary plan.

Because health and nutrition quackery is so common, many other myths also exist. When making choices about your nutrition, follow Health Canada's dietary guidelines. Use information that comes from reliable sources, such as Health Canada, Dietitians of Canada, the Canadian Food Inspection Agency (CFIA), the U.S. FDA, the Canadian Medical Association, the Canadian Heart and Stroke Foundation, and the Canadian Cancer Society.

Nutrition Advertising Strategies and Tactics

You might know about strategy and tactics in games and sport. A strategy is a general plan of action for reaching a specific goal; in sport, a strategy is an overall plan to help win a game, match, or other competition. After the first level of planning—outlining a strategy—tactics are devised to help reach a goal. Tactics are specific actions taken to implement the strategy and reach the goal. Some food manufacturers have adopted a strategy of selling to the youth market (children and teens). This strategy is designed not to sell foods that are healthy but simply to sell more food. One tactic used by marketers is

to concentrate television advertisements for sugared cereals at times when children are out of school and shows are directed at children. Another tactic is to include toys with meals in fast food restaurants to boost interest in fast food among children.

Today, teens represent one of the largest groups of consumers in Canada. Using the "merchants of cool" strategy is one way companies target the teen market. In this approach, companies (merchants) try to make their products seem cool to teens. This strategy is used to sell, among other things, clothing, electronics, energy drinks, sport drinks, and soda. One specific tactic used to carry out this strategy is to feature movie stars and entertainers promoting a brand. Nutrition scientists and dieticians want to make you aware of these strategies and tactics so you can make informed decisions when you choose foods and drinks.

Eating Before Physical Activity

Most people can do moderate activity after a meal if they wait about 30 minutes to an hour. People who have problems doing activity after eating may have to wait longer or modify when and what they eat. You may also have to modify your eating pattern if you plan to do vigorous physical activity or participate in a highly competitive athletic event. Use the following guidelines for eating before physical activity.

- **A special diet is usually not necessary before an athletic competition.** Some athletes think they need a steak before they compete. Steak, however, is high in protein and fat, both of which are digested slowly. As a result, eating steak within two hours of the event might interfere with your performance. In general, you can eat what you like as long as it doesn't disagree with you.

- **Allow extra time between eating and a vigorous competitive event.** Eat one to three hours before competing. Allow more time if you're eating food that's difficult to digest (for example, large servings of meat, spicy foods, and high-fibre foods).

- **Before competition, reduce meal size.** Small meals are easier to digest than large ones. If you get very nervous or often have an upset stomach before competition, limiting meal size can be helpful.

- **Before competition, avoid snacks that are high in simple carbohydrate (simple sugar).** Some people think that having a candy bar or drink that's high in simple carbohydrate before competition will provide quick energy. In fact, taking a big dose of simple carbohydrate right before an event causes blood sugar to go up, but a drop in blood sugar level often follows after exertion. This can cause lack of energy and even dizziness, and it may negatively affect performance and increase risk of injury.

- **Drink before, during, and after activity.** Whether you're competing or not, it's important to drink water. You don't usually need added salt or sugar, except for during especially long events and events occurring in high heat and humidity. Using drinks with too much sugar can even detract from your performance for reasons explained in the previous bulleted item. Drinking too much before activity can cause a side stitch in some people. These people should drink fluids well before the activity and in several small amounts. They should not drink a large amount right before the activity.

Lesson Review

1. How can the FIT formula help people meet their nutritional needs?
2. What are three examples of information you can find on a food label?
3. What are some nutrients that should be limited in your diet?
4. What are two common food myths? How are they incorrect or misleading?

TAKING CHARGE: Saying No

Sometimes the simple act of saying no is the best way to avoid a potentially harmful situation. However, while it may seem easy, saying no can actually be very difficult to carry out successfully. Here's an example.

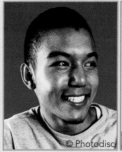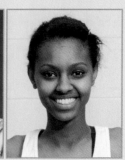

© Photodisc

Many cultures celebrate holidays with special meals and foods. On one such occasion, Manny was invited to spend the Cinco de Mayo holiday with his girlfriend's family. Plans were made to spend the afternoon water-skiing at a nearby lake, then have a big party. Manny's girlfriend Rita warned him that her mother always prepared huge amounts of food for this special day. The family did not normally eat so much, but on this special day it was their tradition to feast on traditional foods. She told him to make sure he came with a big appetite. Unfortunately, Manny's doctor had just instructed him to restrict his intake of salt, fat, and calories.

Manny arrived at the party just as Rita's mother was setting out the food. The table was loaded with tortilla chips, guacamole, beef and bean burritos, chiles rellenos, and fresh corn, as well as cakes, pies, and cookies. Manny knew that he faced a difficult situation as Rita came forward with a plate piled high with cookies.

"Manny, you're just in time," she said. "The food is great!" Manny was concerned about the salt and fat in the food and wanted to avoid consuming too many calories, but he did not want to hurt Rita's feelings. So he replied, "Everything looks good, but I have to watch my diet."

Rita offered him a cookie, knowing they were Manny's favourite. "But you've got to try my mother's cookies. Everyone says they're the best. You'll hurt my mother's feelings if you don't eat one." Manny felt pressured to eat something he didn't really want.

For Discussion

In what way does the party put Manny in a difficult situation? How can Manny say no to Rita without embarrassing her or hurting her feelings? What can he do so that his refusal won't hurt Rita's mother's feelings? What could he have done to prepare for the situation before going to the party? What are some other situations in which saying no would be the best response? Consider the guidelines presented in the Self-Management feature when answering the discussion questions.

SELF-MANAGEMENT: Skills for Saying No

Most of us try to eat well, do regular physical activity, and live a healthy lifestyle. But sometimes the situation we're in or the people we're around make it difficult to stick with healthy behaviours. We're tempted to do things that we wouldn't normally do. You can take steps to make it easier to say no when you're in situations that encourage you to engage in behaviours you know are not best for you. The following guidelines will help you say no to eating food that you don't want or need. You may also be able to use these strategies to help you say no in other situations involving choices about health-related behaviour.

- **Say no to food offered on special occasions.** Eat a light meal before a holiday event so that you don't arrive hungry. Practice ways to refuse food so that you don't hurt the host's feelings. For example, talk to the host or hostess ahead of time to explain why you may limit your food intake. Prepare statements ahead of time that you can use if you're pressured to eat.

- **Use strategies to avoid temptation.** Avoid standing near food. If you feel the urge to eat, talk to someone or find something else to do.

- **Say no to extra food when eating out.** Plan in advance what you will eat. Resist ordering foods that are advertised or that others eat. Choose small servings—avoid big orders such as large burgers and fries. Say no to special deals that include foods you don't want; instead, order single items you do want. Say no to extra sauces, toppings, and condiments such as mayonnaise.

- **Shop with a strategy.** Prepare a list ahead of time and stick with it to help you say no to foods that are high in empty calories. Use food labels and avoid foods that are high in calories per serving. Look for better choices. Eat before you shop so that you're not hungry while making choices.

- **Consume healthy snacks.** Eating vegetables and fruits for snacks can help you say no to snacks that are high in empty calories, such as potato chips, cookies, and candy. Avoid sugared soft drinks and sport drinks; instead, carry a water bottle.

- **Eat healthy foods at school.** Prepare your own lunch and snacks for school to help you say no to unhealthy food offered in snack machines. If you have free time, find a way to be active to avoid thinking about eating things you don't really want or need. If you eat school food, ask for small servings to avoid eating too much. If you have free time with friends, bring healthy snacks to share.

- **Say no to large servings and seconds.** Tell family members and friends not to offer seconds. Limit dessert servings.

- **Eat slowly and avoid eating while studying or watching television.** Some experts recommend that you limit your eating to the kitchen or dining room to help you say no to unwanted food.

TAKING ACTION: Burn It Up Workout

All types of activity included in the Physical Activity Pyramid use calories and therefore help you balance your calorie expenditure with your calorie intake. Moderate-intensity activity can be beneficial because it can be performed over a long span of time. Vigorous-intensity activity is also good because it uses more calories in a given amount of time. For example, a 54-kilogram (119-pound) person burns about 85 calories by walking for 20 minutes (a moderate activity) but 125 calories by jogging for 20 minutes (a vigorous activity). You can also boost your energy expenditure fairly easily by adding bursts of higher-intensity effort to your exercise routine. Muscle fitness exercises also expend calories, as well as building muscle mass that causes you to expend more calories even at rest. In addition to burning calories, weight-bearing exercise like muscle fitness exercise, walking, jogging, running, and jumping also strengthen your bones.

Take action by trying the Burn It Up workout delivered by your physical educator. This workout includes activities of various types and intensities. During the workout, moni-tor your overall effort to see if the intensity is moderate or keeps you in the target heart rate zone for vigorous physical activity.

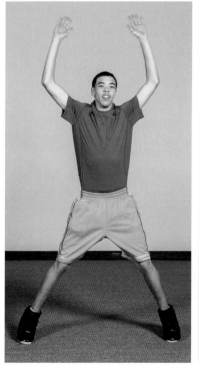
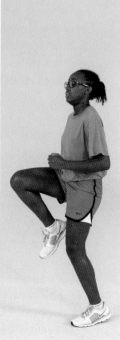

Take action with the Burn It Up workout.

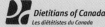 **GET ACTIVE WITH DIETITIANS OF CANADA**

Who We Are

Dietitians of Canada is the national professional association for dietitians, representing 6,000 members at the local, provincial, and national levels. As the voice of the profession, Dietitians of Canada promotes health through food and nutrition.

What We Do

Dietitians of Canada provides easier access to trusted food and nutrition information from dietitians. Through our public website, our annual Nutrition Month Campaign, and our online dietitian referral systems, we facilitate access to dietitians for the public, the media, and other health professionals.

Dietitians translate scientific research into practical solutions. Dietitians play a major role in health care, industry, government, and education. They influence policy development, direct nutrition programs, manage high-quality food services, and conduct nutrition research. To become a dietitian, you need to complete a degree at an accredited university program plus at least 1,250 hours of supervised, hands-on training.

Get Involved

Want to track your eating and activity patterns and compare them to national standards? Then download the eaTracker app from the Apple Store or Google Play. It's from Dietitians of Canada, so it's Canadian and it's free. You'll find more tips from dietitians at www.dietitians.ca in the Your Health section.

Visit Dietitians Views at www.dietitians.ca to learn about key food and nutrition issues facing Canadians. Thinking of dietetics as a career choice? Check out the Become a Dietitian section.

Reviewing Concepts and Vocabulary

Complete the following in order to show your growing understanding of fitness, health, and wellness. Answer items 1 through 5 by correctly completing each sentence with a word or phrase.

1. _____ are nutrients that provide energy.
2. Foods that are high in calories but low in nutrients are said to contain _____ calories.
3. _____ are food substances that make up protein.
4. A portion of food is the amount of a specific food on your plate; it differs from a _____, which is the recommended amount for a specific food.
5. _____ obesity refers to gradual weight gain as a person grows older.

For items 6 through 10, match each term in column 1 with the appropriate phrase in column 2.

6. carbohydrate
7. protein
8. fibre
9. saturated fat
10. mineral

a. major source of energy
b. regulates cell activity
c. solid at room temperature
d. cannot be digested by the body
e. building block for your body

For items 11 through 15, respond to each statement or question.

11. Describe your body's need for fat and the best types to include in your diet.
12. Describe the four groups depicted in Canada's Food Guide.
13. Explain how side-of-box food labels can help you eat well.
14. Describe several guidelines about eating before physical activity.
15. Describe several guidelines for saying no in situations when you might feel pressured to do something you don't want to do.

Thinking Critically

Your friend asks for your advice about her diet. She wonders whether the food choices she makes are important or whether she needs only to count calories. She has also started to increase her physical activity and wonders how that will affect her caloric and nutritional needs. Write a paragraph explaining the advice you would give her. Remember to try to connect it back to concepts from this chapter.

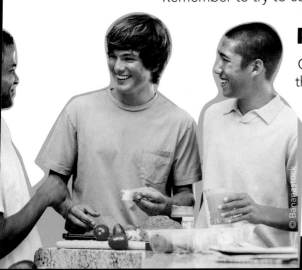

Project

Compare Canada's Eat Well Plate with MyPlate from the United States. What could each country learn from the other (i.e., what are the pros and cons of each)?

Alternatively, create a poster that compares Canadian and U.S. food labels. How do they differ and why are they different? What could each country learn from the other?

15

Making Good Consumer Choices

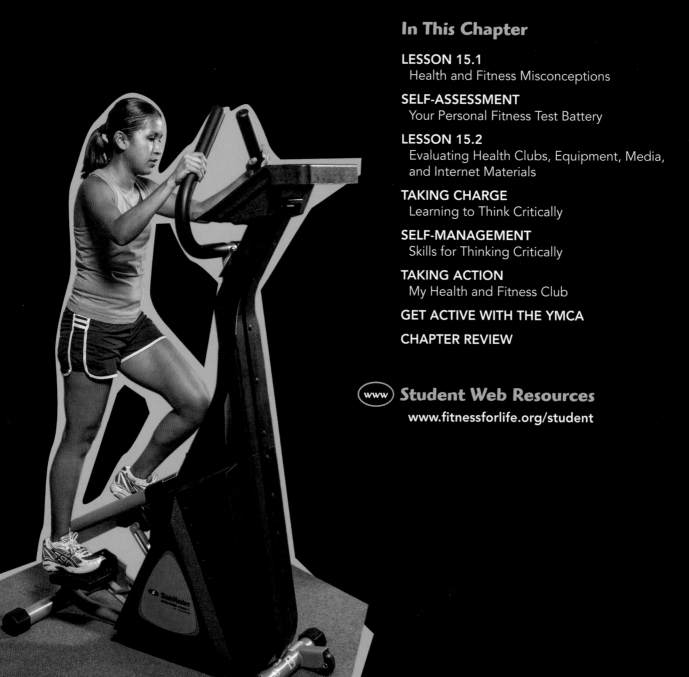

In This Chapter

(www) **Student Web Resources**
www.fitnessforlife.org/student

Lesson 15.1
Health and Fitness Misconceptions

Lesson Objectives

After participating in this lesson, you should be able to

1. explain the difference between quackery and fraud;
2. explain the importance of being an informed consumer in the area of fitness, health, and wellness;
3. name some reliable sources of health- and fitness-related information; and
4. give some examples of health and fitness misconceptions and quackery.

Lesson Vocabulary

con artist, electrolyte, fraud, passive exercise, quack, quackery

You've probably come across ads for health and fitness products and services in newspapers and magazines and on radio, television, and the web. Is a product or service effective simply because it is advertised? Would you buy the product advertised in figure 15.1? In this lesson, you'll learn how to become a wise consumer (purchaser) of health and fitness products.

What Is Quackery?

Some people are in a hurry to lose body fat or gain muscle. Often, people who want quick results are persuaded to purchase useless health or fitness products or services. In other words, they become victims of **quackery**—a method of advertising or selling that uses false claims to lure people into buying products that are worthless or even harmful. Some people who practice quackery actually believe their products work; thus they may have good intentions but still do harm. A person who practices quackery is sometimes referred to as a **quack**.

Some people who practice quackery are guilty of **fraud**. People who practice fraud try to deceive you and get you to buy products or services that they know are ineffective or harmful. A person who practices fraud is called a **con artist**. Because what they do is often illegal, con artists may be

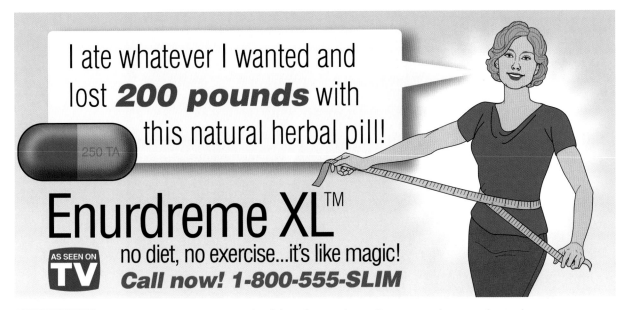

I ate whatever I wanted and lost **200 pounds** with this natural herbal pill!

250 TA

Enurdreme XL™

AS SEEN ON TV

no diet, no exercise...it's like magic!
Call now! 1-800-555-SLIM

FIGURE 15.1 Some advertisements make false claims about fitness products and supplements.

convicted of a crime. The common saying, "If it seems too good to be true, it's probably untrue" cautions buyers that con artists are good at making you believe they're offering you a good deal. But deals that seem exceptionally good are often not as good as the con artist makes them seem.

> " Modern health quacks are super-salesmen. They play on fear. They cater to hope. And once they have you, they'll keep you coming back for more . . . and more . . . and more. "
>
> —Stephen Barrett and William T. Jarvis of the Quackwatch website

Detecting Quackery and Fraud

People who commit quackery and fraud use a variety of deceptive practices to get you to buy their products or services or use products they endorse. Separating fact from fiction can be difficult. Use the guidelines presented in the following sections to help you spot health and fitness quackery and fraud.

Check Credentials

Be sure that the person you think is an expert really is an expert. A con artist might claim to be a doctor or to have a college or university degree. However, the degree might be in a subject unrelated to health and physical fitness. It might also come from a nonaccredited school; it might even be falsified. You can verify credentials by checking with your local or state health authorities or with professional organizations.

If you have questions about health or fitness, ask a real expert's advice. For example, physical education teachers have a college degree that requires them to study all branches of kinesiology. Some other fitness leaders are certified by a group such as the Canadian Society for Exercise Physiology (CSEP). For medical advice, talk to a physician (MD or DO) or a registered nurse (RN). For questions about general health, ask a certified health education teacher. For questions about using exercise to rehabilitate from injury, consult a physiotherapist. All of these experts have college degrees and relevant training in their area of specialization.

For questions about diet, food, and nutrition, consult a registered dietician (RD). Be aware that a person who uses the title of nutritionist is not necessarily an expert. Similarly, staff members in health clubs are often not required to hold college degrees. Practitioners certified by a well-respected organization are more qualified than those without certification, but certification without a degree is not adequate to allow someone to be considered an expert. Neither nutritionists nor health club employees are considered reliable sources of health

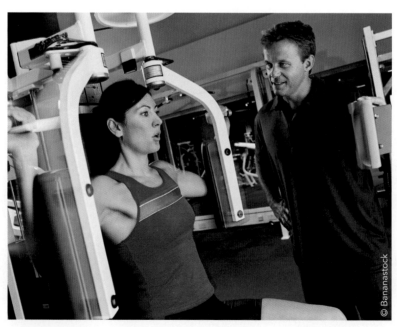

Check credentials to make sure that "experts" are really experts.

or fitness information unless they hold the credentials described here.

FIT FACT

"Buyer beware" is a saying used to remind people that they have to be responsible and knowledgeable when making a purchase of anything, and that includes fitness, health, and wellness products. People who commit fraud make promises that they know they cannot or will not keep, and buyers must beware of people trying to sell fraudulent products. However, if a seller makes a promise (warranty) for a product, it must be fulfilled.

Check the Organizations of the Experts You Consult

Quacks and con artists sometimes try to get you to believe that they know more than experts from well-known organizations such as those listed in the Consumer Corner feature. Be wary of people who claim they know more than well-known experts or who try to discredit respected organizations.

Quacks and con artists also use names and initials of phony organizations with important-sounding names that are similar to the names of well-known organizations. But anyone can form an organization and use it to try to impress you. Check the background of anyone who claims to be a member of an organization whose name you've never heard.

As a consumer, you need to be informed about the products and services you use. Do not assume that every advertised product is safe and effective. Corporations do not always live up to their claims for their products. For example, a "fat-burning" product called West Pharma Lean was recalled by Health Canada because it did not have a Natural Product Number (NPN) and there was reasonable probability that the use of, or exposure to, the product could cause serious adverse health consequences or death. In another example, a study by the American Council on Exercise found so-called hologram bracelets, commonly worn by many famous athletes, to be ineffective. The bracelets' maker falsely claimed that they improved fitness in areas such as strength, flexibility, and balance.

So remember: *The fact that a famous person uses a product does not mean that it is safe or effective.* Agencies such as the ones named in the Consumer Corner feature can provide accurate information, but they do not police all products. In many cases, *you* are the one who has to make the final decision about buying a product or service. Being informed can help you stay safe and avoid spending money on worthless products.

Guidelines for Preventing Quackery and Fraud

Consider the following guidelines before purchasing a product or service.

CONSUMER CORNER: Reliable Consumer Groups

Many organizations work to protect consumers from misleading advertising and quackery. Canadian governmental agencies that do this type of work include the Competition Bureau; the Canadian Food Inspection Agency; Advertising Standards Canada; the Consumer Measures Committee; federal, provincial, and territorial Consumer Affairs; and the Financial Consumer Agency of Canada. Better Business Bureaus and consumer groups and alliances exist across the country and can be accessed on the Canadian Consumer Handbook website as well as Canadian government websites. There are some

great resources for health information in the United States including the National Institutes of Health, the Centers for Disease Control and Prevention, and the National Center for Complementary and Alternative Medicine.

The groups listed here maintain websites that provide reliable health information. However, some other popular websites are unreliable. As a consumer, you need to be able to accurately evaluate potential sources of health and fitness information, as well as the quality of products and services offered for purchase.

Be Wary of Advisors Who Sell Products

People who sell products make money by selling them, and salespeople often have little training in health, fitness, and wellness. For example, people who sell exercise equipment or food supplements may know less about their products than their customers do. In addition, salespeople are often willing to stretch the truth in order to make a sale. With this in mind, consult a true expert before you make a purchase.

Be Suspicious of Sales Pitches That Promise Results Too Good to Be True

Look for words and phrases such as "miracle," "secret remedy," "scientific breakthrough," and "endorsed by movie stars." A quack or con artist is likely to use these or similar terms in a sales pitch for an item that is useless. Be suspicious if a salesperson promises immediate, effortless, or guaranteed results.

Be Cautious About Mail-Order and Internet Sales

You cannot examine mail-order and Internet-marketed products before buying them. Money-back guarantees may seem to protect you, but a guarantee is only as good as the company that backs it. Unlike a traditional store, where you can take a product back and talk to someone in person, mail-order and Internet-based companies may not offer this opportunity. Some have staff members to help you with returns and questions, but many do not. Some also require you to pay return mail costs. Before buying from any source, know the company's return

SCIENCE IN ACTION: Sport and Energy Drinks

Exercise physiologists, dieticians, and medical scientists work together to investigate heat-related conditions that can result from physical activity, especially during hot weather. In fact, regardless of the weather, you need to keep your body hydrated during exercise to prevent conditions such as heat stress and heatstroke. To replenish the body, researchers have developed flavoured "sport drinks" that contain important minerals called **electrolytes**. When appropriate ingredients are used, these drinks can help adults keep their body hydrated during exercise. "Energy drinks" are also popular, but they are not intended primarily to replace fluids lost during exercise. They may contain ingredients similar to those in sport drinks, but they often also contain large amounts of sugar and relatively large amounts of caffeine.

The Canadian Paediatric Society cautions against the overuse of sport drinks and recommends their use for young athletes only when they are exercising in intense heat and humidity or for longer than 60 minutes. Canada's Food Guide recommends limiting the intake of sport drinks. Health Canada states that sport drinks are not appropriate for everyone and that if you are exercising for under an hour or at a low intensity, plain water will enable you to perform at your best. The Dietitians of Canada agree with this view and state that for most teens who perform the amount of activity recommended by national guidelines, plain water is best.

Health Canada has also issued a strong warning with respect to energy drinks: "Energy drinks are not recommended and should not be sold or provided to children and youth." In fact, Health Canada has a proposed plan of attack to limit the consumption of energy drinks due to potential health risks of ingesting too much caffeine, with children and youth being the most at risk. Children are at increased risk of experiencing behavioural effects from consuming caffeine. Other suspected health problems, as reported by Health Canada, that are associated with energy drinks are irregular heartbeat and nervousness. As well, common problems caused by too much caffeine include fast heart rate, inability to sleep, stomach upset, anxiety, and headache.

Student Activity

Research one sport drink and one energy drink. Find out about its key ingredients, benefits, and side effects. Prepare a visual display about the possible benefits and dangers associated with the drinks for teens.

policy. Internet-based companies are usually rated for reliability and quality of service, and you should check a company's rating before buying from it.

Be Wary of Product Claims

A favourite trick of some con artists is to claim that a product is "brand new" or is just now being offered for the first time. Others may claim that a product is "available in Canada for the first time." They try to make you think that you're getting something special. Quacks and con artists may also try to get you to believe their product is popular in Europe, Asia, or some other location. This technique is usually used to impress you. It does not provide any useful information.

Be Wary of Untested Products

Using untested products can be risky. Quacks do not subject their products to thorough scientific testing. Their products are often rushed to market in order to make money as quickly as possible. One way to tell whether a product or service is a good one is to see whether information about it has been published in a respected journal. If so, the study was conducted by a qualified expert.

Health Quackery

The market is flooded with health products, many of which are useless. Although some of these products may not be harmful, false advertising claims give people unrealistic expectations about the benefits they can provide. Indeed, many advertisers promote myths about health and fitness.

FIT FACT

Cellulite is a term often used for fat that causes the skin to look rippled or bumpy. Con artists would have you believe that cellulite is a special kind of fat that can be eliminated with creams or other special products. In fact, cellulite occurs when fat cells become enlarged. It is best reduced by expending more calories than you consume.

Food Supplements

A food supplement is a product that is not part of the typical diet. Supplements are often produced as syrups, powders, or tablets (figure 15.2). Generally, they are sold in health food stores or through the mail. Common supplements include protein (amino acids), vitamins, minerals, and herbs. The Canadian government applies the term "Natural Health Products" to common supplements and regulates them differently than medicine and food.

Health Canada's Canadian Food Inspection Agency (CFIA) is responsible for ensuring the safety, effectiveness, and quality of Natural Health Products (i.e., supplements). If a product has an eight-digit Natural Product Number (NPN), the product has been reviewed and approved by Health Canada. However, there are so many supplements sold in Canada that the CFIA has not been able

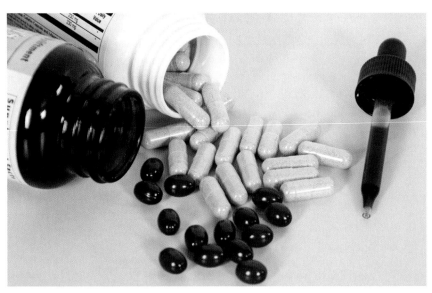

FIGURE 15.2 Food supplements are regulated by the government as Natural Health Products.

to review all of them for safety, effectiveness, and quality. Many supplements sold in Canada do not have an eight-digit NPN. As a consumer you need to protect yourself from false and misleading claims and ineffective and even dangerous products on the market. More than a few people have died from taking supplements that were contaminated or contained ingredients that were not supposed to be in the supplement. Many people have also suffered illness and even death as the result of taking supplements marketed as causing fat loss or enhancing performance.

Some other supplements are not harmful but simply do not provide the benefits promised by those who sell them. In recent years the sale of supplements has increased dramatically. Many people are wasting money on products that don't work. All Canadians can access more information on Natural Health Products by visiting Health Canada's website.

Some supplements can be beneficial if used according to a physician's recommendation. For

FIT FACT

Using a Canadian-developed chemical analysis technique called DNA bar coding, University of Guelph researchers showed that nearly 60 percent of herbal products analyzed contained unlabelled plant ingredients, and more than 20 percent contained "fillers" such as rice and wheat, also not listed on the labels.

example, a vitamin B_{12} supplement is recommended for strict vegetarians (vegans), and a folic acid supplement is recommended for expectant mothers. But even vitamins can be dangerous if taken in amounts that are too large. Before you take any supplement, consult with your parent or guardian, as well as your family physician.

Sport Supplements

One continuing trend, even in light of potential health risks and dangers, involves the use of sport supplements or sport vitamins—products sold to enhance athletic performance. These supplements are also called ergogenic aids. Many supplements sold as ergogenic aids are actually quack products. Many supplements can also be harmful to your health.

Fad Diets

"Lose pounds a day on the ice cream diet!" "The rice diet works wonders!" "Fruit diet dissolves fat!" How many similar weight loss claims have you seen? Each of these claims is false and involves an example of a fad diet. Although fad diets are popular because they usually promise fast results, nearly all are nutritionally unbalanced. They often restrict eating to only one or two food groups, or even one specific food. As you've learned, the only safe and effective way to reduce body fatness and lose weight is to combine physical activity with eating fewer calories. Eating healthy, low-calorie foods can help you control your calorie intake.

Restricting Fluids

It is possible to lose weight in a short time as a result of dehydration. If you do not drink enough fluid, or if you lose excessive water through sweating, you will become dehydrated, thus losing water weight. Some people think this weight loss is permanent. It is not! Restricting fluid intake and taking products that cause water loss do not help you lose body fat, and as soon as you replace the fluids, your weight will return to normal. In addition, these practices can be dangerous to your health.

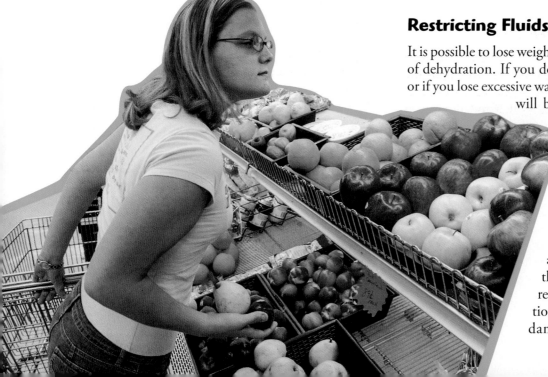

FITNESS TECHNOLOGY: Quack Machines

You've learned in other chapters about many technological innovations that can make our lives better. However, not all technological devices are safe and effective. Some unscrupulous people sell devices that not only are ineffective but also can be quite dangerous.

One example is a device with electrodes that are placed on the abdominal muscles. Electrical current is sent through the electrodes, thus stimulating the muscles. People who advertise these devices claim that you can use them to build strong abdominal muscles without doing any regular abdominal exercises, such as crunches or curl-ups. But studies show that these devices do not build fitness. In addition, because the electrodes are placed on the abdomen, they can cause the heart to beat irregularly and result in serious health problems.

Physiotherapists do use muscle stimulators to help restore normal muscle function in people who have been injured or who are recovering from illness. These machines can be effective when used by experts for very specific therapeutic purposes. They are not the same as muscle stimulators sold with claims of building abdominal muscle. Be wary of sellers who promise fitness without exercise.

> **Using Technology**
>
> Check with a physiotherapist to see how a muscle stimulator works and how it helps people with injury or illness. Also ask for more information about the dangers of using an abdominal muscle stimulator.

Dehydration can lead to physical problems such as headache and fatigue, mental problems such as lack of concentration and mood changes, and heat illnesses such as heat exhaustion and heatstroke.

Fitness Quackery

Many useless products claim to improve fitness and reduce body fat. Claims for these products are false. Be alert to the following worthless fitness devices and methods.

Passive Exercise Machines

Passive exercise refers to the use of machines or devices that move your body for you and supposedly promote fat reduction and weight loss. Examples include machines with rollers that roll along your hips or legs; vibrating machines that shake certain body areas and are said to "break up" fat cells; and motorized belts, cycles, tables, and rowing machines. The claims made for these products are

false. These passive exercise programs are ineffective because your body is moved by outside forces rather than your own muscles.

Figure Wrapping

Figure wrapping involves the use of bandages or nonporous garments to compress body parts. The wraps are sometimes soaked in fluid, or the person may soak in a bath after being wrapped. The wraps are advertised for weight loss or as a method of losing "inches" from the body. In reality, they are not effective for either fat loss or size reduction. They can, however, cause overheating and dehydration and can be extremely dangerous to your health.

An unqualified fitness instructor might recommend that you perform "spot" fat loss exercises. Those who promote spot fat loss claim that people can remove fat from specific spots in the body by performing exercises in those particular locations. Research shows, however, that no type of exercise causes fat loss at one specific location.

Lesson Review

1. What are quackery and fraud, and how do they differ?
2. Why is it important to be an informed consumer in the area of fitness, health, and wellness?
3. What are some of the more reliable sources of health-related and fitness-related information?
4. What are some examples of health and fitness misconceptions and quackery?

As you've worked your way through this book, you've had the opportunity to take many physical fitness tests. The tests available to you are listed in table 15.1. After you finish this class, you would be wise to continue assessing your fitness, but it's not reasonable to perform all the tests you've done here. To simplify things, you can prepare your own fitness test battery that includes tests from each of the four categories (cardiorespiratory endurance, body composition, muscle fitness, and flexibility) listed in table 15.1. A test battery comprises several tests designed to measure all parts of fitness. Use the following guidelines in choosing tests for your test battery.

- For cardiorespiratory endurance, choose at least one test.
- For flexibility, choose at least two of the three tests available.
- For body composition, choose at least one test.

- For muscle fitness, choose at least one test for the arms and upper body, one test for the trunk and abdominal muscles, and one test for the lower body. Consider including tests for different parts of muscle fitness (muscular endurance, strength, power).
- Choose tests for which you have adequate equipment.
- Choose tests that you think you're likely to actually do.
- Use a chart similar to table 15.1 to select tests for your battery.

Perform the tests in class, then retest yourself from time to time to see how you're doing and to help you set future fitness and physical activity goals. If you're working with a partner, remember that self-assessment information is personal and considered confidential. It shouldn't be shared with others without the permission of the person being tested.

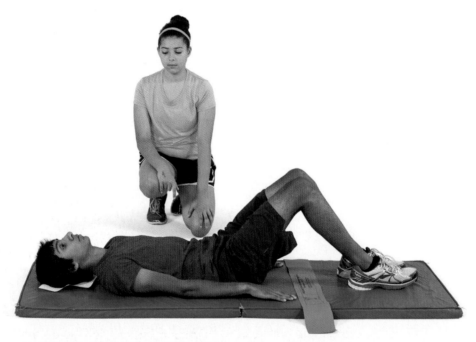

Create your own fitness test battery to track your fitness over time and help you prepare future personal plans.

TABLE 15.1 Choices for Your Personal Fitness Test Battery

Self-assessment	Place a ✔ to select a test
Cardiorespiratory endurance	
PACER	
Step test	
Walking test	
One-mile run	
Muscle fitness	
Curl-up	
Push-up	
Side stand	
Sitting tuck	
Arm press 1RM (per kilogram of body weight)	
Leg press 1RM (per kilogram of body weight)	
Grip strength (right)	
Grip strength (left)	
Standing long jump	
Medicine ball throw	
Body composition	
Height–weight (based on BMI)	
Skinfold measures	
Waist-to-hip ratio	
Waist girth	
Flexibility	
Back-saver sit and reach	
Trunk lift	
Arm, leg, and trunk flexibility tests	

Lesson 15.2

Evaluating Health Clubs, Equipment, Media, and Internet Materials

Lesson Objectives

After participating in this lesson, you should be able to

1. evaluate health-related and fitness-related facilities,
2. describe the proper equipment for physical activity,
3. evaluate printed materials and video resources related to health and fitness, and
4. describe the guidelines for choosing a good website for health and fitness information.

Lesson Vocabulary

spa, web extension

Where do you get your health, fitness, and wellness information? Have you ever considered how that information is created? People in developed countries are more interested in health and fitness now than at any other time in history, and they look to many sources to get relevant information. As a result, many magazines are now totally dedicated to health and fitness, but the leading source of health information throughout the world is the web. In fact, there has been an explosion of health and fitness information, but not all of it is accurate. In this lesson, you'll learn how to evaluate printed material and web resources. First, however, you will learn about health and fitness clubs, where many people seek information delivered in person, as well as exercise equipment.

Evaluating Health Clubs

You do not need to join a health club, **spa**, or gym to attain or maintain fitness. Health clubs do offer their members special equipment and personnel; and modern spas offer saunas, whirlpool baths, and other services such as massage and hair and skin care. In addition, some people find that joining a club helps motivate them to exercise and remain physically active. But these services are expensive, and well-educated people can save money and still get the benefits of regular exercise by designing their own fitness and activity programs without using special facilities or equipment.

Many low-cost programs are offered through community centres, universities, churches, and other groups (if you or your classmates completed the project from chapter 6, you'll already have a list started). In addition, your school may be among the many that have built their own fitness centres, sometimes called wellness centres. Such programs can give you the same benefits and motivation as more expensive clubs. Still, if you feel that it would help you stay active, you may be interested in join-

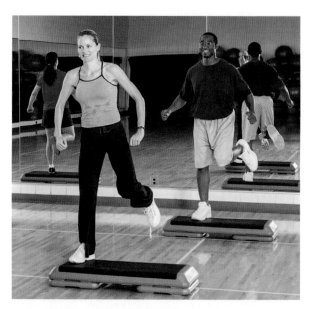

When choosing a health club, be sure to pick a well-established club that includes activities you enjoy.

ing a commercial club, spa, or gym at some point. Some schools have made cooperative arrangements with fitness clubs that allow their students to work out at special rates or allow school classes to use club facilities. Use the following guidelines when deciding whether to join a health club.

- **If possible, join on a pay-as-you-go basis.** If you sign a contract, make it a short-term one. Read the fine print carefully. Do not sign a contract right away. Too often, people pay a lot for a long-term contract, then stop using the facility. It's best to pay for a short membership until you're sure that you'll stick with it. The fine print may contain special clauses that will cost you money. For example, do you still have to pay if you move? Often, the salesperson pressures you to sign a contract on your first visit, but it's best to think about it for a while before signing.

- **Choose a well-established club.** Such a club is less likely to go out of business. Make sure the facility employs qualified fitness experts such as those discussed in this chapter. Be alert for signs of fitness quackery; if you see them, consider choosing a different club.

- **Make a trial visit to the club.** Visit at a time when you would normally use the club. Make sure you feel comfortable with the employees and other patrons. Also make sure that the equipment and facilities are available for you to use at that time.

- **Choose a club that meets your personal needs.** For example, a person with joint pain might prefer to avoid harsher activities such as jogging and decide instead to swim for cardiorespiratory endurance. Such a person, of course, should choose a facility that includes a swimming pool.

- **Avoid clubs that cater primarily to bodybuilding for adults.** Research shows that clubs frequented mostly by adults interested in bodybuilding are more likely to sell unproven supplements and even illegal products. Some people who frequent these places subscribe to their own theories and reject scientific evidence developed by experts. Furthermore, practices that may be acceptable for adults are often not appropriate for teens. Find a club that is appropriate for families and teens and employs qualified experts on its staff. Avoid advice from so-called experts with theories that are not consistent with the information provided in this book.

- **Consider any medical needs.** If weight loss is your primary goal, consider joining a program recommended by your physician or sponsored by a hospital rather than joining a health club. If you have a special medical need, you may need the help of a physical therapist.

FIT FACT

The Government of Canada recalled the Basis Peak fitness watch in the summer of 2016 because it was found that the watch could overheat, posing a burn hazard to the consumer.

Evaluating Exercise Equipment

Some people choose not to join a club but to buy home exercise equipment instead. If you're considering home exercise equipment, use the following guidelines.

- **Consider inexpensive home equipment.** For resistance exercise, you can use homemade weights, inner tubes, or rubber or latex bands. To build cardiorespiratory endurance, you can use jump ropes, stepping benches, or stairs. If you're interested in fitness for health and wellness, this equipment may be all you need.

- **Consider your personal needs before buying equipment.** If you're interested in a higher level of fitness for sport or a high-performance job, you might choose to purchase machines or other equipment for use at home. For building muscle fitness, you can use free weights and home exercise machines. For cardiorespiratory endurance, you can use home exercise machines such as treadmills, bicycles, and stair steppers. A regular bicycle is also a good choice if you have a safe place to ride. Exercise equipment is often quite expensive, so it's important to choose well. Rather than depending on the advice of a salesperson, consult an expert or Consumer Reports. Buy from a well-established company that honours the warranty, services the product, and sells replacement parts.

- **Be sure before you buy.** Avoid investing money in exercise equipment until you're sure you'll use it. Many people buy equipment, then don't use it after the first few months. You can see evidence of this behaviour in the many ads for slightly used equipment. Some of the high-tech equipment described in this book, such as pedometers and heart rate watches, can be useful. However, some equipment can be quite expensive, and you

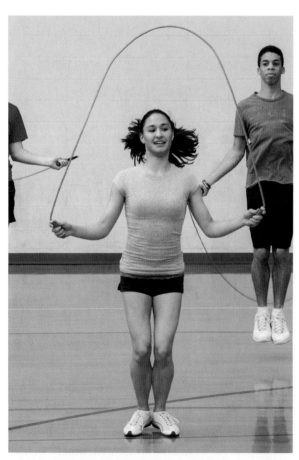

Equipment does not need to be expensive to be helpful in promoting fitness.

may find that you won't use it regularly. See if you can try equipment owned by a friend or by your school before deciding to buy the product. In addition, some high-tech products simply are not worth the cost. For example, expensive electrical devices for measuring body fat level are not worth the personal investment when an inexpensive calliper can give you accurate fat measurements.

- **Make sure you have enough space for the equipment.** One of the main reasons people fail to use the exercise equipment they buy is that they don't have a good place to keep it. If you have to get the equipment out each time you use it or move it from place to place, you're less likely to use it than if you have a room or another location where you can set it up permanently.

> " If you order health products from unreliable sources, you have no guarantee that they will be safe, effective, and of high quality. Certain NHPs promoted online for weight loss have posed serious health risks because they have been mixed with prescription drugs or contaminated with heavy metals. "
>
> —Government of Canada

Evaluating Books and Articles

The growing emphasis on health and fitness has led to the publication of many books and articles on weight control and exercise. Unfortunately, much of the information presented through the media is misleading or incorrect. How can you evaluate health and fitness information that you read, view, or hear? Use the following guidelines to help you decide which information sources are worthwhile.

- **Consider the author's credentials.** The author or consultant should be a registered dietician, should have completed advanced study in nutrition, or should hold an advanced degree in an exercise-related field such as exercise science, kinesiology, or physical education.

- **Check for sound information.** The book or article should provide information about a balanced diet and physical activity that is consistent with the information presented in this book or by Health Canada. Books that promise quick and easy fitness or fat loss are not good sources. The information in the book or article should not support techniques used by quacks and con artists (see the first lesson in this chapter). Exercise discussions should address the principles of overload, progression, and specificity, in addition to the FIT formula for each type of physical fitness.

- **Recommended exercises should be safe and effective.** The exercises should require you to use your own muscles (effortless devices should not be recommended). Make sure that the exercises are performed with proper biomechanics.

Evaluating Exercise Videos

You've probably noticed exercise videos for sale and television shows featuring exercises you can perform.

Exercise videos are also available for web viewing. Use the following guidelines to help you evaluate an exercise video or show.

- **Check the creator's credentials.** The creator is the person who prepares the exercises, which may then be performed by someone other than the creator. Check to see that the creator has a degree or certification from a reputable institution or organization. Check to see that the person performing the exercises is doing them properly; this book provides you with some insights into how to do exercises properly.

- **Choose a video that includes appropriate warm-up and cool-down exercises.** The warm-up and cool-down should be consistent with guidelines provided in this book.

- **Make sure the video contains only safe exercises.** This book provides you with information about safe exercises, as well as dangerous exercises to avoid.

- **Choose a video that rotates muscle groups and addresses all parts of fitness.** For example, use arms, then legs, then back, then abdominal muscles, and so on. If the video claims to be a total fitness program, make sure it includes activities for all parts of fitness.

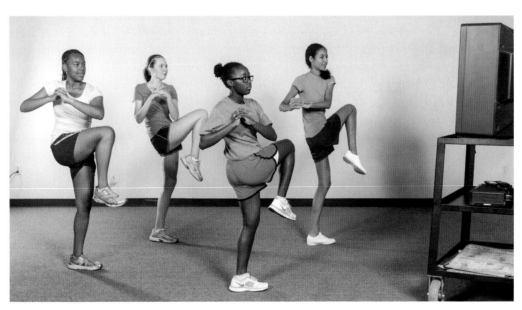

Video exercise routines should be appropriate for your skill and fitness level.

- **Choose a video that is appropriate for you.** Make sure that the activities on the video are appropriate for your skill and fitness level. For example, if the video is said to be for beginners, are the exercises really for beginners?

- **Make sure the exercises start gradually and progress in intensity.** If the first part of the exercise program is moderate in intensity, it may serve as the warm-up.

- **Choose a video with a fun and interesting routine.** Review the video to see if it includes exercises that you would enjoy doing on a regular basis.

- **If the video does not meet all of these guidelines, modify it.** For example, change the order of the routine presented in the video to make it safe and effective.

Evaluating Internet Resources

We depend on the web more than any other source for health and fitness information. Yet research shows that many web sources provide incorrect information. If you use the web to locate information about health, fitness, and wellness, ask yourself the following questions.

FIT FACT

Be wary of advertisements for lotions or creams to improve muscle tone. *Tone* is a term created by advertisers and something that cannot be easily measured. For this reason, it's easy to claim that creams or lotions can improve tone, but it's very hard to prove. There are no creams or lotions that can improve muscle fitness as measured by legitimate tests of muscle fitness. Place your trust in experts who help you build muscle fitness using sound exercise programs rather than quack products.

- **Who developed the website?** Websites with the best information are developed by government agencies, professional organiza-

tions, and educational institutions, and their websites end with standard **web extensions**. Governmental health agencies' web addresses end with .gc.ca in Canada and .gov in the United States; professional organizations' web addresses end with .ca or .org in Canada and .org in the United States; and education institutions' web addresses end with .ca in Canada and .edu in the United States. Choose websites presented by well-known agencies, organizations, and institutions such as those listed in the Consumer Corner feature in this chapter or the student section of the Fitness for Life Canada website. Remember, however, that any organization can now obtain a .ca or .org web address, so that alone does not guarantee that the information on the site is reliable. At the same time, some websites with an address ending in .com or .net do provide good information.

- **Is the web article a research document, or is it really an advertisement?** Governments have cracked down on companies that post web articles falsely appearing to be scientific research. These "fake news" articles are really advertisements. They are not based on real science, and they advertise products that do not work as claimed. Examples include articles on dietary supplements, products that supposedly provide fitness without exercise, and weight loss products. Several companies have paid fines for deceptive practices and have been banned from mounting future promotions. Unfortunately, such companies often make a lot of money before they are caught, and the fines they pay are much smaller than their profits. In light of these practices, you need to make sure that you use information from reliable news sources and scientific journals rather than the fake news articles that often appear in ads and pop-up screens on your computer. You can visit the Government of Canada's Competition Bureau to get consumer alerts that will protect you from deceptive marketing practices, misleading advertising, and scams.

To reduce your chances of being deceived by a website, ask yourself the following questions:

- **Does the website sell products?** Websites that sell products are more likely to provide false information than those that do not.
- **Do you recognize any techniques that seem suspicious?** Be wary of websites using the techniques associated with quacks and con artists as described in this chapter.

- **Do experts find the website credible?** The site should be recommended or highly regarded by genuine health and fitness experts.

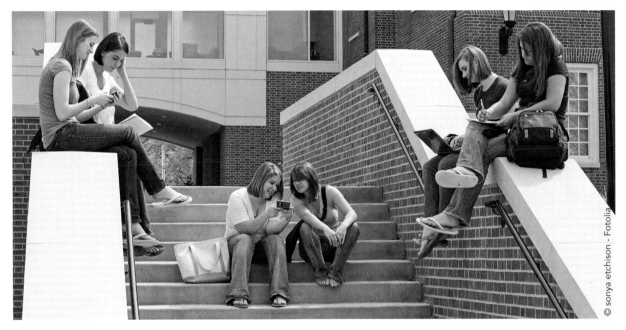

Be critical consumers when you and your friends evaluate online fitness and health information.

Lesson Review

1. What are some guidelines for evaluating health and fitness clubs?
2. What should you consider before buying exercise equipment?
3. What are the guidelines for evaluating exercise videos and books and articles about health and fitness?
4. What are the guidelines for choosing a good website for health and fitness information?

TAKING CHARGE: Learning to Think Critically

A misconception is a belief based on incorrect or misunderstood information or lack of facts. The best way to counter a misconception is to increase your knowledge so that you can recognize and interpret facts correctly. Here's an example.

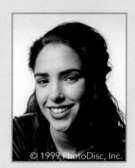
© 1999 PhotoDisc, Inc.

Amy Kay had tried several exercise programs but had not found one that she felt would help her meet her goal of developing muscle fitness. She had never even considered progressive resistance exercise (PRE) because she believed it would cause her to develop big, bulky muscles.

One day, Amy Kay's physical education teacher took her class to the fitness room. There, the teacher explained how to use the free weights and resistance machines for the best benefit. Over the next several weeks, the class practiced the correct use of the PRE equipment. As a class assignment, Amy Kay's teacher had each member of the class find one news article about PRE and write a report on it. In doing her report, Amy Kay learned that muscles do not become bulky if weight training is done properly.

With this new knowledge, Amy Kay realized that the correct PRE program would give her exactly what she was looking for. She began working out with PRE on three days each week. The knowledge she gained about PRE dispelled her original misconceptions. Now Amy Kay is trying to help others change their irrational beliefs about PRE. When friends ask her why she is trying to build big muscles, she tells them, "I'm not trying to build big muscles, I'm trying to increase my lean muscle and bone strength so that I'll be healthier."

For Discussion

What misconception did Amy Kay have? How was she able to build knowledge to dispel her misconception? What are some other misconceptions people have about physical activity? Why do you think people have misconceptions about PRE? Consider the guidelines provided in the Self-Management feature when answering the discussion questions.

SELF-MANAGEMENT: Skills for Thinking Critically

Thinking critically means using a problem-solving process before making important decisions. You can use several steps to solve problems and make good choices. These steps are similar to those used in applying the scientific method. The steps are listed here with examples for using each one to help you select exercise equipment. You can use the same steps to solve problems and make decisions about other important topics.

- **Step 1: Identify the problem to be solved or clarify the decision that must be made.** If you know that you want to improve your muscle fitness but are not sure how to do it, you have to define the problem more clearly. Do you want to do your exercises at school, join a health and fitness club, buy exercise equipment, or use inexpensive equipment? You also need to clarify your reasons for

wanting to build muscle fitness. Do you want to improve your health, improve your appearance, or get fit for sport performance? For this discussion, let's assume that you want to decide what equipment to use in order to build your muscle fitness for good health. Thus the problem has been clearly defined.

- **Step 2: Collect information and investigate.** One way to collect information relevant to the defined problem is to perform self-assessments for muscle fitness. Knowing your current status will help you learn about areas of personal need so that you can select exercises to meet your needs. You can also consult experts and explore reliable websites, such as those described in this chapter's Consumer Corner feature or in the student section of the Fitness for Life

Canada website. In this case, you would also want to try out several equipment options, perhaps by using the school exercise room, visiting local health and fitness clubs, or trying out machines on display at a sporting goods store. You could also try several of the inexpensive equipment options you've learned about in this book. Focus on finding information that will help you solve the specific problem you've identified in step 1.

- **Step 3: Develop a plan of action.** Use the information gained from your investigation to formulate a plan. For example, your results from step 2 might indicate that the school exercise room is not open when you are free to use it, and perhaps the health and fitness clubs are too far from your home and cost too much. In addition, exercise equipment available in stores can be quite expensive. After rejecting these options, then, you might decide to do elastic band exercises. The equipment is inexpensive, and you can

do all the exercises necessary to meet your goal. You might decide to choose several of the exercises described in this book. You could then make a written plan specifying the days of the week on which you'll do each exercise and how many sets and reps you'll do each day.

- **Step 4. Put your plan into action.** For a plan to be effective, you must use it. The sooner you begin to act after preparing your plan, the more likely you are to change your behaviour. In this example, you would use the plan developed in step 3 to get started with the elastic band exercises.

- **Step 5. Evaluate the effectiveness of your plan.** Use self-monitoring to keep records and use self-assessments (reassessments) to chart your progress. As you go forward, you can continue using the five critical thinking steps presented here to solve problems that arise and make effective decisions about your health, fitness, and wellness.

TAKING ACTION: My Health and Fitness Club

You've learned how to plan a personal physical activity program, and by now you're performing it regularly on your own. But you may also enjoy being active with others. Using school facilities and equipment, you can create your own health and fitness club for use during class time. Work with the other students in class to survey the types of activity that class members enjoy.

When putting together a workout for others, consider their current fitness, their skill levels, and their interests. Prepare several exercise stations for which equipment is available. Balance the workout so that a variety of activities are offered and all the parts of health-related fitness are addressed. Have a class member describe the purpose of each exercise station to the rest of the class as a fitness instructor would at a community or commercial health or fitness club. Take action by having all class members use the health and fitness club to perform a physical activity workout that meets their personal goals. Evaluate the effectiveness of your health and fitness club.

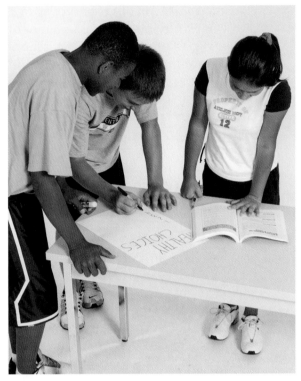

Take action by creating your own health and fitness club.

▼ GET ACTIVE WITH THE YMCA

Reprinted, by permission, from YMCA-Canada.

Who We Are

People, places, and programs come together at the YMCA. From the day the first YMCA opened in Canada—more than 165 years ago—we've been passionate about the health and well-being of Canadians. From coast to coast, the Y offers a unique blend of programs specifically suited to each community. Ask anyone involved and they'll say that being part of this supportive network helps them achieve their personal development goals.

What We Do

Whether you want to run, jump, swim, dance, shoot some hoops, or train with weights, you can take your pick. Our fitness centres and camps give you a place to feel comfortable and free to be yourself. We offer hundreds of high-quality programs that build confidence, improve social skills, and foster independence and leadership. There are tons of opportuni-ties to do what you already love and to try something new.

Our expert staff and volunteers are always available to support and guide you to positive outcomes every step of the way. And when you choose the Y, you get the added benefit of being part of our community because it's important to feel safe and welcome while improving your health.

Get Involved

You want to get more active, and we can help. When you're active, all aspects of life are better: mental, emotional, social, and physical. Come with your friends, or make some new ones—there's always something to check out at the Y. Come to your local YMCA! Join our movement to make Canada the healthiest place on earth. Find us at ymca.ca, ymcacanada on Facebook, or @ymca_canada on Twitter.

Reprinted, by permission, from Angela de Burger, YMCA-Canada.

Reviewing Concepts and Vocabulary

Complete the following in order for you to determine your growing understanding of fitness, health, and wellness. Answer items 1 through 5 by correctly completing each sentence with a word or phrase.

1. A method of advertising or selling a health product or service that uses false claims is called _____.
2. Selling a health product one knows to be worthless is called _____.
3. A _____ is a product added to the diet rather than being part of the regular diet.
4. _____ exercise uses machines or outside forces to move your muscles.
5. The extensions .gc.ca and .gov indicates that a website is associated with the _____.

For items 6 through 10, match each term in column 1 with the appropriate phrase in column 2.

6. medical doctor
7. certified health education teacher
8. physiotherapist
9. dietician
10. nutritionist

a. may not be an expert
b. provides medical advice
c. offers advice about diet and nutrition
d. has information about exercises
e. provides general health information

For items 11 through 15, as directed by your teacher, respond to each statement or question.

11. Discuss three ways to recognize quackery.
12. What would you do if you identified a case of quackery?
13. Explain why you selected each of the tests in your personal fitness test battery.
14. Describe the five steps for critical thinking that you can use to solve problems and make decisions about physical activity and good health.
15. How can understanding these five steps help you make informed choices?

Thinking Critically

Write a paragraph to answer the following question.

Your friend Lee visited a health food store and got interested in taking a supplement. He says that he can make his own decision because the products must be safe and must work or they wouldn't be on the shelves of the store. What advice would you give your friend? Explain your reasons.

Project

Choose one of the following: Visit a local health club, choose an article about exercise from a popular magazine, view an exercise video, or visit a health or fitness website. Use the guidelines presented in this chapter to evaluate its quality. Write a blog or do a video blog on your evaluation.

UNIT VI

Creating Positive and Healthy Experiences

Self-Assessment Features in This Unit
- Healthy Lifestyle Questionnaire
- Identifying Signs of Stress
- Developing Leadership Skills

Taking Charge Features in This Unit
- Positive Self-Talk
- Managing Competitive Stress
- Conflict Resolution

Self-Management Features in This Unit
- Skills for Positive Self-Talk
- Skills for Managing Competitive Stress
- Skills for Conflict Resolution

Taking Action Features in This Unit
- Your Healthy Lifestyle Plan
- Relaxation Exercises for Managing Stress
- Team Building

Canadian Sport and Health Organization Features in This Unit
- Get Active With Canadian Parks and Recreation Association
- Get Active With Canadian Yoga Alliance
- Get Active With Coaching Association of Canada

16

Choosing Healthy Lifestyles

 Student Web Resources
www.fitnessforlife.org/student

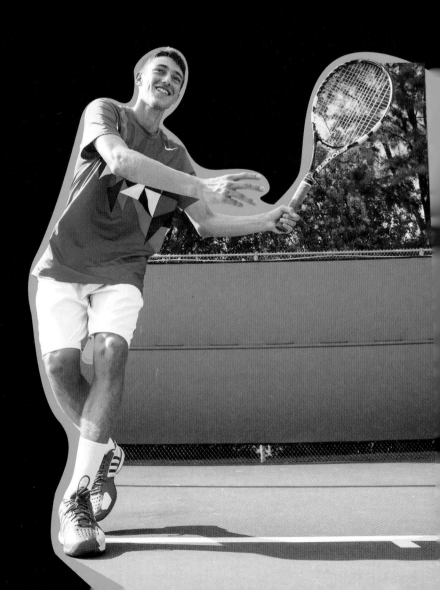

Lesson 16.1
Lifestyle Choices for Fitness, Health, and Wellness

Lesson Objectives

After participating in this lesson, you should be able to

1. describe several lifestyle choices—other than priority healthy lifestyle choices—that contribute to fitness, health, and wellness;
2. describe factors associated with the physical environment that affect fitness, health, and wellness; and
3. describe factors associated with the social environment that affect fitness, health, and wellness.

Lesson Vocabulary

accelerometer, built environment, controllable risk factor, lifestyle, sleep apnoea, uncontrollable risk factor

Everyone you know would probably like to have good health and wellness. But how many are aware of all the things they can do to achieve it? In this lesson, you'll learn about healthy lifestyle choices and how they can help you achieve good fitness, health, and wellness. You'll also learn about environmental and social factors that can influence your fitness, health, and wellness.

As you can see in figure 16.1, four major factors contribute to early death. Most early deaths result from unhealthy lifestyle choices. This means that these problems could be prevented if people changed the way they live. Making healthy lifestyle choices not only reduces the risk of disease and death from disease but also enhances wellness. For example, not smoking greatly reduces your risk of heart disease and cancer and also increases your quality of life. You can breathe better, you have a keener sense of smell, and you save the money you would have spent on tobacco and medical care.

Healthy Lifestyle Choices and Risk Factors

You know by now that the term **lifestyle** refers to the way you live. A healthy lifestyle is a way of living that helps you prevent illness and enhance wellness. Healthy lifestyle choices are ways that you can reduce **controllable risk factors**—the risk factors that you can act upon to change. Healthy lifestyle choices are in your control, and if you choose well you reduce your risk of many major health problems. For example, one controllable risk factor is sedentary living; simply by being active, you can reduce your health risks.

Other risk factors—such as age and sex—are not in your control and thus are called **uncontrollable risk factors**. Because you cannot do anything about these risk factors, focus instead on those that you can control. This chapter discusses several healthy lifestyle choices over which you do have some control.

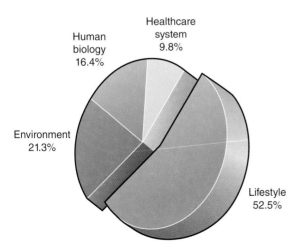

FIGURE 16.1 Four main factors contributing to early death.

Healthcare system 9.8%
Human biology 16.4%
Environment 21.3%
Lifestyle 52.5%

Making Healthy Lifestyle Choices

This book focuses on three priority lifestyle choices: regular physical activity, healthy eating, and stress management. These lifestyle choices are considered to be most important because they can improve the fitness, health, and wellness of virtually all people. However, they are not the only lifestyle choices you can make to promote fitness, health, and wellness.

FIT FACT

The prevalence of youth ever having smoked a cigarette is at an all-time low since it was first monitored among Canadian youth. In 1994, nearly half the students in grades 6 to 9 (45 percent) reported having tried smoking a cigarette; in 2012-2013, that number decreased to 13 percent. Among students in grades 6 to 12, the prevalence of ever having smoked a cigarette also decreased since it was first recorded, from 33 percent in 2006-2007 to 24 percent (approximately 603,000 youth) in 2012-2013. In 2012-2013, 4 percent of students in grades 6 to 12 were current cigarette smokers: 2 percent daily smokers and 2 percent occasional smokers.

This lesson outlines other lifestyle choices you can make to maximize your fitness, health, and wellness.

Adopt Good Personal Health Habits

In elementary school, you most likely learned about personal health habits, such as regular tooth brushing and flossing, good grooming (for example, hair and fingernail care), hand washing before meals and after bathroom use, and a healthy amount of sleep. But how many of these habits have you adopted? Practicing good health habits is one way you can prevent illness and promote optimal quality of life.

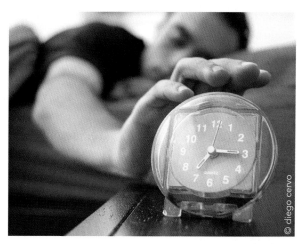

Getting enough sleep and practicing other simple personal health habits enhance health and wellness.

 ## FITNESS TECHNOLOGY: Sleep Tracking

Considerable evidence indicates that insufficient sleep can lead to health problems. Teens need about nine hours of sleep each night, but 9 out of 10 teens report getting less than that, and 10 percent get less than six hours. But the number of sleep hours is not the only issue; your sleep patterns are also important. People who wake up numerous times, or toss and turn frequently during the night, are not getting restful sleep.

For years, scientists have used sophisticated machines to detect **sleep apnoea** and other serious sleep disturbances. Now, **accelerometers** (such as those worn to count steps) called *sleep trackers* can be used to determine movement patterns during the night. Experts caution against overgeneralizing the results from a sleep tracker because it is possible that a person sleeps well most of the time but still has periodic restless nights. They also point out that sleep trackers do not sense different levels of sleep (light vs. deep sleep). While sleep-tracking devices cannot directly determine the quality of sleep that a person gets, they can be used to screen for sleep problems in people who frequently feel tired or suspect that they have a problem.

Using Technology

Investigate sleep-tracking apps and evaluate the pros and cons of using one. Check to see if activity-tracking devices cost more when they also include sleep-tracking functionality.

For example, if you have an illness that could have been prevented by means of proper health habits, you'll feel bad and will have at least a temporary reduction in your quality of living. Adopting good personal health habits is important throughout your life, and it can help you look and feel your best.

Avoid Destructive Habits

Just as adopting healthy habits contributes to good health, practicing destructive habits detracts from your fitness, health, and wellness. Examples include, among many others, smoking and other tobacco use, legal and illegal drug abuse (including steroids), and alcohol abuse. These destructive habits can impair your fitness; detract from your performance of physical activities; and result in various diseases, lowered feelings of well-being, and reduced quality of life.

FIT FACT

Texting while driving is a major source of automobile accidents. In fact, doing so makes you 23 times more likely to crash. More generally, cell phone conversations during driving increase collision risk by 4 to 6 percent.

Adopt Good Safety Practices

Reports of injuries and deaths caused by motor vehicle accidents fill the news each day. Other common causes of death and injury include falls, poisonings, drownings, fires, bicycle accidents, and accidents in and around the home. Many of these injuries and deaths might have been prevented if simple safety rules had been followed. In order to reduce the number of deaths and injuries resulting from accidents, you can make a number of healthy lifestyle choices to reduce your risk of accidents, including wearing a seat belt; wearing a helmet when riding a bike, doing in-line skating, skateboarding, snowboarding, or skiing; making sure that poisons are properly labelled; installing and maintaining smoke detectors; practicing water safety; and keeping your home in good repair. And remember—being physically fit can also help you prevent accidents.

Learn Cardiopulmonary Resuscitation

Cardiopulmonary resuscitation (CPR) is a first aid procedure that is performed when the heart or breathing has stopped, and it saves many lives each year. The procedure uses chest compressions to keep blood flowing, preventing brain damage and death until expert medical help arrives. Cardiopulmonary resuscitation training is strongly recommended, and many schools and several national organizations offer CPR classes and certification. The Canadian Red Cross and Canadian Heart and Stroke Foundation suggest that you can perform compression-only (i.e., hands-only) CPR on someone who suddenly collapses even if you are untrained. However, hands-only CPR is *not* recommended for use with children.

The Canadian Red Cross recommends two basics steps to help save a life. First, call 911 or direct someone else to call 911. Second, start chest compressions—push hard and fast at the center of the chest. The technique for chest compression is shown in figure 16.2. When two people are available, both mouth-to-mouth breathing and chest compression can be used.

Cardiopulmonary resuscitation techniques and procedures are often revised based on new research and findings. For this reason, a regular check of the Canadian Red Cross or the Canadian Heart and Stroke Foundation website for the latest information is recommended.

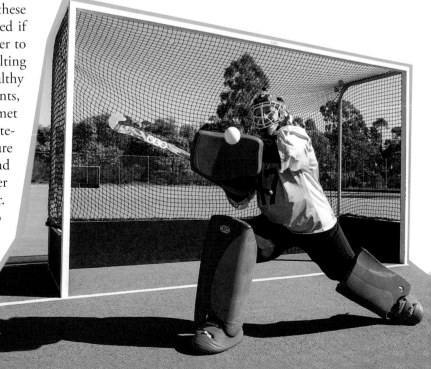

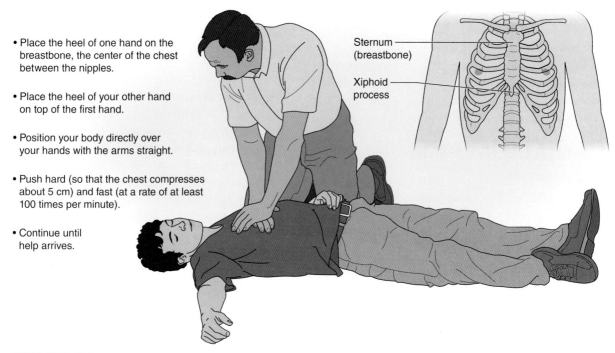

- Place the heel of one hand on the breastbone, the center of the chest between the nipples.

- Place the heel of your other hand on top of the first hand.

- Position your body directly over your hands with the arms straight.

- Push hard (so that the chest compresses about 5 cm) and fast (at a rate of at least 100 times per minute).

- Continue until help arrives.

Sternum (breastbone)

Xiphoid process

FIGURE 16.2 Technique for performing hands-only CPR.

Learn the Heimlich Manoeuvre (Abdominal Thrusts)

The Heimlich manoeuvre (also called abdominal thrusts) is performed when an object blocks a person's windpipe (air pathway). As shown in figure 16.3, the person administering the manoeuvre stands behind the person who is choking with his or her arms around the person's waist. The fist of one hand is placed just above the choking person's navel, with the thumb side of the fist against the body. The other hand is held over the fist. Pulling upward and inward causes pressure to force the object from the windpipe. As with all first aid procedures, training in the Heimlich manoeuvre is highly recommended. Do *not* perform the Heimlich manoeuvre unless you are certain the person is choking.

Learn Other First Aid Procedures

Even people who make healthy lifestyle choices and adopt good safety practices can have accidents. Because accidents can happen to anyone, all people should maintain a first aid kit and know how to

 SCIENCE IN ACTION: The Evolution of CPR

Over the past 50 years, new methods of CPR have been developed, resulting in thousands of saved lives. Mouth-to-mouth resuscitation was first used in France in the 1700s, and medical doctors used chest compression to revive people in the late 1800s.

Later, "artificial respiration" was modified to use a back-pressure arm-lift method, which in turn was replaced by chest compression and mouth-to-mouth breathing in the 1960s. Later, one-person CPR alternated chest compression with mouth-to-mouth breathing. Doctors started using these procedures before they were recommended to the general public.

In recent years, CPR has changed considerably. As shown in figure 16.2, the hands-only method (chest compression) is now used for helping adults and teens in distress. This procedure is easier to do, and experts feel that it will be used more often as a result.

Student Activity

Do a search to determine which local organizations offer CPR classes and for which purposes (e.g., lifeguarding, babysitting, firefighting). If possible, take a class and get certified.

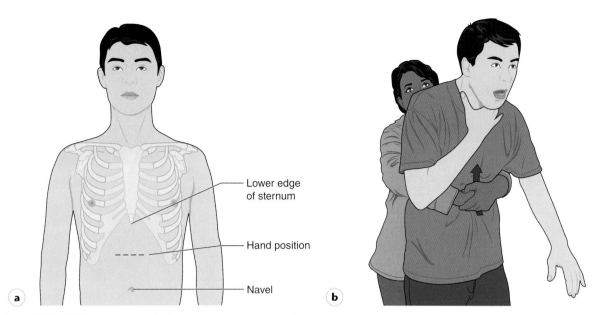

The Heimlich manoeuvre: *(a)* hand placement; *(b)* action—pull upward and inward.

Lower edge of sternum

Hand position

Navel

a **b**

FIT FACT

Among adults, the most common reasons for not seeing a doctor include excuses such as "I'm too busy," "It's only a minor problem that will go away on its own," "I can't afford it," and "I don't like to go to doctors." Sometimes children and teens will not tell anyone when they aren't feeling just right because they think it will go away, their families can't afford it, or they are scared of doctors and hospitals. In reality, putting off a doctor visit for the prevention and treatment of minor problems can result in more serious problems that will require more time for treatment, more time for recovery, and more money for medicine and supplies.

administer first aid. In addition to learning how to perform CPR and the Heimlich manoeuvre, you should also learn how to apply pressure to prevent bleeding, how to clean and treat cuts and open wounds, how and when to use the RICE formula (rest, ice, compression, and elevation) to treat sprains and strains, and how to use other accepted first aid techniques.

Seek and Follow Appropriate Medical Advice

Even if you make healthy lifestyle choices, you may occasionally become ill. In those cases, seek and follow appropriate medical advice. In fact, for best results, get regular medical and dental checkups to help you prevent problems before they even start. Consult your physician and dentist to determine how often you should be seen and what services are provided under your provincial medical and dental plans. Some people avoid seeking medical help, but as noted in the Fit Fact, this practice can be dangerous because early detection of health problems is often important to an ultimate cure.

The Environment and Fitness, Health, and Wellness

The second leading contributor to early death (see figure 16.1) is an unhealthy environment. An environment is unhealthy if it causes health problems or detracts from personal wellness. Your physical and social environments are both important to your health and wellness.

> " Earth provides enough to satisfy every [person's] need, but not every [person's] greed. "
>
> —Mahatma Gandhi, human rights leader

Physical Environment

The physical environment refers to the air, land, water, plants, and other physical things that exist around you. We know that certain physical environments can be very harmful to your health. For example, people who live in polluted cities are at greater risk than those who live in the countryside, where the air is often cleaner. Similarly, people who work in a coal mine or an area in which smoking is allowed have a higher risk of illness than those who work in less polluted areas. Your work environment is sometimes referred to as your vocational environment, and it can have serious consequences for your health. If your job requires you to sit all day and your work environment doesn't allow you to get up and move around frequently, you will have higher health risks. Similarly, many school environments require students to sit all day and don't allow you to get up and move around frequently, which may affect your overall fitness, health, and wellness. You are in control of what you do in your nonschool time; it's important for you to choose physical activity as one of your spare time activities.

You may not be able to change some physical environment factors, such as the place where you live. You can, however, take action to improve your environment. For example, you can avoid or minimize exposure to smoke-filled places, excessive exposure to the sun, and exposure to pollutants, such as weed killers and insecticides. To avoid excessive air pollution, exercise away from heavily traveled streets. You can also take certain steps to improve the physical environment—for example, recycling household materials and conserving water and electricity. You can also help people in your community who are making efforts to improve what is called the **built environment**—the physical characteristics of our neighbourhoods. Improvements in the built environment—such as adding sidewalks and bike paths and improving street lighting and street crossings—have been shown to increase healthy physical activity such as walking and biking in neighbourhoods.

Social Environment

Your social environment refers to the settings in which your social interactions take place. Social interactions refer to your contacts, conversations, and activities with friends, teachers, work colleagues, and others in leisure-time situations.

Researchers have shown that teens whose friends make unhealthy lifestyle choices are more likely to

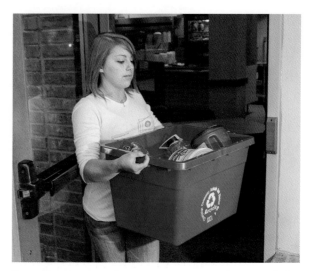

Recycling is something everyone can do to aid the environment.

try risky behaviour such as abusing tobacco, drugs, or alcohol. In contrast, teens whose friends and family members make healthy lifestyle choices are more likely to practice healthy behaviours such as being physically active and eating well. With these two scenarios in mind, choosing supportive friends is important to your health and wellness.

Even if you make good choices, you, like most people, will probably be exposed to unhealthy social environments at some point in your life. If this does happen to you, consider using some of the self-management skills described in this book to help you make good choices in the heat of the moment. For example, learn to think critically, learn relapse prevention strategies, and practice ways to say no so that you can stick with your healthy behaviours. There is absolutely no need to be embarrassed about or apologize for practicing healthy behaviours.

Building a practice of gratitude is the best way I know to create an optimistic approach to life. Start each day by lying in bed for five minutes and mentally acknowledging what you are grateful for. **"**
—Silken Laumann, Canadian Olympic rower

Lesson Review

1. What are several lifestyle choices—other than priority lifestyle choices—that contribute to fitness, health, and wellness? How do they affect fitness, health, and wellness?
2. What factors associated with the physical environment affect fitness, health, and wellness?
3. What factors associated with the social environment affect fitness, health, and wellness?

SELF-ASSESSMENT: Healthy Lifestyle Questionnaire

Wellness is the positive component of good health. The five components of wellness include physical, emotional–mental, social, intellectual, and spiritual wellness. Complete the questionnaire to assess your current wellness. (Your teacher may give you a worksheet to use.) Remember that this information is personal and confidential. You can choose not to share it with others.

1. Read each wellness statement and decide whether you strongly agree, agree, disagree, or strongly disagree.

2. Record your results in order to assess your wellness.

3. Calculate your score for each wellness component by adding your results for the three questions in that component.

4. Add all five component scores to get your overall wellness score.

5. Use table 16.1 to determine your rating for each component and overall score.

Healthy Lifestyle Questionnaire

Wellness statement	Strongly agree	Agree	Disagree	Strongly disagree
1. I am physically fit.	4	3	2	1
2. I can do the physical tasks needed in my work.	4	3	2	1
3. I have the energy to be active in my free time.	4	3	2	1
Physical wellness score =				
4. I am happy most of the time.	4	3	2	1
5. I do not get stressed often.	4	3	2	1
6. I like myself the way I am.	4	3	2	1
Emotional–mental wellness score =				
7. I have many friends.	4	3	2	1
8. I am confident in social situations.	4	3	2	1
9. I am close to my family.	4	3	2	1
Social wellness score =				
10. I am an informed consumer.	4	3	2	1
11. I check facts before making health decisions.	4	3	2	1
12. I consult experts when I'm not sure of health facts.	4	3	2	1
Intellectual wellness score =				
13. I feel a sense of purpose in my life.	4	3	2	1
14. I feel fulfilled spiritually.	4	3	2	1
15. I feel strong connections to the world around me.	4	3	2	1
Spiritual wellness score =				
Total wellness score =				

Adapted from C. Corbin et al., 2013, *Concepts of fitness and wellness: A comprehensive lifestyle approach*, 10th ed. (St. Louis, MO: McGraw-Hill).

TABLE 16.1 Rating Chart: Wellness

Wellness rating	Three-item score	Total wellness score
Good	10–12	≥50
Marginal	8 or 9	40–49
Low	≤7	≤39

Planning for a Healthy Lifestyle

Lesson Objectives

After participating in this lesson, you should be able to

1. describe the five steps involved in planning for health behaviour change and
2. describe several career options in fitness, health, and wellness.

 Lesson Vocabulary

consumer community, professional

In other chapters of this book, you've learned about healthy lifestyle planning and had the opportunity to prepare several types of physical activity plans. It's also important to plan for the healthy lifestyle choices discussed in this chapter.

Healthy Lifestyle Planning

The same five steps you've used to plan physical activity can be used to prepare plans for eating better, reducing stress in your life, and adopting other behaviours described in this chapter's first lesson. We'll use the example of Lila, who was already implementing her physical activity plan but also wanted to make some other changes. To plan these changes, she used the five-step approach.

Step 1: Determine Your Personal Needs

As part of SMART goals, Lila learned that it's important to make goals realistic. If she was going to be successful in adding to her current plan, she knew she shouldn't try to make too many changes at once. She reviewed some of the healthy lifestyle choices described in this chapter's first lesson, then decided to start by choosing one area in which she needed improvement. As indicated by the checkmark in the following list, she chose to eat more healthfully.

> **"** Don't dig your grave with your own knife and fork. **"**
>
> —English proverb

Check one or more areas of personal need in which you want to plan a change.

✔ Eat healthier	___ Adopt safety habits
___ Reduce stress	___ Seek and follow medical advice
___ Adopt personal health habits	___ Learn first aid
___ Avoid destructive behaviours	___ Learn CPR

When studying nutrition earlier, Lila did a daily self-assessment of her eating habits, based on Canada's Food Guide, that best reflected her needs. She found that she could improve in several areas. Specifically, her diet included too much fat; she ate more calories than she should; and she didn't eat the recommended amount of fruits and vegetables.

Step 2: Consider Your Program Options

Based on her needs and nutrition assessments, Lila's options included changing her eating habits to be healthier.

- Cut the fat in her diet
- Eat more fruits
- Eat more vegetables
- Consume fewer calories

Step 3: Set Goals

To help her eat more healthfully, Lila set some SMART goals. That is, she set specific, measurable, attainable, realistic, and timely goals for changing her diet.

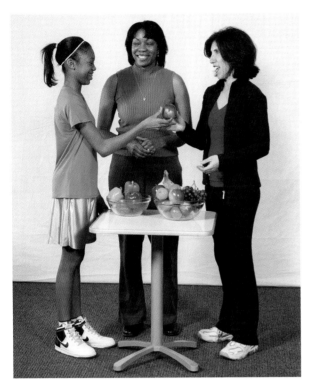

Dietary planning can help you eat more healthfully.

- Goal 1: Eat at least two servings of vegetables every day for two weeks.
- Goal 2: Eat at least two servings of fruits every day for two weeks.
- Goal 3: Eat at least five total servings of fruits and vegetables every day for two weeks.
- Goal 4: Drink two glasses of skim milk rather than whole milk each day.

Step 4: Structure Your Program and Write It Down

Lila prepared a written plan (see figure 16.4) that included each of her SMART goals and a calendar showing each day of the week. She posted the chart

on the refrigerator (for the second week, she posted a clean copy of the same chart).

Step 5: Keep a Log and Evaluate Your Program

Lila used checkmarks on her written plan (see figure 16.4) to track whether she met each of her daily goals. Her results? She did meet her goal for fruits and her goal for vegetables on all of the days, but on two days she did not eat five total daily servings of fruits and vegetables. She met her goal of drinking two glasses of skim milk on five of the seven days. During the second week, she was able to meet all of her goals on every day of the week.

When the two-week period ended, Lila evaluated her results. She thought she had done pretty well. She was eating more fruits and veggies and had reduced the fat in her diet by drinking skim rather than whole milk. She decided to renew the plan for two more weeks just to be sure she kept on track. After that, she would consider making other healthy lifestyle changes based on new circumstances in her life. In the Taking Action feature, you'll have the opportunity to prepare your own healthy lifestyle plan using the same steps as Lila. You can also use the planning steps to make changes later in life as circumstances change (for example, moving away from home to attend college, get a job, or start a family of your own).

Careers in Fitness, Health, and Wellness

In this book, you've learned about various scientists who do research related to fitness, health, and wellness. Scientists do research to find new knowledge. In many ways, what they do is like finding pieces of a puzzle. But new information is not of much value

Goal	Mon.	Tues.	Wed.	Thurs.	Fri.	Sat.	Sun.
Eat at least 2 daily servings of vegetables.	✔	✔	✔	✔	✔	✔	✔
Eat at least 2 daily servings of fruit.	✔	✔	✔	✔	✔	✔	✔
Eat at least 5 total daily servings of vegetables and fruit.	✔	✔		✔		✔	✔
Drink 2 daily glasses of skim milk rather than whole milk.	✔	✔		✔		✔	✔

FIGURE 16.4 Lila's weekly plan and log.

👥 CONSUMER CORNER: Consumer Communities

How do you get good consumer information? One way is to consult a book like *Fitness for Life Canada.* You can also consult experts at your school or high-quality websites such as those described in this book. Another method is to establish a **consumer community** for finding and disseminating good information. Some schools have consumer communities that review scientific information and answer student questions related to fitness, health, and wellness. Some consumer communities provide a newsletter or contribute articles to the school newspaper. Others use the web or the school's intranet (local network) to provide information. Consumer communities with web access may also offer a website devoted to consumer

issues. The site may feature articles by students, provide sources of good consumer information, and answer questions from students. Some high school consumer communities have also used social media, such as Facebook.

Just as the work of scientists has to be reviewed by peers before it can be published, consumer communities must review the information they provide to make sure that it is accurate and responsibly reported. They typically have older members who assume leadership roles and guide the review of information presented by the group. A consumer community provides a great opportunity to learn and serve for teens who are interested in a career in fitness, health, and wellness.

unless it is made available to the general public. This is where **professionals** come in. They deliver and apply the research knowledge developed by scientists; in other words, they put the pieces of the puzzle together so that the public can use the information. Professionals go through an extended education, typically a bachelor's degree or higher,

and often they must also be certified by a professional organization or governmental agency.

Now that you're nearing completion of this course, you may want to consider a career in fitness, health, and wellness. Table 16.2 lists various science and professional careers, as well as some examples (the table is not meant to be comprehensive).

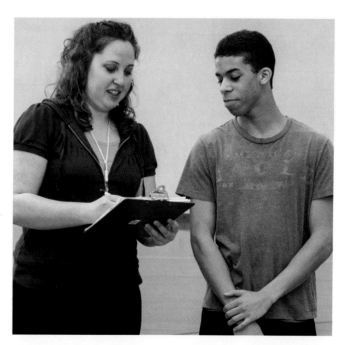

Qualified professionals are a good source of fitness, health, and wellness information.

TABLE 16.2   Selected Careers in Fitness, Health, and Wellness

Science career	Description	Professional career	Description
Kinesiology	Biomechanics Exercise anatomy Exercise physiology Exercise sociology Motor learning and control Sport and exercise psychology Sport pedagogy	Physical educator Coach Fitness management Fitness leader Personal trainer Sport management Sport psychologist Athletic trainer Physiotherapist Occupational therapist Strength coach Dance educator Recreation leader-therapist	Teaches physical education Coaches sport Manages corporate and commercial fitness Leads exercises at clubs and worksites Assesses and prescribes personal exercise Applies business principles in sport settings Helps athletes achieve optimal performance Provides health care for athletes Provides preventive and rehabilitative health care related to musculoskeletal problems Provides rehabilitative health care related to musculoskeletal problems; helps people with tasks of daily life Helps athletes and exercisers build muscle fitness Teaches dance in schools, studios, other settings Organizes programs and treats problems through recreation
Nutrition	Food science Food services Food technology Sport nutrition	Clinical dietician Community dietician Management dietician	Works in hospitals and nursing facilities Works with organizations Works in schools, health care facilities, and institutions such as prisons
Health	Environmental health Epidemiology Health statistics Public health	Health educator School health Public health Worksite wellness	Teaches health concepts in schools Provides healthy school environment Works in public health agency Conducts programs in businesses
Medical and life sciences	Genetics Immunology Medical technology Microbiology Pathology Virology	Medical doctor Nurse Dentist Veterinarian Medical technician Physician's assistant Chiropractor	Provides health care (diagnoses and treats) Provides health care as part of health care team Provides dental health care Provides animal health care Performs laboratory analysis Helps physicians provide health care Provides health care focused on musculoskeletal system

Lesson Review

1. What are the five steps involved in planning for health behaviour change?
2. What are several career options in fitness, health, and wellness?

TAKING CHARGE: Positive Self-Talk

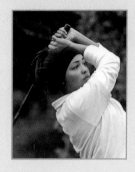

Alexis was not on the school golf team, but she did like to play golf. She thought about trying out for the team, but she wasn't sure that she was good enough. When she played with her family, she did well, but when she played with people she didn't know, she didn't do as well. Sometimes she talked to herself while playing, saying things like "Why did you do that, dummy?" or "Oh, no—I'm starting to play badly again." Sometimes she even talked to herself out loud, saying things like "I got a 7 on that hole? Now I don't even have a chance for a good score!"

After one particular round in which she didn't play as well as she would have liked, Alexis asked her mother, "Why do things always go wrong when I play with people I don't know?" Her mother said that she had read a book by a sport psychologist who recommended avoiding negative self-talk (saying negative things to yourself, which affects your self-confidence and leads to poor play). The key is to replace the negative self-talk with positive self-talk. As Alexis' mom said, "If you expect bad things to happen, they probably will. Next time you play, try to cut the negative talk and focus on positives. If you have a bad hole, say to yourself, 'It's just one hole—I'm going to do better on the next one.'"

For Discussion

What are some examples of negative self-talk common in sport and other activities? What are some examples of positive self-talk that can be used to replace negative self-talk? What other suggestions do you have for Alexis and other people who are in sporting situations? In crafting your advice, consider the guidelines presented in the Self-Management feature.

SELF-MANAGEMENT: Skills for Positive Self-Talk

You know that some people are considered pessimists and others optimists. A pessimist thinks bad things are going to happen, and an optimist believes good things are sure to come. Experts in exercise and sport psychology have found that with practice, you can develop "learned optimism." Specifically, you can replace negative thoughts and negative self-talk with positive thoughts and positive self-talk. Follow these guidelines to use positivity to improve your performance.

- **Learn the ABCs. A** stands for adversity, which can lead to negative thoughts and negative self-talk. Learn to recognize when you're facing adversity. **B** stands for beliefs. If you believe that you're going to do poorly when you face adversity, you probably will. Learn to recognize negative beliefs when you face adversity. **C** is for consequences. Learn to recognize your feelings about the consequences of adversity. A pessimist might say, "If I do poorly on one

hole in golf, I have no chance to get a reasonable score." Learning to reassess consequences and be more realistic can help you become more optimistic.

- **Accept adversity as a challenge rather than a sure cause of failure.** Adversity causes negative self-talk only if you let it.

- **Alter your beliefs about adversity.** If you accept adversity as a challenge, you can tell yourself to avoid negative thoughts and replace them with positive ones. Experts suggest that replacing negative comments (such as "That was a dumb decision!") with positive ones (such as "I know I can do it!") leads to better performance. So when you're faced with adversity, respond with positive self-talk. Tell yourself, "I believe I can do this!"

- **Don't overdramatize the consequences of adversity.** Think realistically about adversity. Ask yourself if your view of the potential consequences is pessimistic.

If so, replace it with a more realistic or even positive view.

- **Put the past behind you.** Failing at a task or doing less well than you'd like doesn't necessarily mean you'll fail next time. For example, in golf, don't let one bad hole get you down. You can't change the past—only the future. Worrying about the last hole leads to negative thoughts when you play the next one. Playing a hole badly creates adversity, but positive thinking and positive self-talk can turn the last bad hole into the next good one.

- **Practice creating a positive circle of success.** Pessimists think negatively when faced with adversity. Negative beliefs lead to poor performance, which contributes to more negative thoughts, thus creating a negative circle. Work instead to create a positive circle of success. Every time you face adversity, remember the ABCs (recall the first item in this list) and practice them. Recognize adversity when it arises and establish positive beliefs ("I know I can do this."). This can lead to positive consequences (improved performance).

- **Be realistic.** In learning about SMART goals, you've seen that being realistic is important to setting effective goals. Setting unrealistically high goals can lead to feelings of failure even when you're doing quite well. Remember that practice is necessary for success.

In the second lesson of this chapter, you read about Lila's plan for adopting a healthy lifestyle. Use the same five steps that Lila used and take action by selecting at least one of the healthy lifestyle choices presented at the beginning of this lesson and preparing a plan to make a positive change in that area. You won't be able to take this action in class; it will be something that you do on your own.

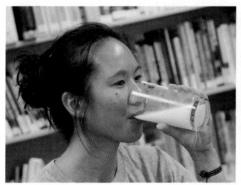

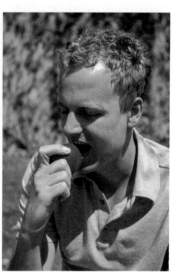

Take action by making a positive change to a lifestyle, such as eating more healthfully.

 GET ACTIVE WITH CANADIAN PARKS AND RECREATION ASSOCIATION

©Canadian Parks and Recreation Association (CPRA)

Who We Are

Canadian Parks and Recreation Association (CPRA) is a national organization dedicated to realizing the full potential of parks and recreation as a major contributor to individual and community health. CPRA membership includes the 13 provincial and territorial recreation associations and their extensive network of recreation and sport leaders.

What We Do

CPRA collaborates with a host of other national organizations operating in the recreation, parks, physical activity, facilities, sport, public health, and social services arenas. In addition to our communication activities on the benefits of parks and recreation, we provide our members with the information, resources, and professional development they can use to make a difference in their own community.

Get Involved

CPRA is a leader in the sector with the co-development of the Framework for Recreation in Canada. Working with the Interprovincial Sport and Recreation Council (ISRC), the framework was developed to provide a new vision for recreation and suggests some common ways of thinking about the renewal of recreation based on clear goals and underlying values and principles. The framework is currently being implemented by communities, individuals, and municipal and provincial governments across Canada. Check out www.cpra.ca for more information.

CPRA Professional Development Certification program (www.cprapdc.ca) opened its virtual doors in September 2015. Since then, recreation and parks practitioners from across the country have taken the opportunity to invest in their professional development. Together, they are contributing to a growing network of programmers, policy makers, supervisors, and educators dedicated to strengthening their contribution to the sector.

Follow CPRA on Facebook (Canadian Parks and Recreation Association) and Twitter (@CPRA_ACPL) and contact us (info@cpra.ca) about how you can become involved in parks and recreation today.

©Canadian Parks and Recreation Association (CPRA)

CHAPTER REVIEW

Reviewing Concepts and Vocabulary

Complete the following in order to determine your growing understanding of fitness, health, and wellness. Answer items 1 through 5 by correctly completing each sentence with a word or phrase.

1. Risk factors that you can change are referred to as _____ risk factors.
2. _____ is another name for mouth-to-mouth breathing and chest compression.
3. A technique to prevent choking is called _____.
4. Changing the physical environment to make it easier to walk or ride a bicycle is referred to as changing the _____ environment.
5. A _____ helps athletes achieve optimal performance.

For items 6 through 10, match each term in column 1 with the appropriate word or phrase in column 2.

6. career in kinesiology   a. veterinarian
7. career in nutrition   b. athletic trainer
8. career in health   c. frequent cause of accidents
9. career in medical or life science   d. dietician
10. texting   e. epidemiologist

For items 11 through 15, respond to each statement or question.

11. Describe several healthy lifestyle changes that can be made to improve a person's fitness, health, and wellness.
12. Explain the difference between controllable and uncontrollable risk factors. Give examples.
13. Identify one healthy lifestyle choice and explain how it contributes to fitness, health, and wellness.
14. Explain how a person's environment relates to personal wellness.
15. Discuss career options in one of the areas of science identified in this chapter.

Thinking Critically

Interview several people who are currently active in careers covered in this chapter. Ask how their time is spent in a typical day and what roles and responsibilities they enjoy or struggle with. Keep either a written or electronic record of their comments. Based on the information in this chapter and your interview record, identify a career that interests you. In one to three paragraphs, describe why this career might be a good option for you.

Project

Many schools have a wellness committee that includes students, teachers, parents, and other school staff. Wellness committees often schedule special events such as wellness weeks or monthly wellness activities during which a schoolwide effort is made to promote fitness, health, and wellness. If your school has a committee, attend a meeting, interview a committee member, prepare a questionnaire, or check out the committee's social media site in order to prepare a report of its activities. Indicate how students can become involved. If your school doesn't have a committee, explore ways for getting one created and construct a detailed plan in order to get one up and running in your school.

17

Managing Stress

In This Chapter

 Student Web Resources
www.fitnessforlife.org/student

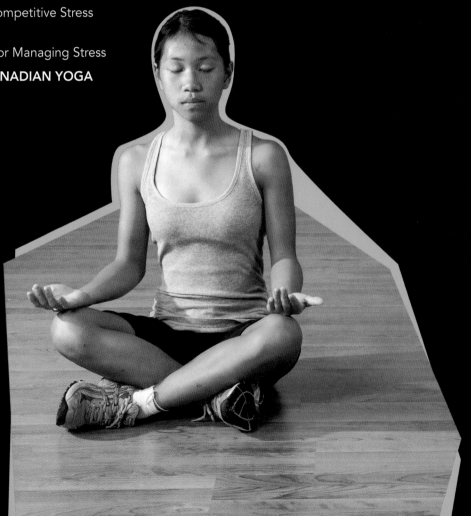

Lesson 17.1
Facts About Stress

Lesson Objectives

After participating in this lesson, you should be able to

1. define *stress* and *stressor*,
2. explain the three stages of general adaptation syndrome,
3. describe the five steps in the Stress Management Pyramid, and
4. discuss some causes and effects of stress.

 ## Lesson Vocabulary

alarm reaction, coping, coping skill, depression, distress, eustress, general adaptation syndrome, stage of exhaustion, stage of resistance, stress, stressor

Have you ever given a speech or performance in front of a lot of people? Did it make you anxious? If so, your heart rate may have increased and your muscles may have gotten tense. Stressful situations can bring these changes about by causing your body to release a chemical called adrenaline. The changes are part of what is called the stress response—your body's way of preparing you to deal with a demanding situation. Dealing with stress effectively helps people live happier and healthier lives.

You probably face stressful situations every day that affect you both physically and emotionally. Two-thirds of Canadians report feeling "stressed out" on a regular basis. Canadians are some of the most "stressed-out" people in the world. In this lesson, you'll read more about stress, how your body responds to it, and stress management. Along with regular physical activity and good nutrition, stress management should be a priority in your healthy lifestyle. This lesson teaches you about the Stress Management Pyramid and its five steps (see figure 17.1).

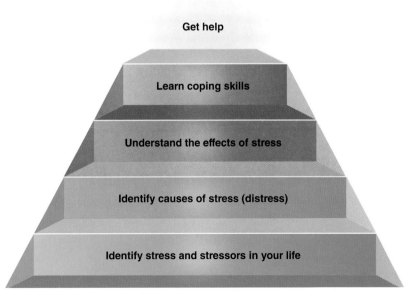

Get help

Learn coping skills

Understand the effects of stress

Identify causes of stress (distress)

Identify stress and stressors in your life

FIGURE 17.1 The five steps of the Stress Management Pyramid.

Adapted from Physical Activity Pyramid for Teens, source: C.B. Corbin.

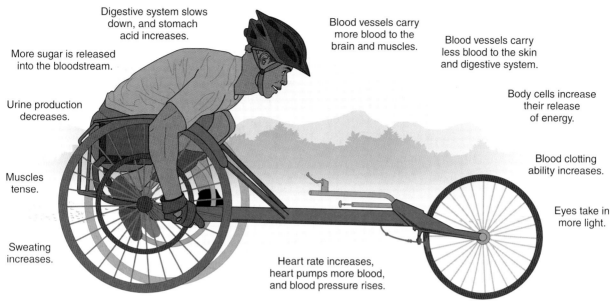

Digestive system slows down, and stomach acid increases.

More sugar is released into the bloodstream.

Urine production decreases.

Muscles tense.

Sweating increases.

Blood vessels carry more blood to the brain and muscles.

Blood vessels carry less blood to the skin and digestive system.

Body cells increase their release of energy.

Blood clotting ability increases.

Eyes take in more light.

Heart rate increases, heart pumps more blood, and blood pressure rises.

FIGURE 17.3 The stress response: your body's way of preparing.

(figure 17.4*a*). (The prefix *eu* is taken from the word "euphoria," which means a feeling of well-being.) Situations that can produce eustress include riding a roller coaster, successfully competing in an activity, passing a driving test, playing in the school band, and meeting new people. Eustress helps make your life more enjoyable by helping you meet challenges and do your best.

Negative stress is sometimes called **distress**, which is produced by situations that cause worry, sorrow, anger, or pain (figure 17.4*b*). A situation that causes eustress for one person can cause distress for another. For example, an outgoing person might

FIT FACT

The prefix *eu* in the word "eustress" is taken from the word "euphoria," which means a feeling of well-being.

look forward to joining extracurricular activities at school or attending social events, whereas a shy person might dread the same situations. In addition, the same experience can be eustressful for you at one time and distressful at another. For example, taking a test for which you're well prepared can

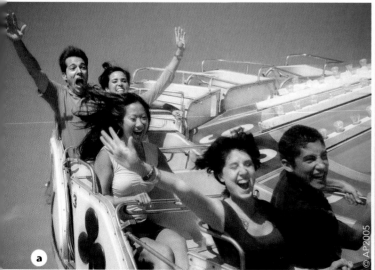
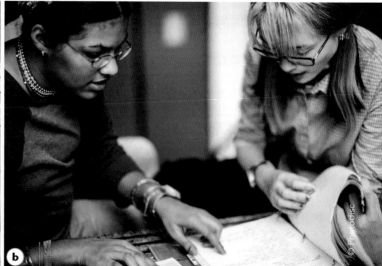

FIGURE 17.4 Stress can be positive or negative. *(a)* Eustress is positive stress; *(b)* distress is negative stress.

cause eustress, but taking a test for which you are not prepared might cause distress. You'll learn more about identifying stressors in your own life in the Self-Assessment feature that follows this lesson.

FIT FACT

Sometimes being in controlled stressful situations can help you prepare for more stressful situations in the future. For example, doing physical activity may be a stressor, but regular physical activity can help you become fit, healthy, and better able to handle stress in the future.

Distress can negatively affect your total health and fitness (more on this in a moment). To control stress in your life, you need to understand the cause of the stress you're experiencing. Some causes of stress are described in the following sections.

Physical Stressors

Physical stressors are conditions in your body or environment that affect your physical well-being. Examples include thirst, hunger, overexposure to heat or cold, lack of sleep, illness, pollution, noise, accident, and catastrophe (such as a flood or fire). Even excessive exercise can be a stressor, as in the case of athletes who overtrain. However, healthy people who follow good exercise principles and achieve good fitness are better able to adapt to the changes produced by physical stressors.

Emotional Stressors

Emotions such as worry, fear, anger, grief, depression, and even falling in love are powerful stressors that can strongly affect your physical and emotional well-being. Another cause of emotional stress is overload—taking on more tasks than you can accomplish in the time available. To prevent or correct overload, learn to say no and develop your time management skills.

Social Stressors

Social stressors arise from your relationships with other people. Each day, you have experiences that involve your family members, friends, teachers,

employers, and others. As a teenager, you're probably exposed to many social stressors. Think about the stressors you experience in social situations in your life; these stressors can cause much of the stress you experience.

Step 3: Understand the Effects of Stress

Stress—particularly high levels or prolonged periods of stress—can lead to both physical and emotional changes. Physical effects include increased stomach acid, which can aggravate ulcers. High blood pressure can also be related to stress and can lead to serious cardiovascular diseases and disorders. Prolonged stress can also lower the effectiveness of your body's immune system, making you more susceptible to certain diseases. The following lists these and other physical signs of stress:

- Acne flare-ups
- Allergy flare-ups
- Backaches
- Blurred vision
- Constipation
- Diarrhoea
- Difficulty sleeping
- Extreme fatigue
- Headaches
- Hyperventilation
- Increased blood pressure
- Indigestion
- Irregular heartbeat
- Light-headedness
- Muscle spasms
- Muscle tension
- Neck-aches
- Perspiring
- Shortness of breath
- Tightness in throat or chest
- Trembling
- Upset stomach
- Vomiting

SCIENCE IN ACTION: Depression Among Teens

Psychologists and public health scientists have done considerable research about **depression** among teens. As many as one in four teens reports feeling sad for as long as two weeks at some time during the high school years. While feeling sad is something that we all experience from time to time, extended bouts of sadness can be a sign of depression. Other feelings that we all experience such as anxiousness, restlessness, guilt, and irritability can also be signs of depression when they occur in excess. Other more serious signs of depression include feelings of emptiness and hopelessness. The risk of teen suicide is higher among depressed teens than among those who are not depressed. The Canadian Mental Health Association offers the following suggestions for helping a friend who shows signs of depression.

- If you're concerned about someone else, talk with the person. Ask directly if he or she is thinking about suicide. Talking about suicide won't give the person the idea. If someone is seriously considering suicide, he or she may be relieved to be able to talk about it.

- If someone you love says he or she is thinking about ending his or her life, it's important to ask if he or she has a plan. For someone who has a plan and intends to end his or her life soon, connect with crisis services or supports right away. Many areas have a crisis, distress, or suicide helpline, but you can always call 911 if you don't know who to call. Stay with the person while you make the call, and don't leave until the crisis line or emergency responders say you can leave.

- The two most important things you can do are to listen and to help the person connect with mental health services.

Student Activity

Interview a school guidance counsellor or school nurse. Ask what your school offers to help reduce stress and depression among teens. Ask what students can do to help. Write a summary of the interview.

Some doctors think that many health problems in Canada requiring medical attention are stress related, which should give us all the motivation we need to deal effectively with stress, especially distress.

Emotional effects of stress include feelings of nervousness; anger, anxiety, or fear; frequent criticism of others; frustration; forgetfulness; difficulty paying attention; difficulty making decisions; irritability; lack of motivation; boredom, depression, or withdrawal; and change in appetite.

Step 4: Learn Coping Skills

Once you've learned about the causes and effects of stress, you can move to the next level in the pyramid—learning **coping skills**. **Coping** means attempting to deal with problems, and coping skills are techniques that you can use to manage stress

and address problems. The next lesson describes five types of coping skills.

Step 5: Get Help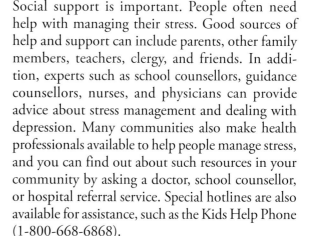

Social support is important. People often need help with managing their stress. Good sources of help and support can include parents, other family members, teachers, clergy, and friends. In addition, experts such as school counsellors, guidance counsellors, nurses, and physicians can provide advice about stress management and dealing with depression. Many communities also make health professionals available to help people manage stress, and you can find out about such resources in your community by asking a doctor, school counsellor, or hospital referral service. Special hotlines are also available for assistance, such as the Kids Help Phone (1-800-668-6868).

Mental Health Is Important

According to the Canadian Mental Health Association, approximately 10 to 20 percent of Canadian youth are affected by a mental illness or disorder. That's 1 out of every 5 to 10 students in your class! Suicide is the second leading cause of death for 15- to 24-year-old Canadians. Nearly half of those affected by a mental disorder never seek professional help. If we broke a bone in our body, would we not seek professional help? Why are we more reluctant to get help for broken mental health than we are for broken bones? When we avoid dealing with our stress, it can lead to serious mental health issues. Mental health issues can lead to physical health issues because mental and physical health affect one another. Take care of your heart and your mind!

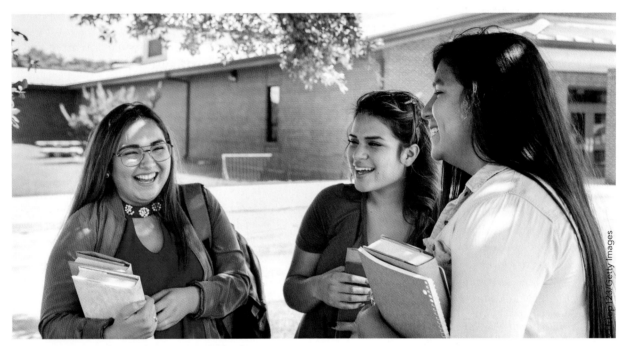

Your mental health is just as important as your physical health. Take care of both! Having fun with friends can help you deal with stress, which improves mental health.

Lesson Review

1. What is meant by the terms *stress* and *stressor*?
2. What are the three stages of general adaptation syndrome?
3. What are the five steps in the Stress Management Pyramid?
4. What are some causes and effects of stress?

All people experience some negative stress in their lives, and when you experience distress, your body sends off certain signals. You'll learn to identify some of these signals in this self-assessment.

Table 17.1 lists some common signs of stress. You may notice some of these signs when you are not under excessive stress, but they're often especially apparent in times of great stress.

One way to determine whether an activity is stressful to you is to self-assess for signs of stress before and after the activity. Working with a partner, use the following steps to look for the signs of stress included in table 17.1. Record results as directed by your instructor. Remember that self-assessment information is personal and considered confidential. It shouldn't be shared with others without the permission of the person being tested.

1. Lie on the floor, close your eyes, and try to relax. Have your partner count your pulse and your breathing rate. Ask your partner to observe you for irregular breathing and unusual mannerisms. Then ask your partner to evaluate how tense your muscles seem using the list in table 17.1. Report to your partner any feeling of butterflies in your stomach or other indicators of stress. Record your results. Then have your partner lie down while you make the same assessments for her or him.

2. When directed to do so by your instructor, all members of the class should write their names on a piece of paper and place the papers in a hat or box. The teacher will then draw names until only three remain in the container. The students whose names remain will each give a one-minute speech about the effects of stress. During and after the name drawing, observe your partner. Look for signs of stress. Also, notice your own feelings during the drawing. Finally, observe the people who were required to make a speech. Write down your observations about stress symptoms in you, your partner, and other class members. Refer to table 17.1 as needed.

3. Finally, walk or jog for five minutes after the second one-minute speech delivered by a student. Then, once again, work with a partner to assess your signs of stress. Notice that the exercise causes your heart rate and breathing rate to increase. At the same time, however, it may help reduce earlier signs of the emotional stress related to the possibility of performing in front of the class. Record your observations.

TABLE 17.1 Signs of Stress

Heart rate	Is it higher than normal?
Muscle tension	Are your muscles tighter than usual? • Arms and shoulders • Back and neck • Legs
Mannerisms	Are unusual mannerisms present? • Frowning or twitching • Hands to face (nail biting)
Nervous feelings	Do you feel different than you normally do? • Feeling of butterflies in stomach • Tense or anxious feelings
Breathing	Is your breathing different than usual? • Irregular • Rapid or shallow

Lesson 17.2

Stress Management

Lesson Objectives

After participating in this lesson, you should be able to

1. describe five types of coping strategies,
2. explain some guidelines for using the five coping strategies, and
3. explain why avoidance is often an ineffective method of coping.

Lesson Vocabulary

competitive stress, runner's high

We all get "stressed out" at times. What stresses you? How do you react to stress? Do you have strategies for dealing with your stress? Are they healthy strategies? Distress in life is unavoidable. Perhaps you feel overwhelmed by the many causes of distress and its effects. The first three steps in the Stress Management Pyramid require you to know and understand stress and the stressors that cause it. The fourth step refers to coping skills that you can use to manage stress. As described in the previous lesson, coping means attempting to overcome problems. Table 17.2 presents five types of coping skills.

Physical Coping

As shown in table 17.2, the first type of coping skill involves taking physical steps to deal with stress. Here are some examples.

- **Do regular physical activity.** Regular physical activity can help you reduce your stress. Noncompetitive physical activity can help you get your mind off of stressful situations. For example, people who jog regularly report experiencing a **runner's high**. The runner's high refers to feelings of eustress experienced during or after a run. Similar feelings of eustress are experienced during or after other forms of vigorous aerobic exercise. Certain specific exercises, such as those described at the end of this lesson, are especially useful in helping you to relax. Yoga, tai chi, stretching exercises, and deep breathing exercises also can be useful in managing stress.

- **Reduce your breathing rate.** Sit or lie quietly. Take a long slow breath, breathing in through your nose for four to six seconds.

TABLE 17.2 Five Types of Coping Skills

Coping skill	Description and examples
Physical coping	Using physical techniques: exercising, reducing muscle tension, eating well, and getting enough sleep
Intellectual coping	Using your thought process: using problem-solving techniques, establishing priorities, managing time effectively
Emotional coping	Altering your emotions, especially in stress-producing situations, can help you cope. Laughing and seeking fun activities can help reduce tension and anxiety. Using intellectual coping skills, such as thinking positive thoughts (thinking that you will do well) and avoiding negative thoughts, can be useful in controlling emotions. Being flexible and having a willingness to adjust to the situation can also help.
Social and spiritual coping	Using positive social and spiritual situations and guidance: seeking social support, seeking spiritual support, seeking professional help
Coping by avoidance	Pretending the problem doesn't exist or putting off taking action to solve it: ignoring, avoiding, and escaping

Exhale slowly through your mouth, again for four to six seconds. Repeat several times.

- **Reduce muscle tension.** Relaxing your muscles can help you reduce distress. You'll learn helpful relaxation techniques for reducing muscle tension in this chapter's Taking Action feature.

- **Rest in a quiet place.** Relax indoors or outdoors. Read. Listen to peaceful music. Take time out to relax in a quiet place (figure 17.5).

- **Eat a nutritious, well-balanced diet.** Good nutrition contributes to good health, which can help you handle stress better. On the other hand, foods or drinks high in caffeine may cause you to be irritable and restless.

- **Get enough sleep.** Lack of sleep can contribute to distress; in fact, lack of sleep is itself a stressor. Some problems may be easier to handle when you feel rested. Try to sleep at least eight hours a night.

- **Pay attention to your body.** Notice how your body reacts in different situations. If you experience physical signs of distress, use some of the stress management techniques described in this lesson.

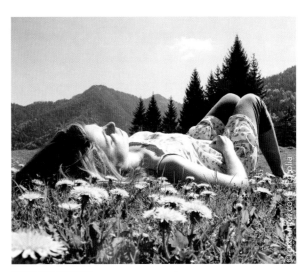

FIGURE 17.5 Sometimes taking a moment to rest in a quiet place can help you manage stress.

" I find that I get a little depressed if I don't move my body each day, so sometimes it's just as simple as walking, and other times it's training for a marathon or some kind of personal goal that I'm trying to meet. "

—Ryan Reynolds, actor and producer

Intellectual Coping

The second type of coping skill, intellectual coping, involves using your thought processes to manage stress. Here are some examples.

- **Use problem solving.** You can use the scientific method to solve problems that cause stress. Rather than worrying about a problem, try to solve it. Make decisions and carry them out. When making a decision, look at several choices, consider the likely results of each, and choose the best one.

- **Establish your priorities and tackle one thing at a time.** If several problems pile up, ask yourself which is most important and which can wait.

- **Manage your time effectively.** Prioritize your activities so that you have time for the most important things. Learn to say no to new responsibilities and activities if you can't give them the time required.

- **Reduce your mental activity.** In stressful situations, imagining pleasant circumstances can help you relax. Try imagining a pleasant outdoor scene before a test or when you have thoughts that make you feel anxious. Some athletes listen to relaxing music before a competition to help reduce mental activity.

- **Write down your worries.** A recent study discovered that those with high exam anxiety significantly improved their test scores by simply taking 10 minutes before the exam to write down everything that was worrying them. Expand on this practice by writing down what is worrying you and then writing down the steps you have taken to deal with the worry. For example, if you wrote "I don't test very well," you would follow this up with a true statement such as "I am more prepared for this test than tests in the past." This practice helps you acknowledge your worries and address them.

❤ FITNESS TECHNOLOGY: Prevention of Cyberbullying

Cyberbullying is illegal! Many websites are designed to prevent bullying. In addition to defining bullying, these websites discuss who is at risk of bullying, how to prevent bullying, methods of responding to bullies, and how to get help regarding bullying. Teens more likely to be targeted for bullying include those who are perceived as different from their peers, as weak or unable to defend themselves, or as having few friends; but all teens can be subjected to bullying at one time or another. Others who face higher risk for bullying include teens who are lesbian, gay, bisexual, or transgender and those with a disability.

Many of the websites discuss cyberbullying— bullying that involves electronic technology. Cyberbullying includes bullying using devices such as cell phones, computers, and tablets. This type of bullying often uses social media, text messages, and chat rooms. Cyberbullying is different from other forms of bullying because it can be done 24/7; it often reaches teens when they are alone and without social support; and messages can be posted anonymously and distributed to many people very quickly. New technology also makes it relatively easy to take and post embarrassing photos to be used in cyberbullying.

Some of the better websites, including those described in the student section of the Fitness for Life Canada website, offer content designed to help schools assess bullying and create effective anti-bullying rules and policies.

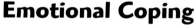

Using Technology

Investigate your school to see if it has anti-bullying policies. Assess the extent of bullying and cyberbullying in your school. Assessment tools are available on anti-bullying websites.

Emotional Coping

The third way to manage stress is to use emotional coping skills. Here are some examples.

- **Have fun.** Laughter can help reduce distress. Take time to laugh and do things that are fun for you. Enjoy your life!

- **Change the way you think.** Not all problems can be solved as you would like, but you can still deal with them effectively. For example, suppose you're asked to trim the hedges at home. You do the job, then find that you did it incorrectly. You can't change what you've already done, but you can deal with the stress by recognizing that all people make mistakes. You can also learn from your mistake and make sure you understand the directions next time so that you can do a better job.

- **Think positively.** Positive thoughts can help you reduce distress. For example, try thinking that you will get a hit in the softball game instead of worrying about striking out. In softball,

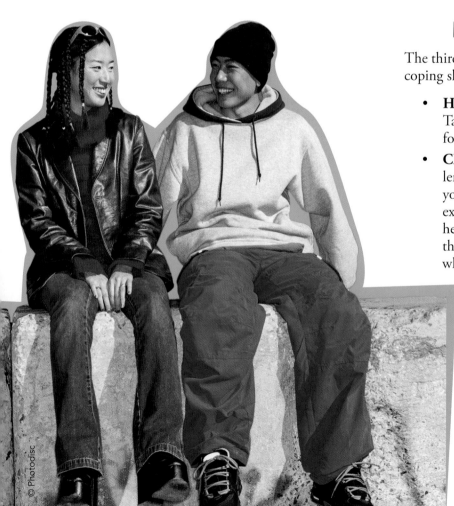

© Photodisc

and all activities of life, success does not come with every attempt you make. Even the best hitters get a hit only about 30 percent of the time. A positive thinker would have confidence that she or he will get a hit the next time at bat. Making an effort to perceive a stressor as a challenge rather than as a problem can help you think positively.

- **Try not to let little things bother you.** Many events in life are simply not worth stressing over. For example, if you're disappointed, remind yourself that a situation might be better the next time.

- **Be flexible.** In stressful situations, be willing to bend a little, or adjust to changes as the situation demands.

> " Adopting the right attitude can convert a negative stress into a positive one. "
>
> —Hans Selye, stress researcher

FIT FACT

Bullying is a major source of stress among teens. The Royal Canadian Mounted Police describe bullying as follows: Bullying happens when there is an imbalance of power; where someone purposely and repeatedly says or does hurtful things to someone else. Bullying can occur one-on-one or in one or more groups of people. There are many different forms of bullying: physical, verbal, and social bullying.

Social and Spiritual Coping

You can also manage stress by using social and spiritual coping skills. The following list gives some examples, all of which relate to getting help—the top step in the Stress Management Pyramid.

- **Seek help from friends and family.** When you feel down, don't keep it to yourself. Talk to family members and friends you trust. Just talking about problems can often help reduce distress.

- **Seek spiritual guidance.** Again, just talking to others often helps reduce stress, and trusted spiritual advisors may be able to offer additional help.

- **Seek professional help.** Sometimes it's necessary to seek professional help.

FIT FACT

When faced with a stressor, your body initiates a process called the "fight-or-flight" response. In earlier times, when people were hunter-gatherers, they had to fight wild animals or flee from them. We don't typically have that problem today, but when faced with a stressor our bodies still engage in the same fight-or-flight response, which results in the stress symptoms described in this chapter.

Coping by Avoidance

The final type of coping is called avoidance, which involves pretending that the problem doesn't exist or putting off action to solve it. In some cases, avoidance can work; sometimes, if you know a situation will be stressful, you can avoid it. For example, you can choose to avoid an event at which alcohol might be served. However, avoiding or ignoring a problem often just lets it get more serious, and the other coping strategies described in this chapter are typically much more effective.

Similarly, trying to escape a problem is rarely effective. For example, using drugs may be a method of trying to cope by escaping, but it both is ineffective and comes with serious long-term consequences.

Lesson Review

1. What are the five types of coping strategies?
2. What are some guidelines for using the five coping strategies?
3. Why is avoidance often an ineffective method of coping?

RELAXATION EXERCISES FOR STRESS MANAGEMENT

Did your self-assessment indicate that you have a high level of stress? Most people need to deal with stress at one time or another. In this activity, you will get the opportunity to perform several exercises that are useful in reducing stress. You will also get the opportunity to practice a muscle relaxation procedure called contract–relax.

Notice that you can do some of these exercises at almost any time and almost any place. You might do them when you are sitting and studying or while you are riding or waiting for a bus. You can do most of them lying down or from a sitting position. You can even adapt some of these exercises to do them while standing.

RAG DOLL

1. Sit in a chair (or stand) with your feet apart. Stretch your arms and trunk upward as you inhale.

2. Then exhale and drop your body forward. Let your trunk, head, and arms dangle between your legs. Keep your neck and trunk muscles relaxed. Remain relaxed like a rag doll for 10 to 15 seconds.

3. Slowly roll up, one vertebra at a time. Repeat the stretch and drop.

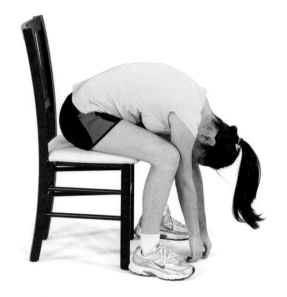

NECK ROLL

1. Sit in a chair or on the floor with your legs crossed.
2. Keeping your head and chin tucked, inhale as you slowly rotate your head to the left as far as possible. Exhale and slowly return your head to the centre.
3. Repeat the movement to the right.
4. Rotate three times in each direction, trying to rotate farther each time so that you feel a stretch in the neck.
5. Now drop your chin to your chest. Inhale as you slowly roll your head to the left shoulder, and then exhale as you roll it back to the centre. Repeat the movement to the right shoulder.

Caution: Do not roll your head backward or in a full circle.

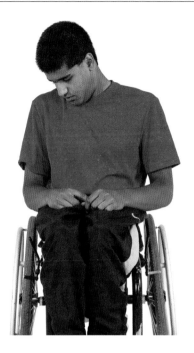

BODY BOARD

1. Lie on your right side. Hold your arms over your head.
2. Inhale and stiffen your body as if you were a wooden board. Then exhale as you relax your muscles and collapse completely.
3. Let your body fall without trying to control whether it tips forward or backward.
4. Lie still as you continue letting the tension go out of your muscles for 10 seconds. Then repeat the exercise starting on your left side.

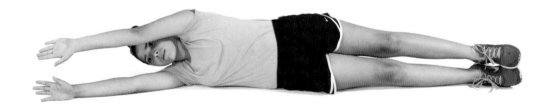

JAW STRETCH

1. Sit in a chair or on the floor with your head erect and your arms and shoulders relaxed.

2. Open your mouth as wide as possible and inhale. (This may make you yawn.) Relax and exhale slowly.

3. Open your mouth and shift your jaw to the right as far as possible; hold for three counts.

4. Repeat the movement to the left. Repeat it on both sides 10 times.

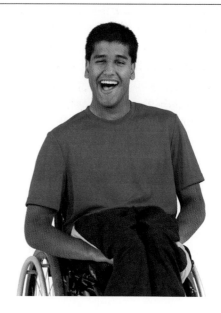

CONTRACT–RELAX METHOD OF MUSCLE RELAXATION

Lie on your back with a rolled-up towel placed under your knees. Contract your muscles in the order that they are named in the following instructions. Hold each contraction for 3 counts. Then relax the muscles and keep relaxing for 10 counts. Each time you contract, inhale; each time you relax, exhale.

Do each exercise twice. Try this routine at home for a few weeks. With practice, you should eventually progress to a combination of muscle groups and gradually eliminate the contracting phase of the program.

1. Hand and forearm: Contract your right hand, making a fist. Relax and continue relaxing. Repeat the exercise with your left hand. Repeat it with both hands simultaneously.

2. Biceps: Bend both elbows and contract the muscles on the front of your upper arms. Relax and continue relaxing. Repeat the exercise.

3. Triceps: Bend both elbows, keeping your palms up. Straighten both elbows and contract the muscles on the back of the arm by pushing the back of your hand into the floor. Relax.

4. Hands, forearms, and upper arms: Concentrate on relaxing these body parts all together.

5. Forehead: Make a frown and wrinkle your forehead. Relax and continue relaxing. Repeat the exercise.

6. Jaws: Clench your teeth. Relax. Repeat the exercise.

7. Lips and tongue: With your teeth apart, press your lips together and press your tongue to the roof of your mouth. Relax. Repeat the exercise.

8. Neck and throat: Push your head backward while tucking your chin. Relax. Repeat the exercise.

9. Relax your forehead, jaws, lips, tongue, neck, and throat. Relax your hands, forearms, and upper arms. Keep relaxing all of these muscles.

10. Shoulders and upper back: Hunch your shoulders to your ears. Relax. Repeat the exercise.

11. Relax your lips, tongue, neck, throat, shoulders, and upper back. Keep relaxing these muscles all together.

12. Abdomen: Suck in your abdomen, flattening your lower back to the floor. Relax. Repeat the exercise.

13. Lower back: Contract and arch your lower back. Relax. Repeat the exercise.

14. Thighs and buttocks: Squeeze your buttocks together and push your heels into the floor. Relax. Repeat the exercise.

15. Relax your shoulders, upper back, abdomen, lower back, thighs, and buttocks. Keep relaxing these muscles all together.

16. Shins: Pull your toes toward your shins. Relax. Repeat the exercise.

17. Toes: Curl your toes. Relax. Repeat the exercise.

18. Relax every muscle in your body all together and keep relaxing.

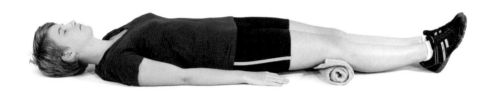

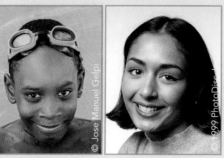

A little stress can give you more energy and help you meet a challenge. However, the effects of too much stress can interfere with your performance, especially during a competition. To do your best, you need to recognize the symptoms of **competitive stress** and know how to manage them. Here's an example.

Shelly watched from the bottom row of the bleachers as Willie shook his shoulders and arms. Shelly knew that swimmers did that to help them stay relaxed.

"You're the best, Willie! You're going to win!" Shelly had to yell so that Willie would hear her because the crowd was cheering so loudly.

Willie thought to himself, *I'm not so sure.* He shook his shoulders and legs again.

"You can do it!" Shelly screamed. "You're faster than anyone! We're all behind you!" She wasn't sure whether Willie heard her.

Willie had heard, and he thought, *That's the problem! The whole school is watching! My parents, too! If I don't get at least second place, our team might not go on to the region-* *als. The way my stomach feels, these people are more likely to see me throw up than win the 200.*

Willie knew it was just stress. He'd felt the same way at the last meet. And Shelly had told him she felt the same kind of stress during a debate last week. The debate coach had shown her how to slow down her breathing to help her relax, and she had shown Willie how to do it.

Shelly stood up and took a deep breath. Willie saw her and did the same thing, and then he grinned to let her know he felt better. Willie was ready.

For Discussion

How were Willie's muscles affected by the stress he felt? What were his other symptoms? How was Willie's stress similar to the stress Shelly had felt before her debate? What advice would you give Willie and Shelly (or anyone who is in a similar situation)? Consider the guidelines presented in the Self-Management feature when answering the discussion questions.

In lesson 17.2, you learned that doing regular, noncompetitive physical activity can help you reduce stress. On the other hand, stress can be caused or increased by competitive sports and other competitive activities, such as performing a music solo or giving a speech. Factors that can make these activities stressful include competition, being evaluated by others, performing in front of a crowd, and feeling that the outcome is important. If you get involved in situations that cause competitive stress, use the following guidelines to help you manage your stress.

- **Learn to identify signs of stress.** You can learn this skill by using the self-assessment included in this chapter.

- **Avoid competitive stress.** One way to prevent competitive stress is to avoid competitive situations and other situations in which you perform for others. This approach could, however, cause you to miss participating in activities that are fun. You might also fail to accomplish things that you're capable of doing.

- **Use muscle relaxation techniques.** Use the muscle relaxation techniques presented in this chapter's Taking Action feature.

- **Get experience.** Remember that most people feel stressed the first few times they compete or perform in public. With experience, competing and performing do become easier.

- **Practice and prepare.** Practice and preparation help you experience eustress when competing and performing, thus helping you achieve your full potential. When you practice, try to simulate the real event. Competitive practices with an audience can help you prepare.

- **Use mental imagery.** Some people do well in practice but not in actual competition. One method used by experienced competitors to address this issue is mental imagery. During the real event, they imagine themselves as they are in practice—relaxed and confident.

- **Use a routine.** For example, golfers find a regular putting routine very helpful. Following a routine before and during a competitive event can help you stay focused and avoid being affected by factors around you.

- **Take a deep breath and slow your breathing.** For example, take a deep breath before shooting a free throw or performing a solo. If you find yourself becoming tense, slow down your breathing—it can help.

- **Use other effective stress management procedures.** Use the effective ways of managing stress discussed earlier in this lesson.

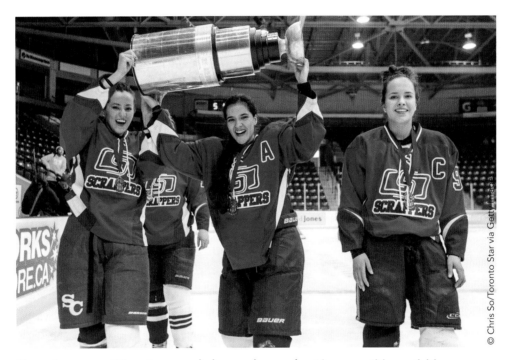

Managing competitive stress can help you do your best in competitive activities.

Did your self-assessment indicate that you have a high level of stress? Even if it didn't, you will have to deal with stressful situations from time to time. One way to manage the effects of stress on your body is to learn how to perform relaxation exercises, such as deep breathing, meditation, guided imagery exercises, and simple stretching techniques. Relaxation exercises may not seem beneficial the first time you try them because they may be unfamiliar or even uncomfortable. But as with any skill, you can learn to use them effectively if you perform them properly and practice them regularly. The more you practice using the techniques, the more successful you'll become in using them to manage your stress. You may have the opportunity to take action by performing relaxation exercises and trying muscle relaxation procedures such as the contract–relax method in class.

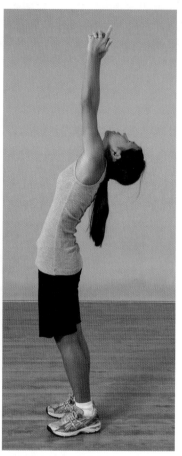

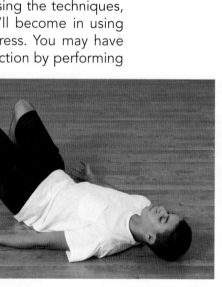

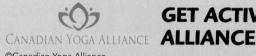
Take action to manage your stress levels by doing relaxation exercises.

GET ACTIVE WITH CANADIAN YOGA ALLIANCE

CANADIAN YOGA ALLIANCE
©Canadian Yoga Alliance

Who We Are

Canadian Yoga Alliance fosters an environment that encourages individuals to take charge of their lives, spirituality, minds, and bodies.

What We Do

Canadian Yoga Alliance provides the public with an online database resource of Canadian Registered Yoga centres, schools, and individual teachers who are certified and insured. Visit our website at www.canadianyogicalliance.com.

Get Involved

Take action! Empowerment, health, wellness, and happiness belong to everyone! Find training across Canada by searching our website for yoga schools and join a growing number of Canadians taking action in a proactive wholesome approach to living!

E-mail us at admin@canadianyogicalliance.com to ask how we can help with your yoga training.

©Canadian Yoga Alliance

Reviewing Concepts and Vocabulary

Complete the following in order for you to determine your growing understanding of fitness, health, and wellness. Answer items 1 through 5 by correctly completing each sentence with a word or phrase.

1. _____ is the body's reaction to a demanding situation.
2. The first phase of general adaptation syndrome is called the _____.
3. _____ is defined as positive stress.
4. Coping that includes physical activity and reducing your breathing rate is called _____ coping.
5. Problem solving is a type of _____ coping.

For items 6 through 10, match each term in column 1 with the appropriate phrase in column 2.

6. Stress Management Pyramid step 1   a. identify causes of stress
7. Stress Management Pyramid step 2   b. understand effects of stress
8. Stress Management Pyramid step 3   c. find help
9. Stress Management Pyramid step 4   d. identify signs of stress
10. Stress Management Pyramid step 5   e. learn coping skills

For questions 11 through 15, respond to each statement or question that follows.

11. What is the difference between eustress and distress?
12. What are some guidelines for helping a friend who is depressed?
13. How can physical activity help you deal effectively with stress?
14. What is cyberbullying, and why is it a problem?
15. Describe some negative effects of competitive stress and explain how to manage it in a positive manner.

Thinking Critically

Write a paragraph to answer the following questions.

You've been asked to give a speech to your class. You're concerned that if you refuse the opportunity, you may feel disappointed in yourself. However, you're also afraid that you'll be too nervous to speak in front of a large group. What are the positive and negative consequences of each choice? What decision would you make? How could you manage the stress associated with whichever decision you made?

Project

Create a brochure to help teens manage stress or to prevent bullying or cyberbullying.

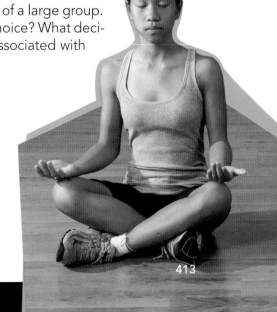

18

Lifelong Leadership and Physical Activity

In This Chapter

LESSON 18.1
Leadership Skills in Physical Activity

SELF-ASSESSMENT
Developing Leadership Skills

LESSON 18.2
Active Living Opportunities

TAKING CHARGE
Conflict Resolution

SELF-MANAGEMENT
Skills for Conflict Resolution

TAKING ACTION
Team Building

GET ACTIVE WITH COACHING ASSOCIATION OF CANADA

CHAPTER REVIEW

 Student Web Resources
www.fitnessforlife.org/student

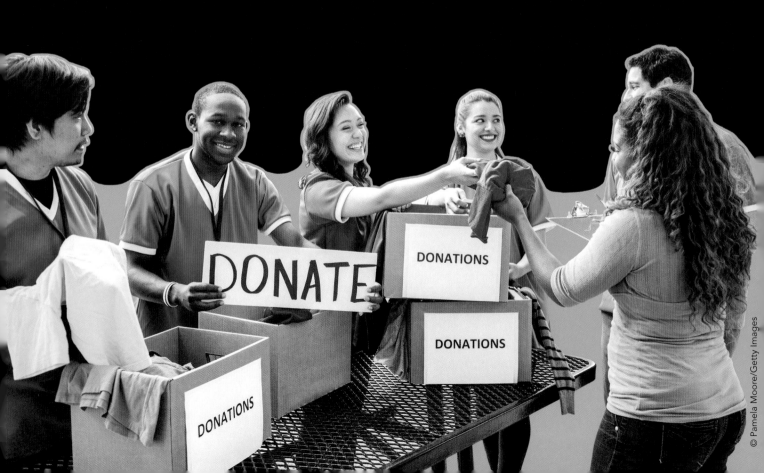

© Pamela Moore/Getty Images

Lesson 18.1
Leadership Skills in Physical Activity

Lesson Objectives

After participating in this lesson, you should be able to

1. describe five leadership skills,
2. define *team* and *teamwork* and describe five guidelines for becoming an effective team member,
3. define *group cohesiveness* and factors that develop it, and
4. describe *team building* and its benefits.

Lesson Vocabulary

group cohesiveness, leadership, team, team building, teamwork

Have you ever been part of a team or a group such as a sport team, a group for a school project, a volunteer team or group, a band, or other kind of team or group? If you answered "yes" to any of these questions, what role did you play, and how comfortable were you in that role? Did the team or group have good chemistry, or were there issues that kept the group members distant from each other, making it difficult to reach the final goal?

One purpose of this book is to help people move from dependence to independence, whether in working out to get fit, making decisions about what to eat, or becoming increasingly responsible for themselves and others. This growth involves not only engaging in positive social interactions in school but also developing skills that will help you outside of school now and in the future. In school, teachers and coaches often appoint leaders, and rules are often made and enforced by others. This chapter provides guidelines for helping you make responsible choices and developing leadership skills, especially in physical activity settings.

> " Whether it is with friends or family, I expect them to set a great example for me, and hopefully I will do the same for them. And that is all part of being a leader. "
>
> —Steve Nash, two-time NBA MVP

Leaders and Leadership

A leader guides or directs a group of people, such as a sport team or club. **Leadership** involves actively assuming the role of a leader. You can't be a leader just because you want to. Becoming a leader requires leadership skills that can be developed, and some of the most important are presented in table 18.1. Like all skills, leadership skills must be practiced in order to be mastered.

Physical activity contexts provide a wide range of possible leadership experiences. For example, one way to get leadership experience is to play sports and games. Another way is to participate in physical education class. Approaches to physical education such as the Teaching Personal and Social Responsibility model, Peer Teaching, Cooperative Learning, and Sport Education are designed to support the growth of leadership skills. For example, Teaching Personal and Social Responsibility uses physical activity settings as a place to practice personal responsibility in order to eventually extend that to others within and beyond the physical education setting. Cooperative Learning requires students to take on a variety of roles such as leader, reporter, recorder, errand monitor, and time keeper in order to learn with, for, and from each other, not just beside each other. Peer Teaching supports leadership skill development by focusing on helping students assume both leader and follower roles in groups of two. Sport Education provides opportunities to develop leadership skills by grouping students in teams with roles such as leaders, team members,

TABLE 18.1 Leadership Skills

Skill	Description	How to build
Integrity	Integrity means being fair; for a leader, it means directing while adhering to rules and standards of the group. Not all leaders have integrity, but good leaders do.	Integrity is built over time. You establish a reputation based on your actions.
Communication	Good leaders are good listeners. They listen in order to understand the group's needs, then speak clearly to be understood. Good leaders also inspire and persuade.	Practice listening even when you have much to say. Keep track of what others say. Ask whether what you think they said is what they meant. Ask what they heard you say to see if they got your message. Get the facts to help you make good arguments.
Strategy and planning	Creating a strategy requires creating a clear vision of your goals. It also involves developing tactics for carrying out the plan.	Practice using the steps for developing a strategy and carrying out a plan. Get the facts before planning.
Management	Leaders help group members work together to meet goals. Keys include building teamwork (group unity) and building trust based on integrity. Relevant skills that can be learned include directing and supervising others, resolving conflicts, and negotiating.	Study the information presented in this chapter about teamwork and conflict resolution.
Other	Other characteristics of a good leader include self-confidence, optimism, enthusiasm, decisiveness, and being proactive. Good leaders can also accept criticism and are willing to learn better ways to reach group goals.	Most of these characteristics are built through experience. It also helps to practice the self-management skills presented in this book.

and referees. In the workplace, companies often use cooperative games to train their leaders (in this case, managers and executives).

Ultimately, leadership is not about glorious crowning acts. It's about keeping your team focused on a goal and motivated to do their best to achieve it, especially when the stakes are high and the consequences really matter. It is about laying the groundwork for others' success, and then standing back and letting them shine.

—Chris Hadfield, first Canadian astronaut to walk in space

Teams and Teamwork

A **team** is a group of people who band together or are assigned to work together. Therefore, for the purposes of this text the word "team" is used to refer to any group of people, not just a sport team. Ideally, team members work together to achieve a common goal. Sometimes, however, not all team members are committed to the team's goal; in fact, some members may even work to undermine the team's efforts. **Teamwork** is effective, combined work by all team members toward achieving a common goal. In order to experience teamwork, group members often have to sacrifice personal recognition in favour of team goals. For this reason, sport teams often use the slogan "There is no I in TEAM" to emphasize that individual goals are secondary to team goals (figure 18.1).

Hayley Wickenheiser on Leadership Styles

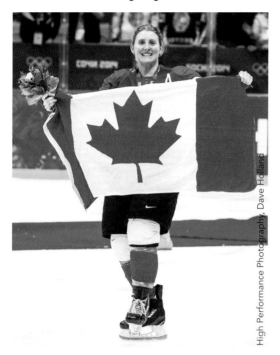

High Performance Photography, Dave Holland

Hayley Wickenheiser, five-time Olympic medalist and one of the best female hockey players in the world.

During the course of my career I have had the opportunity to meet and work with some of the best leaders in the world, and each has had their own style. This chapter will discuss many different components of leadership and styles of leadership and, with some thought, I am sure you will be able to draw a correlation in any group to identify, and identify with, a true leader.

If you look around at work, in a sports environment, among your classmates, and even in your own family group you will begin to notice traits of a leader. But don't assume they are always the loudest voices—often they are not. In fact, in some cases, such as my own, they tend to lead in nonvocal ways. I think at different points in my career, different styles of leadership were required of me, and I found two that felt natural to me and hopefully to my teammates.

I believe early on in my career I was a lead-from-behind kind of leader on our team. That is to say, when I was the youngest or the rookie on the team, I tended to lead my team by supporting those with more seniority or experience. I tried to be an open ear and someone they could trust to put in the work, pull my weight, and always be at the highest level of competition possible.

As the years went on and some of the best leaders I have ever worked with moved onto different phases in their lives, I found that my own leadership style adapted to the role I had on the team. I became more of a lead-by-example captain. I wasn't the loudest cheerleader in the dressing room but gave space to those who were, for those of my teammates who responded best to that leadership style. I did always work to be an example of what I expected of my teammates.

I worked hard to have the best fitness scores, the strongest work ethic, the fastest feet, the hardest shot, and the most empathy and desire to help my teammates. In short, I expected nothing of my teammates that I wasn't willing to do myself. I didn't demand respect because of the role of captain, I worked to earn it by being the best possible athlete I could be. As the years on the National Team have gone on, I believe I have gone back to a lead-from-behind style.

There is one thing I have learned with any leadership style I have employed, or seen in others, that is for certain: In a sports team setting, particularly on teams as large as a hockey team, there are those who respond differently to styles of leadership. You have to have the courage to allow people to step into the leadership roles that aren't as natural to you in order to reach the whole team. That can define a team.

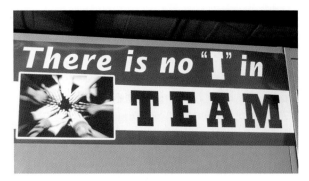

Motivational slogans are sometimes used to promote teamwork.

Aristotle, the Greek philosopher, stated, "The whole is greater than the sum of its parts." The implication is that if people work together, they can accomplish things that they could not accomplish working independently. Consider the following guidelines about teamwork. They can be useful in helping groups to function effectively.

- **Learning your role.** What tasks are you best able to perform that will help the team? A team has a few common goals but many different roles. While some roles are more prominent (for example, pitcher on a softball team), all roles must be performed well for the team to succeed.

- **Accepting your role.** The role you want may not be the role you get. A person who accepts the role assigned is more likely to help the team than one who does not. In addition, carrying out a role that you don't prefer can lead to more desirable roles in the future. As illustrated in this chapter's Science in Action feature, teams can function effectively even if a member does not like his or her role—and even when team members don't get along well—as long as members *accept* their roles. Of course, being on a team is more fun if team members like each other and work well together.

- **Practicing your role.** As with being a leader, being an effective team member requires practice. Every role requires specific skills. For example, the pitcher on a softball team must have motor skills suited to that position but may not be an especially good hitter. For this reason, the pitcher may be called on to perform a sacrifice bunt to move a runner into scoring position. This pitcher practices bunting more than other players because this is an assigned role. Of course, roles are often assigned by leaders on the basis of special skills that individuals possess. In an example from a school setting, one grade 11 student council president, named Hideko, sought artists to make posters, computer specialists to prepare websites, and other people with special skills for specific roles.

- **Carrying out your role.** It's one thing to practice your role but another to carry it out effectively. Even when everyone does his or her job as practiced, success may not follow. For example, the opposing team may use a tactic that overcomes your team's tactic. Or the other team may simply have players who are very good. Thus, carrying out your role may not always get the desired result, but it does give your team the best chance for success. For this reason, it's important not to get discouraged if you and your team are not successful every time you perform your roles well.

- **Adapting as necessary.** Again, even if all team members work hard and perform their roles well, success may not follow. If the team's strategy and tactics are not working,

FIT FACT

Developing skills required to assume roles that you do not prefer, and taking a step back to bring out the best in a team, are also signs of a great leader. Being the "boss" is not the same as being a leader, although a boss can also be a leader. For instance, leaders establish equal relationships by listening, motivating, teaching and learning, taking part, and also stepping back and letting others step up. In contrast, bosses are characterized as getting things done by ruling, commanding, and terrifying; not sharing in the group responsibilities; and ultimately creating an unequal relationship that reduces group satisfaction and production.

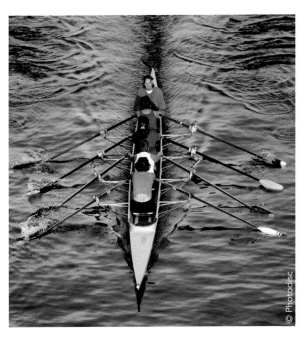

Group cohesiveness occurs when team members work together toward a common goal.

adjustments need to be made, and those adjustments could mean a change in some team members' roles.

Team Building

Team building is a collective term that is used in many contexts such as educational and business settings. Teams must work cooperatively and collaboratively, within defined roles, to solve problems. Within a physical activity context, teams would be supported in developing teamwork and cohesion in order to solve a challenge requiring physical, cognitive, and social skills. One of the goals of this type of team building is to build leadership skills such as sharing ideas, accepting the ideas of others, praising and encouraging others, gaining confidence in one's own abilities and skill set, and respecting and supporting others physically, cognitively, and emotionally.

⚛ SCIENCE IN ACTION: Group Cohesiveness

Cohesion means sticking together tightly. In chemistry, it means uniting particles to form a single mass. When applied to groups of people, cohesion is referred to as **group cohesiveness**, which occurs when group or team members stick together in working toward common goals. Scientists have studied group cohesiveness in a variety of sports and found that several factors help groups stick together; these include small group size, friendship among members, commitment to the group's goals, group success or failure, and competitiveness of group members.

It's easier to achieve group cohesiveness in small groups because fewer people have to coordinate their efforts. For example, it's easier for 4 people on a curling team to work together than for 11 people on a soccer team to do so. It's also easier for small groups to agree on goals.

In addition, if team members know and like each other, it's easier for them to agree on goals and work together. However, studies also show that some teams win championships despite dissension among their members because team members are strongly committed to the group's

goals. Several studies of rowers, for example, show that personal feelings can be overcome if team members want strongly enough to win. Thus competitiveness is also a factor that creates desire among team members to work together, though it can cut both ways: Winning a competition can help members get along, but losing sometimes leads to disagreements between team members (see this chapter's Taking Charge feature).

Research also shows that it's important for group members to recognize that everyone makes mistakes sometimes. This acknowledgment reduces blaming when the team does poorly and increases the chances for achieving group cohesiveness in the future. It's crucial to support fellow team members when they're down.

Student Activity

Search websites, social media, magazines, or newspapers to find a true story about group cohesiveness. Describe how the group members worked together to achieve a common goal.

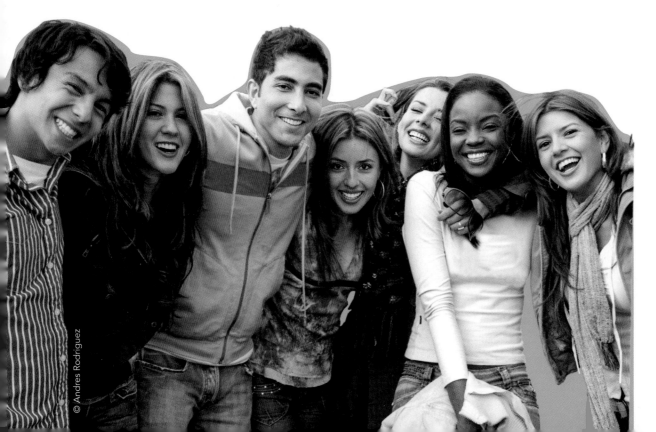

Successful team building requires supporting each other physically, cognitively, and emotionally.

Diversity: Respect for Others

The word "society" refers to a large group of people who have a history of working and living together.

FIT FACT

Team building has many benefits, such as improved communication, motivation, and cohesiveness; the development of leadership skills; and increased self-confidence. Supporting and practicing team building also builds a strong and positive community through the development of a positive environment and a reduction in negative influences.

It can refer to a neighbourhood, a community, a nation, or an even larger group (for example, Western society). Characteristics of a society include traditions, organized laws and rules, and standards for living and conduct (social etiquette).

Societies provide for the common interests of their members and protect them from outside threats. One common interest in a society is that of providing for all members of the group, not just the biggest and strongest. Diversity in a society refers to the inclusion of different types of people, and the great diversity in many modern societies makes social sensitivity and responsibility necessary. Specifically, it requires sensitivity to others regardless of race, ethnicity, age, disability, culture, socioeconomic status, sex, or gender identity. To achieve the goal of treating all members equally and fairly, it is

© Andres Rodriguez

helpful to consider all people when selecting leaders; to follow the rules of the social group (such as a team or school); and to practice good etiquette in daily activities. In 1971, Canada became the first country to adopt multiculturalism as an official policy. By doing so, Canada affirmed the value and dignity of all Canadian citizens regardless of their racial or ethnic origins, language, or religious affiliation. The 1971 Multiculturalism Policy of Canada also confirmed the rights of Aboriginal peoples and the status of Canada's two official languages.

> " Diversity is Canada's strength. "
>
> —Justin Trudeau, 23rd
> prime minister of Canada

Sensitivity, Trust, and Respect

Sensitivity refers to paying attention to the feelings and concerns of others. Ways to build sensitivity include listening (for example, hearing what others have to say rather than only telling others what to do) and communicating in nonthreatening language (for example, giving positive comments rather than harsh criticism). Trust refers to the belief that others are honest and reliable. Demonstrating honesty and reliability in your actions helps others learn to trust you. Trustworthy people keep their promises and are sensitive to the needs of others. People who are trustworthy and sensitive (including leaders) typically have the respect of others.

Lesson Review

1. What are the five leadership skills?
2. What is teamwork, and what are the five guidelines for becoming an effective team member?
3. What is group cohesiveness, and what are some factors that develop it?
4. What is team building, and what are the benefits of team building?

This self-assessment will give you insight into the importance of assuming and carrying out teamwork roles. Follow the steps listed next to complete this self-assessment. Remember that self-assessment information is personal and considered confidential. You do not have to share your self-assessment with anyone.

Applying *leadership, teamwork, group cohesiveness, respect for others,* and *sensitivity, trust,* and *respect* concepts from this chapter, complete the following tasks:

1. Cooperatively form a group of four to six people.

2. Respectfully decide who will assume and carry out the five cooperative learning roles (see table 18.2). If there are four in the group, one person may have to assume two roles, but be respectful of the expectations of each role so that this person does not have an unbalanced portion of the work. If there are six in the group, two people will have to share a role. Discuss which roles would benefit the most from having two people share the responsibility.

3. Imagine that your group is developing and implementing a new physical activity program at the community centre for preteens.

   a. Remember, the goal of this self-assessment is to accept and assume your roles (e.g., the time keeper should ask the instructor for a time frame for completion; the recorder is responsible for recording the information in such a way that the reporter can easily and clearly report the major points of the discussion).

   b. Discuss group and individual behaviours that would make it difficult for a team to reach the goal of developing and implementing a new physical activity program for preteens.

   c. Discuss how these group and individual behaviours could realistically be changed to support greater group success and ultimately the successful implementation of a much needed preteen physical activity program.

4. Answer the following questions individually and privately.

   a. In what ways did you support the group by
      - quickly and easily finding a group?
      - assuming a role?
      - carrying out that role?

   b. In what ways could you have improved your leadership skills in these areas?

   c. In your role, what did you do to support the group?

   d. How could you make improvements in your leadership skills within a group next time?

   e. Given these and other factors that have come to mind, which leadership skills (i.e., actively assuming your role and guiding the group within the responsibilities of your role) do you feel confident in?

   f. In what leadership skill areas do you still need practice to improve?

   g. What will you do to improve these skills?

TABLE 18.2   Cooperative Learning Roles

Role	Responsibilities	Sound bites
Leader	Makes sure that every voice is heard. Focuses work around the learning task.	• *"Let's hear from ____ next."* • *"That's interesting, but let's get back to our task."*
Recorder	Compiles group members' ideas on collaborative graphic organizer. Writes on the board for the whole class to see during the presentation.	• *"I think I heard you say_____; is that right?"* • *"How would you like me to write this?"*
Time keeper	Encourages the group to stay on task. Announces when time is halfway through and when time is nearly up.	• *"We only have five minutes left. Let's see if we can wrap up by then."*
Presenter	Presents the group's finished work to the class.	• *"How would you like this to sound?"*
Errand monitor	Briefly leaves the group to get supplies or to request help from the teacher when group members agree that they do not have the resources to solve the problem.	• *"Do you think it's time to ask the teacher for help?"* • *"I'll get an extra graphic organizer from the shelf."*

ABC Bookmaking Builds Vocabulary in the Content Areas lesson by Laurie Henry, provided by ReadWriteThink.org, a website developed by the International Reading Association and the National Council of Teachers of English.

Lesson 18.2
Active Living Opportunities

Lesson Objectives

After participating in this lesson, you should be able to

1. define *autonomy* and explain how it relates to decision making about healthy lifestyles,
2. describe five or more sources of information about opportunities for physical activity,
3. explain three guidelines for organizing for participation in physical activity, and
4. define *extrinsic motivation* and *intrinsic motivation* and explain the difference between them.

Lesson Vocabulary

autonomy, extrinsic motivation, intrinsic motivation, optimal challenge, self-reward system

Do you feel as though you have the power to make your own decisions in life? How do you feel when you have a choice compared with when you don't? Consider the following scenario.

Two years after graduating from high school, a group of friends gathered at a social. Hal hosted the party at his house. He was now married and worked full-time. He'd gained quite a few kilograms since high school and wasn't as active as he had been when he played football in school. His wife, Fatima, had been a cheerleader in school but was also less active now because she also had a full-time job. Hal and Fatima stayed in touch with their friends, but some were off at college, and others were busy working.

Other people attending the social event included Kris, who had also played on the football team. He was now attending a local community college and working part-time. Like Hal, he knew he was less active than he should be. Jennifer was attending the local university, where she played on the soccer team. She was very active but missed interacting with her friends. Will was also attending the university, where he played some intramurals and worked out at the campus recreation centre. Coretta and Josh had not gone to school with the others but were now neighbours of Hal and Fatima. Josh played slow-pitch softball, and Coretta used some home exercise videos. They had a 4-year-old daughter named Clara.

The seven friends decided that it would be good if they could all be more active (except, of course, for Jennifer, the soccer player). They also wanted to spend more time together socially. They decided to do some type of physical activity together to help them be more active and have fun at the same time. The rest of this lesson describes some of the steps

that the friends used to investigate opportunities for their group.

FIT FACT

Self-determination theory is one theory of human motivation. It places high importance on autonomy and intrinsic motivation. It is often used in the study of sport and physical activity. Students report that physical education classes are more enjoyable when they are given an opportunity to choose (to have autonomy in) some of the activities in their classes.

Autonomy

Autonomy refers to self-direction or the ability to make decisions for yourself. One goal of this book is to help teens move from having others make decisions for them (dependence) to making decisions for themselves (independence). Hal, Fatima, and their friends are at a stage of life in which they make their own decisions. In elementary school, and even in middle school, many decisions had been made for them. Even in high school, they were somewhat dependent on others (such as parents, teachers, and coaches) for many things. Now, however, they have the autonomy to make their own decisions.

The friends applied some of the self-management skills they had learned in junior high and high school to their search for active living opportunities in their community. For example, they had learned about the self-management skill of finding social support from friends, but they did have some barriers to overcome. For one thing, to be active together they would have to find activities that they were all interested in and find times when they would all be available. To solve this and other problems, they used elements of the scientific method and critical thinking skills. Like Hal, Fatima, and their friends, you can practice self-management skills and use the scientific method to become more autonomous in making decisions about healthy lifestyles.

Finding Opportunities to Participate

One of the first steps in finding ways to be active is to find out what's available. Options in most communities include government agencies, community organizations, worksite programs, commercial options, and places of worship. Table 18.3

TABLE 18.3 Finding Opportunities for Physical Activity in the Community

Type	Examples	How to contact
• Government agencies • Youth programs • Sport leagues • Facilities (tennis courts, bike trails, golf courses, hiking trails, parks) • Community centres • Cultural centres • Museums	• Local parks and recreation department • Provincial parks and recreation department • Local public school programs	Use a phone book or do a web search to locate agencies. Search for a specific department or facility.
National and provincial sport organizations	• Canadian Olympic Committee (Team Canada) • National Sport Organizations (Government of Canada) • Special Olympics Canada • Canadian Paralympics • Provincial sport organizations (e.g., wheelchair rugby SK) • Sport and recreation by province (e.g., Sport and Recreation Government of Nunavut)	Do a web search to locate the organizations. For sites such as Government of Canada National Sport Organizations, links are provided to specific sport pages.
Community organizations	• YMCA and YWCA • Boys & Girls Clubs Canada • Easter Seals Canada (or by province, e.g., Easter Seals NL) • Activity-specific clubs (e.g., walking, jogging, and tennis clubs) • Local sport organizations • Park organizations (for bike and walking trails, swimming)	• Do a web search for the organization name or sport and your town or city name (e.g., YMCA Grande Prairie, AB, or Minor Baseball Riverview, NB). Contact the organization by phone or in person. • Find the city or town website for dropdown menus of sporting and recreation opportunities.
Worksite programs	• Company wellness programs • Company fitness centres • Company sport leagues and teams	Check with the human resources office at your worksite to see what's available.
Commercial options	• Health and fitness clubs and spas • Private sport facilities (sport fields, ice rinks, skating rinks or parks, golf courses, leagues) • Dance, yoga, martial arts studios • Youth activity centres • Physical therapy centres	Do a web search for the activity and your town or city name (e.g., dance classes Whitehorse, YT). Contact the facility by phone or in person.
Places of worship (e.g., church, gurdwara, mosque, synagogue)	• Sport leagues • Exercise groups • Summer camps • Social groups	Check with religious organizations' offices.

summarizes multiple types of opportunity for being active in your local area.

Organizing for Participation

After investigating opportunities, Hal and his friends decided to join a co-rec volleyball league sponsored by their community's parks and recreation department. They needed at least 10 people because a team requires 6 people every time it plays and they knew that not everyone would be able to make every game due to their busy schedules. They also needed their group to be evenly split between men and women because three of each had to be on the court during every game. The group elected Hal as captain and coach and recruited another couple (Nancy and Cole) who lived nearby. Jennifer also asked her friend Jasmine to join, which brought their total to 10: 5 women and 5 men.

Not all people have such a ready-made social group. Here are some good guidelines for finding or forming a group for physical activity participation.

- **Consider nonleague participation as a start.** Joining a club or league can be quite intimidating for some people. If you're just learning an activity, you may want to join recreational sessions or take a class at a local club before joining a league. For example, Coretta had not played much volleyball, so she joined with others in the group to practice at the park before the league started. Will went to the rec centre at his university and played in some pickup volleyball games to get some practice.

- **Check with friends at school or work.** Start with a few people; then each can recruit others with similar interests to participate. You might want to start with noncompetitive games before moving on to league play.

- **Check out your work wellness program or school recreation centre.** See if there's a list of people interested in the same activity that you can recruit to join you. There might even be an existing club or exercise group that you can join. Club members often get to know each other and then form teams for leagues after starting with recreational play.

- **Check with the organizations listed in table 18.3.** See if they have opportunities for individuals or small groups to join larger teams.

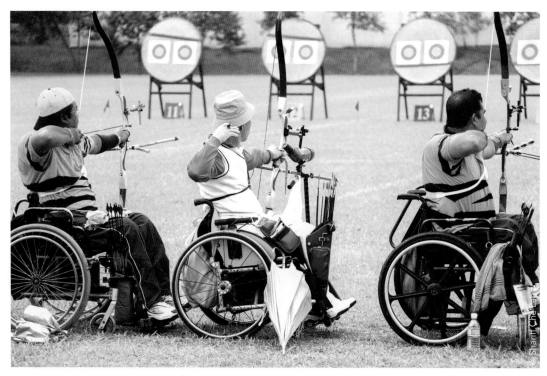

Community recreation, commercial, and worksite wellness programs provide good opportunities for lifelong participation.

Daring to Try

Sometimes one of the hardest things to do is simply to dare to try. This can be especially true when you're starting something new and don't have others to do it with. Coretta had friends to support her, so joining them on a volleyball team was not as threatening as it might have been. Still, she lacked confidence, so before the volleyball league began she joined with others to practice. She was initially motivated by her desire to please her friends in the group; she didn't want to let them down.

Coretta's initial motivation for playing is called **extrinsic motivation**. Extrinsic motivation is motivation that comes from outside the individual (for example, pressure from others, external rewards). In this case, Coretta wanted to be on the team not because she particularly enjoyed volleyball but because the team needed another player. Even after trying recreational volleyball, she felt very nervous when she first played on the competitive team. As she practiced, however, she found success in serving and digging, which encouraged her to keep trying.

As she got better, she started to look forward to the games. She was not playing to please someone else (extrinsic motivation); she was now playing because she enjoyed it (**intrinsic motivation**). Intrinsic motivation comes from within the individual; the rewards for participation are personal and internal (for example, fun, joy of participation).

In school, Coretta had learned about **optimal challenge** (see figure 18.2). In her practice group, she tried to do things that were neither too easy nor too hard. Because the challenge was reasonable, she found success rather than failure. In turn, this success encouraged her to keep trying. Gradually, she started to enjoy herself, and that made her want to keep participating.

Coretta also learned to reward herself for her performance rather than rely on praise from others. If she had gone right into the volleyball league without practicing first, she might have become frustrated and quit trying.

Kris had a very different experience. He became bored with the volleyball team. Although he liked being with his friends, his volleyball skills were

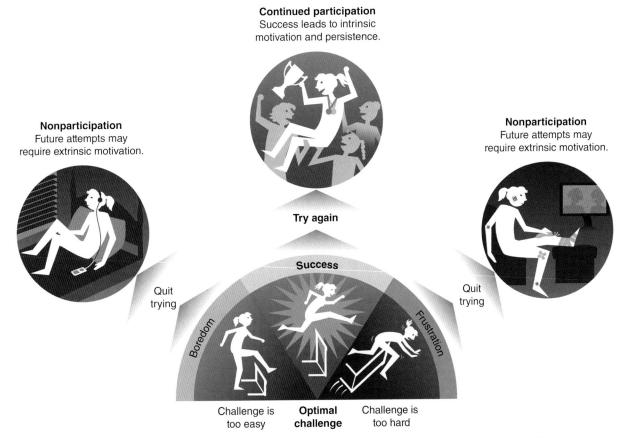

Continued participation
Success leads to intrinsic motivation and persistence.

Nonparticipation
Future attempts may require extrinsic motivation.

Nonparticipation
Future attempts may require extrinsic motivation.

Try again

Quit trying

Quit trying

Success

Boredom

Frustration

Challenge is too easy

Optimal challenge

Challenge is too hard

FIGURE 18.2 Finding an optimal challenge helps you achieve success and intrinsic motivation.

better than his friends' skills, and he lost interest in the games. It took encouragement and even pleading from his friends (extrinsic motivation) to keep him coming to the games. Ultimately, he dropped out of the league, and the team finished with nine players.

Sometimes you need a little extrinsic or external motivation to get you going. But researchers have shown that long-term participation requires intrinsic motivation. People who have intrinsic motivation (such as Coretta) are more likely to stick with participation than people who are extrinsically motivated (such as Kris). Being able to gradually build your skills and find success and ultimately intrinsic motivation is called having a **self-reward system**. You reward yourself rather than expecting others to reward you for your efforts.

FIT FACT

Video game creators use the concept of optimal challenge. To ensure success, they design games that start players at a low level. This success creates intrinsic motivation that keeps players' interest high and encourages them to keep participating. Indeed, evidence shows that gamers play for hours with no extrinsic rewards.

 ## FITNESS TECHNOLOGY: Social Support

As noted in chapter 5, social support is important in helping people adopt and stick with healthy lifestyle changes. Weight Watchers is an organization that uses social support to help people maintain a healthy weight throughout life. Meetings allow group members to support each other and receive support from program leaders. Weight Watchers also uses the web to provide social support through interactive tools that help members self-monitor their eating and activity habits. Optimal challenges are provided to encourage success and intrinsic motivation. Even people who are intrinsically motivated benefit from the support of others, and Weight Watchers messages are sent periodically to provide support and encouragement. New apps and electronic trackers are being developed daily that integrate social support to help people attain their health goals whether they be activity, nutrition, or sleep based (e.g., FitBit, Lose It!). Even some doctors are starting to provide messages to encourage patients.

You can use the web and social media to encourage others and help them be successful in making healthy lifestyle choices. You can do this through e-mail messages and tweets to support group members with similar goals. For example, Hal and his friends could use e-mails, text messages, phone calls, or tweets to encourage each other to come to practices and games.

Messages from others can also be harmful if not done properly. You've learned that autonomy is important and that we all want to make decisions for ourselves. Messages that encourage a person to stick with his or her plan encourage autonomy. On the other hand, messages or comments that treat people as if one is trying to control their behaviour do not encourage autonomy and may be ignored. For example, if someone misses a practice, a good message of support might be, "Missed you at practice—hope to see you next time." A not-so-good message might be, "If you keep missing, you will never get better." This message suggests that the person should attend in order to please someone else.

Appropriately supportive personal messages delivered via phone or the web have been shown to help people who are trying to stop smoking, maintain a healthy weight, or be active for health and fitness.

Using Technology

Get a group of friends together to form a support network. Discuss ways in which the group will use social support technology to help each other meet their goals.

Helping Others in Physical Activity

In this book, you've learned many self-management skills designed to help you be active for the rest of your life. In the years ahead, you'll find that having active people around you helps you be more active. You'll also have the opportunity to help others be physically active. A few of these opportunities are described in the following list.

- **Family activities.** A popular slogan says, "Families that play together stay together." You can use the skills you've learned in this class to help family members be active. Examples include family outings (such as camping, fishing, and biking trips), family exercise sessions (such as walks and hikes), and family activity nights (such as bowling or skating night). Because not all family members will always like the same activities, you can also support each other's activities.

Family support is a type of social support that can help family members stick with their exercise—for example, watching a family member's team play or praising the jogger in the family for sticking with it over time.

- **Coaching.** When you were younger, you may have played a sport such as soccer or tee ball. If so, someone coached your team. You can give back by volunteering to coach children in your neighbourhood. Training for volunteer coaches is provided by many organizations.

" You can motivate by fear, and you can motivate by reward. But both those methods are only temporary. The only lasting thing is self-motivation. "

—Homer Rice, football coach

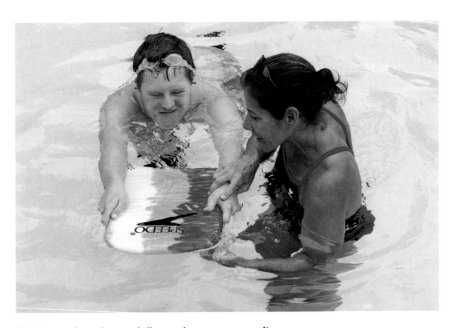

Helping others learn skills can be very rewarding.

Lesson Review

1. What is autonomy, and how does it relate to decision making about healthy lifestyles?
2. What are some sources of information about opportunities for physical activity?
3. What are some guidelines for organizing for participation in physical activity?
4. What are extrinsic and intrinsic motivation, and how do they differ?

TAKING CHARGE: Conflict Resolution

Conflict can be a barrier to participation; it can be the reason that a person doesn't stick to a physical activity plan. Here's an example. Monica and Juana developed a plan to walk to school five days a week for one month. Unfortunately, their friend Miguel kept offering them a ride to school. The third time Miguel offered, Monica accepted and left Juana to walk alone. Juana did not accept because she wanted to walk as planned. Juana then felt mad at both Monica and Miguel and didn't speak to them at school. The next day, Monica didn't

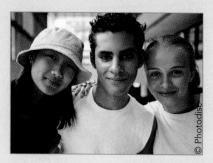

© Photodisc

stop by to walk with Juana—she just rode with Miguel. The friends did not speak at school. In fact, Monica said something to other friends about Juana that upset her.

For Discussion

What could the friends have done to avoid the conflict? What steps should they take to resolve it? List possible solutions. Consider the skills in the Self-Management feature when answering the discussion questions.

SELF-MANAGEMENT: Skills for Conflict Resolution

At times, all of us have disagreements with our friends. The disagreements are usually over small things and can be easily resolved. A conflict is typically bigger than a disagreement. When a conflict occurs, one or more of the people involved come to feel threatened, whether physically or emotionally. In sport, for example, one player may get angry with another, and strong emotions may lead to angry words. In extreme cases, the anger can result in fighting. Whether the conflict occurs in sport or daily life, the following steps can help you resolve it.

- **Consider the three Bs.** When working with others to resolve conflict, remember to *be calm, be patient,* and *be respectful.* Keeping emotions under control is essential.

- **Communicate.** To resolve a conflict, you need good communication. Be willing to listen to what the other person has to say. Watch what you say. Words can hurt, and it's crucial not to make the conflict worse.

- **Recognize that there is a conflict.** Don't ignore it. Avoiding a conflict can cause it to get worse.

- **Consider a meeting.** While a conflict can sometimes be resolved on the phone, by e-mail, through social media, or in other ways, it's often best to meet face to face. Meeting in person makes harsh words less likely. The meeting should

be held in a neutral and safe setting for all involved.

- **Set the scene.** Define the problem, and restate it if necessary. Using the three Bs, each person should describe the problem without interruption. After each person has done so, the parties can try to find a statement of the problem that all can agree to.

- **List possible solutions.** Make a list of possible solutions based on ideas from people on all sides of the conflict.

- **Consider the options.** Once options have been proposed, communicate respectfully to find the options that best meet the needs of all parties concerned.

- **Compromise.** If the people involved have very different ideas about the conflict, it may be necessary for each person to give up something in order to find a resolution.

- **Seek help.** Another way to resolve a conflict is through arbitration. If the parties involved cannot resolve the conflict on their own, an independent arbitrator may be used. In sport, a coach or referee can resolve some conflicts, and others may be resolved with the help of a common friend, but difficult conflicts may call for a professional arbitrator (such as a lawyer).

TAKING ACTION: Team Building

The TEAM concept (Together Everyone Achieves More) can help you succeed in all aspects of your life. It's an exciting challenge to build a team of individuals who work well together in pursuit of a common goal. Team-building activities are easily accessible on the Internet. Take action by finding a team-building activity that can be performed in your physical education or health education class.

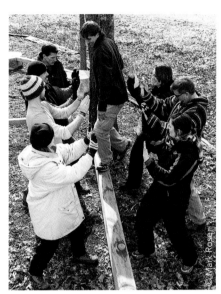

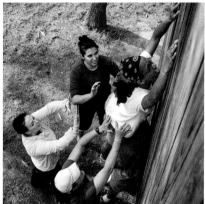

Take action by trying team-building activities.

REACH *HIGHER*

© Coaching Association of Canada

GET ACTIVE WITH COACHING ASSOCIATION OF CANADA

Who We Are

The Coaching Association of Canada (CAC) unites stakeholders and partners in its commitment to raising the skills and stature of coaches and ultimately expanding their reach and influence. Through its programs, the CAC empowers coaches with knowledge and skills, promotes ethics, fosters positive attitudes, builds competence, and increases the credibility and recognition of coaches.

What We Do

The National Coaching Certification Program (NCCP) is the CAC's flagship program and has been identified as a world leader in coach education. It is currently the largest adult continuing education program in Canada. The CAC is committed to ensuring that all coaches receive training based on best practices in instructional design and ethical decision-making and with content that is relevant, is current, and leads to the development of competent coaches. The NCCP is designed in collaboration with 66 national sport organizations (NSOs) in Canada and the 13 recognized provincial and territorial coaching representatives.

Get Involved

Many great coaches learn their skills by assisting other coaches—where they can watch, ask questions, learn, and eventually lead athletes and coach a team of their own. Here are some of the many ways to get information and get involved in coaching!

- Take a National Coaching Certification Program (NCCP) training workshop.
- Take our Get Coaching! e-activity to prepare for your first practice.
- Sign up to coach with a friend and help each other learn.
- Talk to someone who is already coaching—a friend, a neighbour, another coach. People are always willing to share.
- Sign up to assist a team, or ask the coach for more information.
- Volunteer with a local amateur club or community team.
- Ask your local club or provincial sport organization for resources (books, videos, guidance).

Every child deserves a certified coach. If you are ready to begin your training, visit Coach.ca today and learn more.

© Coaching Association of Canada

Reviewing Concepts and Vocabulary

Complete the following in order to determine your growing understanding of fitness, health, and wellness. Answer items 1 through 5 by correctly completing each sentence with a word or phrase.

1. _____ is effective, combined work by all team members toward achieving a common goal.
2. Sticking together when working toward a common goal is called _____.
3. _____, unlike leaders, are said to rule, command, and terrify in order to get things done.
4. People who have _____ are self-directed and make their own decisions.
5. People who need an external reward to do a behaviour have _____ motivation.

For items 6 through 10, match each term in column 1 with the appropriate phrase in column 2.

6. self-determination theory
7. diversity
8. optimal challenge
9. leader
10. intrinsic motivation

a. places importance on autonomy
b. inclusion of different types of people
c. person who guides or directs
d. comes from within
e. neither too hard nor too easy

For items 11 through 15, respond to each statement or question.

11. List and describe several leadership skills.
12. Explain some factors that contribute to good teamwork.
13. Develop a team-building challenge with the goal of navigating one group member who is hearing impaired, and another who is vision impaired, to the finish line.
14. Describe groups that provide opportunities for physical activity in a community.
15. Describe the guidelines for resolving conflict.

Thinking Critically

You've been asked to form a lunchtime physical activity initiative at your school. Write a paragraph to describe the steps you would take to get a team organized that would best be able to respond to the request in a positive way.

Project

Work with a group to develop a directory of physical activity for your community. Include a list of agencies and businesses offering various kinds of physical activity. Consider the following categories and list the activities they provide: local government agencies, community sport organizations, work-site activity programs, commercial options (local businesses), places of worship, and other types. Use table 18.3 for ideas.

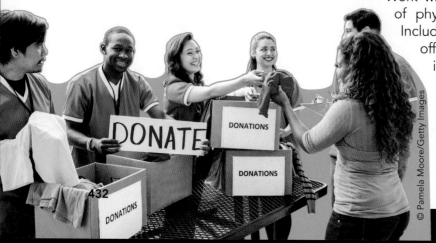

© Pamela Moore/Getty Images

UNIT VII
Making Lifestyle Choices

● ●

Self-Assessment Features in This Unit
- My Alcohol Knowledge
- Sexuality Survey
- Rate Your Relationships

Taking Charge Features in This Unit
- Building Strong Refusal Skills
- Improving Social Self-Perception
- Dating Coercion and Violence

Self-Management Features in This Unit
- Skills for Strong Refusal
- Skills for Improving Self-Perception
- Skills for Reducing Your Risk of Experiencing Dating Coercion and Violence

Taking Action Features in This Unit
- Raising Your Awareness About Alcohol, Drug, and Tobacco Abuse
- Sexual Well-Being
- Taking Dating Violence Seriously

Canadian Sport and Health Organization Features in This Unit
- Get Active With MADD Canada
- Get Active With SexandU
- Get Active With WAVAW Rape Crisis Centre

The authors acknowledge the significant contributions of David E. Corbin, Terri D. Farrar, and Karen E. McConnell to chapters 19, 20, and 21.

19

Alcohol, Drugs, and Tobacco

(www) **Student Web Resources**
www.fitnessforlife.org/student

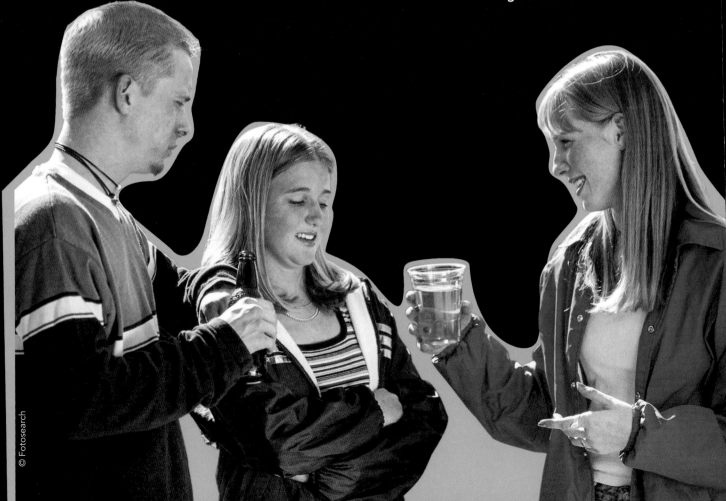

© Fotosearch

Lesson 19.1
Alcohol Use and Abuse

Lesson Objectives

After participating in this lesson, you should be able to

1. define what alcohol is,
2. list two health problems associated with drinking alcohol,
3. identify two reasons for the differences in alcohol tolerance between males and females,
4. list what constitutes binge drinking for males and for females, and
5. list at least three predictable effects of blood alcohol content (BAC) on driving.

Lesson Vocabulary

acute alcohol poisoning, addiction, alcoholism, alcohol tolerance, binge drinking, blood alcohol content (BAC), DriveCam, driving under the influence (DUI), empty calories, heavy drinking, ignition interlock

Alcoholic drinks, such as wine, beer, or cocktails, are enjoyed by many for their taste and their ability to alter a person's state of mind. Alcohol is often used to complement a gathering of friends, to enhance a meal, or to enliven a celebration (e.g., wedding, special accomplishment). Alcohol is also something that people may drink excessively (and then make bad choices), or drink too often and become addicted. It is estimated that Canadians spend more than $12 billion per year, or about $1.4 million every hour of every day, on alcohol. In addition, Canadians spend more than $14 billion dealing with alcohol-related costs including death, injury, lost wages, and rehabilitation from alcohol-related addiction. That's nearly $500 every second of every day spent on alcohol-related problems.

> **"** I'm very serious about no alcohol, no drugs. Life is too beautiful. **"**
>
> —Jim Carrey, actor and comedian

Alcohol is created when grains, fruits, or vegetables are fermented. When alcohol is consumed it is absorbed in the bloodstream, and from there it affects the brain and nervous system functioning. Alcohol is a depressant but has the initial effect of making drinkers more animated and less reserved. It alters brain chemistry so that your brain activity slows down. This calming effect can be pleasant in a safe environment—or catastrophic if a person is in a situation in which quick reaction time is necessary (driving a car or boat) and good judgment is required (resolving conflicts and problem solving). We need to ask ourselves, What are healthy and unhealthy levels of alcohol consumption? What are the short- and long-term health impacts of alcohol consumption?

Overconsumption of Alcohol Is Dangerous

If alcohol is consumed rapidly and in large amounts, it can depress the part of the brain that controls breathing and heart rate, which can result in coma or death. Or, people who drink a large amount of alcohol in a short time period—as in a drinking contest or game—can potentially suffer from fatal **acute alcohol poisoning**, which occurs almost once a week in Canada. Fortunately, in most circumstances, the body automatically reacts to too much alcohol by causing the drinker to vomit or lose consciousness ("pass out"). Vomiting protects the body by getting rid of some of the alcohol.

In this situation it is important to remember that if someone passes out due to alcohol consumption, you should contact 911 immediately. Do not induce vomiting in a person who has passed out because he or she has lost control over the structures (e.g., tongue) and functions (e.g., swallowing) of the mouth and is at risk of choking on the vomit. This can result in death. In addition, it is never a good idea to leave someone alone who has passed out from drinking too much. Passing out, of course, stops a person from drinking more. However, if people drink too much too fast, they can bypass the safeguards of vomiting or passing out, and the alcohol can kill them.

A common misperception is that drinking coffee will speed up the sobering process. If a person is thirsty, permit him or her to drink water, as this will help hydrate the body and reduce the effect of the alcohol. Taking a shower might feel good and clean a person up but does nothing to speed up the sobering process.

Contrary to popular belief, being able to drink more than other people is not a good sign, because people who can drink a lot often think that alcohol can do them no harm. Furthermore, as people become more experienced drinkers, they develop an **alcohol tolerance**, which means that it takes more and more alcohol for them to feel the effects that they used to get when drinking less. This process can lead to a cycle of drinking more and increases the likelihood of alcohol poisoning and many other health risks associated with binge drinking.

Binge drinking involves consuming many drinks on a single occasion, typically five or more drinks within two hours for males and four or more drinks within two hours for females. Sixty-two percent of Ontario students between grades 7 and 12 reported drinking at least once in the last year (which means that a third abstain—probably none are of legal age), and 25 percent of males and 20 percent of females reported binge drinking in the past month.

In Canada a standard drink contains about 13.6 grams of pure alcohol. That means that one standard drink comprises 341 millilitres of beer, a 142-millilitre glass of wine, or a 43-millilitre serving of distilled alcohol like rum (see figure 19.1).

Heavy drinking refers to the average number of drinks a person has on a daily basis over a long time period (i.e., months to years). **Alcoholism** is a disease in which a person is dependent on alcohol. Symptoms include strong cravings for alcohol, loss of control over how much alcohol is consumed, high tolerance for alcohol, and physical dependence on alcohol. Young people who begin drinking before the age of 15 are five times as likely to have alcohol-related problems, and four times more likely to become addicted, compared to those who start drinking later. Why do you think this is the case? How do we prevent ourselves becoming one of those statistics, and how can we help others to not become one of those statistics?

FIT FACT

One in 10 Canadians deals with an addiction to alcohol at some time in his or her life.

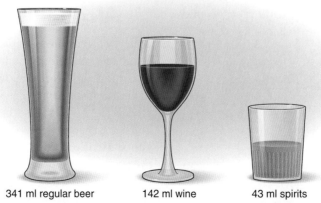

341 ml regular beer   142 ml wine   43 ml spirits

Each of these types of alcohol contains 13.6 g of alcohol.

FIGURE 19.1 Examples of what constitutes a standard drink for different beverages.

What Are the Differences in Alcohol Tolerance Between Males and Females?

For several scientific reasons, males and females tolerate alcohol differently. The most obvious reason is that the average adult female is smaller than the average adult male. The smaller a person's body is (whether male or female), the less alcohol it takes to raise **blood alcohol content (BAC)** (expressed as a percentage of ethanol in the blood in units of mass of alcohol per volume of blood).

The second and dominant physiological reason is that the average female has a higher percent of body fat than the average male at the same age. Body fat contains little water, so most females have less body water than most males. Alcohol is not absorbed into body fat; therefore, BAC is increased in those with more body fat. Of course, there are many males who have more body fat than females at the same age, and they will also be more quickly and dramatically affected by alcohol.

There are also two more reasons. First, women have less alcohol dehydrogenase (an enzyme) than men, which allows more of what women drink to enter the bloodstream as pure alcohol. Finally, the level of the hormone estrogen varies with the female menstrual cycle (and in women who take birth control pills), and increased estrogen can result in a higher level of blood alcohol.

FIT FACT

Forty-six percent of Canadian boys and 42 percent of girls in grade 10 indicated that they had been "really drunk" at least twice.

Immediate Health Risks of Alcohol Consumption

Excessive drinking has immediate effects that increase your risk of many harmful health conditions. These immediate effects, which result most often from binge drinking, include the following:

- Unintentional injuries increase, including traffic-related injuries, falls, drownings, burns, and firearm injuries. People who drink before they are 15 are six to seven times more likely to be involved in a motor vehicle crash or a physical fight after drinking.

- Violent acts increase, including intimate partner violence and maltreatment of children. In fact, alcohol use is associated with two out of three incidents of intimate partner violence.

- Risky sexual behaviour increases, including unprotected sex and sex with multiple partners, as does the risk of sexual assault. These behaviours can also result in unintended pregnancy and sexually transmitted infection. Alcohol can impair your judgment and reduce your level of consciousness.

- Miscarriage and stillbirth increase among pregnant women, along with the risk of physical and mental birth defects in their children.

- The risk increases for acute alcohol poisoning—a medical emergency resulting from a high blood alcohol level that suppresses the central nervous system and can cause loss of consciousness, low blood pressure, low body temperature, coma, respiratory depression, and death.

FIT FACT

Excessive alcohol use accounts for about 6,700 deaths each year in Canada.

Long-Term Health Risks of Heavy Alcohol Consumption

Those who drink heavily over an extended period (months or years) can develop a range of chronic health problems. Heavy drinkers increase their risk of heart disease, cancer, high blood pressure, and liver disease. Heavy drinkers can also experience disruptions in their social structure and livelihood. Common results of chronic drinking include family problems, broken relationships, job and career difficulties, and an increased risk of unintentional injury (e.g., in firearm and automobile accidents).

Alcohol and Calories

Because overweight and obesity are increasing in Canada, people need to know that alcoholic beverages are high in calories and low in nutrients. For example, alcohol contains 7 calories per gram (a gram is the weight of an average paper clip), whereas carbohydrate and protein each contain only 4 calories per gram (fat contains the most, at 9 calories per gram). If a person drinks sweetened drinks (e.g., wine coolers) or mixes alcohol with sweetened pop, then the number of calories is further increased. People who are trying to lose weight or maintain their current weight are often advised not to consume the "empty calories" that come from alcoholic beverages. **Empty calories** are foods such as sugar that supply energy but few or no vitamins and minerals. For example, there are approximately 100 to 150 calories per bottle of beer or small glass of wine. Furthermore, recent studies suggest that drinking alcohol stimulates appetite, so when we drink alcohol we tend to eat more.

 SCIENCE IN ACTION: What Happens When We Combine Caffeinated Drinks and Alcohol?

Alcohol is a depressant, while caffeine is a stimulant. When alcohol is mixed with caffeine or another stimulant, as in a rum and coke, the combination can make people feel less intoxicated than they really are. Drinking alcohol with caffeinated beverages can also cause drinkers to drink more because they feel less intoxicated. The result is that drinkers make poor judgments about what they can do while intoxicated.

Recently, drinkers have been combining alcohol with other caffeinated drinks, or energy drinks. Energy drinks have been available in Canada for only about 15 years. Originally Health Canada categorized this type of drink as "a product for natural health" but more recently changed the categorization to "a product to limit because of caffeine." Health Canada determined, through a national survey, that young people are four to five times more likely to consume caffeinated alcoholic beverages (CABs) than older Canadians. Health Canada has also added warnings to energy drinks stating that these drinks should not be combined with alcohol.

However, people do combine these drinks regularly. In a study of over 400 university students, these were the top five reasons students listed for using CABs:

1. Taste
2. Energy boost
3. Stay awake when drinking
4. Party longer
5. Hide the taste of the alcohol

Two of the most common places to drink CABs were at parties and at the homes of friends. When consumers of CABs were interviewed, they did describe common negative symptoms including dehydration, bad hangover, and vomiting. Furthermore, after drinking CABs, drinkers have a higher likelihood of being sexually assaulted or committing sexual assault, riding in an automobile with a driver who is under the influence of alcohol, driving while under the influence of alcohol themselves, being hurt or injured, and requiring medical treatment. People who became intoxicated by drinking CABs were four times more likely to drive while intoxicated than people who were intoxicated but had not consumed caffeinated drinks. Drinking CABs is associated with even more problems than drinking alcohol alone because CABs mask the effects of alcohol but do not reduce the physiological effects of alcohol on the body.

Student Activity

Reducing alcohol-related diseases, violence, disability, and death is an important public health concern. In 2012, a study conducted by the Canadian Centre on Substance Abuse reported that public and school-based educational initiatives about alcohol were not very effective. Survey five students and ask them why they think public and school-based initiatives to reduce the harm associated with alcohol and CABs aren't very effective or successful.

Alcohol Use and Pregnancy

According to Health Canada, there is no known safe amount of alcohol consumption during pregnancy. Therefore, the best advice is "NO exposure equals NO risk." This doesn't mean that drinking during pregnancy will definitely cause problems in a newborn. It does mean that drinking increases the chance of something going wrong—and the more the mother drinks, the greater the risk. Potential problems include miscarriage, stillbirth, and increased risk of foetal alcohol spectrum disorders (FASD) (figure 19.2). Of course, many women don't immediately know that they're pregnant, and most women quit drinking once they do know. However, a woman who is a drinker and is not yet aware of being pregnant will continue drinking, thus increasing health risks for the embryo. Therefore, for the health of a potential child, a woman who is sexually active and not using reliable birth control should not drink alcohol.

> " Water is the only drink for a wise man. "
>
> —Henry David Thoreau, author

Alcohol Laws

Due to the risk for people to make bad choices and do harm to themselves or others while under the influence of alcohol, most countries in modern society restrict alcohol access only to adults.

Alcohol laws govern the sale, distribution, advertisement, and use of alcohol. Federal alcohol laws apply to everyone across the country; other alcohol laws vary by jurisdiction (city, county, or province). All of these laws govern where and when alcohol can be sold and when it can be consumed in public. Open container laws make it illegal, as the name indicates, to have an open container of alcohol in certain areas, even if you're not actively drinking. If police have a reason to believe you are underage and are in possession of alcohol, they have the right to search you.

Minimum Drinking Age Act

Despite the cultural influences and advertisements that promote drinking among teens, the Canadian provinces and territories make it illegal to drink under the age of 18 or 19 anywhere in Canada (with the exception that parents are allowed to serve alcohol to their own children in their own home). It is illegal for minors to drink at home without their parents present, and it is also illegal for parents to provide alcohol to minors other than their own children. These laws also make it illegal to sell alcohol to minors or purchase alcohol for minors. In addition, laws in many provinces are getting stricter regarding adults who purchase alcohol for minors and for people who use fake identification cards to purchase alcohol. If police find you, as an underage person, in possession of liquor, in a bar, trying to

When a woman drinks alcohol during pregnancy, her baby may suffer the consequences. Here are some of the major complications of drinking during pregnancy.

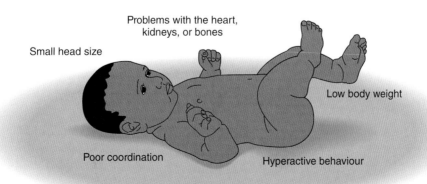

FIGURE 19.2 Problems related to drinking alcohol during pregnancy.

purchase liquor, or using false ID to purchase liquor, the typical fine is over $200. If an adult purchases alcohol for a minor who is then seriously injured or dies due to an alcohol-related cause, the adult may receive a long jail sentence.

Alcohol and Driving

Laws also regulate the use of alcohol with respect to driving for people of all ages. Currently, people violate the Canadian Criminal Code when they have a BAC of 0.08 percent or over and drive. Blood alcohol content is the percentage of alcohol in the bloodstream. A BAC of 0.08 percent indicates that a person has 0.8 parts alcohol per 1,000 parts of blood in the body. However, British Columbia, Manitoba, Newfoundland and Labrador, Nova Scotia, and Ontario have a limit of 0.05 percent at which licence suspensions can take place, and in Saskatchewan it is 0.04 percent during driving. For those under a graduated licensing program (often lasting until the age of 21), there is no tolerance and the BAC level is 0.00 percent.

Table 19.1 summarizes the physiological and psychological effects of selected BAC levels. The table shows the BAC level at which each effect is usually first observed. Getting behind the wheel with a BAC above the legal limit is known as **driving under the influence (DUI)**, impaired driving, or driving while intoxicated. Most deaths and injuries related to alcohol consumption result from vehicle crashes. In Ontario, approximately 13,000 drinking and driving convictions are recorded annually. In Canada, an estimated 1,000 individuals die from alcohol-related crashes each year—about 19 per week, or almost 3 people per day! According to a study conducted by MADD Canada (Mothers Against Drunk Driving), the statistics for motor

TABLE 19.1 Psychological and Physical Effects of Selected Blood Alcohol Content (BAC) Levels

BAC	Typical effects	Predictable effects on driving
0.02	• Some loss of judgment • Relaxation • Slight body warmth • Altered mood	• Decline in visual functions (e.g., rapid tracking of a moving target) • Decline in ability to perform two tasks at the same time (divided attention)
0.05	• Exaggerated behaviour • Possible loss of small-muscle control (e.g., focusing the eyes) • Impaired judgment • Lowered alertness • Release of inhibition	• Reduced coordination • Reduced ability to track moving objects • Difficulty steering • Reduced response to emergency driving situations
0.08	• Poor muscle coordination (e.g., for balance, speech, vision, reaction time, hearing) • Impaired detection of danger • Impaired judgment, self-control, reasoning, and memory	• Reduced concentration • Short-term memory loss • Greatly reduced coordination • Reduced information-processing capability (e.g., signal detection, visual search) • Impaired perception
0.10	• Clear deterioration of reaction time and control • Slurred speech, poor coordination, and slowed thinking	• Reduced ability to maintain lane position and brake appropriately
0.15	• Far less muscle control than normal • Vomiting (unless this level is reached slowly or the person has developed a tolerance for alcohol) • Major loss of balance	• Substantial impairment in vehicle control, attention to driving task, and visual and auditory information processing

Reprinted, by permission, from Human Kinetics, 2009, *Health and wellness for life* (Champaign, IL: Human Kinetics), 398.

vehicle crashes and impairment-related crashes among young drivers are alarming.

- Young people have the highest rates of traffic death and injury per capita among all age groups and the highest death rate per kilometre driven among all drivers under 75 years of age. More 19-year-olds die or are seriously injured than any other age group.

- Motor vehicle crashes are the leading cause of death among 16- to 25-year-olds, and alcohol or drugs (or both) are a factor in 55 percent of those crashes.

- Persons aged 16 to 25 years constituted 13.6 percent of the population in 2010 but made up almost 33.4 percent of the impairment-related traffic deaths.

Studies conclude that young drivers are overrepresented in road crashes for two primary reasons: inexperience and immaturity. Although young people are the least likely to drive impaired, the

An Alcoholic and a Cyclist Meet Twice

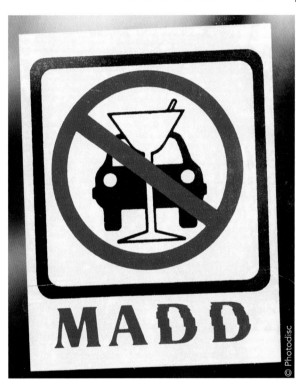

Mothers Against Drunk Driving is an organization that works to stop drunk driving.

A man had a challenging life. He married young; his first and only child died shortly after birth; his wife died of cancer. He used alcohol to medicate feelings of loneliness, sadness, and depression.

Another man also had a challenging life. Work and family kept him busy and provided support but caused stress. He valued fitness and he loved to bike but had not done it for a while. He invested in a new bike and began to ride. He rode for the fitness and psychological benefits and began to discover other benefits as well (enjoying the beauty of nature).

One morning he "met" the alcoholic when he was riding; he had just cycled a kilometre. The next thing he remembered (about three hours later) was lying in a hospital bed getting X-rayed. He had been hit by the truck driven by the alcoholic with a blood alcohol level of 0.18. He recovered in the hospital for about a week; after two months he began to walk unassisted again, and after six months his cranial nerve was healed and he could see properly again. But he could not perform his normal work and family duties because he had forgotten almost everything. Years later he resumed much of his work and battled daily; he would battle for the rest of his life with forgetfulness and constant headaches.

Fifteen months after the collision, the alcoholic and the cyclist met a second time. This time it was in court. It was an opportunity for the cyclist to read a victim impact statement (describing how the collision had changed his life) to the court and to the alcoholic. The judge sent the alcoholic to jail for nine months and took away his license for 10 years. The cyclist went home with lifelong injuries. There are no winners when it comes to drinking and driving.

ones who do are at very high risk of collision; and some young people will choose to drive with someone under the influence rather than preventing a person with a BAC over 0.08 percent from driving or calling 911.

Fortunately, recent years have brought decreases in both the total number of traffic deaths per kilometre driven and the number of alcohol-related crash deaths. Organizations such as Mothers Against Drunk Driving (MADD) have helped raise awareness and increase penalties for drinking and driving. In addition, roads and vehicles have become safer, and more people wear seat belts and use child safety seats. Despite these improvements, far too many alcohol-related traffic deaths still occur. Consider contacting a MADD chapter in your area and asking how you can help reduce drinking and driving and save lives.

Alcohol Dependence and Treatment

Some people who drink alcohol develop a physical dependence (**addiction**). They crave alcohol and don't feel right unless they drink it. What this means is that for some people, drinking gets out of control. They are alcoholics. Many programs are available to help people stop drinking. They include treatment centres, counselling, behaviour modification, medication, Alcoholics Anonymous (AA) groups, online Alcoholics Anonymous (e-AA) groups, other support groups, and even technology (e.g., smartphone apps and text messages). Groups also exist to help family members and friends of problem drinkers; examples include Al-Anon and Alateen. These groups are self-help groups or support groups, in which people with similar problems work together

 FITNESS TECHNOLOGY: Alcohol Safety Apps and Electronics

Technological developments related to alcohol consumption include smartphone apps that can help people with various needs. Some, for example, help adult drinkers count their calories (people are often unaware of how many calories alcoholic beverages contain). Other apps estimate an adult drinker's blood alcohol level based on height, weight, and what drinks were consumed.

In addition, some auto insurance companies offer driver cameras (one brand is **DriveCam**) for use in cars driven by teenagers. These cameras monitor for erratic driving and send notifications to a parent's or guardian's computer. Some insurance companies even monitor the cameras themselves and raise the insurance rate if a teen driver often drives dangerously or erratically. Other companies leave it to parents and guardians to decide how to deal with bad driving.

Another form of technology that is growing in popularity is the **ignition interlock**, which tests drivers' BAC before allowing them to drive. This technology can be court-ordered for people who are found guilty of alcohol-related driving offences. The device is installed in the vehicle at

the offender's expense (in Nova Scotia the cost is approximately $150 for installation; then there is a monthly monitoring fee of approximately $100 and a removal fee of $50). Before the person can start the vehicle, he or she must breathe into the device, which determines the blood alcohol level. If it is above the legal limit, the car will not start. Some of the more sophisticated ignition locks include a camera to ensure that the proper person is blowing into the device. The intent, of course, is to keep people from driving under the influence of alcohol.

Using Technology

With a partner, select a free app on your phone or tablet that calculates your BAC. Select one drink and determine for yourself the number of drinks you would need to consume to have a BAC over 0.08. Discuss with the class your app's features (or lack of features) and what you learned from using the app to help each other. Group support offers help for people with alcohol addiction. People who have taken control of their own alcohol problems help others who are trying to quit. In AA, a person who helps another person is called a sponsor. Because the sponsor has experienced similar problems and challenges, he or she serves as a guide for the person who is trying to stop drinking.

It is difficult to change addictive behaviour. Whenever possible, problem drinkers should seek help from others and know their options. Your school counsellor or school nurse can inform you about local groups that help people with alcohol problems as well as their family members and friends. Make no mistake about it, quitting drinking for an alcoholic is very difficult, but with the right treatment, people can and do overcome their addiction. Most alcohol treatment programs believe that alcoholics should completely refrain from drinking because if the person starts to drink even small amounts, the drinking is likely to escalate to being out of control again.

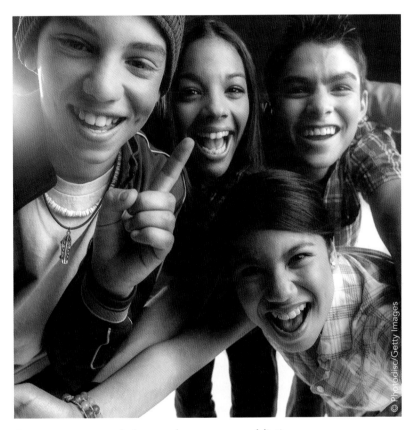

Group support can help people overcome addiction.

Lesson Review

1. What is the definition of alcohol?
2. What are two health problems associated with drinking alcohol?
3. What are two reasons for the differences in alcohol tolerance between males and females?
4. How is binge drinking defined for males and for females?
5. What are three predictable effects of BAC on driving?

Answer true or false to the following questions. For a variation, compare your answers with those of a few friends or fellow students. See if you can all agree on the right answers.

1. Alcohol is a mood-altering stimulant.
   a. true
   b. false

2. Drinking coffee or taking a cold shower will sober a person up.
   a. true
   b. false

3. Alcohol's effects on the body vary according to the individual.
   a. true
   b. false

4. The most serious consequence of consuming alcohol is a hangover in the morning.
   a. true
   b. false

5. Blood alcohol charts that help you estimate your BAC, based on your weight and the number of drinks you have had, provide a safe and accurate means of determining how much alcohol is circulating in your bloodstream.
   a. true
   b. false

6. If an intoxicated person is semiconscious, you should encourage vomiting.
   a. true
   b. false

7. Women and men respond differently to alcohol.
   a. true
   b. false

8. Alcohol increases your sexual functioning.
   a. true
   b. false

9. If a person is passed out from drinking, he or she should be put in bed to "sleep it off."
   a. true
   b. false

10. The legal blood alcohol limit for driving for people under age 19 is 0.08 percent.
    a. true
    b. false

Here are the correct answers: 1b, 2b, 3a, 4b, 5b, 6b, 7a, 8b, 9b, and 10b. If you got 9 or 10 answers right, you're very knowledgeable about alcohol. If you got seven or eight right, you're above average in your knowledge. If you got six or fewer right, spend some time learning about alcohol to protect yourself and your family and friends.

Lesson 19.2
Drugs and Tobacco

Lesson Objectives

After participating in this lesson, you should be able to

1. explain the difference between prescription and over-the-counter drugs,
2. list three guidelines for taking prescription medications,
3. list three dangers that can arise from using illicit drugs,
4. list three long-term health problems caused by cigarette smoking, and
5. describe two negative effects of smoking on pregnancy.

Lesson Vocabulary

chronic obstructive pulmonary disease (COPD), depressant, drug addiction, drug dependence, drug tolerance, illicit drug, muscle dysmorphia, opioids, over-the-counter (OTC) drug, prescription drug, secondhand smoke, smokeless tobacco, stimulant, sudden infant death syndrome (SIDS), withdrawal

Similar to the situation with alcohol, drug and tobacco use and abuse have been around almost as long as people have existed. Many cultures and religions use drugs and tobacco in ceremonies. You may have read about leaders of First Nations passing the "peace pipe" or calumet, which contained tobacco. However, recreational drug use (i.e., using drugs for fun) is common in Canada and can lead to serious health problems, reduce your quality of life, and even lead to death. It is important to gain knowledge about drugs and tobacco if you plan on making healthy lifestyle choices. In this chapter you will learn about the dangers of over-the-counter and illicit drugs as well as the negative health consequences of using tobacco.

 Let food be thy medicine. ""

—Hippocrates, Greek physician
and originator of modern medicine

Prescription Drugs

The purpose of **prescription drugs** is to help people treat illnesses or symptoms, such as pain and discomfort. Prescription drugs are drugs that can be obtained only by means of a physician's prescription. These drugs help millions of people suffering from a wide range of diseases and disorders, and they save millions of lives, but no drug is free of potentially harmful side effects. A prescription should always

do more good than harm; if it doesn't, it should be discontinued or replaced by a different one.

These medications include the following:

- Opioid pain relievers such as those containing oxycodone, hydromorphone, fentanyl, morphine, and codeine
- Stimulants such as those containing dextroamphetamine, methylphenidate, and amphetamines
- Sedative hypnotics such as those containing benzodiazepines like diazepam and alprazolam
- Medications used to treat addiction and pain such as methadone and buprenorphine

Prescription drugs can also be abused, particularly when they are used for nonmedical purposes. According to Health Canada, 80,000 Canadian teenagers used prescription drugs to get high, even though this can be very dangerous. The most commonly misused and abused prescription drugs are called **opioids** (used for pain relief), central nervous system **depressants** or benzodiazepines (used to treat anxiety disorders), and **stimulants** (used most often to treat attention-deficit/hyperactivity disorder [ADHD]). But are North Americans (i.e., Americans and Canadians) taking too many prescription drugs? The U.S. National Institute on Drug Abuse notes that enough painkillers were prescribed in the United States to medicate every

American adult around the clock for a month, and that prescriptions for opioids and stimulants have increased steadily since 1991. After people in the United States, Canadians are the second largest group of users of prescription opioids in the world. How might exercise, different eating patterns, or stronger friendships help us deal with some of the health issues that we now use drugs for?

FIT FACT

North Americans consume approximately 80 percent of the world's opioids (i.e., medications that relieve pain).

There is a cost to too much drug use. In Ontario, deaths related to prescription opioid use doubled in just over 10 years, from 13.7 deaths per million people in 1991 to 27.2 deaths per million people in 2004. That is approximately one person dying every two days in Canada from opioid use. Approximately three people die every day in Ontario from drug overdoses. Some First Nations communities in Canada have taken a progressive stance on prescription drug use by declaring prescription drug overuse and the associated health problems a community crisis.

According to Health Canada, teenagers may choose prescription drugs over illegal drugs for a number of reasons:

- They may have a misperception that prescription drugs are less dangerous when abused than illegal drugs because they are prescribed by a doctor.
- Compared to illegal drugs, prescription drugs may be seen as more attractive for youth because these drugs are legal.
- Young people might also think that getting prescription drugs is easier than getting illegal drugs. The abuse of prescription drugs by youth often involves obtaining these drugs from a friend, from a relative, or from home.

Guidelines for Taking Prescription Medicines

Although experts are far from solving the problem of prescription drug use, people can follow certain good practices to help prevent problems associ-

ated with prescription drugs. First, remember that prescription drugs are intended to help people who have medical problems. Prescription drugs should not make people feel worse or be used for recreational purposes. The following guidelines represent some of the most important practices you can follow to prevent problems with prescription medicines.

- Make sure you understand why your medicine has been prescribed.
- Make sure you get complete instructions about how and when to take the medication. If you don't understand the instructions, ask your doctor or pharmacist to explain them in simpler terms.
- Know the common side effects of your medicine. Ask your doctor or pharmacist to explain them. If you don't understand the wording on the package insert, ask the doctor or pharmacist to give you a printout in language that is easier to understand.
- Always tell your doctor and pharmacist about any other medications (prescription or otherwise) that you take so they can account for any possible drug interactions.
- Don't improvise on your dosage—if you start to feel better, don't stop taking the medication without consulting your doctor or pharmacist.
- Don't share your prescription with anyone else. Doing so is dangerous and against the law.
- Make sure the medication is current. Don't save old medications after they have expired. Many communities have prescription drug take-back events; you can drop off unused or expired drugs and they will be disposed of properly.
- If you have to take more than one medication, develop a system for keeping track of them.
- Find out whether your medication requires you to avoid or limit certain foods or beverages. If so, there is often a warning on the bottle or package insert. That's not always the case, so you should ask your doctor or pharmacist to be sure.
- Alcohol reacts badly with many of the most commonly prescribed drugs. Not only is it illegal for minors to consume alcohol (except

in states where it is legal to consume it in your own home under the supervision of a parent or guardian); in many cases it is also dangerous to consume alcohol along with prescription drugs.

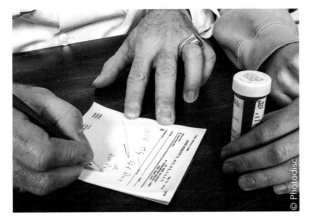

To help prevent problems with prescription drugs, always follow your doctor's instructions, and don't share your prescription or improvise on your dosage.

Over-the-Counter Drugs

Over-the-counter (OTC) drugs are available on the shelf in stores, rather than by prescription, because they are less likely to cause harm and less likely to need close monitoring. Over-the-counter drugs can be helpful in treating minor disorders, aches, and pains. They are generally indicated for short-term use, but that doesn't mean they can't be harmful. Any drug can be harmful if not taken for the intended purpose, or according to the instructions provided, or in the recommended dosage.

Abuse of OTC drugs is most common among teens between the ages of 13 and 16. Because OTC medicines are easily accessible, it is more likely that young people could experiment with them than with prescription drugs. This type of experimentation may seem less harmful than abusing prescription drugs or using illicit drugs, but it carries real risks. It also often leads to the use and abuse of more addictive drugs.

👥 CONSUMER CORNER: Selecting and Using Over-the-Counter Drugs

Over-the-counter drugs include a range of familiar medicines, such as aspirin, decongestants, antacids, nonsteroidal anti-inflammatory drugs (NSAIDs; e.g., ibuprofen), sleep aids, and antihistamines. When purchasing OTC medications, you need to be a wise consumer. All OTC medications should be used only for their intended purpose, according to the directions provided, and in the recommended dosage. When buying and using OTC drugs, use the SAFER guidelines:

- **S**peak up (if the drug doesn't work or seems to be producing bad side effects).

- **A**sk questions (about what the drug can be expected to do).

- **F**ind the facts (ask your doctor or health care professional if he or she recommends this drug).

- **E**valuate your choices. (Is the OTC drug you want to buy the best way to treat your condition?)

- **R**ead the label (make sure this drug is appropriate for you and that it won't interact with any other medication you're taking).

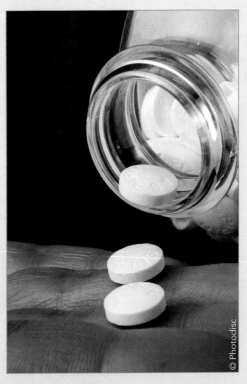

Use the SAFER guidelines when selecting and using OTC drugs.

Illicit Drugs

Illegal drugs are generally referred to as **illicit drugs**. These drugs are often the focus in TV shows and movies—for example, heroin, cocaine, and methamphetamine (meth). In Canada, laws make it illegal not only to use certain drugs but also to give illicit drugs (or your own prescription drugs) to another person, to manufacture or grow illicit drugs, to sell or buy illicit drugs, or to possess illicit drugs.

Using or distributing illicit drugs not only poses potential legal and health problems; there is also a good chance that an illicit, or "street," drug does not contain what the buyer intends to obtain. Studies have found that street drugs are often "cut" with dangerous substances or replaced by other drugs. For example, cocaine has been found to be cut with substances such as flour, powdered milk, ground drywall, rat poison, and battery acid. As a result, if a user has an adverse reaction (bad experience) with the drug, emergency room staff will not know how to treat the person properly because they don't know what the person has ingested.

Risks of Illicit Drugs

Illicit drug use poses many other dangers. For one thing, loss of inhibition can lead a person to take risks that he or she normally wouldn't take—for example, engaging in risky sexual behaviour (which might result in pregnancy or a sexually transmitted infection), driving while impaired, getting in a car with someone who is impaired, taking other drugs, and sharing infected needles. Teens who use illicit drugs have most likely obtained them from friends or siblings. According to the Canadian Centre on Substance Abuse, nearly as many drivers die in road crashes after using drugs (34.2 percent) as drivers who had been drinking (39.1 percent). Basically, and sadly, drugs and alcohol each cause three deaths per day in Canada.

Drug use can also result in drug dependence, which means a person needs a drug in order to function. A person with **drug dependence** typically exhibits signs and behaviour changes such as withdrawing from school activities, being easily aggravated, and being physically sloppy and unclean. Drug addiction, on the other hand, is the compulsive use of a substance despite negative or dangerous effects. A person can be physically dependent on a substance without being addicted to it.

Addiction often includes **drug tolerance**—needing an increasingly high dose to attain the same effect. And, of course, once a person is addicted to a drug, he or she must also deal with emotional and physical withdrawal symptoms when quitting.

Despite all of the possible dangers of using illicit drugs, millions of Canadians do use them, including a significant proportion of teens. For some reason, people often believe they will experience only the positive aspects of drug use—that the negative aspects happen only to other people. However, just as many people don't know they have an allergy until they use a certain substance or eat a certain food; there is no way to know how any given person will respond to a specific drug, dosage, or mixture of drugs and alcohol until it happens.

Marijuana

Marijuana laws are changing because there are disagreements, even among experts, about the medical value of marijuana. Some people believe that the possible harms from marijuana use are less than those from already legal drugs (e.g., tobacco and alcohol for adults). Canada legalized marijuana in 2014 for use in certain medical conditions, like treating the symptoms of cancer and the nausea that chemotherapy might cause. Some people believe the use of marijuana should be a personal choice for adults. Others argue that marijuana has not been subjected to the rigorous testing that is required in order for other drugs to be approved by the Food and Drugs Act (FDA). The Canadian Medical Association believes there is "insufficient scientific evidence available to support the use of marijuana for clinical purposes."

Suffice it to say that marijuana is not suitable for use by young people, whose bodies are still growing and developing and should not be exposed to any known or unknown harms that marijuana use can cause. Research suggests that marijuana use—particularly chronic use—can negatively affect mental and physical health, brain function (memory, attention, and thinking), and driving performance. Marijuana can also harm the cognitive development of children born to women who use marijuana. Yet Canadian youth had the highest rate of marijuana use in 2009-2010 (28 percent) compared to students in other developed countries. Why do we do that to ourselves?

Drug Use to Enhance Performance

Muscle dysmorphia is a condition in which a person sees his or her own body very differently from its actual appearance. As a result, the person may resort to using steroids or other substances to gain muscle mass. "Bulking up" in this way to look more muscular or gain a performance advantage is tempting to many athletes, but it is also dangerous, illegal, and unethical. Most people agree that taking performance-enhancing drugs violates the spirit of good sporting behaviour—sort of like having a secret motor in a sailboat race. It's just not fair, and it's not right. The International Olympic Committee and most sport organizations have strict rules against the use of performance-enhancing drugs such as steroids.

Why Do People Use Illicit Drugs?

Drugs occurring in nature (e.g., in plants or animals) were probably originally consumed by accident a long time ago. Someone ate the bark of a tree, accidentally ingested mold in a food item, or picked up a frog (thus getting a particular substance on his or her hand), and later put the hand in his or her mouth—and as a result experienced an altered state of consciousness. Many people in various cultures viewed such experiences as supernatural, allowing them to talk to the gods.

We now know that most psychoactive drugs distort people's judgment. These are generally the drugs that people take for thrill seeking, consciousness raising (i.e., people believe they have special insights into the meaning of life), or mood elevation. People who take psychoactive drugs may think they are stronger, braver, or more intelligent, but to outside observers this is not so. Still, some people are attracted to the prospect of an altered state of consciousness, and drugs offer a relatively easy—but often unsafe—way to experience it.

Many factors are known to influence a person's likelihood of using illicit drugs. For example, there is a strong connection between drug use and mental illness, especially for people with depression, bipolar disorder, anxiety disorder, and schizophrenia.

Young people often feel invincible and believe that bad things happen to other people but not to them. These types of beliefs may contribute to risky behaviour. In addition, young people may be tempted to take "dares," thinking that they will be perceived as weak if they don't do something dangerous for the benefit of impressing their friends. People are also more likely to use drugs if they have easy access to drugs, if their parents use drugs, if they have low self-esteem, if they are in stressful economic or emotional circumstances, or if they live in a culture with high acceptance of drug use. So why do teens try drugs? According to the Canadian Centre for Addictions, teens use drugs to express their independence and as a way to escape from stress and boredom. But is drug choice really expressing independence and contributing to quality of life? How might you improve your quality of life now and in the future other than by using drugs? How might you deal with stress and boredom more constructively than by using drugs?

Some people think that the attraction of drugs is similar to the lure of magic potions described in fairy tales. People may believe that a substance can make them happier, more beautiful, stronger, more likable, thinner, or more lovable. Drugs are sometimes used to provide a temporary sense of escape or to produce the sensations and feelings they bring. In other words, people often look for external solutions to their problems rather than working to solve problems internally.

You may have heard of famous artists who used drugs and even attributed some of their creativity to their drug use. But drugs do not teach people how to play a musical instrument, write a book, or

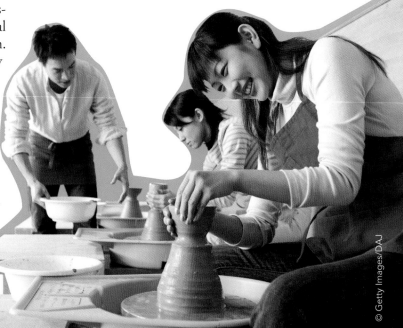

be a good actor or dancer. Talented people practice their art over and over. Alcohol and drugs didn't make Amy Winehouse, Michael Jackson, or Prince great musicians. In fact, drugs made it harder for them to perform and ultimately contributed to their deaths. Other stars who have recently died from drug overdoses include Lisa Robin Kelly, Philip Seymour Hoffman, and Cory Monteith. Unfortunately, people who are dependent on drugs may deceive themselves into thinking that the drugs are essential to their performance. Add to this the addictive nature of drugs, and it's easy to explain why some people keep taking more and more drugs despite the risk of disease, injury, and death.

Drug Fads and Fantasies

Drug use tends to go in social cycles, and the rise of social media (e.g., YouTube, Vimeo, Twitter, Facebook) enables fads to catch on faster and spread farther than ever before. Fads range from drinking cough medicine to using newer, more exotic-sounding substances, such as bath salts, K2, and Spice. Some people even post online videos of drug use, for example taking "eyeball shots" of vodka, which does not get a person drunk but can permanently damage the eye. All of these practices can be very dangerous, but since people see them online or on TV shows, they tend to think of them as safe and even funny.

In fact, there seems to be no end to the various substances that some people try to sell or convince others to use with the promise of happiness, bliss, enlightenment, or just plain fun. It would take several books to discuss all of the fads and fantasies associated with drugs, but the usual pattern involves big promises, followed by experimentation, followed by disappointment (including adverse side effects), and then followed by the next fad that comes along.

Perhaps some people will always believe that a magic potion somewhere out there will make them live happily ever after. In reality, no substance can live up to this expectation in the long run, and experimenting with fad drugs often leads to use of even harder and more dangerous drugs—and to addiction.

Drug Treatment

Just as different drugs can affect different people in different ways, some treatments work for some people but not for others. As discussed in the previous lesson on alcohol, it is difficult to overcome drug dependence or addiction. **Drug addiction** is often recognized on the basis of the drug user's developing a drug tolerance and thus craving more and more of the drug to get the same feeling. If the user is deprived of the drug, he or she goes through **withdrawal**, which can be emotional and physical. These are difficult problems to solve. Even if a person is not drug dependent or addicted, it can still be difficult to change or reverse a drug habit.

For people who are physically dependent or addicted, treatment can involve a range of responses, including counselling, medical intervention, behaviour therapy, support groups (e.g., Narcotics Anonymous), and participation in a rehabilitation program. Some communities have drug courts in which minor drug offenders are assigned to a rehabilitation program to help them stop using drugs instead of going to jail. Treatment can be complicated by dependence on more than one substance and by other medical problems. Despite these various challenges, hundreds of thousands of people in Canada have been able to return to a life free of drug dependence, misuse, and abuse. Of course, it is better to prevent drug problems than to have to treat them.

Tobacco

According to Health Canada, nicotine is the chemical that makes tobacco products so addictive. Tobacco is prepared with the nicotine-rich leaves of tobacco plants, which are cured by a process of drying and fermentation for smoking or chewing. As you introduce nicotine to your body, you will begin to crave more. The use of cigarettes and other forms of tobacco that contain nicotine (such as electronic cigarettes, cigarillos, cigars, pipes, chewing tobacco, and snuff) may lead to addiction. Nicotine is easily absorbed through the lungs and then moves quickly through the bloodstream and into the brain (in less than 10 seconds) and other organs of the body. When nicotine enters a person's bloodstream, it immediately stimulates the

FIT FACT

Studies suggest that 7 out of 10 teenagers will not date someone who smokes.

adrenal glands to release the hormone epinephrine (adrenaline). Epinephrine, in turn, stimulates the person's central nervous system and increases blood pressure, respiration, and heart rate. In addition, glucose is released into the blood, and insulin output from the pancreas is suppressed. These effects result in chronically higher blood sugar among nicotine users. Nicotine is addictive, so stopping smoking and stopping the use of nicotine products is very difficult.

Why Do People Choose to Start Smoking?

According to the 2005 Youth Smoking Survey from Health Canada, the two main reasons teens start to smoke are the perception that it is "cool" (60 percent) and the behaviour of friends or peer pressure (57 percent). Young Canadians (12-24 years) are most at risk of taking up smoking. The same is true in the United States. Most Americans who smoke started before the age of 18 years. The drugs in cigarettes tend to stimulate you when you are down and calm you when you are under stress. In addition, some studies indicate that nicotine might improve the brain functioning of very old people with Parkinson's. However, for most people, the negative effects of tobacco strongly outweigh the positive.

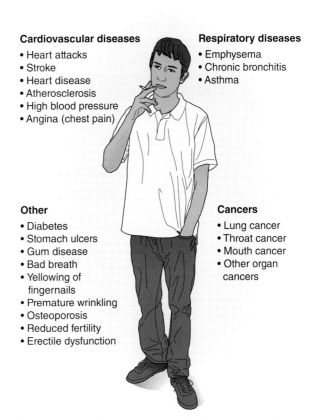

Cardiovascular diseases
• Heart attacks
• Stroke
• Heart disease
• Atherosclerosis
• High blood pressure
• Angina (chest pain)

Respiratory diseases
• Emphysema
• Chronic bronchitis
• Asthma

Other
• Diabetes
• Stomach ulcers
• Gum disease
• Bad breath
• Yellowing of fingernails
• Premature wrinkling
• Osteoporosis
• Reduced fertility
• Erectile dysfunction

Cancers
• Lung cancer
• Throat cancer
• Mouth cancer
• Other organ cancers

FIGURE 19.3 A partial list of diseases and disorders associated with or made worse by smoking.

Health Risks of Tobacco Use

As cool as smoking appears to some, there are well-known immediate and long-term negative health effects. If you have ever smoked, you may recall your first cigarette and how you experienced some or all of these immediate effects: coughing, dizziness, and a dry, irritated throat. Other immediate effects may include nausea, weakness, stomach cramps, headache, coughing, or gagging. As people begin to smoke more regularly they develop a tolerance to nicotine and don't experience those immediate negative health effects. However, the long-term effects of smoking are very serious (figure 19.3).

" Oh, I did stop smoking a long time ago. "

—Mario Lemieux, Hall of Fame hockey player

The science on cigarette smoking is clear. Cigarette smoking is the number one cause of death in North Americans. Cigarette smoking harms nearly every organ in the body. It can cause cardiovascular disease, can cause cancer of the lungs and almost any organ in your body, can make it harder for a woman to get pregnant, and can harm a baby's health before and after birth. Cigarette smoking can also affect men's sperm and increase the risks for birth defects and miscarriage.

Chronic obstructive pulmonary disease (COPD) includes emphysema, bronchitis, asthma, and chronic airway obstruction. About 10,000 Canadians die per year from COPD—more than one person each hour. Smoking causes irreversible decreases in lung function for those with COPD. If it is not difficult enough to have asthma, decreasing your lung function by choosing to smoke tobacco will decrease the length and quality of your life even more.

FIT FACT

Lung cancer is the leading cause of cancer deaths in Canada for both men and women. Eighty-five percent of all lung cancer cases are attributed to cigarette smoking. On average, two Canadians die every hour from lung cancer.

Types of Tobacco

Tobacco is legally available to adults in Canada in many different forms. Manufactured cigarettes are the most commonly used form, followed by cigars (large cigars, cigarillos, and little cigars), smokeless tobacco (chewing tobacco and snuff), pipes, and hookahs (water pipes). Other forms include bidi cigarettes (hand rolled in special leaves) mostly from India and Kreteks (cigarettes containing cloves and tobacco). None of these modes of tobacco use are considered to be safe with long-term use.

Other Tobacco Products

Secondhand smoke is also very harmful. Second-hand smoke is smoke that is inhaled involuntarily from tobacco being smoked by another person. Nonsmokers exposed to secondhand smoke breathe in the same harmful chemicals as smokers. No exposure to secondhand smoke is safe. Third-hand smoke, smoke that lingers in carpets, sofas, clothes, and other materials hours or even days after a cigarette is put out, is a health hazard for infants and children. Using **smokeless tobacco** products, such as chewing tobacco or snuff, can also affect your health. These products increase the risk for different types of cancer and can lead to gum disease, high blood pressure, heart disease, and stroke.

A relatively new product has been introduced to the market—electronic cigarettes, or e-cigarettes. These products liquefy and vaporize nicotine into an aerosol mist. Users puff (sometimes called "vape") on the e-cigarette to get the nicotine that they crave. The e-cigarette looks like a cigarette and has the approximate feel of a cigarette, but the vapour is not smelly to the user or to those nearby. E-cigarettes have helped many people cut back on traditional cigarettes, but because there is not enough research on their possible harmful effects, there has been considerable debate among experts regarding what to do about these new nicotine delivery systems. Some experts want to ban or regulate e-cigarettes until more is known about the possible harmful effects. Others believe that e-cigarettes are valuable for harm reduction. This means they believe that e-cigarettes are safer than traditional cigarettes. It is important to note that there have been instances when e-cigarette devices have malfunctioned, resulting in serious facial burns to the smoker. Aside from the possible levels of harm that may be found, no health or medical experts recommend the use of e-cigarettes by people who do not currently use nicotine products.

Are Light Cigarettes Safer?

Sometimes people are tricked into believing that light cigarettes are safer than regular cigarettes. This is not true. In fact, there is no established safe level of tobacco smoking. Side-stream smoke, or secondhand smoke, can be more dangerous than smoke that is directly inhaled from a cigarette, cigar, or pipe because the particles in the secondhand smoke are smaller. Most people are not exposed to secondhand smoke as often as smokers are exposed to direct smoke, though. Of course, smokers breathe in both direct and secondhand smoke.

FIT FACT

As you begin to smoke more, your fingers and teeth become nicotine stained, your clothes smell like smoke, and, unless you brush your teeth and wash your hands, face, and clothes often, you smell awful to nonsmokers.

Nicotine and Addiction

Nicotine in cigarettes and nicotine in smokeless tobacco are both harmful. Nicotine from smoking may enter the body faster than nicotine absorbed through the mouth or gums. If a given amount of nicotine enters the body, regardless of the source, the harm is the same. Because people tend to use tobacco products at a level that satisfies them, the blood levels of nicotine in smokeless and smoked tobacco users tend to be very similar over the period of a day.

Like cocaine, heroin, and marijuana, nicotine increases a person's level of the neurotransmitter dopamine, which affects the brain pathways that control reward and pleasure. For many tobacco users, long-term brain changes induced by continued nicotine exposure result in addiction—a condition of compulsive drug seeking and use even in the face of negative consequences. Nicotine is actually more addictive than drugs like cocaine, but cocaine has a much greater potential for causing immediate harm than nicotine.

Costs of Smoking

One cigarette costs about 50 cents. An average youth smoker (8.8 cigarettes per day) spends about $5.00 per day, $35.00 per week, $1,820 per year, and $109,200 in a lifetime (if a 15-year-old smoked until the age of 75 years). You could purchase a brand new MINI Cooper every 15 years or make a significant dent in purchasing a home for that kind of money. But what about costs to Canada and Canadians? The Alberta government estimated that the annual health care cost to treat people in Canada for damages caused by smoking is approximately $4.5 billion—or that nearly $1,300 is paid each year by you and every Canadian for the health costs incurred by those who smoke. In addition, about 3,500 fires each year are caused by smokers. The cost for that is approximately $43 million per year. Just think of what else we could do with all of that money!

FIT FACT

If you choose to smoke, you are choosing to live with more disability, a lower quality of life, and a more painful death.

Smoking and Pregnancy

Smoking during pregnancy is not a good idea. A pregnant mother who smokes has a higher risk of having a baby with a low birth weight. Low birth weight is one of the main causes of illness and disability in babies and also increases the risk of a baby's being stillborn. Furthermore, smoking in pregnancy increases the risk of **sudden infant death syndrome (SIDS)** by four times if the woman has between

Women who smoke during pregnancy are more likely to have vaginal bleeding or problems with the placenta.

Babies born to women who smoke during pregnancy are more likely to be born with birth defects such as cleft lip or palate or be underweight or still-born.

Babies exposed to secondhand smoke are more likely to die from SIDS (sudden infant death syndrome); be at greater risk for asthma, bronchitis, pneumonia, ear infections, and respiratory symptoms; or experience slow lung growth.

FIGURE 19.4 Effects of smoking on infant health.

one and nine cigarettes a day. This rises to an eight times higher risk of SIDS if she smokes 20 cigarettes or more a day. Other harmful effects include miscarriage, premature labour, placental abruption, and vaginal bleeding. Smoking may also affect the child's mental development and behaviour, leading to a short attention span and hyperactivity—and the list goes on. If someday you are pregnant and smoking, for the sake of the child you need to stop smoking (see figure 19.4).

Policies and Laws

In recent years, many policies and laws have dramatically changed how people view smoking in Canada. It is now hard to believe that at one time people could smoke on airplanes, in movie theatres, in school teachers' lounges, and even in hospitals. Smoke-free laws have been implemented in most of Canada. Many workplaces have created their own smoke-free policies—for example, banning smoking in company vehicles or even anywhere on the organization's property. Not surprisingly, most hospitals have also banned smoking on their property—inside or outside. Your school probably does not allow smoking on school property.

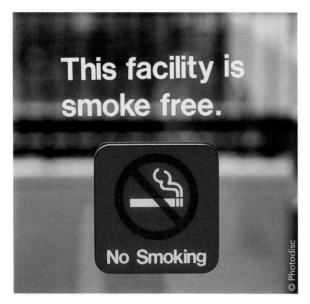

This facility is smoke free.

No Smoking

© Photodisc

Where there are fewer places for people to smoke, more people quit smoking.

Smoking bans have been passed for several reasons. Probably the most important one is to protect others from secondhand smoke, especially the children of smokers. Just as construction companies require their workers to wear helmets to protect them from injury, policies and laws have been passed to protect workers from the dangers of secondhand smoke. Physicians for a Smoke-Free Canada estimates that 1,000 (and perhaps as many as 7,800) deaths per year in Canada are related to secondhand smoke.

When children are exposed to secondhand smoke at home, they are more likely to suffer severe asthma attacks and other respiratory conditions, such as bronchitis, coughing, and sneezing. Smoking bans reduce the risks of heart attack in both smokers and nonsmokers and thus are considered an effective mechanism for creating a healthier society.

Another reason for laws and policies against tobacco use is the fact that nonsmokers greatly outnumber smokers. The greater the gap grows between nonsmokers and smokers, the more likely communities are to enact policies and laws restricting smoking. Nonsmokers find it unfair to have to inhale secondhand smoke at work or in restaurants and other public places.

As you might expect, where there are fewer places for people to smoke, more people quit smoking. With the passage of more and more smoking bans, the habit of smoking is becoming increasingly difficult for people to maintain.

Legal Age for Buying Tobacco Products

The legal age to purchase tobacco products in Canada is either 18 or 19 years, depending on the province you live in. Stores are not allowed to sell to people under the legal age. Many communities conduct compliance checks by having people under the legal age try to buy tobacco in order to see if the business operator properly checks identification rather than selling the product to a minor. Businesses that sell to minors are often fined, and many times the employee who sold to the minor is fired. If a business repeatedly sells tobacco to minors, it may lose its license to sell tobacco products. It is also illegal for adults to purchase tobacco for minors.

Depending on provincial law, minors who try to purchase tobacco products could also be fined or assigned to perform community service. Purchasing tobacco (or alcohol) with a fake ID is a much more serious offence, and it is also illegal to make, manufacture, or sell fake IDs; doing so can result in a felony conviction and a large fine.

Time to Quit?

If you have been smoking for a few months or years, you may have started noticing that it's costing a lot of money. Maybe it's making your body feel unhealthy. Maybe it's getting harder to find a comfortable place to smoke, and you'd rather not hang out in the cold and rain. Maybe your friends are making unwelcome comments about how you smell, or maybe there's a special person you like and you think he or she won't care for the habit or the smell. You are past the precontemplation (not thinking about quitting) stage and are contemplating how to stop smoking. You might want to stop smoking by gradually cutting back on cigarettes, or you may want to quit "cold turkey" (quit right away). You might have strategies in place like chewing gum when you want a smoke or going for a walk when you want a smoke. You might also get a nicotine patch. Whatever methods you choose, it is usually best if you quit with the social support of someone you trust and are close with. School counsellors and professional counsellors might be able to provide support to help you successfully quit smoking.

The Smokers' Helpline provides a number of fun challenges to help you stay focused, complete with e-mail messages. It also has quitting coaches to

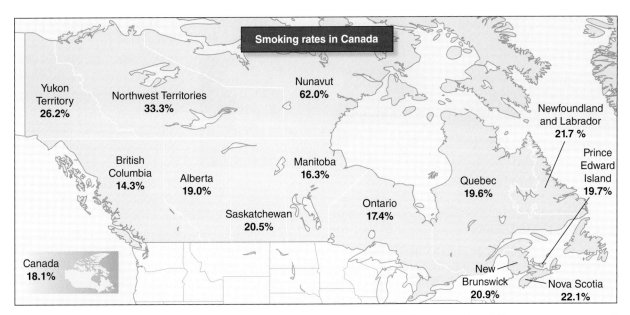

Smoking rates in Canada

Yukon Territory 26.2%

Northwest Territories 33.3%

Nunavut 62.0%

Newfoundland and Labrador 21.7 %

Prince Edward Island 19.7%

British Columbia 14.3%

Alberta 19.0%

Manitoba 16.3%

Quebec 19.6%

Saskatchewan 20.5%

Ontario 17.4%

Canada 18.1%

New Brunswick 20.9%

Nova Scotia 22.1%

FIGURE 19.5 What are some reasons you think the rates are so different in the different provinces and territories?

help you. Just call for free at 1-877-513-5333. The personnel are there to help you increase your health and quality of life by quitting smoking.

As with most behaviour change strategies, no single program works for everyone. There are enough options, though, that one is bound to work for you. It may take several tries, but persistence pays off. Just as you can't become a great athlete or musician (or anything) without making lots of mistakes, you can't stop smoking without facing some setbacks. But each setback you overcome makes it more likely that you'll eventually succeed.

The Good News: Fewer People Are Smoking

The number of people smoking tobacco has been declining for the last number of years. Only one out of five students in grades five through nine has ever tried any type of tobacco product. The average age for Canadian youth to start smoking is 12. The 2012 current smoking rate was 8 percent for males and 6 percent for females. Four percent of youth aged 15 to 17 smoked daily, consuming an average of 8.8 cigarettes per day. Smoking rates vary across Canada (see figure 19.5). The statistics are moving in a positive direction as fewer and fewer teens turn to cigarettes as a way to be cool—in fact, smoking is considered by most to be uncool. Nevertheless, smoking is addictive. According to research on North Americans, about 80 percent of high school students who smoke will smoke into adulthood.

> " Quitting smoking is easy, I've done it 1,000 times. "
>
> —Mark Twain, author

FIT FACT

According to Health Canada, in 2012, the smoking rate among youth aged 15 to 17 years was 7 percent, representing about 93,000 youth, the lowest ever recorded.

Lesson Review

1. What is the difference between prescription and OTC drugs?
2. What are three guidelines for taking prescription medications?
3. What are three dangers that can arise from using illicit drugs?
4. What are three long-term health problems caused by cigarette smoking?
5. How does smoking negatively affect pregnancy? Provide two examples.

⚡ TAKING CHARGE: Building Strong Refusal Skills

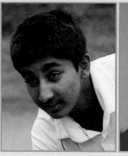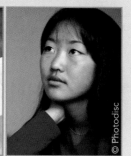

Everyone says no to something at least once in a while, but sometimes it's more important than at other times. Being able to say no—that is, having strong refusal skills—helps you navigate risky or complicated situations with better results. Saying no may seem like a simple skill, but doing it effectively and comfortably requires confidence and practice. It's important to be able to say no without feeling guilty or self-conscious.

Emily was invited to her new friend Amelia's house after school. She liked Amelia and was excited to go, but when they got to the house she quickly realized that things weren't right. Amelia's parents weren't home, and her older brother was drinking beer and seemed to be on some sort of drug. When she asked Amelia about it, Amelia said, "Yeah, my brother scores marijuana from a guy at work, and we light up out back when no one else is home." Emily immediately felt nervous because she didn't agree with using drugs for recreation. Her stomach was in knots, and she felt really uncomfortable when she saw Amelia get a small package out of her brother's bag.

Charles was working hard to lose some weight and get in better shape. So far, he had lost approximately 3 kilograms (6.5 pounds) in just under three weeks. Then a few of his buddies invited him over to watch the Super Bowl, and they were all bringing food with empty calories. He knew that they'd be eating a lot and that food would be a big part of the event. As part of his diet, however, Charles was eating only lean meats, fruits, vegetables, and whole grains, and he was drinking only water and tea. Last time the guys had watched a game together, they had all gotten sick on chicken wings, nachos, chili, and soda. Charles knew that his friends would pressure him to join the party and tell him he could just take some diet pills the next day.

For Discussion

Both Emily and Charles need to use refusal skills. Emily is in a dangerous situation and is feeling uncomfortable. Charles isn't in danger, but he doesn't want to wreck his hard work or feel bad about his choices the next day. What strategies can Emily use to say no? What strategies can Charles use? What might some of the long-term consequences be if Emily can't develop effective refusal skills? What about Charles?

➡ SELF-MANAGEMENT: Skills for Strong Refusal

Being able to say no is a key part of building refusal skills. Throughout your life, you'll be presented with opportunities and choices that may require you to say no in order to be true to your beliefs and values and maintain your health and safety. Use the following tips to help you say no when necessary.

- **Know what you believe and stick to it.** Having a strong and clear sense of your personal values goes a long way in helping you say no when you need to.

- **Be assertive.** When you say no, do it with conviction. You don't need to be

mean or aggressive. Instead, stand tall, make eye contact with the person or people you're talking to, and simply say "No, thank you" or "No, that is not something I am willing to do."

- **Don't apologize for saying no.** If you feel strongly about a choice you're making, don't apologize for it. Apologizing makes it easier for others to talk you out of your decision. Rather than saying, "I'm sorry, guys, but I don't want to do that," say, "I understand that you want to do this, but I don't want to, and I am saying no."

© Photodisc

- **Offer alternatives.** If someone pressures you to do something you don't want to do, say no and also consider offering an alternative choice. If you don't want to smoke, suggest going for coffee instead. If you don't want to be alone with someone else, suggest meeting in a public place like a park.

- **Support others when they say no.** If you offer your support when a friend or family member refuses something, that person will likely support you when you do so. You often get the same treatment from others that you give them.

- **Have a plan.** If you're going out with friends, know what your plan is and stick to it. Making spontaneous decisions may seem fun, but it often leads to situations in which you feel pressured or uncomfortable. Having a plan for healthy living also makes it easier to say no to unhealthy food choices and to choose an active pursuit rather than a sedentary one.

TAKING ACTION: Raising Your Awareness About Alcohol, Drug, and Tobacco Abuse

Unfortunately, alcohol, drug, and tobacco abuse is common in Canada and even common among teens. Becoming aware of a problem is the first step to solving that problem. Fortunately, numerous and easily accessible resources can help you identify the signs and symptoms; learn about the health effects; understand some of the psychological issues; and access support for alcohol, drug, and tobacco abuse. These resources are also created for and cater to teens. Take action by searching the Internet to access the following free and confidential resources to become aware and develop the tools to support your friends, family, and loved ones:

- Alateen
- Kids Help Phone
- Smokers' Helpline
- Government of Canada: Healthy Canadians (healthycanadians.gc.ca)

madd* GET ACTIVE WITH MADD CANADA

Saving Lives, Supporting Victims
Used courtesy of MADD Canada.

Who We Are

MADD Canada (Mothers Against Drunk Driving) is a national charitable organization committed to stopping impaired driving and supporting the victims of this violent crime. At the heart of MADD Canada are our volunteers; they include not only mothers but fathers, friends, business professionals, experts in the anti-impaired driving field, and concerned citizens who want to make a difference in the fight against impaired driving.

What We Do

MADD Canada strives to offer support services to victims and survivors and their families and friends, heighten awareness about the dangers of alcohol- and drug-impaired driving, and save lives and prevent injuries on our roads. Our key program areas include victim and survivor services, youth services, public awareness and education, public policy, and technology.

Get Involved

MADD Canada is always looking for youth leaders who want to take action and join the fight to end impaired driving. Get involved with your local MADD Canada chapter and help them raise awareness about the dangers of impaired driving. Or get active in your school. Download our *Youth Resource Manual*, which helps schools and youth groups raise awareness about impaired driving. Visit us on the web at www.madd.ca.

Used courtesy of MADD Canada.

Reviewing Concepts and Vocabulary

Complete the following in order to determine your growing understanding of fitness, health, and wellness. Answer items 1 through 5 by correctly completing each sentence with a word or phrase.

1. Two natural physiological responses to drinking that protect people from acute alcohol poisoning are _____ and _____.

2. Two diseases that can be caused by smoking are _____ and _____.

3. When a person who drinks alcohol regularly over a long time no longer gets the same effect from drinking the same amount, she or he has developed an _____.

4. A drug requiring a physician's approval is called a _____ drug.

5. _____ drugs are generally the ones that people take for thrill seeking, consciousness raising, and mood elevation.

For items 6 through 10, match each term in column 1 with the appropriate phrase in column 2.

6. BAC
7. drug addiction
8. binge drinking
9. withdrawal
10. 45,000

a. compulsive use of a substance
b. consuming a large amount of alcohol in a short time
c. deaths each year by cigarette smoking
d. the concentration of alcohol in the blood
e. physical and emotional condition that occurs when a drug is stopped

For items 11 through 15, respond to each statement or question.

11. Identify two things that make underage drinking unhealthy or dangerous.
12. What does the acronym SAFER stand for, and what does it help you understand?
13. Give two reasons why people use illegal drugs.
14. List two treatments for alcohol dependence.
15. List two reasons why a person might start smoking.

Thinking Critically

Write a paragraph in response to the following questions.

Do you think that people who break the law while under the influence of drugs or alcohol should be required to go to jail or should be required to enrol in mandatory treatment? Explain your answer and use specific facts to support your position.

Project

Prepare an attention-grabbing poster that informs teens about the dangers associated with one of the following:

- Alcohol
- Drugs
- Prescription drugs
- Tobacco

On the poster, be sure to identify at least one resource that helps teens deal with addictions for the substance you chose.

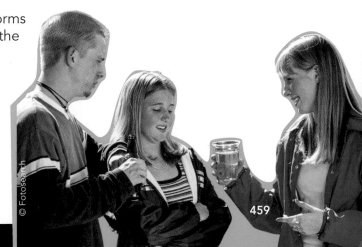

© Fotosearch

20

Reproductive and Sexual Wellness

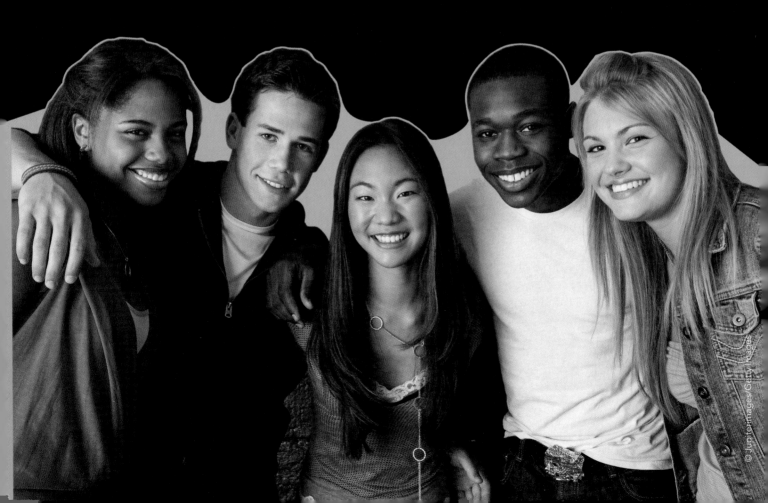

© Jupiterimages/Getty Images

Lesson 20.1
Sexuality and Sexual Orientation

Lesson Objectives

After participating in this lesson, you should be able to
1. explain (define and describe) sexuality,
2. explain the various influences on an individual's sexuality, and
3. explain what sexual orientation is.

Lesson Vocabulary

abstinence, age of consent, bisexual, celibacy, contraception, gay, HIV, lesbian, questioning, sexual assault, sexuality, sexual orientation, transgender

Sexuality is an important part of the life of human beings. It is described in this chapter as the feelings, thoughts, identities, sensuality, intimacy, and reproduction of people. The terms *sex* and *sexuality* are often used interchangeably and can also include being attracted by and attractive to others, in a relationship, and in love. Given the importance of sexuality, young people should be taught factual and complete information about it and have access to confidential reproductive and sexual health services. Young people should be treated with respect; they should be involved in decisions about what they learn and should have input about policies that affect them. Even so, sex education in school is a controversial topic, one that should be discussed in a mature, factual manner.

The basis for much of the information presented in this chapter was developed by young people, teachers, and medical and public health experts over a two-year period and was presented in the Canadian Guidelines for Sexual Health Education. In this first lesson, you'll learn about sex and sexuality, media influence on people's views of sexuality, and sexual orientation.

Sex and Sexuality

The word "sex" is used in different ways. Most commonly it refers to your biological classification, the state of being male or female. The word "sex" is also used to refer to a sexual relationship or sexual contact with someone (act of having sex). At other times it is used as a shortened version of the word "**sexuality**." In this chapter we refer to sexuality education. However, both "sex" and "sexuality" are used as they relate to various concepts in this chapter.

Sexuality has been the topic of literature and dramatic performances for hundreds of years. In modern society, it has also been a frequent topic of television shows, popular songs, and movies. And now, of course, we can add the Internet and smartphones to the list of ways in which messages

FIT FACT

The more people know about human sexuality, the more likely it is that their sexual relationships will be positive. Information provides the basis for making good decisions that support individual beliefs. Not all people share the same beliefs about human sexuality, and not all people will use the information they learn about human sexuality in the same way. Once you are informed about the facts, you can use the information to make decisions that are consistent with your values and beliefs. In fact, study after study has revealed that students who participate in comprehensive sex education classes are much more likely than others to have good sexual health and stronger sexual relationships when they choose to become sexually active. Effective sex education can help you understand that sexual development is a normal, natural, healthy part of your human development.

about sexuality are communicated. In one way or another, sexuality affects many aspects of life—for example, love, communication, relationships, law, health, media, and culture.

Most wellness issues involve both positive and negative aspects. Drugs, for example, can heal us or harm us, depending on how they are used. The same is true of human sexuality. Sexual relationships can be loving, fulfilling, and life affirming. They can also be manipulative, degrading, or, as in the case of **sexual assault**, dangerous.

Am I Normal?

Young people often ask, "What is normal sexual development and sexual behaviour?" Believe it or not, that's a difficult question to answer. Statistics, like some given in this chapter, can let you know what is average or what is common, but "normal" is a value-laden word. For example, if a person chooses a life of **celibacy** (i.e., refrains from sexual activity), is that normal? One could reasonably say that it is normal, respected, and even expected among certain religious leaders and their followers. Most adults, however, choose to engage in sexual relationships, though the age at which they do so

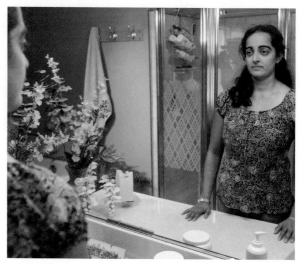

Most people wonder if they are normal when it comes to sexual behaviour and sexual development.

varies widely. Many health experts and religious leaders believe that certain types of sexual behaviours should be reserved for adults, but people can hold different views even on the question of when a person becomes an adult. Also, puberty, which affects sexual development, happens anywhere from about the age of 10 to 16, with some individuals beginning puberty earlier and some beginning puberty later. There isn't an exact time in which sexual development takes place, as it is truly an individual experience.

In Canada, the **age of consent** for sexual activity is 16. This applies to all forms of sexual activity ranging from sexual touching (e.g., kissing) to sexual intercourse. However, there are also many exceptions depending on what is being done and who it is being done with. For example, sexual activity with someone under the age of 18 is illegal if the other person is in a position of trust or authority, if it involves exploitation such as prostitution or pornography, and if anal sex occurs. Legal age of consent is just one example of the potentially confusing aspects of human sexuality. Others include laws and policies addressing birth control and abortion access, which are equally complex and varied. Even school policies vary widely on a number of topics—for example, how students

SCIENCE IN ACTION: Growth and Development, or Puberty

Hair growth in new places, menstruation (a period), body odour, lower voices in both girls and boys, breast changes in both boys and girls—these are just some of puberty's telltale signs. What is the science behind it all? The hypothalamus in the brain begins to release a hormone for the first time. This hormone travels

to the pituitary gland where even more hormones are released, but this time to many different parts of the body. What happens next depends on whether you are boy (e.g., sperm and testosterone are produced) or a girl (e.g., eggs mature and are released; estrogen production begins maturing the body in preparation for pregnancy).

Student Activity

Pimples and acne are a common concern during puberty. Search for ways to "treat" and help reduce pimples and acne (i.e., search the Internet or ask the school health nurse, a doctor, or other knowledgeable person). What advice could you give to someone trying to "treat" or reduce the occurrence of pimples or acne? Be careful of the myths that are circulating out there.

are allowed to dress, access the Internet, dance at school functions, hold hands or kiss on school property, and hold after-school meetings of organizations such as LGBTQ+ (**lesbian**, **gay**, **bisexual**, **transgender**, queer/**questioning**, and others) clubs. As a result, it's always a good idea to find out the rules, policies, and laws in your school, community, and country. Of course, they may be changed over time to reflect ongoing developments in societal values.

Influences on Human Sexuality

Our views of sexuality are affected by a wide range of influences—for example, family, friends, school, culture, society, religion, and the media. Thus we don't learn about sexuality only from formal institutions, such as schools or religious groups. Sometimes, in fact, these influences are weaker—and other influences are stronger—than we think. Between 2006 and 2008, for example, among teens aged 15 to 19 years, 93 percent had received formal instruction about sexually transmitted infections (STIs), 89 percent about human immunodeficiency virus (**HIV**), and 84 percent about **abstinence** (i.e., refraining from sex). But only about 67 percent had received formal instruction about **contraception**, and fewer males (62 percent) had received it than females (70 percent). In addition, although a large majority of students may receive certain types of sex

education, they likely spend more time receiving messages about sexuality from other sources, such as family, friends, religious groups, television, movies, advertising, and using the Internet for information.

What's more, the information you receive about sexuality—whether online, from a friend, or from

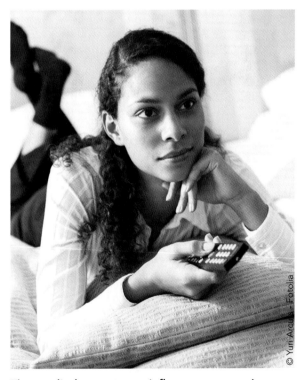

The media has a strong influence on our views on sexuality, but much of the information can be incorrect or incomplete.

a parent—is sometimes incorrect or incomplete. Not even all medical professionals have been well educated about sexuality issues. Therefore, you need to develop the skills to find reliable information and communicate effectively with others about sexuality. To do so, you can use some of the principles in the Taking Charge sections in this book. Unlike what is suggested in popular TV shows, music, and movies, relationship problems in real life don't always get solved quickly and easily. You'll get better information if you seek out knowledgeable adults, such as school counsellors and health professionals who specialize in sexual wellness and communication skills. You can also find reliable information on the web pages of the Public Health Agency of Canada, Health Canada's Sexual Health and Promotion, SexandU, KidsHealth, and other reputable agencies, organizations, and websites.

How much do you think the media influences teenagers' understanding of sex and sexuality? What are some of the sexuality-related messages you've seen presented in media sources? How might these messages influence your behaviours and choices?

Most people would like to believe that we're not influenced by advertising or other mass media, but research shows that we are. The same is true for the influence of our friends and family; in fact, we often underestimate the influence that family members and friends exert on us. Our culture also greatly influences how people dress, act, date, and recreate. Even people who know a lot about sexuality often make poor decisions when they are sexually aroused or under the influence of alcohol or other drugs. The emotional parts of the human brain tend to dominate the more logical parts at times.

For example, hundreds of thousands of teens have taken a vow not to have sex before they get married. These teens are sincere and well intentioned, but when they are faced with sexual temptation or the opportunity to have sex with someone they really like or love, their resolve may weaken. In addition, evidence shows that when students who participate in abstinence-only programs (which don't provide full sexuality education) do have sex, they are less likely to use a contraceptive, which means that they face an increased risk of unintended pregnancy and STIs. On the other hand, when students are taught how to prevent pregnancy and STIs, they are more likely to be prepared to properly practice safer sex than those who believe they will always be able to abstain. Of course, some people can and do remain abstinent until marriage, yet surveys indicate that about 70 percent of teens have had sex by age 19.

Changing Cultural Norms

Cultural norms change over time, including norms related to sexuality. For example, according to Statis-

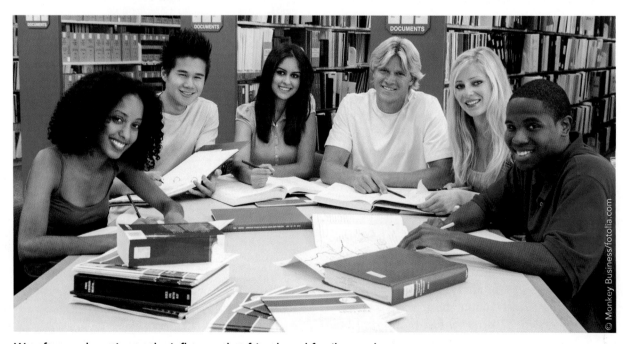

We often underestimate the influence that friends and family members exert on us.

tics Canada, the average age of marriage in Canada is 31 for men and almost 30 for women. Changing norms also affect who can get married; specifically, same-sex couples can now marry in Canada. In another area of sexuality, the Canadian teen birth rate has decreased by 68 percent since 1996, even though more than half of unmarried teens (ages 15 to 19) reported that they had had sex. Of course, the phrase "having sex" can mean different things to different people, ranging from sexual intercourse to oral sex and other types of sexual interaction. Yet young people who are sexually active—whatever their definition of sex—make up more than their share of new cases of STIs, which are discussed later in this chapter.

Sexual Orientation

According to Parents and Friends of Lesbians and Gays (PFLAG), Canada's only national organization that helps all Canadians with issues of sexual orientation, gender identity, and gender expression, **sexual orientation** "represents an important part of each of us, as individuals, and defines who we are naturally attracted to." Sexual orientation refers to the sexuality of each of us, straight (heterosexual), gay or lesbian (homosexual), bisexual, or asexual. Despite much research, professionals and scientists have not reached an agreement about the reasons that individuals develop a heterosexual, gay or lesbian, bisexual, or asexual orientation. However, many researchers do think both that nature and nurture play a role in an individual's sexual orientation, as most individuals experience little or no sense of choice in their sexual orientation.

It's common today to hear the term *LGBTQ+* as a group noun referring to people who are lesbian, gay, bisexual, transgender, queer/questioning (questioning people are unsure of their sexual orientation or gender identity), and others (e.g., two-spirited:

traditionally referring to a respected leader in some Aboriginal communities as having both a male and female spirit). As with other issues involving human sexuality, people's views vary, and some people raise moral or religious concerns about being lesbian, gay, bisexual, transgender, queer/questioning, and other. In addition, people sometimes disagree about the very terms used to talk about sexuality. For example, some people find the phrase "sexual preference" problematic; they argue that people do not choose their sexuality and thus it is similar to handedness (being left- or right-handed). Do people choose to be right- or left-handed? Do straight people choose to be straight? There was a time when parents and teachers tried to force left-handed people to be right-handed, but ultimately people came to believe that it is best for naturally left-handed people to be left-handed and naturally right-handed people to be right-handed. Of course, sexual orientation is more complex than handedness, but some people find that the comparison can help us understand individual differences.

People who are lesbian, gay, bisexual, transgender, queer/questioning, or other may experience prejudice and discrimination that can have negative psychological effects. As a result, many schools, universities, and government entities have established antidiscrimination policies or laws. Many private organizations also work to prevent discrimination against lesbian, gay, bisexual, transgender, queer/

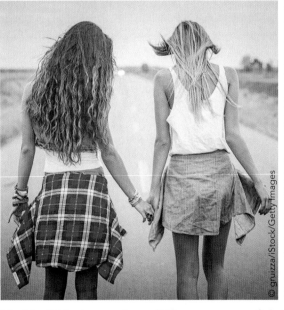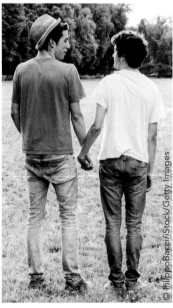

Most individuals experience little or no sense of choice in their sexual orientation.

questioning, and other people. At the same time, many others work against equal rights for LGBTQ+ people and believe that gays and lesbians should be encouraged to become heterosexual. The American Psychological Association's statement on that approach is as follows: "To date, there has been no scientifically adequate research to show that therapy aimed at changing sexual orientation (sometimes called reparative or conversion therapy) is safe or effective."

While there may always be some prejudice and discrimination regarding people who are lesbian, gay, bisexual, transgender, queer/questioning, or other, it is important to be accepting of everyone. Regardless of whether it is sexual orientation, religious views, political views, or any other controversial topic, there may be disagreement based on personal opinions. Learning to be tolerant of others regardless of their sexual orientation is of great importance to each individual's dignity and self-esteem. Being respectful of an individual's sexual orientation doesn't mean you necessarily agree with it, but you do respect the individual and the values he or she holds as a person.

Being Transgender

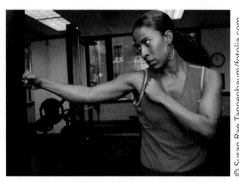

© Susan Rae Tannenbaum/fotolia.com

LGBTQ+ groups, found in more schools every year, offer a healthy and supportive environment for adolescents questioning their sexuality.

My name is Kelly, and I am transgender (a word referring to instances in which a person's inner sense of gender does not correspond to his or her biological sex as male or female). From the time I was little, I knew that I was meant to be a girl although everyone else thought of me as a boy. My body didn't match my feelings. I remember wanting to be like my sister Lisa, and I remember feeling confused and self-conscious about it. I wanted to wear her clothes, grow my hair like hers, and play with her tea sets and toys.

When I started going through puberty, it was unbearable. I hated the way my body was changing, and my feelings kept getting stronger. One day my mom confronted me—she asked me if I was gay. I said no. I told her that I was attracted to boys but that I didn't want to be one—I told her I was a straight girl and not a gay guy. She didn't understand, and we fought about it for years. Luckily, I found support in my school's LGBTQ+ (lesbian, gay, bisexual, transgender, queer/questioning, and others) support group, and I kept bringing home pamphlets and information from my school counsellor. Over time, we started to talk openly about it, and when I was in college I started hormone therapy and transitioned into living as a girl full-time. I was lucky to have really supportive friends in college.

For the first time in my life, I feel whole, and I am finally beginning to feel comfortable in my skin. I worry that I will never find love or have a family of my own, but for now I am happy to finally just be me.

Lesson Review

1. What is one definition of sexuality?
2. Explain the various influences on an individual's sexuality.
3. What is sexual orientation?

You've now learned some information about a variety of sexuality topics. To test your knowledge, answer true or false to questions 1 through 7. Record your results and compare your answers with the correct ones given at the end of the survey. After lesson 2, do the same for questions 8 through 14.

1. Menstruation is the process in which an unfertilized egg and the lining of the uterus leave the female body.
   a. true
   b. false

2. Sexuality is described as the feelings, thoughts, identities, sensuality, intimacy, and reproduction in people.
   a. true
   b. false

3. Male condoms are 99 percent effective in preventing STIs and pregnancy.
   a. true
   b. false

4. LGBTQ+ stands for lesbian, gay, bisexual, transgender, queer/questioning, and others.
   a. true
   b. false

5. A transgender person's inner sense of gender does not match his or her biological sex (male or female).
   a. true
   b. false

6. Sexual orientation primarily involves the heterosexual and bisexual categories.
   a. true
   b. false

7. The words "sex" and "sexuality" are often used interchangeably but can differ in meaning as well.
   a. true
   b. false

8. The birth control pill often includes a combination of estrogen and testosterone.
   a. true
   b. false

9. In the acronym LGBTQ+, the + includes "others" such as two-spirited.
   a. true
   b. false

10. Conception, or fertilization, is the union of an ovum and a sperm.
    a. true
    b. false

11. Female and male sterilization are the only contraceptive methods considered permanent.
    a. true
    b. false

12. Once your body begins puberty, you are ready to engage in sexual intercourse.
    a. true
    b. false

13. Celibacy (refraining from sexual activity) is the most effective means of achieving birth control and protection against sexually transmitted disease.
    a. true
    b. false

14. Sexting involves sending electronic messages with sexual photos or other sexual content.
    a. true
    b. false

Here are the correct answers: 1a, 2a, 3b (correct answer: 85 percent), 4a, 5a, 6b (correct answer: heterosexual, gay, lesbian, and bisexual), 7a, 8b (correct answer: estrogen and progestin), 9a, 10a, 11a, 12b (correct answer: physically your body is getting ready to reproduce, but you are most likely not emotionally ready for sexual intercourse), 13a, and 14a. If you got 12 to 14 answers right, you really know your stuff. If you got 9 to 11 right, you still have some things to learn. If you got eight or fewer right, seek out more information.

Lesson 20.2

Birth Control, Pregnancy, and Sexually Transmitted Infections

Lesson Objectives

After participating in this lesson, you should be able to

1. describe the four stages of the menstrual cycle;
2. describe the three stages of childbirth;
3. define contraception and describe at least one form of contraceptive; and
4. list four sexually transmitted infections and describe their causes, symptoms, treatment, and prevention.

Lesson Vocabulary

AIDS, conception, female sterilization, menstrual cycle, placenta, pornography, semen, sexting, sexually transmitted infection (STI)

Decisions about your sexual health are among the most personal ones you make—and among the most difficult. When should you become sexually active? When you do, how will you protect yourself against disease or unwanted pregnancy? What type of contraceptive is right for you? Who in your sexual relationship needs to take responsibility for birth control? Nobody can answer these questions but you. This lesson gives you information to clarify the pros and cons of your options so that you can make the best decisions possible for you. Before you can make good decisions, you must know the facts. First, you will learn about the physiology of the reproductive system. This is followed by a discussion of menstruation, conception, pregnancy, and childbirth. The final sections describe methods of birth control and sexually transmitted infections (STIs).

Reproductive System

The human reproductive system allows for the menstrual cycle and sperm development. It differs, of course, between males and females but ultimately serves the overall purpose of reproduction. In the male reproductive system, sperm is produced in the testicles for release through the penis during sexual activity (figure 20.1). The female reproductive system includes the uterus, ovaries, fallopian tubes, vagina, and external genitalia (figure 20.2).

The female menstrual cycle is a monthly cycle that results in the release of a mature egg and prepares the walls of the uterus to implant the egg if it is fertilized by sperm. If fertilization does not occur, the lining of the uterus is shed through menstruation, and the cycle begins again.

Menstrual Cycle

The **menstrual cycle** is a monthly series of changes involving ovulation, the uterine lining, and menstruation (also referred to as a "period"), in which the unfertilized egg and the lining of the uterus leave the body in a menstrual flow. The menstrual cycle consists of four stages (figure 20.3) and lasts for an average of 28 days, though some women have longer or shorter cycles. Menstrual flow usually lasts about five days but can vary from woman to woman.

Stage 1 of the menstrual cycle is the menstrual flow, in which the endometrium (the uterine lining that has thickened during the cycle) is partially shed and expelled through the vagina. The menstrual cycle consists of dark-coloured blood mixed with mucous secretion from the uterine lining and secretion from the vagina. This stage lasts about five days and ends when the shedding is completed.

Stage 2 of the cycle includes days 6 through 12, during which an egg, or ovum, matures. The maturation process of the ovum includes the ovum's being released from the follicle where it developed

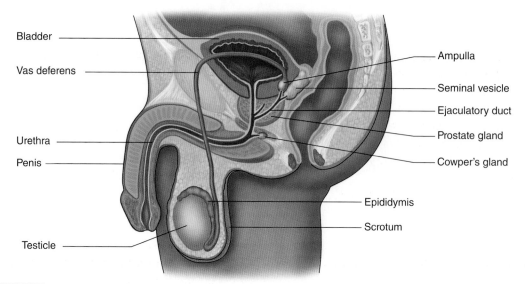

FIGURE 20.1 Cross section of the male human reproductive anatomy.

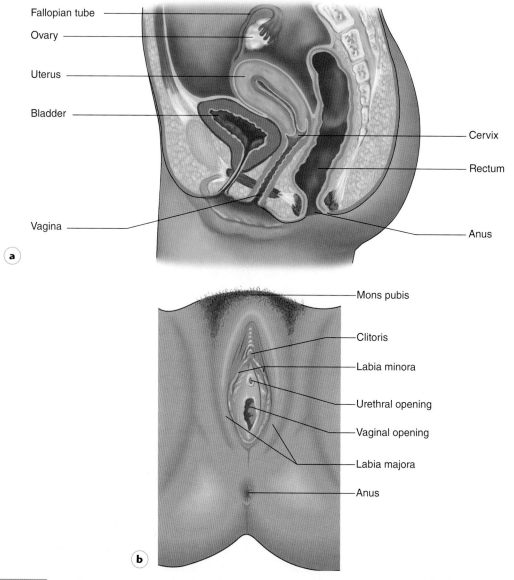

FIGURE 20.2 *(a)* Cross section of the female human reproductive anatomy and *(b)* front view (supine) of the female reproductive anatomy.

and the secretion of progesterone. Progesterone is a steroid hormone secreted by the ovary and is necessary for pregnancy. The uterine lining or endometrium begins to thicken, and the uterus prepares for ovulation and the possibility that an ovum will be fertilized. During this time the cervix also begins to secrete a thick mucus, which will assist in the passage of sperm.

Stage 3 of the cycle includes days 13 and 14, which are marked by ovulation—the release of an egg from one of the fallopian tubes. After release, an egg lives for only 24 hours; if it isn't fertilized, it deteriorates and leaves the uterus during the next menstrual cycle.

Stage 4 consists of days 15 through 28. During this stage, if an egg has been fertilized, it moves from the fallopian tube into the uterus and attaches itself to the endometrium. Progesterone continues to be secreted throughout the pregnancy to support the fertilized ovum. If an ovum has not been fertilized, the ovum disintegrates and the woman begins her next menstrual period, and the cycle begins again. Figure 20.3 illustrates the complete menstrual cycle.

Conception

Conception, or fertilization, is the union of an ovum (figure 20.4) and a sperm (figure 20.5). When ovulation occurs (usually on day 13 or 14 of the menstrual cycle), an ovum is released into a fallopian tube. If sperm are present in the fallopian tube, the ovum can be fertilized. One ejaculation by the male releases about 200 to 500 million sperm, which may seem like a very high number, but many are irregular and never make it to the ovum's location. Sperm enter the uterus through the cervix, where they move into either the right or left fallopian tube in search of an ovum. Once an ovum is found, the sperm work to penetrate it; if a sperm succeeds in doing so, the ovum changes so that no other sperm can get in. Conception has thus been completed. The fertilized ovum now begins cell division and

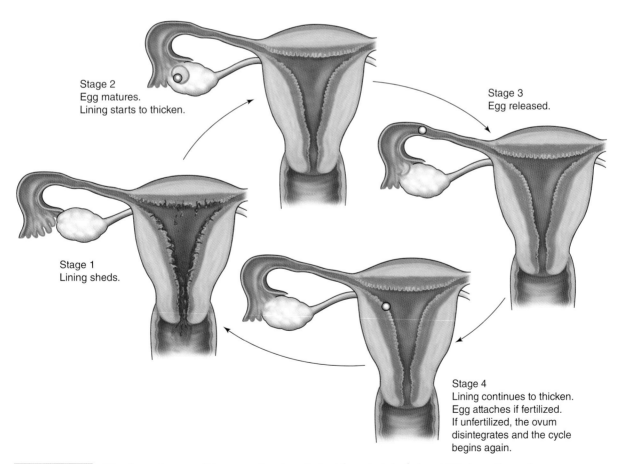

Stage 2
Egg matures.
Lining starts to thicken.

Stage 3
Egg released.

Stage 1
Lining sheds.

Stage 4
Lining continues to thicken.
Egg attaches if fertilized.
If unfertilized, the ovum disintegrates and the cycle begins again.

FIGURE 20.3 The four stages of the menstrual cycle last for a total of about 28 days, though some women have shorter or longer cycles (shown in a cross section of the uterus: one fallopian tube and one ovary).

continues to travel down the fallopian tube to the uterus, where it implants itself into the endometrium about 10 to 12 days after conception. This entire process is illustrated in figure 20.6.

Pregnancy

From the time of conception, human pregnancy lasts about 38 weeks, or nine months, and it is often viewed as consisting of three-month increments known as trimesters. During the first trimester (the first three months), the fertilized ovum becomes an embryo (i.e., a developing baby through approximately the first six weeks after conception). The embryo begins to develop within the amniotic sac, which is a sac of fluid that surrounds the embryo. The amniotic sac protects the embryo from damage and helps maintain a steady temperature. The embryo receives oxygen and nourishment through the umbilical cord, which connects the embryo to the **placenta** (i.e., an organ that anchors the embryo to the uterus). By the third month of the

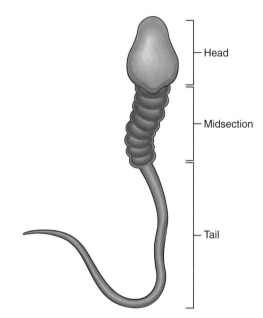

FIGURE 20.5 A mature sperm cell, or spermatozoon (magnified).

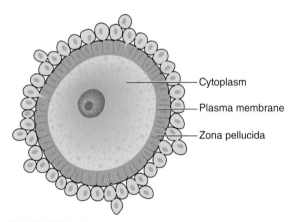

FIGURE 20.4 An ovum, or egg.

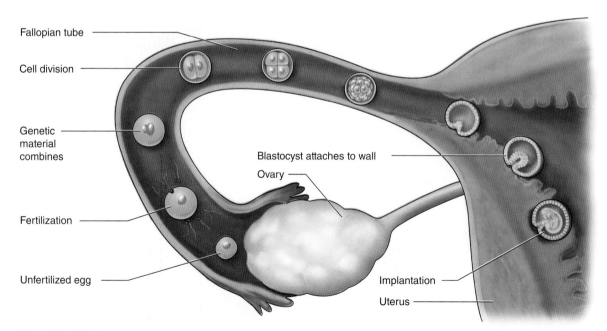

FIGURE 20.6 During conception and implantation, an egg becomes fertilized, undergoes cell division while traveling through the fallopian tube, and implants itself in the uterus. Note: The unfertilized egg is greatly magnified in the figure.

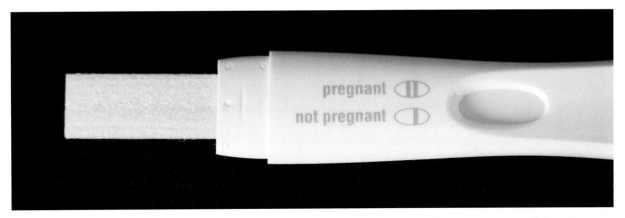

Over-the-counter pregnancy tests can be done at home. It's important to follow the instructions carefully to increase the chances of an accurate reading. If the test indicates pregnancy, you should follow up with a visit to the doctor.

first trimester, the term used to refer to the developing baby changes from *embryo* to *foetus.* This marks the end of the embryonic period during which time the brain, arms and legs, heart, lungs, and internal organs begin to form. Also, the foetal period begins, which is more about growth and development.

At this time, the foetus begins showing male or female genitalia; in addition, limbs, eyebrows, and fingernails begin to become distinguishable by the end of the third month. At the end of the first trimester, the foetus measures approximately 5 centimetres (2 inches).

During the second trimester—months 4 through 6—the foetus begins to breathe the amniotic fluid, organs continue to develop, and brain waves can be detected. During the second trimester, the foetus may be startled by loud noises and can start to hear and recognize voices. Lungs continue to develop as the foetus is inhaling and exhaling small amounts of amniotic fluid. Brain wave activity measured in a developing foetus shows different sleep cycles. It is also during this trimester that the mother begins to gain weight and feels the baby move. By the end of the second trimester, the baby weighs approximately 0.9 kilograms (2 pounds) and is 30 centimetres (12 inches) in length.

The third trimester begins with month 7 and ends at childbirth. During these last three months of pregnancy, the baby has a fully formed brain and nervous system and begins to build up fat, which will provide energy and help keep the baby warm—all in preparation for birth. At birth, the average baby weighs approximately 3 kilograms (7 pounds) and is 45 to 50 centimetres (18 to 20 inches) in length.

Childbirth

In preparation for birth, the foetus usually turns and positions his or her head against the mother's pelvic bone (figure 20.7). In addition, the cervix begins to dilate, and the amniotic sac may rupture (this is also known as "water breaking").

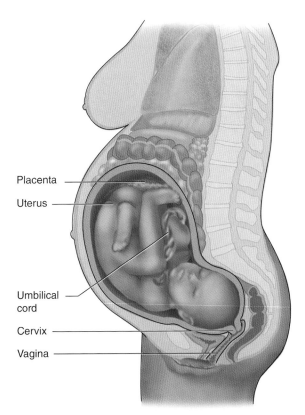

Placenta

Uterus

Umbilical cord

Cervix

Vagina

FIGURE 20.7 Near the end of pregnancy, the foetus positions his or her head against the mother's pelvic bone.

Childbirth includes three stages of labour (figure 20.8). The first stage is the longest, lasting anywhere from a couple of hours to an entire day. During this stage, contractions begin, initially lasting 20 to 40 seconds and occurring every 10 to 20 minutes, then progressively getting stronger and lasting longer. The cervix continues to dilate (to up to 8 to 10 centimetres wide), and the baby begins to move into the birth canal or vagina.

The second stage of childbirth lasts from a few minutes to a couple of hours. During this stage, the woman begins to push during contractions to help the baby move through the birth canal, or vagina.

Once delivered, the baby can breathe on his or her own, and the umbilical cord is cut.

The third stage of childbirth is the delivery of the placenta, which happens very shortly after delivery of the baby and lasts only about 10 minutes.

Contraception

Contraception, or birth control, includes a variety of methods used to prevent an egg from being fertilized by a sperm cell. Many men and women who are sexually active use some type of birth control, but no single contraceptive method is best for everyone.

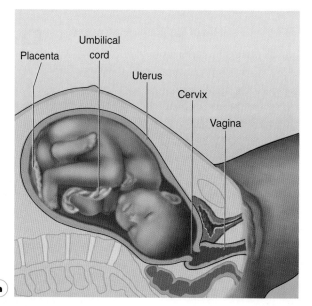

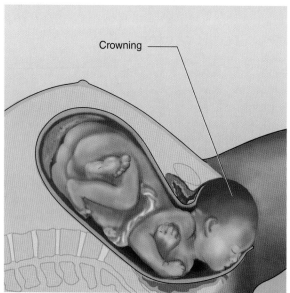

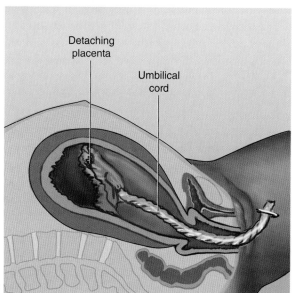

FIGURE 20.8 During childbirth, the mother goes through three stages of labour: (*a*) stage 1, (*b*) stage 2, and (*c*) stage 3.

Facts About Teen Pregnancy

- Each year, about 28,000 teens aged 15 to 19 become pregnant in Canada.
- Teen pregnancy poses increased health risks to both the mother and child.
- Risk factors for adolescent pregnancy include poor school performance, economic disadvantages, and greater risk for developing health problems (e.g., anaemia, hypertension, depressive disorders).
- Adolescents who are pregnant are less likely to finish high school than teens who do not become pregnant.
- Children of teen mothers are more likely to have low birth weights, to be preterm, to have an increased mortality rate, and to have a greater likelihood of developmental problems such as learning difficulties, hearing and visual impairments, and chronic respiratory problems.

Decisions about contraceptive use should take into account many factors, including cost, side effects, effectiveness, convenience, ease of use, and protection against both pregnancy and STIs. The only contraceptive that is 100 percent effective against both pregnancy and STIs is abstinence—refraining from vaginal sex, oral sex, anal sex, and naked genital-to-genital rubbing ("outercourse"). Before using any contraceptive, make sure to read all of the directions and information on the packaging. If you have further questions, contact a medical care provider.

At different stages of people's lives, they may have different needs for contraception. Some people, for example, choose a particular method (e.g., condom use) because they wish to prevent both STIs and pregnancy. Surgical methods (male or **female sterilization**), on the other hand, are generally chosen by people who already have the size of family they want.

Given the importance of your decisions about whether and when to use contraception, you should make them in consultation with someone who is knowledgeable about the pros and cons of each method. That person might be a parent, teacher, school counsellor, older sibling, medical professional, or other trusted individual. Of course, it is also extremely important for you to communicate with your sexual partner about your wants, needs, and expectations. Becoming sexually active shouldn't be determined by statistics or by what others do; it should be determined by your

Teen Sexual Activity and Contraception Use

- About 30 percent of 15- to 17-year-olds have had sex. This jumps to almost 70 percent for 18- to 19-year-olds. Teens are waiting longer these days to be sexually active. In 1996-1997, some 32 percent of Canadian youth aged 15 to 17 years had been sexually active; in contrast, in the years 2003 through 2009-2010, 30 percent of this same population had been sexually active. Youth ages 18 to 19 are also waiting longer to have sex, with a drop from 70 percent to 68 percent from 1996-1997 to 2009-2010.
- With the average age of the first sexual encounter being just 17 years and most individuals remaining single until at least their mid-20s, young adults may face increased risk of unintended pregnancy and STIs for 10 years or more.
- Among teens, 80 percent aged 15 to 17 years and 74 percent aged 18 to 19 years reported using condoms during their last intercourse.
- The most common contraceptive method used during intercourse is the male condom (reported by 70 percent of females and 71 percent of males).

values, your relationship with your partner, and other factors that are important to you and your partner. After all, it's your health and your future that are at stake.

Unfortunately, much inaccurate information is available on the web, in the media, and from friends and peers; therefore, you need to be careful about where you get your information. The Consumer Corner features in chapters 9 and 15 offer you some guidelines for finding reliable and useful information.

Sexually Transmitted Infections

There are many kinds of **sexually transmitted infections (STIs)**, also known as sexually transmitted diseases (STDs). Though not limited to young people, these conditions are common among teens. Sexually transmitted infections have various causes, and treatment is specific to the infection. Proper use of condoms can help prevent most of them; but, just as seat belts and airbags are not foolproof in car accidents, condoms are not 100 percent protective. The only completely effective method of preventing an STI is abstinence.

Some facts about STIs may surprise you. For example, it is possible to have more than one STI at a time, and having an STI does not make a person immune to getting it again. In addition, a person can transmit an STI even if he or she has no symptoms.

As you may know, some STIs can be deadly, such as acquired immune deficiency syndrome (**AIDS**) and untreated syphilis. Thus, if you are sexually active, you should know how to decrease your risk of getting or transmitting an STI. Of course, if you abstain from sexual activity, you can't give or get an STI.

Chlamydia

This common STI affects both men and women and can seriously and permanently damage a woman's reproductive organs. It is the most frequently reported bacterial STI in North America and occurs most often among young people.

Chlamydia can be transmitted through anal, vaginal, or oral sex and can also be spread from an infected woman to her baby during childbirth. In women, the cervix and urethra are infected first, and

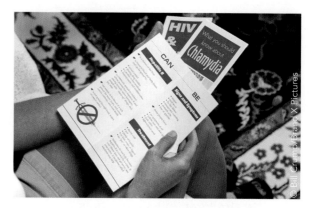

Being educated about STIs is the first step in prevention.

if the infection is left untreated it can spread to the uterus and fallopian tubes.

Most infected people do not have symptoms, but some do. Infected women may experience abnormal vaginal discharge or a burning sensation when urinating. Men may experience discharge from the penis or a burning sensation when urinating.

Fortunately, chlamydia is easily treated and cured with antibiotics. However, repeated infection is common, and persons with sex partners who have not been appropriately treated are at high risk for reinfection. The risk of getting or giving chlamydia can be reduced by correct and consistent use of latex male condoms.

Gonorrhoea

This bacterial STI grows easily in the warm, moist areas of the female reproductive tract and in the urethra in both women and men. It can also grow in the mouth, throat, eyes, and anus. It can be transmitted through anal, vaginal, or oral sex and can also be spread from an infected woman to her baby during childbirth.

Most women with gonorrhoea do not have symptoms. If symptoms do appear, they may include vaginal discharge or bleeding and a painful or burning sensation when urinating. Some men with the infection may also have no symptoms. When symptoms do occur, they may include a burning sensation when urinating or a white, yellow, or green discharge from the penis.

Gonorrhoea is treated with antibiotics, which will stop the infection but will not repair any permanent damage done by the disease. Untreated gonorrhoea can cause serious and permanent health problems. The risk of getting or giving gonorrhoea can be reduced by correct and consistent use of latex male condoms.

Syphilis

Syphilis is a highly contagious disease transmitted by direct contact with a syphilitic sore known as a chancre. Chancres are primarily found on the external genitals, vagina, anus, in the rectum, on the lips, and in the mouth and are transmitted during vaginal, anal, or oral sex. Pregnant women who have syphilis can also transmit the disease to their unborn child. Pregnant women with syphilis have a higher rate of having a stillbirth and of having a baby who dies shortly after birth.

It may be common for an infected person to be initially unaware of the disease because it takes approximately 21 days between infection and the start of the first symptom of syphilis to be recognized. Syphilis follows a progression of three stages. The first or primary stage consists of single or multiple chancre marks. The chancre is usually painless and appears at the location where syphilis entered the body, thus the individual may be unaware he or she has a chancre. The initial chancre or chancres typically last three to six weeks and will heal whether the individual gets treatment or not. If the individual is not treated, the infection will progress to the second stage. The secondary stage is primarily composed of skin rashes or sores in the mouth, vagina, or anus. Again, the symptoms will disappear with or without treatment. If left untreated, the infection will progress to the third or latent and late stages of the disease. In the latent stage the individual will continue to have the syphilis infection in their body and will generally not have any signs or symptoms of the disease. The latent stage may last for many years. The late stage of syphilis can appear 10 to 20 years after the first infection. In this stage, the disease may begin to damage the brain, nerves, eyes, and heart along with multiple other organs, which can cause long-term complications including death.

Syphilis is treatable with penicillin and curable if caught early. The use of penicillin in the primary or secondary stage is very effective in curing an individual with syphilis. It may also be effective in a higher dose for curing syphilis in the latent phase as well as preventing further damage. The transmission of syphilis can be reduced by correct and consistent use of latex male condoms, yet the risk of getting or giving syphilis by direct contact with a chancre can still occur if the chancre is in an area not covered by a condom.

Genital Herpes

This STI is caused by types 1 and 2 of the herpes simplex virus (HSV). Both types can cause sores or blisters on or around the mouth and genitals. These viruses remain in the body for life and can cause periodic outbreaks. About 14 percent of people in Canada have genital herpes, but 94 percent of them are unaware of it due to not having any of the symptoms or not recognizing the symptoms.

The virus can be transmitted through anal, vaginal, or oral sex. Infected individuals can transmit the virus even if they do not have a visible sore and do not know they are infected.

Symptoms of genital herpes may include an itching or burning sensation in the genitals and small, painful blisters on or around the genitals, rectum, or mouth. The blisters break and leave painful sores, along with flu-like symptoms that may last two to four weeks. Repeated outbreaks are common.

There is no cure for herpes, but antiviral medications can prevent or shorten outbreaks, and daily use of antiviral medication can reduce the likelihood of transmission. The risk of getting or giving genital herpes can be reduced by correct and consistent use of latex male condoms. However, when herpes sores or other symptoms are present, individuals should abstain from sexual activity. And remember that even if an infected person has no symptoms, he or she can still infect a sex partner.

Genital HPV Infection

Genital human papillomavirus (HPV) is the most common STI; in fact, more than 40 types of HPV can infect the genital areas, mouth, and throat in both men and women. Human papillomavirus can cause serious health problems, including certain cancers (e.g., cervical, vaginal, anal, oropharyngeal, and penile). It can be transmitted through anal, vaginal, or oral sex even when the infected person has no signs or symptoms.

Other health problems caused by HPV include genital warts and recurrent respiratory papillomatosis, in which warts grow in the throat. Each of these health problems has its own symptoms to be contended with.

There is no treatment for the HPV itself, but treatments do exist for each of the health problems caused by it. In addition, the HPV vaccine can protect males and females against some of the most common types of HPV. The risk of getting HPV may also be lowered by proper use of a male condom.

❤ FITNESS TECHNOLOGY: Sexting and Pornography

Modern technology enables various activities—such as web surfing, **sexting**, and ever-changing birth control approaches. Sexting is sending or receiving sexually explicit or sexually suggestive images or video, usually via a cell phone. People in general, but especially students, need to understand that those messages and especially the photos do not always stay with the person they were sent to. Sexting messages and photos are often sent on to other people or are posted on social media sites for the world to see. Approximately 20 percent of teens have sent naked or semi-nude images of themselves or posted them online. This practice is more common among females than males, with 61 percent of girls saying they were pressured to engage in it and only 9 percent not indicating this as a factor in their sexting. Boys tend to send more sexually explicit texts than girls. Between 24 percent and 33 percent of high school and college students, respectively, have said they have sent nude or semi-nude photos to another person. One in six teens between the ages of 12 and 17 has received a naked or nearly nude picture via text message from someone they know. There are many stories of teens who have been bullied and harassed when their sexting pictures have been sent schoolwide or posted on social media sites.

Before sending an inappropriate sexual picture of yourself or someone else, or an inappropriate text or post to a social media site, think about the consequences of your actions. You cannot control who may ultimately see your picture, text, or post or where else it may end up. Never send images or messages that you wouldn't want everyone to see. If you send inappropriate pictures or messages, you may end up getting fired from a job, getting removed from a team or organization, being humiliated, losing educational opportunities (as colleges are monitoring social media sites), and even getting in trouble with the law. In Canada, sending nude photos of teens under 18 over an electronic device is a criminal offense.

Another technology example is easy access to **pornography**, often via the web, which may expose young people to sexual images that they don't want to see or don't understand. These images may also portray exploitive sexuality as normal or healthy. Be well aware that people who produce pornography are not generally trying to represent what is actually normal, typical, or safe. To the contrary, just as scenes in "reality television" are often manipulated to keep viewers interested or even shock them, pornography and other sexually explicit materials are often exaggerated, contrived, or manipulated. Videos are not reality. Reality is reality, and you should be able to create your own reality that is safe, healthy, and fulfilling.

Using Technology

Do you think that sexting is an acceptable use of technology? What about videotaping sexual activity (consensual or not), or taking revealing photographs and sharing them via social media? There are an increasing number of court cases worldwide involving technology and social media used in these ways. Go online to see what your responsibilities and rights are with respect to the use of technology for activities such as sexting and taking photographs and videos, as well as sharing this content.

Trichomoniasis or Trich

This infection, caused by a protozoan parasite, is the most common curable STI. It is more common in women than in men. It is transmitted through vaginal sex; and the most commonly infected body part in women is the lower genital tract, whereas in men it is the inside of the penis.

About 70 percent of infected people do not have signs or symptoms. Among those who do, both men and women may experience itching or irritation in the genitals, discomfort or burning with urination, and a discharge from either the vagina or penis. Symptoms may come and go.

Treatment is a single dose of an antibiotic medication, which can cure the infection. People who have been treated can get the infection again if all of the symptoms have not gone away or if they are with a partner who has not been treated for the infection. Using male latex condoms correctly and consistently may reduce the risk of getting or spreading trichomoniasis, but because condoms don't cover everything, it is possible to get or spread the infection even when using one.

Pelvic Inflammatory Disease (PID)

This STI infects only women—specifically, the uterus, fallopian tubes, and other female reproductive organs. Pelvic inflammatory disease can lead to infertility, ectopic pregnancy (pregnancy in the fallopian tube or elsewhere outside the uterus), and chronic pelvic pain. It occurs when bacteria move upward from a woman's vagina or cervix into her reproductive organs. PID is not always caused by a STI; however, many cases of PID are associated with chlamydia and gonorrhoea. A woman's risk of developing PID also increases with the number of sex partners she has due to the increased exposure to STIs, especially chlamydia and gonorrhoea.

Because the symptoms of PID are often vague, it frequently goes untreated. The most common symptom is lower abdominal pain.

Pelvic inflammatory disease can be cured with antibiotics, but any damage already done to the reproductive organs cannot be reversed. The risk of PID can be reduced by consistent and correct use of latex male condoms.

Human Immunodeficiency Virus and Acquired Immune Deficiency Syndrome

Human immunodeficiency virus (HIV) is the virus that causes acquired immune deficiency syndrome (AIDS). Once you have HIV, you have it for life. Human immunodeficiency virus affects T cells, which fight infection. It can be transmitted through blood, **semen**, preseminal fluid (i.e., a clear, colourless, sticky fluid that emits from a man's penis when he is sexually aroused; it is similar in composition to semen), rectal fluid (i.e., a lubricating mucus that is secreted from the rectum during anal intercourse), vaginal fluid, and breast milk. For transmission to occur, the infected fluid must come in direct contact with a mucous membrane or damaged tissue. Transmission occurs primarily through unprotected anal, vaginal, or oral sex; through needle sharing; through blood-to-blood contact; or between mother and child during pregnancy, birth, or breastfeeding. Human immunodeficiency virus is *not* spread through general day-to-day contact or through the air; nor does it live for very long outside of the body.

Symptoms of HIV infection can include flu-like ailments and opportunistic infections that take advantage of a weakened immune system; AIDS-defining illnesses include certain cancers, dementia, and progressive and extreme weight loss.

There is no cure for HIV or AIDS; therefore, treatment of both is symptomatic. Treatment for HIV primarily includes antiretroviral therapy, which helps to prolong the duration and quality of survival in people and may help to restore and preserve the function of the immune system. The antiretroviral drugs suppress the virus even to undetectable levels, but they do not completely eliminate HIV from the body. Through suppression of the amount of virus in the body, people infected with HIV can lead longer and healthier lives. A person infected with HIV is diagnosed with AIDS when his or her immune system is seriously compromised and signs of HIV infection are severe. Signs may include *pneumocystis carinii pneumonia*—an extraordinarily rare condition in people without HIV infection—and *opportunistic infections,* which rarely cause harm in healthy individuals. Once an individual has been diagnosed with AIDS, antiretroviral drugs may continue to be used and opportunistic infections are treated as they arise.

The risk of HIV and AIDS can be reduced by consistent and correct use of latex male condoms, as well as female condoms; during oral sex, use a dental dam. A dental dam is a barrier contraceptive made of thin latex rubber and is placed over the labia for oral or vaginal intercourse.

Lesson Review

1. Describe the four stages of the menstrual cycle.
2. Describe the three stages of childbirth.
3. Define contraception and describe at least one form of contraceptive.
4. List four STIs and describe their causes, symptoms, treatment, and prevention.

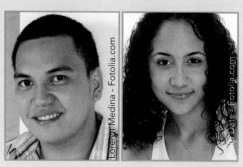

Jack is a shy guy who generally doesn't like social situations. Still, when the time came for prom, he got up the nerve to ask Brianna, a girl he liked who was really smart and funny, to go with him. When she said yes, he felt pretty good about himself.

At the dance, however, Jack noticed that a few of Brianna's friends were standing in a corner watching them. To Jack, it looked as if they were laughing at him, and he began to feel self-conscious. He excused himself and went to the restroom to check his appearance. He thought his hair looked a little messy but otherwise couldn't figure out what they might be laughing about. When he came out of the restroom, Brianna was with the other girls, and they were all laughing loudly. Jack felt insecure for the rest of the night, and things got more awkward. Jack ended up cutting the evening shorter than he'd planned. He just didn't feel good about himself, and he worried that any-

thing else he did would be gossiped about and made fun of later. He felt very self-conscious, and his self-perception crashed. The next year, Jack decided to skip the prom so that no one would be able to make fun of him.

In reality, the girls had simply been laughing about a video that a friend of theirs had taken of her brother doing something funny. The girls had wanted to share it with Brianna because they knew she would get a good laugh out of it, but Jack never knew that.

For Discussion

What initially contributed to Jack's having a positive self-perception? What then contributed to Jack's feeling less sure of himself? What generalization did Jack make that influenced a later decision? Use the information in the Self-Management feature to help you when answering these questions.

SELF-MANAGEMENT: Skills for Improving Self-Perception

The way you see yourself is called your self-perception. When you're young, your self-perception derives largely from how other people react to you—for example, how your parents and other caregivers handle and care for you. As a teen, you're likely to both watch other people's responses to you and look inward at yourself. Whether or not you realize it, you're also weighing whether other people's thoughts, attitudes, actions, and reactions are acceptable to you. Thus your self-perception is influenced by social comparisons.

Self-perception also depends on your experiences. If you have positive experiences that you view as successful, you tend to see yourself in a positive way. Conversely, negative experiences can decrease the likelihood of your viewing yourself in a positive way. At some point, then, you begin to see yourself in your own way.

Your self-perception and your perceptions of the world are so closely related that they are often difficult to separate. How you look at the world depends on what you think of yourself, and what you think of yourself is influenced by how you look at the world. Even though your self-perception is considerably influenced early in your life, it will continue to be shaped as you accumulate life experiences. As you move through your life, consider the following tips to help you build a positive self-perception.

- **Don't ignore or attempt to "delete" experiences.** We can all learn from negative and unpleasant experiences. Instead of just feeling bad, acknowledge the experience and try to identify and remember what you can learn from it.

- **Check your perceptions.** Sometimes our own judgment is inaccurate, and these inaccuracies can influence our self-perception. Check your perceptions—both of yourself and of situations—with trusted people and, if needed, reframe your thinking.

- **Be specific.** If you have a negative experience with a particular person or event, try not to generalize it. For example, if one boy says something negative or cruel to you, don't assume that all boys think the same way. Or, if you do poorly at a drawing assignment, don't assume that you'll always be bad at art. Learning to be specific in your perceptions will help you be more precise in them as well.

- **Stay healthy, get rest, and exercise.** Make every effort to come to the world as healthy, well rested, and sufficiently exercised as possible. Perception depends in part on your senses, and the better condition your senses are in, the more likely it is that they will serve you effectively.

- **Be patient.** Take your time when considering how to think about a situation. Doing so will help you develop a more accurate perception of the situation, whereas rushing to judgment about yourself or others rarely helps.

The World Health Organization defines sexual well-being as "a state of physical, emotional, mental and social wellbeing in relation to sexuality; it is not merely the absence of disease, dysfunction or infirmity [physical or mental weakness]. Sexual health requires a positive and respectful approach to sexuality and sexual relationships, as well as the possibility of having pleasurable and safe sexual experiences, free of coercion, discrimination and violence. For sexual health to be attained and maintained, the sexual rights of all persons must be respected, protected and fulfilled."

With this definition in mind, as well as the information presented in this chapter and other trustworthy and reliable information you have found from other sources (e.g., SexandU, a trusted adult), you can take action toward sexual well-being. Where are you with respect to sexual well-being? This will require you not only to come up with an answer but also to think about the reasons why you feel this way or believe this to be true.

Draw a line that shows sexual well-being on a continuum from low (or negative) sexual well-being to high (or positive) sexual well-being. Where would you position your (a) physical, (b) emotional, (c) mental, and (d) social well-being in relation to sexuality? How certain are you that you are free from (e) disease and (f) dysfunction? How positive or negative is your approach to sexuality and sexual relationships? Remember to always be asking yourself why you believe this to be the case and questioning why these are your answers. To what degree are your sexual experiences safe (i.e., free of coercion, discrimination, and violence)? To what extent do you (g) respect, (h) protect, and (i) fulfill the sexual rights of others?

The next step is to use this information to attain and maintain sexual well-being now and in the future. Other chapters in this book can provide support for setting and meeting personal goals.

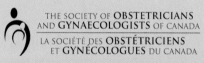

GET ACTIVE WITH SEXANDU

© Society of Obstetricians and Gynecologists of Canada

Who We Are

SexandU (www.sexandu.ca) is a website developed by the Society of Obstetricians and Gynecologists of Canada (SOGC) to provide accurate, credible, and up-to-date information on sex and how to maintain good sexual health.

What We Do

SexandU tackles many of those tough-to-talk-about topics, including contraception choices, sexually transmitted infections, and coming out.

Get Involved

It's often important to speak to a trusted adult about concerns you have regarding your health or your safety. Visit our website to find lots of factual information to inform you and to help start those conversations with friends, your family, or your health care provider. We also provide resources on menstruation, puberty, sexual orientation, sex and the law, and much more. Make SexandU your go-to website at www.sexandu.ca.

© Society of Obstetricians and Gynecologists of Canada

Reviewing Concepts and Vocabulary

Complete the following in order to determine your growing understanding of fitness, health, and wellness. Answer items 1 through 5 by correctly completing each sentence with a word or phrase.

1. A _____ is the most commonly used contraceptive.
2. The letter "Q" in LGBTQ+ stands for _____.
3. HIV is the virus that causes _____.
4. The sending of sexual messages or photos via a cell phone is called _____.
5. _____ is a person's sexual identity in relation to the gender of the people to which he or she is attracted.

For items 6 through 10, match each term in column 1 with the appropriate phrase in column 2.

6. conception   a. monthly changes involving ovulation, uterine lining, and menstruation
7. bisexual   b. refraining from sexual activity
8. semen   c. person who is attracted to both females and males
9. celibacy   d. union of ovum and sperm
10. menstrual cycle   e. fluid containing sperm that is discharged during ejaculation

For items 11 through 15, respond to each statement or question.

11. How could using a condom help prevent STIs and pregnancy?
12. Why isn't there one treatment for all STIs?
13. List two facts about teen pregnancy in Canada.
14. Briefly describe the three trimesters of pregnancy.
15. What is the view of Parents and Friends of Lesbians and Gays (PFLAG) on sexual orientation?

Thinking Critically

Write a paragraph in response to the following questions.

Your friend Sally tells you that she had unprotected sex last night, but she doesn't want you to tell anybody else. She regrets what she did and feels worried that she might get pregnant. She doesn't mention STIs. What advice would you give Sally? What resources would you recommend? What agencies or organizations might be able to help? How do you feel about keeping this secret?

Project

Ask your parents, guardians, or other trusted adults how they learned about human sexuality. What are their views about sex education in school? Ask them if they think it was easier or harder to learn about sexuality when they were young compared to today. Do they think there is too much access to sexual information nowadays? Do you?

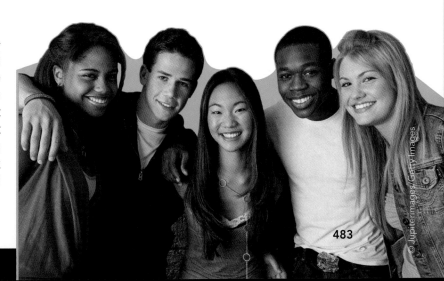

21

Healthy Relationships

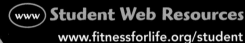 **Student Web Resources**
www.fitnessforlife.org/student

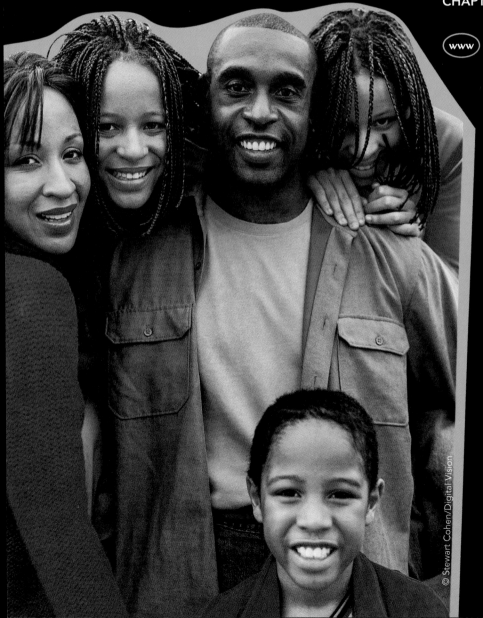

© Stewart Cohen/Digital Vision

Lesson 21.1
Family Life and Family Structure

Lesson Objectives

After participating in this lesson, you should be able to

1. describe the types of families in contemporary society,
2. define gender roles and explain how they have changed over time,
3. explain three factors that contribute to marriage success, and
4. explain the difference between divorce and separation.

Lesson Vocabulary

blended family, culture, divorce, empty nest, extended family, family role, gender, marriage, nuclear family, role model, separation, sex, traditional family

The family has historically been viewed as the most important force in shaping human development. Family offers a place of security and stability for people, each with their own roles. In this lesson, various types of families and the roles fulfilled by family members are described. Marriage, parenting, and family dynamics are discussed as well.

Family and Family Types

Family is defined in many different ways. Definitions include a group of people who are related to each other and a group of people living under one roof. Extending beyond this is the view of family as people who you love and who love you back; they are not necessarily blood or biological relations, but you trust them and they trust you, and they take care of you and you take care of them. Many definitions exist, and we'll explore some of them.

The term **nuclear family**, sometimes referred to as a **traditional family**, is commonly defined as a father and mother with children. In this family unit, the mother was often seen as the primary caretaker of the children who stayed at home to care for the household while the father went to work each day. The most recent census indicates that less than half of all households now have both a husband and wife, and not all households have children. Roles have changed over the years for many reasons, one of which is the fact that in many families, both parents now work full-time outside of the home. This arrangement means that the caretaking of children is often a shared responsibility between parents and others, such as **extended family** members (e.g., grandparents, aunts, uncles), as well as babysitters, day care providers, neighbours, friends, and after-school program providers.

Today more than a quarter of all households are households where a person lives alone. Also, many households have only two people under the same roof (without children), but those in the household consider themselves to be a family. People in one- or two-person family households are typically part of an extended family, but those other family members do not live under the same roof. These people may include those older in age with grown children, those who have no children, or those who have children who do not live with them.

Families with children now have a variety of different forms, including single-parent, adoptive (i.e., with at least one adopted child), divorced, blended (formed when a parent remarries), and LGBTQ+ families (lesbian, gay, bisexual, trans-identifying, queer, two-spirited, questioning, and asexual). Thus the term *family* has broadened and now refers not only to bloodlines but also to an individual's living and social arrangements, which often consist of more than those people who are related by blood.

Families with children, regardless of type, tend to cycle through four stages of development: beginning, parenting, **empty nest**, and retirement (see figure 21.1). The beginning stage is the time when the newly united couple, or the individual, creates the home and adjusts to the new personal and social status. In this stage, people plan their future and move forward to realize their dreams. The parenting stage begins, of course, with the birth or adoption of the first child and never truly ends but instead extends into parenting children no longer living in the same dwelling. Today many parents stay in this stage for a longer time than was traditionally the case, because adult children are more often living at home longer or returning home after college. It is now fairly common for sons and daughters to live at home with parents into their young adulthood.

When the last child leaves home, parents find themselves in the empty nest stage. Some parents have difficulty adjusting to this period of their lives, whereas others enjoy their new freedom. In the retirement stage, adults are typically ending their careers and enjoying the freedom of no longer having to be responsible for a job. However, in today's society, more people are continuing to work at an older age, and some even launch second careers. During this stage, a new role as a grandparent is common. Many indicate that being a grandparent has the benefits of a loving bond with grandchildren without the day-to-day responsibilities of parenting.

Whatever family type you find yourself in, a healthy family provides you with love and support. Generally, our first lessons about relating to others come from our family members. Young people tend to model their behaviour on the examples they see most often—those of their parents, siblings, and extended family members, who fulfill similar functions and roles across family types. That is, individuals fulfill child-rearing roles whether they are part of a two-parent family, a single-parent family, a **blended family**, a divorced family, or a LGBTQ+ family.

Family Roles

Positive family relationships consist of teaching family members about love, respect, responsibility, social interaction, communication, and other life skills necessary for living apart from the family, coping with change, and being financially independent. However, roles for each family member vary from family to family. In today's society, **family roles** aren't as clear-cut as they may have been for previous generations. There was a time when society expected only the adult male to work outside the home each day while the adult female stayed home to take care of the house and children.

Today, both adults (in two-parent and blended families) in the household often work outside of the home and share the financial duties, household chores, and child rearing. In single-parent families, of course, one individual is primarily responsible for all aspects of earning money, finances, chores, and child rearing. LGBTQ+ families may also consist of two adults and would function in much the same manner as heterosexual two-parent and blended families. Familial roles and responsibilities will continue to evolve in response to changes in economic conditions, in the definition of family roles, and in society more generally.

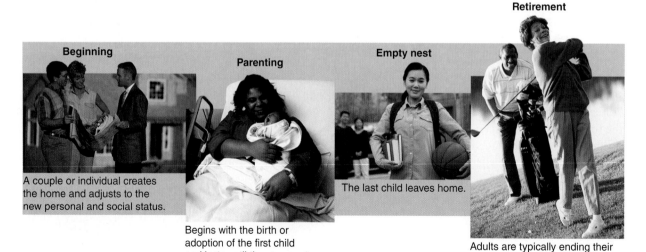

Beginning

A couple or individual creates the home and adjusts to the new personal and social status.

Parenting

Begins with the birth or adoption of the first child and lasts until the youngest child leaves the family home.

Empty nest

The last child leaves home.

Retirement

Adults are typically ending their careers and enjoying the freedom of no longer having to be responsible for a job.

FIGURE 21.1 Four stages of development of families.

Role Models

Parents serve as **role models** who impart values and information to their children. Parenting also requires a set of skills that are learned from experience—for example, patience, emotion management, health promotion, disease prevention, time management, and communication. The lessons that a child needs to learn often come through trial and error; therefore, a parent must have plenty of patience to allow the process to happen. Raising children can be very demanding, and parents must know how to keep their frustration and other emotions in check while setting boundaries and teaching appropriate behaviour.

Parents also need to know how to handle various kinds of hurt—whether it be first aid situations, colds, the flu, bruised feelings, or emotional distress—in their children. They must model a healthy lifestyle for their children to emulate. Many of the diseases and illnesses experienced by average Canadians result directly from poor lifestyle habits (e.g., unhealthy eating, sleeping, and exercise patterns). Parents are called on to provide their children with the best environment possible and to help them develop the necessary tools for facing the ever-changing world around them. One of the most important tools parents can give their children is the ability to communicate effectively. Good communication—both within and outside of the family—can go a long way toward preparing family members for a lifetime of success and happiness.

Parents are not the only role models for children. The learning that takes place outside of the home and the classroom is often the most influential in the lives of young people. This is the case due to the constant flow of information received from friends, peers, and the media. Such sources provide young people with a continuous stream of information that is sometimes questionable. This misinformation is often not discussed fully with parents or educators. As a result, the misinformation is often regarded as accurate when it really is not. The importance of good role models outside the family cannot be underestimated.

In what ways do you model the behaviours and relationships you see in your family? Do you treat your friends or your dating partner in ways that mirror what you see in your home? Overall, are these influences more positive or more negative?

Gender Roles

Our ideas of what it means to be male or female are structured by the messages—both direct and indirect—that we receive from family, friends, and the media. In considering these messages, it is useful to understand the distinction between sex and gender. **Sex** refers to the biological factors (male or female) that influence your fitness, health, and wellness. The word "**gender**" has a similar but slightly different meaning. It refers to social and cultural roles of people (masculine or feminine). For example, in the past, some roles were identified as gender appropriate for males only (masculine) or females only (feminine). Generally speaking, in most societies, males were (traditionally) expected to be independent and physically active, whereas females were traditionally expected to be more social and cooperative. For example, young boys might be encouraged to play sports while young girls might be encouraged to play with dolls. Society asserts and reinforces such expectations even before children are born (e.g., blue for baby boys and pink for baby girls).

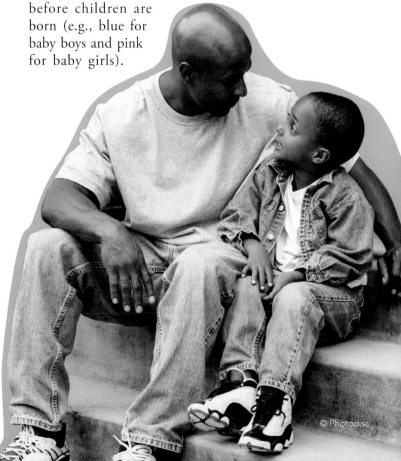

© Photodisc

This type of socialization continues for a lifetime. It is, among other things, the basis for the stereotypes that we see in our **culture**.

> What can you do to promote world peace? Go home and love your family.
>
> —Mother Teresa, religious sister and missionary

Over time, stereotypes have diminished in Western culture. For example, girls and women who often did not have opportunities to participate in sport before the 1970s now are regular participants. Activities previously considered appropriate only for males are now considered to be appropriate for both sexes (male and female).

Roles in a family or social group are influenced by gender stereotype as well. As noted earlier, some roles have traditionally been considered to be masculine (to be fulfilled by males) or feminine (to be fulfilled by females). Some families adhere to strict role expectations, whereas others do not. For example, in some families the man works and the woman stays home. Over time, role expectations have changed, as is the case when parents both work outside the home or the father stays home as the primary caregiver. In today's society, men and women can both pursue most any desired career, educational path, or role (whether in a relationship or in society more generally).

How do you feel about traditional gender roles for males and females? Do you seek relationships in which traditional gender-specific behaviours are expected? Why or why not? Share your perspective with a friend or classmate. Support your perspective with reasons and facts, and be respectful of other opinions.

Family Dynamics and Stability

Marriage plays an important role in most cultures around the world. In Canada, it is a legal bond that typically involves permanence and sexual and emotional exclusivity. Marriage provides stability and fulfills many social, emotional, financial, and sexual expectations and needs. According to a study done by the Pew Research Center to determine why people get married, the top three factors are being in love, making a lifelong commitment, and companionship. Couples who get married are also more likely to live longer compared to their single counterparts.

The term *marriage* was traditionally used to describe only a legal union between a man and a woman, but that is no longer the case. On July 20, 2005, Canada became the fourth country in the world, and the first country outside of Europe, to legalize same-sex marriage nationwide; **marriage**, for civil purposes, is the lawful union of two persons to the exclusion of all others.

Marriage success can be attributed to a variety of factors including the age of the individuals; the length of the relationship and the engagement; the presence or absence of shared interests, values, and goals; the attitudes of each individual's parents or guardians toward the marriage partner; and the individuals' views about having and raising children.

Although marriage is a lifetime commitment for some, the expectations associated with marriage may be difficult to maintain, and married couples may go through periods in which their happiness alternately diminishes and increases. The highest degrees of happiness are typically seen in the beginning stages of the relationship and upon the birth of the first child. Happiness tends to level off as the couple raises adolescents. It increases again as children reach young adulthood and move out and as the retirement years get closer.

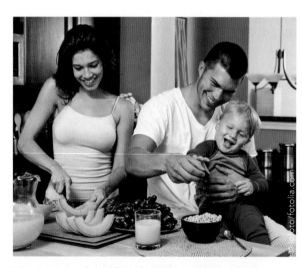

Marriage is a legal bond that provides stability.

SCIENCE IN ACTION: **Strong Relationships Lead to Happier, Healthier Lives**

According to researchers at Harvard University, individuals who have strong relationships with family, friends, and their community experience happier and healthier lives. Such people live longer and experience fewer health problems than others. For example, connecting with others reduces the effects of stress and improves the functioning of the coronary artery, digestive system, and immune system. Research also shows that exhibiting caring behaviour triggers hormones that reduce stress. This means that when people take action to promote social support and express affection, they bring about life-enhancing effects. This is encouraging news for families, because every day provides an opportunity to engage with other human beings and practice this proven strategy for improving the health of both the caregiver and the receiver.

> **Student Activity**
>
> Every day for the next week, tell someone you care about (or a complete stranger if you are brave) why they are important to you. Experience the feelings of happiness, and observe the changes in the person who receives your caring words. Know that you can access these feelings and affect others positively every day.

Some couples who experience trouble in their relationship try separation rather than divorce. The most common type of **separation** is a test period that is not legally recognized. In this approach, any shared property or possessions are still co-owned by the couple. Couples may use a separation to assess their relationship and decide whether they want to work at staying together.

> " Friends are the best to turn to when you're having a rough day. "
>
> —Justin Bieber, singer/songwriter

Though many marriages last, others end in **divorce**, which is a legal termination of the marriage wherein the property, the custody and support of any children, and possibly spousal support are negotiated by the divorcing individuals or decided by a judge or court. According to Statistics Canada, approximately 35 to 40 percent of married Canadian couples divorce, and for people who marry again the divorce rate is even higher. Divorce rates also tend to be higher for younger individuals and those who do not have a strong commitment to marriage.

Most people marry with the intention of having a permanent relationship. When divorce happens, it often results from multiple causes, and it differs for each couple. Divorce also goes beyond the termination of the marriage itself; it often has a ripple effect and influences every aspect of a person's life. People who are divorced often have to establish their individual identity all over again, because changes take place in their financial status, living arrangements, friendships, family relationships, and possibly even work situations. Children are also affected by divorce and may not understand why their parents are divorcing. While children may initially feel fearful of the changes associated with divorce, they can overcome the anxiety and grow up having very positive relationships with both their mother and their father, as well as with a spouse of their own.

Lesson Review

1. Describe the types of families in contemporary society.
2. Define gender roles and explain how they have changed over time.
3. Explain three factors that contribute to marriage success.
4. Explain the difference between divorce and separation.

Think about a family member, friend, or boyfriend or girlfriend you are close to. Select the answer (yes or no) to the following questions. Record your results.

1. This person encourages me to try new things.
   a. yes
   b. no

2. This person is supportive of the things I do.
   a. yes
   b. no

3. We have similar common interests and values.
   a. yes
   b. no

4. It is easy to share my feelings (e.g., happy, sad, frustrated) with this person.
   a. yes
   b. no

5. This person respects me and our relationship.
   a. yes
   b. no

6. This person is not liked very well by the other important people in my life.
   a. yes
   b. no

7. This person gets jealous when I talk with or hang out with other people.
   a. yes
   b. no

8. This person thinks I'm too involved in different activities.
   a. yes
   b. no

9. This person puts me down or criticizes me.
   a. yes
   b. no

10. This person pressures me to do things I don't want to do.
    a. yes
    b. no

Answering "yes" to the first five questions and "no" to the last five is an indicator of a healthy relationship. If you answered "no" to one of the first five questions, what are some actions you could take to improve your relationship? If you answered "yes" to one of the last five questions, what are some actions you could take to improve your relationship?

Lesson 21.2

Building and Supporting Healthy Relationships

Lesson Objectives

After participating in this lesson, you should be able to

1. describe the three main qualities that most people value in their friendships,
2. explain how peer pressure can be both positive and negative,
3. describe the four roles that people may play in a bullying situation, and
4. list at least four healthy dating expectations that you have for yourself.

Lesson Vocabulary

assertive behaviour, bullying, casual friendship, close friendship, cyberbullying, date rape, dating violence, harassment, manipulation, online dating, peer pressure, platonic friendship, refusal skills, sexual coercion

Humans are social beings; we have an innate desire to belong, feel accepted, and be wanted. In fact, your ability to relate with others often determines how happy and successful you will be throughout your life. More specifically, your ability to give and receive love and support is related to your attainment of a healthy and productive life. Relationships can bring much sorrow—and much joy—to your life. Entering into any relationship demands that we take risks. These risks frequently put us outside of our comfort zone, but without them our growth and development would be stunted. In this lesson, you'll learn about different types of relationships and some of the characteristics that define them.

What Is a Relationship?

Relationships are connections between people. They can be strong and last a lifetime (e.g., a parent–child relationship) or short and superficial (e.g., a relationship with a short-term employer). Relationships can involve romance or be based on friendship. A friendship is likely to be based on shared interests and values. Friends play an important role in helping us grow and mature.

Different people look for different qualities in friends. Some of the most valued qualities are trustworthiness (honesty, ability to maintain confidentiality), empathy, and tolerance. Trustworthiness is valued and expected because we want our friends to be fair, sincere, and straightforward. We want to know that we can confide in our friends and not worry that they will disclose information (know that they will keep a confidence). Empathy is the ability to understand how another person feels; without this trait, it would be difficult for friends to understand one another. Tolerance allows friends to remain friends through adversity. Friends do not always get along, but good friends find a way to work through the rough patches.

Longstanding mature relationships provide an opportunity for mutual caring, openness, disclosure, commitment, trust, and tenderness. As people mature, they have more opportunity and capacity for relationships on many levels.

Safe and Healthy Peer Relationships

As you mature, your peer relationships will take on different aspects. Many young people maintain friendships initiated during their school years, while others focus on new relationships as they enter college or the work force. Friendships also vary in commitment and level of significance, and they are dynamic and may continue to evolve over time. Many people enjoy friends that include both males and females, and interacting with a range of peers can enrich your life and encourage your growth and development beyond young adulthood.

Three basic types of friendship are casual, platonic, and close. **Casual friendship** occurs between individuals who share some commonalities (e.g., classmates or coworkers); it is not characterized by the formation of a deep bond. **Platonic friendship** is characterized by affection but no romantic attraction or involvement. **Close friendship** is punctuated by emotional ties and the sharing of intimate personal information. When problems arise, it is generally these close friends that we turn to for support and guidance.

Regardless of the type, positive friendships are built on shared morals and values and common interests. They are characterized by trust, dependability, predictability, and accountability. Maintaining such a friendship requires work and loyalty. Loyal friends are respectful of each other. They encourage and support each other in both easy and difficult times.

Peer pressure can affect one's decisions and actions including relationships with friends. On the positive side, peer pressure can encourage us to try new things and make positive decisions. Our peers can also serve as role models for us to emulate, thus helping us grow. Negative peer pressure, on the other hand, encourages us to make poor decisions and behave badly and thus ultimately leads to negative consequences. People of all ages

can be influenced by negative peer pressure, which is often exerted through **manipulation**—indirect pressure to get you to do something inappropriate or harassing. **Harassment** often includes name calling, teasing, or **bullying**.

Resisting Negative Peer Pressure

One way to address negative peer pressure is to try to avoid it. For example, we know that teens with friends who have destructive health habits (e.g., smoking, use of drugs) are more likely to adopt these habits than people with friends who do not have destructive habits. Finding friends with similar values reduces the chances for negative peer pressure. Whenever possible, try to develop and maintain friendships with people that you know share your values and interests. Be true to yourself and your beliefs by asserting your goals and values; this may reduce your risk of potentially harmful consequences. Nobody is perfect! If you do find yourself in a situation in which you have been affected by negative peer pressure, recognize it and make a positive change.

Being assertive and practicing refusal skills can be very helpful in standing up for yourself if needed. **Assertive behaviour** involves making a firm verbal statement that lets another person know how you

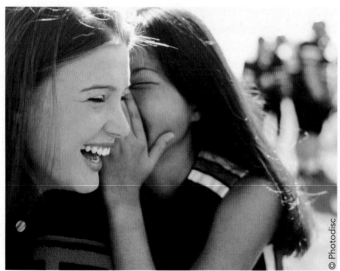
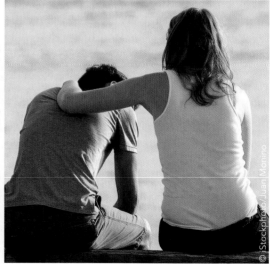

Close friendships are punctuated by emotional ties and the sharing of intimate personal information, allowing friends to turn to each other for support and guidance.

feel. **Refusal skills** are techniques for saying no and sticking with it. The following three steps help you to be assertive and use refusal skills.

- **State your position.** Demonstrate that you mean no. You can do this both verbally and through nonverbal cues. For example, you might say no and state a reason, or you might say no and raise your hand to signify clearly that you are not interested.

- **Suggest an alternative activity.** If you are being pressured to take part in an activity you are not comfortable with, suggest an alternative. You might also provide reasons for doing so.

- **Stick with your position.** Stay positive and firm while you make clear that you are not interested in the suggested activity or behaviour. Use strong words and body language and look your friend in the eye. If this does not work, remove yourself immediately from the situation. In the best-case scenario, your friends will honour your requests. Occasionally, you may have friends who are aggressive and who continue to apply pressure and make you uncomfortable. If your personality tends toward being passive, you may find it difficult to refuse your friends. Assertive behaviour takes practice. With practice, you get better at it, and it will serve you well throughout your life.

Bullying

Bullying involves an imbalance of power between a bully and his or her victim. It is the act of doing or saying something to intimidate or dominate another person. It might involve making threats, spreading rumours, physically or verbally attacking someone, or purposefully excluding someone from a group. Bullying takes three main forms: (1) verbal, in which someone says or writes mean things; (2) social, which involves hurting someone's reputation or relationships; and (3) physical, which includes hurting a person's body or damaging his or her possessions. Furthermore, bullying behaviour includes the use of any physical, verbal, electronic, written, or other means. For those engaged in bullying, there may be legal repercussions. Bullying

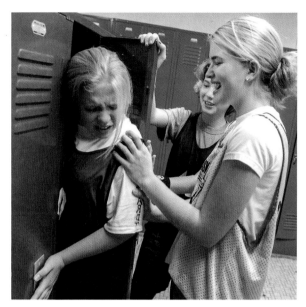

Bullying can take three main forms: verbal, social, or physical.

behaviours fit into Canadian Criminal Codes such as Criminal Harassment, Uttering Threats, Assault, and Sexual Assault, with youth risking adult sentencing depending on the circumstances.

Bullying may involve only the bully and the person being bullied, or other people. Other people can play a variety of roles in bullying, including assistant, reinforcer, bystander, and defender. An individual who assists the bully (assistant) does so by encouraging him or her and perhaps even joining in the act of bullying. A person who reinforces the bully's behaviour (reinforcer) does so by being part of the audience; this person doesn't participate in the bullying itself but does encourage the bully to continue. An outsider neither encourages the bully's behaviour nor defends the individual being bullied. In contrast, a defender helps the person being bullied by comforting him or her and perhaps by coming to his or her defence during the bullying incident itself.

Stopping bullying can be a difficult task, since much of it is subtle and often isn't reported even though an astounding 90 percent of bullying incidents happen in front of people. Youth are left to suffer in silence. However, there are ways to stop bullying. For instance, 60 percent of the time, bullying stops in less than 10 seconds when someone steps in. Aside from actually witnessing an incident of bullying, how can you know when there is a

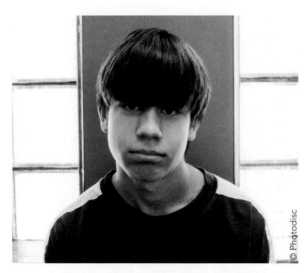

A person who is bullied may not want to go to school—just one of several signs of bullying.

problem? Here are some signs that a person may be getting bullied: unexplainable injuries; lost or destroyed clothing, electronics, or other personal items; changes in eating habits, such as coming home from school hungry (because a bully took one's lunch or lunch money); increased headaches and stomach aches, difficulty with sleeping; decline in grades or desire to go to school; participation in fewer school activities than usual; mental health problems such as self-destructive behaviours (e.g., cutting); and depression and anxiety. These effects do not always end when the bullying does and can last until later in life. There are also signs that a person may be acting as a bully. These include getting into physical or verbal fights; having friends who are bullies; being more aggressive than normal; being sent to the principal's office for being verbally or physically aggressive; having unexplained money or belongings; and blaming others for one's actions. According to the Canadian Institute of Health Research, the following are some statistics about bullying.

- At least one in three adolescent students in Canada has reported being bullied.
- Any participation in bullying increases risk of suicidal ideas in youth.
- The rate of discrimination experienced among students who identify as lesbian, gay, bisexual, trans-identifying, two-spirited, queer, or questioning is three times higher than among heterosexual youth.

- Revenge for bullying is one of the strongest motivations for school shootings in North America.

If you are being bullied, try the following tips.

- If you feel safe, talk to the bullying student and tell the person in a strong, calm voice to leave you alone.
- Walk away from the bully.
- Tell an adult right away about the incident. While this may seem like tattling, it is not (tattling is telling on someone with the purpose of getting the person in trouble when no physical, emotional, or social harm has occurred). Adults can't help unless they know what it is that is happening.
- If possible, try to avoid the bully and make sure you have a friend with you. Many bullies are less likely to bully multiple people.

Cyberbullying

Cyberbullying involves electronic technology, such as cell phones, computers, tablets, and social media sites. It can happen 24/7, since messages and images can be posted anonymously and distributed quickly to a large audience at any time. In addition, once a message or image is posted, it can be difficult or impossible to fully remove.

The signs of cyberbullying are much the same as those for bullying in general. The main difference involves the consistency and amount of bullying that can be done via technology. It isn't done just on the school playground, in the lunchroom, or between classes. Rather, it can happen all day and all night long, and many more people can see the bullying when it is posted to a social media website or distributed electronically. Because it is ongoing, cyberbullying can lead to anxiety, depression, and even suicide. Students must also realize that what they post online can have lasting consequences when they apply for college or a job. Recruiters search for people to see their posts as well as what is posted about them. Cyberbullies and their parents may also face legal charges, as laws are already in place and continue to be formed in several Canadian provinces and territories as part of their Education Act. For more information on bullying, visit the Fitness for Life Canada website.

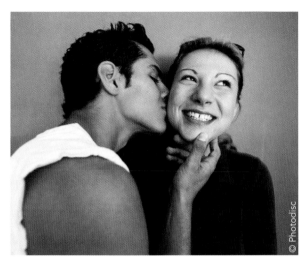

Dating relationships are similar to a friendship-based relationship except for the level of intimacy that is shared.

Dating Relationships

Dating can be described as an extension of a friendship. Dating allows students an opportunity to strengthen self-esteem; being liked by a friend encourages people to gain confidence in how they feel about themselves. Dating also helps to improve social skills and assists students in understanding personal needs.

The dynamics of dating relationships are similar to those of a friendship-based relationship, except for the level of intimacy that is shared. In fact, a dating relationship often begins as a friendship, then develops into a relationship that includes another level of intimacy when two people share a physical attraction. Dating relationships are nonmarital relationships between two people that may or may not include a sexual relationship.

As a dating relationship becomes more serious, trust becomes more and more important. Trust is established over time and is earned as a result of proven commitment. When this kind of trust is experienced by two individuals who are capable of an emotionally mature and physically satisfying relationship, it can be one of the most gratifying experiences in life. When you enter into any type of relationship, your personal values will be questioned, affirmed, and challenged. You must consider your own values when making decisions about relationships. If you decide to behave in ways that conflict with your values, you will cause

yourself distress and feelings of guilt, shame, and loss of self-respect.

Setting Limits

Dating can be an enjoyable experience; it can give you opportunities to develop your social skills and learn more about yourself. Some people, for example, discover new interests and ways of expressing themselves through dating.

FIT FACT

Staying fit and healthy can become more challenging when one is in a relationship. Often there are more trips to the movies, meals out, and time spent socializing that does not involve movement. Plan some dates that involve physical activity as a way to stay healthier physically, mentally, and socially.

Dating can also put you at risk for unwanted peer pressure—for example, pressure to participate in sexual activity. It is important to remember that abstinence in sexual activity is the only method guaranteed to prevent getting pregnant and getting sexually transmitted infections. Abstinence is also the only prevention method that works 100 percent of the time. Before you go on a date, you should determine who else will be present, what time you and your date need to be home, and how you will get from one place to another. Plan for your safety and self-control; first and foremost, avoid places where you will be alone with a date or in an isolated place.

Parents and other caregivers often set limits on where you can go, who you can go with, and how late you can stay out. In most cases, however, it is ultimately up to you and your date to make the final decisions because your parents or caregivers aren't around. As a responsible individual, you will set your own limits about where you will go and what you will do on dates. Communicating these limits to your date before going out helps you avoid risky and sometimes embarrassing situations.

Healthy dating begins with your own expectations. Expect to be treated with consideration and respect. Expect that your partner will respect your values. Expect that you have the courage—and remember that you have the right—to say no to

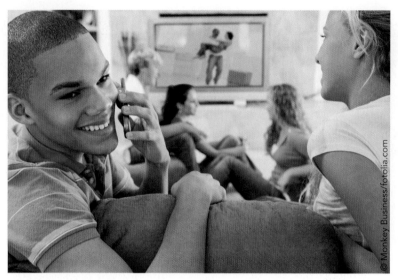

Avoiding being alone with a date is just one limit you could set when dating.

any activity or behaviour for which you are not ready. Remember: No one has the right to force unwanted advances on you. These expectations may seem obvious, but dating can sometimes obscure the obvious.

Satisfying and secure relationships take skill and effort and often share certain identifiable traits. Key traits include trust, predictability, and faith. In fact, trust is punctuated by a sense of predictability, meaning that you can predict your partner's behaviour based on the fact that you have witnessed consistent positive behaviour from him or her in the past. When your partner demonstrates consistent dependability, you know that you can rely on him or her, particularly when you need support the most. Having faith in your partner allows you to feel that you are certain about his or her intentions and principles. These characteristics—trust, predictability, and faith—are crucial to a satisfying relationship, and can be used as a measuring stick for deciding whether a given relationship is a healthy one.

Teens should also consider dating a variety of people as they begin to date. Too often, teens think that they will be with the first person they date for the rest of their life, which is usually not the case. Dating is one part of the high school experience, whether it is for a one-time trip to the movies or a school dance or lasts for an extended period of time. It should not be an all-consuming experience. The person you date should be supportive of you and the activities you are involved with; should

encourage you to be the best person you can be; and should hold values and goals similar to yours. Too many teens "fall in love" only to find that the person they are dating does not share their values and goals for their future. Teens need to understand that while breaking up is difficult to do, many of the dating and friendship relationships they have in high school will change, and the qualities they are drawn to in a partner may also change dramatically as they continue to mature.

Breaking Up

When ending a relationship, break up with the person face to face rather than through texting, social media, or e-mail. While breaking up in person may be more difficult to do, it is also more respectful and less hurtful. It may feel easier to hide behind a phone or computer, but it is also much easier to be hurtful through media than it is in person.

In addition, break up with the person sooner rather than later. You cannot change the other person, and thinking that you can will lead only to arguments and hurt feelings. Breaking up is not the time to pick a fight or blame each other; in fact, it is often just time to move on. Finally, before breaking up, make sure of what both you and the other person need—is it time to talk with each other, or is it time for a clean break to get away from each other?

Also, if someone breaks up with you, it is important to respect his or her decision. While it may be

FITNESS TECHNOLOGY: Dating and Social Media

Social media such as Facebook and teen dating sites are becoming an increasingly popular way to meet people with similar and common interests and values. While traditional dating is the best option for many, **online dating** is an opportunity to meet someone with similar physical activity, health, and fitness interests and values. As always, you need to be very careful about any information you consider providing, and you should talk with a parent, guardian, or other trusted adult before using an online dating site. Online dating can be very risky. Here are some tips to help keep you safe.

- **Protect your personal information.** Never give out your real name, address, or phone number online to a person you don't know. Also do not give out other personal information, such as where you go to school or the names of teams or organizations of which you are a part. Choose an online dating name that cannot be linked to your real name.

- **Read all information available.** Start out slowly by reading all of the profile information about other members along with carefully evaluating the information. Then trust your instincts about what you find. Remember that not everything put on the Internet is the truth. People will exaggerate about themselves as well as lie about who they really are.

- **Protect your privacy.** Create a new e-mail account that you use only for online dating. Make sure that you sign your e-mail only with your dating name.

- **Don't be afraid to stop.** If a conversation ever becomes uncomfortable, terminate it and contact the dating site's administrators about it.

- **Share photos with care.** Use extreme caution if you are asked to share a photo with someone you don't know. If you decide to share a photo, choose one that has no background images that can potentially identify where it was taken. Also, take care that other people are not in the photo. The bottom line is that you have to be okay with the photo you send being shared on all social media, because once you send it, others can resend or post it. Always ask to see a current photo of that person as well, and be aware that he or she may send a fake photo.

- **Use alternate forms of communication.** If you are going to talk on the phone with someone you met online, protect yourself. Do not give out your phone number. Consider using a communication app (e.g., Skype) as a way to avoid using your phone number.

- **Meet in public.** If you get to the point in your relationship where you want to meet face to face, never allow the person to pick you up at home, school, or work. Schedule a meeting during the day in a public place where there are a lot of people around who could help you if needed; in addition, consider bringing a friend with you to the date. Make sure to tell a friend or family member about your date and give this person your phone number, information about the meeting time and place, and a picture of the person you are meeting.

As with any relationship, you need to get to know the person you're talking with before telling too much about yourself. Be cautious about online dating. You never know who may really be at the other end of the computer connection.

Using Technology

Use social media to find out more about people before you go on a date. What is important to them will show up on social media. What pictures have they posted? What do they do for fun?

497

painful, moving on and giving the person the space requested is part of being a mature and responsible person.

Valuing Your Social Health

Dating relationships during the teen years can support healthy growth and development and lead to life-changing experiences. People who enter into such relationships with strong values and morals often fondly remember their first dating relationships. If you can resist the hormone-influenced urges and social pressures that tend to lead people toward high-risk behaviours—including sexual activity and drug and alcohol use—your dating relationships are likely to generate positive feelings of self-respect and self-esteem.

On the other hand, overcoming a bad reputation (whether it is based on real or assumed behaviours) is a difficult task. Teens are often judged not only by their peers but also by their teachers and other adults in the community. Family relationships can also become strained and difficult when parents learn that their children have stepped past the limits set to protect them. When faced with the question of whether or not to become sexually active or participate in other risky behaviours, think critically, evaluate the risks, and ask yourself, "How will this activity affect me and my relationships with people later today, tonight, tomorrow?" or "If I do this, how might it affect my goals for my future?" It is important to remember that remaining abstinent when dating is the only way to ensure that there won't be unintended consequences such as pregnancy and sexually transmitted infections. Your teacher may provide you with more information on this topic. Other resources such as chapter 20 of this text and websites such as Planned Parenthood also provide trustworthy information.

Dating Violence

Dating violence occurs in the form of various kinds of physical, emotional or psychological, and sexual abuse within a dating relationship, and unfortunately it occurs more often than was once assumed. In fact, adolescents and young adults sometimes misinterpret abusive behaviour by a dating partner as a sign of caring. In reality, a dating partner

should never disrespect, dominate, or exert force or excessive control over you. Here are some sobering Canadian statistics about dating violence:

- Dating violence is the highest among the 15 to 24 age group, making up 43 percent of all incidents of dating violence.
- Thirty-one percent of sexual assaults occur in dating and acquaintance relationships.
- One in three youth reports knowing a friend or peer who has been physically abused by a partner.
- Sixty-two percent of youth (age 11-14) who have been in a relationship say they know friends who have been verbally abused.
- Young women between the ages of 15 and 19 experience 10 times more violence in relationships than young men.
- One in five male students surveyed said that forced intercourse was all right "if he spen[t] money on her," "if he [was] stoned or drunk," or "if they had been dating for a long time."
- The results of a 2011 study showed that 61 percent of male participants did not consider forcing sex on an acquaintance to be rape. Rape is any kind of penetration of another person regardless of gender without the victim's consent. **Date rape** is the same as rape except it is committed by a person known to the victim in a dating situation.
- Half of males and females who experience rape or physical or sexual abuse attempt to commit suicide.
- At least half of all violent crimes occur after the offender, the victim, or both have been drinking alcohol.

Basic signs that a relationship may be headed for trouble include manipulation, put-downs, excessive control over the dating partner's behaviour, control over the partner's outside friendships, jealousy and possessiveness, scaring or threatening the partner, and general lack of respect. A healthy relationship should never involve **sexual coercion** (i.e., unwanted sexual penetration that occurs after a person is pressured in a nonphysical way) or sexual violence (i.e., any sexual act that is committed against someone's will). If you find yourself in a situation characterized by one or more of these factors, seek help from parents, teachers, school counsellors, or organizations such as Kids Help Phone. Like all forms of violence, dating violence traumatizes victims and leaves emotional scars. It can also result in unintentional pregnancy and sexually transmitted infections such as HIV.

Myths About Dating Violence

The Public Health Agency of Canada provides a table of myths about dating violence (table 21.1). See what myths you may have believed and the truth behind the myth.

TABLE 21.1 Myths About Dating Violence

Myth	Reality
It will never happen to me.	Dating violence can happen to you. It is not limited to a particular social class, to any ethnic or racial group, or to heterosexual relationships. It is also not simply dependent on you and your values. It also depends on the values of your dating partner.
I can tell if a person is a "hitter" just by looking at them.	Perpetrators of violence come in all shapes and sizes. They do not fit media stereotypes. You can't tell by looking at people.
Things will get better.	Once violence begins in a dating relationship, it usually gets worse unless there is some kind of intervention. Abusers need to learn new strategies for dealing with conflict, and they need to learn new attitudes about violence and relationships.
There is only a problem when my partner is under stress, is drunk or high, or when there is a conflict in our relationship. Otherwise things are fine.	While violence may be more common in these situations, they are not the cause of violence. These things are used as excuses and justifications.
Jealousy is a sign of love.	Jealousy is a common excuse given for using dating violence. Jealousy does not justify the use of violence against a dating partner. In addition, jealousy can be a warning sign of intimate terrorism in which the perpetrator is controlling and will escalate violence to achieve control.
Victims of dating violence provoke the abuse.	Blaming the victim is unacceptable. Even when a person is provocative, using violence in response is not acceptable. It never solves problems, although it often silences the victim.
Sexual abuse in dating relationships happens because we cannot control our sexual urges. If a dating partner sexually arouses the other, they deserve what they get.	We are capable of controlling our sexual urges. That's why forcing sex on another person can be the basis for criminal charges. Dating partners who have agreed to petting or necking still have the right to control their own body. When dating partners say NO or NO MORE, indicating that they want sexual contact to stop, the other person is required by law to stop.
Name calling doesn't hurt.	Name calling hurts; that's why people do it. Psychological or emotional abuse can damage self-confidence. It can be more devastating than other forms of intimate violence.
It's okay for my partner to use violence—that's what my friends say.	If your friends are supporting a partner who is being abusive—excusing or justifying the behaviour—you need to go elsewhere for help. School counsellors can provide support by listening, offering advice, and providing information on support groups and help lines.

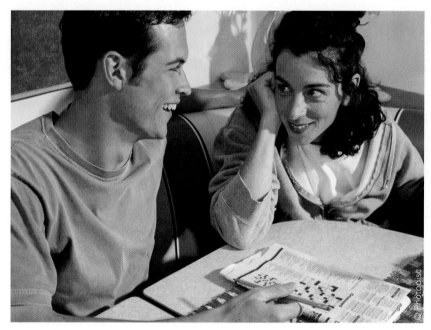

It is possible to have a healthy relationship even if you've been abused.

Overcoming Abuse

For those who have suffered abuse or dating violence, it is important to remember that they have not done anything to justify being treated in an abusive way. All forms of abuse are illegal and should be reported to the authorities. Reporting such an incident can be instrumental in preventing further abuse. The Canadian Child Welfare Research Portal site provides easy access to provincial and territorial contacts in order to facilitate the reporting of abuse. In addition, help for victims of abuse is offered by health care facilities, educational institutions, and places of worship. The Public Health Agency of Canada provides a comprehensive list of where to go for help. Victims should seek out this assistance in order to protect themselves and others from future abuse and to receive emotional and spiritual support.

 You don't develop courage by being happy in your relationships every day. You develop it by surviving difficult times and challenging adversity. **"**

—Epicurus, ancient Greek philosopher

Lesson Review

1. Identify the three main qualities that most people tend to value in their friendships. How can you strengthen these qualities in yourself?
2. Explain how peer pressure can be both positive and negative.
3. Describe the four roles (other than that of the bully) that people may play in a bullying situation.
4. List at least four healthy dating expectations that you have for yourself.

TAKING CHARGE: Dating Coercion and Violence

Skyler has been dating Taylor for three months. They spend a lot of time together and have a lot of fun together. Although they like many of the same things, they have also been trying out things that only one of them has done before and likes. Once Taylor suggested rock climbing and they both had a great time. Another time Skyler invited Taylor to the local museum the one night a month when it was free. There was so much art to see that they agreed to come back another time to see more. Lately however, Skyler has been noticing that even when Taylor agrees to do something Skyler likes, when the time comes, Taylor has an excuse as to why they cannot do that and instead they end up doing something Taylor wants to do. When Skyler spends

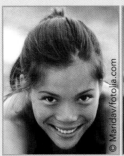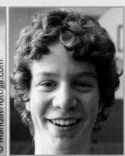

© Maridav/fotolia.com

time with friends, Taylor is constantly texting, making time with the friends less enjoyable. Skyler is beginning to become frustrated by these behaviours but doesn't know where to turn.

For Discussion

If Skyler came to you for advice, what advice would you give? Who would you recommend Skyler talk to—family, teachers, school counsellor, somebody else? If Skyler isn't comfortable talking face to face to anyone, are there organizations that could help Skyler in this situation? What other advice might you give Skyler and why? Consider the skills for reducing your risk of experiencing dating violence presented in the self-management section.

SELF-MANAGEMENT: Skills for Reducing Your Risk of Experiencing Dating Coercion and Violence

Clearly, it is critical to take measures that reduce your risk of experiencing dating coercion and violence. Make sure that your dates take place in well-lit public areas. Encourage your date to invite others. Date as part of a group until you know him or her better. Avoid using alcohol and other drugs on dates, and immediately remove yourself from any situation involving alcohol or drugs—they increase your risk for violence and trouble. Always tell a parent or guardian who you are with and where you intend to go on your date. Bring a cell phone and some extra money in case you need to get home on your own. Here are some tips for reducing your risk of experiencing dating coercion and violence.

- **Acknowledge that dating coercion and violence exist.** Acknowledging that you are supporting or initiating these behaviours is the first step. Seeking help to change these behaviours, or support

for getting out of a relationship where these behaviours exist, is essential. School counsellors, doctors, or other health professionals can support you in developing the skills to eliminate dating coercion and violence from your life.

- **Paying attention to behaviours.** Noticing what people are like when they are disappointed or frustrated can signal potentially dangerous behaviours. If aggression and disrespect and blaming others are how someone responds when things do not go his or her way, you may want to reconsider your relationship with this person. Do not feel guilty if someone has been violent toward you and tries to coerce you by acting sad. You do not owe anything to someone who endangers you. Once you notice such behaviours, ending the relationship is the mature and wise decision.

- **Practice saying no.** Practice refusal skills and using an assertive voice and stance before going on dates. Assertively practice saying "NO" and "I do not want to go out with you." Be prepared to pull away and loudly but calmly say "That is NOT okay. I am leaving now," or "Take me home NOW, my parents (or somebody else) know where I am."

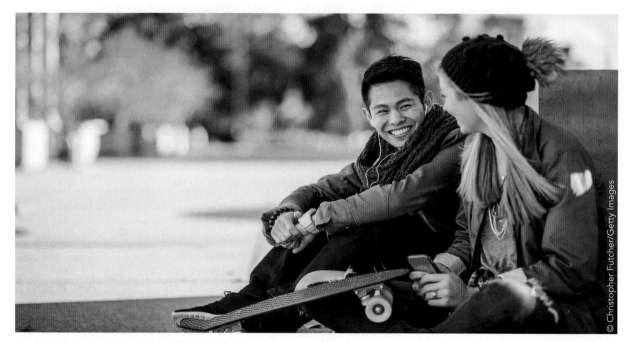

© Christopher Futcher/Getty Images

Healthy dating relationships should never involve coercion or violence.

TAKING ACTION: **Taking Dating Violence Seriously**

If a friend comes to you about dating violence, support and understanding are needed. Demonstrate that you are a trustworthy, empathetic, and tolerant friend. Take the person seriously; acknowledge that the violence is a problem. Do not downplay the violence or blame the victim, as this often leads to an increased risk that the violence will continue. Take action by labelling the behaviour as abusive and wrong and supporting your friend in recognizing that the behaviour is unacceptable. Making this connection often leads victims of abuse to seek the help they need to protect themselves. Provide your friend with contact information for organizations that work to provide support for

youth or find trustworthy organizations in your community by doing online searches.

When people you care about tell you about dating violence, remind them that there are friends, family, and significant adults who respectfully love and care for them and that it is these people they need to trust with their secret. Supporting friends in these ways and ensuring that they understand that this is not their fault—and it is not what they somehow deserve—will serve as a reminder of how a respectfully caring person treats others, and a reminder that they are deserving of this kind of love, caring, and compassion.

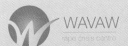 **GET ACTIVE WITH WAVAW RAPE CRISIS CENTRE**

© WAVAW Rape Crisis Centre, Vancouver, BC, Canada.

Who We Are

Women Against Violence Against Women (WAVAW) Rape Crisis Centre was founded in Vancouver, British Columbia, in 1982. We are a not-for-profit charitable organization working in the interests of women who have been victimized by sexual assault.

What We Do

WAVAW Rape Crisis Centre works to end all forms of violence against women. Guided by our feminist anti-oppression philosophy, we challenge and change thinking, actions, and systems that contribute to violence against women. We provide all women who have experienced any form of sexualized violence with support and healing, and engage with youth to develop leadership for prevention of future violence.

Get Involved

WAVAW is a feminist organization committed to doing anti-violence work; we are an inclusive and pro-choice agency. We encourage self-identified women of ALL ages, abilities, colours, sizes, and backgrounds to join us. No matter how you choose to get involved, you

will gain a greater insight into how violence impacts the community and what we can do to end it. You can:

- Visit our website at www.wavaw.ca.
- Join the conversation on Facebook and Twitter.
- Join the WAVAW team and run, walk, roll, dance, or move with us at the Scotiabank half marathon/5K Walk.
- Propose a guest blog post. Pick a topic that bugs, interests, or inspires you about feminism, social justice, or violence against women, and we can work with you to share your thoughts on our site.
- Hold an awareness event at your school or in your community. We can send a speaker or resources.
- Visit our events calendar and join us at a march, rally, or parade. Or let us know about other great events.
- Ask your school to include our Raise It Up youth social justice program in your classes, or invite us for presentations and workshops.
- Organize a fundraiser for WAVAW.

© WAVAW Rape Crisis Centre, Vancouver, BC, Canada.

Reviewing Concepts and Vocabulary

Complete the following in order to determine your growing understanding of fitness, health, and wellness. Answer items 1 through 5 by correctly completing each sentence with a word or phrase.

1. A _____ family—consisting of a mother, a father, and at least one child—is a traditional depiction of "family," but many other family formations are typical today.

2. _____ refers to the biological factors (male or female) that influence your fitness, health, and wellness.

3. _____ behaviour involves making a firm verbal statement that lets another person know how you feel.

4. _____ is a characteristic valued by most people that involves the ability to understand how another person feels.

5. Techniques used to help an individual say no and stick with it are referred to as _____ skills.

For items 6 through 10, match each term in column 1 with the appropriate phrase in column 2.

6. manipulation
7. separation
8. gender
9. online dating
10. platonic friendship

a. relationship, often with a member of the opposite sex, in which there is no romantic involvement
b. social and cultural roles of people
c. searching for a romantic partner on the Internet
d. indirect pressure to get you to do something inappropriate
e. test period for couples that is not legally recognized

For items 11 through 15, respond to each statement or question.

11. List and briefly explain the four stages of development that all families tend to cycle through.
12. What is the primary difference between bullying and cyberbullying?
13. List the factors that predict marriage success.
14. Why do you think the divorce rate is higher among people who get married at a younger age?
15. Explain the three steps for using refusal skills.

Thinking Critically

Write a paragraph in response to the following question.

Have you ever really thought about the characteristics that you value in a partner? List four characteristics that you value the most and write about why they are so important to you.

Project

Talk to a parent, guardian, or other trusted adult about online dating. Make a list of the pros and cons of online dating as compared with traditional dating. Discuss any differences in rules or parameters (e.g., appropriate age to start dating) between the two types.

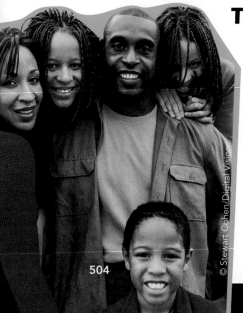

© Stewart Cohen/Digital Vision

Glossary

This glossary contains definitions of all the boldfaced terms throughout the book. You can also find all the vocabulary terms grouped by lesson in the student web resource.

1-repetition maximum (1RM)—Test of muscle strength in which you determine how much weight you can lift (or how much resistance you can overcome) in one repetition.

absolute strength—Strength measured by how much weight or resistance you can overcome regardless of your body size.

abstinence—Voluntarily choosing not to do something or not to be sexually active.

accelerometer—Device that measures movement; frequently used to measure steps, intensity of movement, and duration of physical activity.

acronym—Specific kind of mnemonic in which the first letters of each word in a phrase are combined to form an easy-to-remember word (for example, SMART—specific, measurable, attainable, realistic, and timely).

active stretch—Stretch caused by contraction of your own antagonist muscles.

activity neurosis—Condition in which a person feels overly concerned about getting enough exercise and upset if he or she misses a regular workout.

acute alcohol poisoning—Potentially fatal overdose of alcohol or a medical emergency resulting from binge drinking.

addiction—Physical dependency on a chemical substance such as alcohol, nicotine, or heroin.

Adequate Intake (AI)—Dietary reference intake (DRI) used when there is insufficient evidence to establish a Recommended Dietary Allowance (RDA).

aerobic—Often referring to moderate to vigorous physical activity that can be sustained for a long time because the body can supply adequate oxygen to continue the activity; means "with oxygen."

aerobic activity—Activity that is steady enough to allow your heart to supply all the oxygen your muscles need.

aerobic capacity—The ability of the cardiorespiratory system to provide and use oxygen during very hard exertion over a specific amount of time. The maximal oxygen uptake test measures aerobic capacity.

age of consent—Legal age at which a young person can consent to being sexually active with a person of legal age. The age of consent in Canada is 16 years old.

agility—Ability to change your body position quickly and control your body's movements.

AIDS—Acquired immune deficiency syndrome; AIDS is caused by the human immunodeficiency virus, which can weaken the immune system and exposes the body to other types of infections.

air quality index—Scale used to rate pollution levels ranging from good air quality to very unhealthful.

alarm reaction—First stage of the general adaptation syndrome; occurs when your body reacts to a stressor.

alcoholism—Disease in which a person is dependent on alcohol.

alcohol tolerance—When the body becomes less responsive to alcohol because of continued alcohol use over a long period of time.

amino acid—Building block of protein.

anabolic steroid—Synthetic drug that resembles the male hormone testosterone but that has health risks. It produces lean body mass, weight gain, and bone maturation.

anaerobic activity—Activity so intense that your body cannot supply adequate oxygen to sustain it for a long time.

anaerobic capacity—The ability of the body to perform all-out exercise using the body's high-energy fuel sources (ATP-PC and glycolytic systems); commonly measured using the Wingate Test.

androstenedione—Substance considered to be a steroid precursor because it is converted into anabolic steroids such as testosterone (male hormone) after it enters the body; also called "andro."

anorexia athletica—Eating disorder with symptoms similar to those of anorexia nervosa; most common among athletes involved in sports in which low body weight is desirable (such as gymnastics and wrestling).

anorexia nervosa—Eating disorder in which a person severely restricts the amount of food eaten in an attempt to be exceptionally low in body fat.

antagonist—Muscle or muscle group having the opposite function of another muscle or muscle group.

artery—Vessel that carries blood from your heart to another part of your body.

assertive behaviour—Behaviour that involves making a firm verbal statement letting another person know how you feel.

atherosclerosis—Clogging of the arteries.

autonomy—Self-direction; the ability to make decisions for yourself.

balance—Ability to maintain an upright posture while standing still or moving.

ballistic stretching—Series of gentle bouncing or bobbing motions that are not held for a long time.

basal metabolism—Amount of energy your body uses just to keep you living.

bikeability—A measure of how a community's or neighbourhood's physical spaces support bicycling.

binge drinking—Consumption of five or more drinks by men and four or more drinks by women in a two-hour time span.

bisexual—Relating to a person who is attracted to both men and women.

blended family—Family formed when a parent remarries.

blood alcohol content (BAC)—Percentage of alcohol in the bloodstream. A BAC of 0.08 percent is the legal level of intoxication in Canada. The legal BAC limit is even lower in British Columbia, Manitoba, Newfoundland and Labrador, Nova Scotia, and Ontario (0.05 percent) and Saskatchewan (0.04 percent).

blood pressure—Force of blood against your artery walls.

body composition—The proportional amounts of body tissues, including muscle, bone, body fat, and other tissues that make up your body.

body dysmorphia—A mental disorder that causes people to have a distorted image of their body to the point where it interferes with their life.

body fat level—Percentage of body weight that is made up of fat.

bodybuilding—A competitive sport in which participants are judged primarily on the appearance of their muscles rather than how much they can lift.

built environment—The physical characteristics of a community that either support or are barriers to healthy behaviours.

bulimia—Eating disorder in which a person binges, or eats very large amounts of food within a short time, followed by purging.

bullying—The act of repeatedly doing or saying something to intimidate or dominate another person.

calisthenics—Exercises done using all or part of the body weight as resistance.

calorie—Unit of energy or heat that refers to the amount of energy in a food (the true term is *kilocalorie*).

calorie expenditure—Calories (energy) used in physical activity.

calorie intake—Calories (energy) ingested.

calorimeter—Apparatus used to determine the amount of heat generated by a chemical reaction; also can determine the number of calories in food.

carbohydrate—Type of nutrient that provides you with your main source of energy.

cardiorespiratory endurance—Ability to exercise your entire body for a long time without stopping.

cardiovascular disease (CVD)—A physical illness that affects the heart, blood vessels, or blood. Examples include heart attack and stroke. It's the second leading cause of death in Canada.

cardiovascular system—Body system that includes your heart, blood vessels, and blood; provides oxygen and nutrients to the body.

casual friendship—A friendship between individuals who share some commonalities (e.g., classmates or coworkers) that is not characterized by the formation of a deep bond.

celibacy—Refraining from sexual activity.

cholesterol—Waxy, fatlike substance found in meat, dairy products, and egg yolk; a high amount in the blood is implicated in various types of heart disease.

chronic obstructive pulmonary disease (COPD)—A group of lung diseases that includes emphysema, bronchitis, asthma, and chronic airway obstruction.

circuit training—Performance of different exercises one after another, separated only by brief breaks, with the goal of keeping your heart rate in your target zone and building various components of health-related fitness.

close friendship—A friendship with emotional ties and the sharing of intimate personal information. Close friends provide support and guidance.

colleague—A person you work with at your job, on committees, or in clubs.

compendium—List of physical activities that tells you the intensity of various activities.

competitive stress—The body's reaction to participation in a sport or other activity in which people or teams attempt to outperform an opponent; a stress condition that may be eustressful.

complete protein—Protein containing all nine essential amino acids; derived from animal sources, such as meat, milk products, and fish.

con artist—Person who practices fraud.

concentric—Referring to a shortening isotonic muscle contraction.

conception—Union of an ovum and a sperm.

consumer community—A school group or club that reviews scientific information and answers student questions related to fitness, health, and wellness.

contraception—Any means of preventing pregnancy, such as abstinence, condoms, and birth control pills.

controllable risk factor—Risk factor that you can act upon to change.

coordination—Ability to use your senses together with your body parts or to use two or more body parts together.

coping—Dealing with or attempting to overcome a problem.

coping skill—Technique that you can use to manage stress or deal with a problem.

coronary artery disease (CAD)—Specific kind of cardiovascular disease in which the arteries in the heart become clogged.

CRAC—Contract-relax-antagonist-contract; a type of PNF stretch that requires the muscle or muscles to contract and then relax before being stretched by the contraction of the opposing muscle or muscles.

creatine—Natural substance manufactured in the body by meat-eating animals including humans and needed in order for the body to perform anaerobic exercise, including many types of progressive resistance exercise.

creeping obesity—Slow, gradual weight gain typically caused by consuming empty calories.

criterion-referenced health standards—Fitness ratings used to determine how much fitness is needed to prevent health problems and to achieve wellness.

culture—A set of rules governing behaviour in a society. It is influenced by morals, values, and religious beliefs.

cyberbullying—Bullying that takes place through electronic technology, such as cell phones, computers, tablets, and social media sites.

date rape—Forced sex that occurs between two people in a dating situation.

dating violence—Various kinds of physical, emotional, and sexual abuse that take place in a dating relationship.

depressant—A prescription drug used to treat anxiety disorders.

depression—Mood disorder characterized by extreme sadness and hopelessness that interferes with daily functioning.

determinant—Factor affecting your fitness, health, and wellness.

diabetes—Disease in which a person's body is unable to regulate sugar levels, leading to an excessively high blood sugar level.

diastolic blood pressure—Pressure in your arteries just before the next beat of your heart.

Dietary Reference Intake (DRI)—Amount of a given micronutrient that you should consume daily.

dietician—Expert in nutrition who helps people apply principles of nutrition in daily life; has a college degree and certification by a reputable national organization.

distress—Negative stress stemming from situations that cause worry, sorrow, anger, or pain.

divorce—Legal termination of marriage.

double progressive system—The most-used method of applying the principle of progression for improving muscle fitness, first by increasing repetitions (reps) and second by increasing resistance or weight.

DriveCam—A camera typically installed in a teenager's car to monitor for erratic driving and send notifications to a parent's or guardian's computer.

driving under the influence (DUI)—Operating a vehicle with a blood alcohol content above the legal limit or while under the influence of drugs.

drug addiction—Compulsive use of a substance despite negative or dangerous effects.

drug dependence—State in which a person needs a drug in order to function.

drug tolerance—Condition in which a person who is a regular and excessive user of an addictive drug needs more of the drug to get the same effect as he or she did before with a smaller amount.

dynamic movement exercise—Exercise such as jumping, skipping, and calisthenics that are often used in a warm-up for activities requiring strength, power, and speed. They move the joints beyond normal resting ROM and cause the muscles and tendons to stretch. The stretch caused by dynamic movement exercise is followed by a contraction of the stretched muscle.

dynamic stretching—Slow-movement exercises designed to lengthen the muscles.

dynamic warm-up—A type of warm-up that uses whole-body movements like jogging, skipping, hopping, and sport-related movements that mimic movements used in competition.

dynamometer—Device that measures the amount of force produced by a muscle or group of muscles.

eating disorder—Condition that involves dangerous eating habits and often excessive activity to expend calories for fat loss.

eccentric—Referring to a lengthening isotonic muscle contraction.

electrolyte—A mineral in your blood and body fluids that is important for normal body functioning and prevention of water loss during exercise.

empathy—The ability to understand the thoughts, feelings, or emotions of another person.

empty calories—Calories that provide energy but contain few if any other nutrients.

empty nest—In child-rearing families, situation in which the last child leaves home and parents find themselves at home alone.

energy balance—Balance between calorie intake and calorie expenditure.

ergogenic aid—Anything used to help you generate work or to increase your ability to do work, including vigorous exercise.

ergolytic—Referring to substances that negatively affect performance (*ergo* meaning work and *lytic* meaning destructive).

essential body fat—The minimum amount of body fat that a person needs to maintain health.

eustress—Positive stress.

exercise—Form of physical activity specifically designed to improve your fitness.

extended family—Family that extends beyond the nuclear family, including grandparents, aunts and uncles, and others.

extrinsic motivation—Reason for doing something that comes from an outside source (for example, prizes, approval, or acceptance).

family role—The role that a person plays in a family, including, for example, financial duties, household chores, and child rearing. Roles vary from family to family.

fast-twitch muscle fibre—Fibre that contracts quickly, is white because it receives less blood flow delivering oxygen, and generates more force than slow-twitch muscle fibre when it contracts (thus, muscles with many fast-twitch fibres are important for strength activities).

fat—Nutrient that provides energy, helps growth and repair of cells, and dissolves and carries certain vitamins to cells.

female sterilization—Permanent contraceptive method that blocks the egg's pathway to the uterus; performed by cutting, cauterizing, or blocking the fallopian tubes.

fibre—Type of complex carbohydrate that your body cannot digest.

fibrin—Substance involved in blood clotting.

fitness target zone—Optimal range of physical activity for promoting fitness and achieving health and wellness.

FITT formula—Prescription or recipe (based on the ingredients frequency, intensity, time, and type) for appropriate physical activity.

flexibility—Ability to use your joints fully through a wide range of motion without injury.

food environment—A measure of the availability of healthy foods in a neighbourhood and how easily residents can access those foods.

food label—Nutritional information that appears on food packaging.

force—In physical activity, energy exerted by the muscles to cause movement or resist movement; other uses include military force (ships and troops), violent force (a physical attack), or resistance force (stopping a moving body or object).

fraud—Intentional use of deception to get you to buy products or services known to be ineffective or harmful.

frequency—How often a task is performed; in the FITT formula, refers to how often physical activity is performed.

functional fitness—Capacity to function effectively when performing normal daily tasks.

gay—Referring to a person who is sexually or romantically attracted to people of the same sex. Gay women may prefer to use the word "lesbian."

gender—The social and cultural roles of people (masculine or feminine).

general adaptation syndrome—Body's reaction to stress in three phases: alarm reaction, stage of resistance, and stage of exhaustion.

goal setting—Process of establishing objectives to accomplish; the objectives for lifetime fitness are to achieve good fitness, health, and wellness and to adopt a healthy lifestyle.

graded exercise test—Test used to detect potential heart problems by having you exercise on a treadmill while your heart is monitored by an electrocardiogram.

group cohesiveness—Sticking together in working toward a common goal.

habituate—To get used to something because of repeated exposure to it.

harassment—Behaviour that includes name calling, teasing, or bullying.

health—Freedom from disease and a state of optimal physical, emotional–mental, social, intellectual, and spiritual well-being (wellness).

health education—A school subject, sometimes combined with physical education, focused on learning experiences designed to help individuals and communities improve their health.

health literacy—The ability to access, comprehend, evaluate, and communicate information as a way to promote, maintain, and improve health in a variety of settings across the life course.

health-related physical fitness—Parts of physical fitness that help a person stay healthy; includes cardiorespiratory endurance, flexibility, muscular endurance, strength, power, and body composition.

heart attack—Condition in which the blood supply within the heart is severely reduced or cut off, which can cause an area of the heart muscle to die.

heart rate reserve (HRR)—Difference between the number of times that your heart beats per minute at rest and during maximal exercise.

heat index—Scale that rates the safety of the environment for exercise based on temperature and humidity.

heavy drinking—Consuming two or more drinks per day for men and one or more per day for women over a long period ranging from months to years.

high-density lipoprotein (HDL)—Lipoprotein often referred to as "good cholesterol" because it carries excess cholesterol out of your bloodstream and into your liver for elimination from your body.

HIV—Human immunodeficiency virus, which causes AIDS; can be transmitted via blood, semen, vaginal fluids, or breast milk.

human growth hormone (HGH)—Illegal drug that is exceptionally dangerous, especially for teens; causes premature closure of bones and can have deforming and even life-threatening effects.

humidity—Relative amount of moisture in the air.

hyperkinetic condition—Health problem caused by doing too much physical activity.

hypermobility—Unusually large range of motion in the joints; sometimes referred to as double-jointedness.

hypertension—Condition in which blood pressure is consistently higher than normal.

hyperthermia—Exceptionally high body temperature often associated with exposure to hot or humid environments.

hypertrophy—Increase in muscle fibre size.

hypokinetic condition—Health problem caused partly by lack of physical activity.

hypokinetic disease—Health problem caused by doing too little physical activity.

hypothermia—Abnormally low body temperature often associated with exposure to cold and windy environments.

ignition interlock—Device installed in a motor vehicle that is designed to keep people from driving if they have been drinking. The driver has to blow into a monitor that determines if he or she has been drinking. If so, the vehicle will not start.

illicit drug—Drug that is illegal to use, such as heroin or alcohol; illegal for people under age 21.

incomplete protein—Protein that contains some, but not all, essential amino acids.

intensity—Magnitude or vigorousness of a task; in the FITT formula, refers to how hard you perform a physical activity.

intermediate muscle fibre—Fibre with characteristics of both slow- and fast-twitch fibres.

interpersonal—Between people or between individuals.

interval training—Type of training that uses bouts of high-intensity exercise followed by rest periods.

intrinsic motivation—Reason for doing something that comes from within (for example, enjoyment, desire to be more fit).

isokinetic exercise—Type of isotonic exercise in which movement velocity is kept constant through the full range of motion.

isometric contraction—Contraction in which muscles exert force but do not cause movement at a joint.

isometric exercise—Exercise involving isometric contractions, in which body parts do not move.

isotonic contraction—Muscle contraction that pulls on bone and produces movement of a body part.

isotonic exercise—Exercise involving isotonic contractions, in which body parts move.

kyphosis—Posture problem characterized by rounded back and shoulders.

laws of motion—Rules of physics that help us understand human movements.

leadership—Ability to motivate and help people in a group work toward a common goal.

lean body tissue—All tissue in the body other than fat.

leisure time—Time free from work and other commitments; also called discretionary time.

lesbian—Woman who is sexually or romantically attracted to women.

lifestyle—The way you live.

lifestyle physical activity—Activity done as part of daily life (such as walking to school or doing yard work).

lifetime sport—Sport in which you're likely to participate throughout your life.

lipoprotein—Protein that carries lipids and cholesterol through your bloodstream.

long-term goal—Goal that takes months or even years to accomplish.

lordosis—Posture problem characterized by too much arch in the lower back; also called swayback.

low-density lipoprotein (LDL)—Type of lipoprotein often referred to as "bad cholesterol" because it carries cholesterol that is most likely to stay in your body and contribute to atherosclerosis.

macronutrient—Nutrient that supplies the energy your body needs to perform daily tasks; the three types are carbohydrate, protein, and fat.

manipulation—Indirect pressure used to control someone else's behaviour.

marriage—In Canada, marriage is the lawful union of two persons to the exclusion of all others.

maturation—Process of becoming fully grown and developed.

maximal heart rate—Number of times your heart beats per minute during very vigorous activity; the highest your heart rate can go.

maximal oxygen uptake—Lab measure considered to be the best for assessing fitness of the cardiovascular and respiratory systems; see also *aerobic capacity*.

menstrual cycle—Monthly series of changes involving ovulation, the uterine lining, and menstruation.

metabolic equivalent (MET)—Measure that refers to metabolism (the use of energy to sustain life), with 1 MET representing the energy you expend while resting; multiples are used to describe the intensity of all types of physical activity.

metabolic syndrome—Condition in which a person has high body fat, large girth, and other health risks such as high blood pressure, high blood fat, and high blood sugar.

micronutrient—Nutrient (vitamin or mineral) that your body needs in smaller amounts than it needs carbohydrate, protein, and fat.

mnemonic—A term that is useful in remembering specific information, such as an acronym (for example, SMART).

moderate-intensity physical activity—Activity that requires energy expenditure four to seven times greater than that required by being sedentary (that is, 4 to 7 METs).

motor skill—The learned ability to use the muscles and nerves together to perform a physical task (for example, throwing, running).

muscle bound—Having tight, bulky muscles that inhibit free movement.

muscle dysmorphia—Disorder typically seen in males; involves an intense desire to become more muscular accompanied by excessive exercise, extreme dietary practices, or steroid abuse.

muscle–tendon unit (MTU)—Skeletal muscles and the tendons that attach them to bones.

muscular endurance—Ability to use your muscles many times for an extended period of time without tiring.

natural health product (NHP)—Vitamins and minerals, herbal remedies, homeopathic medicines, traditional medicines (such as traditional Chinese medicines), probiotics, and products like amino acids and essential fatty acids that are safe to use as over-the-counter products and don't need a prescription to be purchased.

nuclear family—A father and mother with children, sometimes referred to as a traditional family.

obesity—Condition of being especially overweight or high in body fat.

online dating—The process of searching for a romantic partner on the Internet. It is also called Internet dating.

opioids—Medications used to relieve pain.

optimal challenge—Activity that is neither too hard nor too easy; activity that isn't too distressful compared to a competitive situation.

osteoporosis—Condition in which bone structure deteriorates and bones become weak.

overexercising—Doing so much exercise that you increase your risk of injury or soreness.

over-the-counter (OTC) drug—Drug that can be bought without a doctor's prescription.

overweight—Condition of having a weight higher than the healthy range.

passive exercise—Use of a machine or device that moves your body for you. Programs using passive exercise are ineffective.

passive stretch—Stretch requiring an assist from an external source (gravity, a partner, or some other source).

peak bone mass—Highest bone density achieved during life; typically occurs in late adolescence or early adulthood.

pedometer—Small battery-powered device that can be worn on your belt to count your steps.

peer pressure—The pressure an individual can feel from peers. It can be positive, with peers serving as role models encouraging us to try new things and be better in some way, or it can be negative, with peers encouraging us to make poor decisions and behave badly, thus ultimately leading to negative consequences.

periodization—Way of scheduling muscle fitness exercise in which you perform a given plan for a while, then alter it to perform different exercises at different frequencies or intensities and for different amounts of time.

personal lifestyle plan—Written schedule of activities designed to improve fitness, health, and wellness.

personal needs profile—Chart listing self-assessment scores and corresponding ratings.

personal program—Written individualized plan designed to change behaviour (the way you live) to improve fitness, health, and wellness.

physical activity—Movement using the large muscles; includes sport, dance, recreational activity, and activities of daily living.

Physical Activity Pyramid—Diagram or model that describes the various types of physical activity that produce good fitness, health, and wellness.

Physical Activity Readiness Questionnaire (PAR-Q)—Seven-question assessment of medical and physical readiness that should be taken before beginning a regular physical activity program for health and wellness.

physical education—A school subject focused on movement experiences designed in part to develop physical literacy among students.

physical fitness—Capacity of your body systems to work together efficiently to allow you to be healthy and effectively perform activities of daily living.

physical literacy—The ability to move with competence and confidence in a wide variety of physical activities, in multiple environments, that benefit the healthy development of the whole person.

Pilates—Form of training, quite popular in recent years, designed to build core muscle fitness; named for Joseph Pilates, who described core exercises and developed special exercise machines for building core muscles.

placenta—An organ that anchors the embryo to the uterus.

platonic friendship—A relationship, often with a member of the opposite sex, in which there is no romantic involvement.

plyometrics—Type of training designed to increase athletic performance using jumping, hopping, and other exercises to cause lengthening of a muscle followed by a shortening contraction.

PNF stretching—Flexibility exercise using proprioceptive neuromuscular facilitation; a variation of static stretching that involves contracting a muscle before stretching it.

pornography—Sexually explicit materials (printed or visual) intended to stimulate erotic feelings.

power—Capacity to use strength quickly; involves both strength and speed.

powerlifting—Competitive sport using free weights and involving only three exercises: bench press, squat, and deadlift.

prescription drug—Drug prescribed by a doctor to help treat illnesses or symptoms, such as pain and discomfort.

principle of overload—The most basic law of physical activity, which states that the only way to produce fitness and health benefits through physical activity is to require your body to do more than it normally does.

principle of progression—Principle stating that the amount and intensity of your exercise should be increased gradually.

principle of rest and recovery—Principle stating that you need to give your muscles time to rest and recover after a workout.

principle of specificity—Principle stating that the type of exercise you perform determines the type of benefit you receive.

priority healthy lifestyle choice—One of the key lifestyle choices (regular physical activity, sound nutrition, and stress management) that help you prevent disease, get and stay fit, and enjoy a good quality of life.

process goal—Goal relating to what you do rather than the product resulting from what you do.

product goal—Goal relating to what you achieve as a result of what you do.

professional—Highly educated person who delivers information and helps people apply it to improve their lives.

progressive resistance exercise (PRE)—Exercise that increases resistance (overload) until you have the amount of muscle fitness you want; also called progressive resistance training (PRT).

protein—Group of nutrients used for building, repairing, and maintaining your body cells.

ptosis—Posture problem characterized by a protruding abdomen.

public health scientist—Expert who studies disease prevention and wellness promotion in communities.

quack—Person who practices quackery.

quackery—Method of advertising or selling that uses false claims to lure people into buying products that are worthless or even harmful.

questioning—Referring to individuals who are unsure of their sexual orientation or gender identity.

range of motion (ROM)—The amount of movement in a specific joint that is considered to be healthy (neither too much nor too little).

range-of-motion (ROM) exercise—Exercise that requires a joint to move through a full range of motion by using either your own muscles or the assistance of a partner or therapist.

reaction time—Amount of time it takes to move once you have recognized the need to act.

Recommended Dietary Allowance (RDA)—Minimum amount of a nutrient necessary to meet the health needs of most people.

recreation—Something you do during your free time.

refusal skills—Techniques for saying no and sticking with it.

relative strength—Strength adjusted for your body size.

reps—Short for *repetitions* (the number of consecutive times you do an exercise).

respiratory system—Body system made up of your lungs and the passages that bring air, including oxygen, from outside of your body into your lungs.

resting metabolism—Number of calories expended by your body for basic functions and typical light activities done during the day.

rhabdomyolysis—Condition in which muscle fibres break down and the bloodstream absorbs muscle fibre elements.

risk factor—Any action or condition that increases your chances of developing a disease or health condition.

role model—A person who imparts values and information to others.

runner's high—The eustress people feel when they run or do exercise that they enjoy.

saturated fat—Fat that is solid at room temperature and is derived mostly from animal products, such as lard, butter, milk, and meat.

secondhand smoke—Tobacco smoke that is inhaled involuntarily or passively by someone who is not smoking. Also referred to as sidestream smoke or environmental tobacco smoke.

sedentary—Not engaging in regular physical activity from any of the steps of the Physical Activity Pyramid.

self-management skill—Skill that helps you adopt a healthy lifestyle now and throughout your life.

self-reward system—System for gradually building skills and finding success and, ultimately, intrinsic motivation; involves rewarding yourself rather than expecting others to reward you for your efforts.

semen—Fluid that is discharged during ejaculation. The fluid contains sperm and other fluids to help maintain the sperm.

separation—A test period for married couples to separate that is not legally recognized.

set—One group of repetitions.

sex—Biological classification; the state of being male or female.

sexting—Sending of sexual messages or photos via cell phone.

sexual assault—Act of knowingly engaging another person in an unwanted sexual act by either force or threat (also known as sexual abuse).

sexual coercion—The use of force, manipulation, or intimidation to get someone to participate in unwanted sexual activity.

sexuality—State of being sexual; includes feelings, thoughts, identity, sensuality, intimacy, and reproduction. Also includes being attracted to and attractive to others, being in relationships, and being in love.

sexually transmitted infection (STI)—Also known as sexually transmitted disease (STD); an infection that is transmitted from one person to another during sexual contact. An STI can be caused by bacteria, viruses, parasites, or other microorganisms.

sexual orientation—People's sexual identity in relation to the gender of the people to whom they are attracted.

short-term goal—Goal that can be reached in a short time, such as a few days or weeks.

skill—Ability to perform a specific task effectively that results from knowledge and practice.

skill-related physical fitness—Parts of fitness that help a person perform well in sports and activities requiring certain skills; the parts include agility, balance, coordination, reaction time, and speed.

skinfold—Fold of fat and skin used to estimate total body fat level.

sleep apnoea—Disorder that results in poor sleep or inability to sleep, characterized by pauses in breathing or shallow breathing during sleep.

slow-twitch muscle fibre—Muscle fibre that contracts at a slow rate, is usually red because it has a lot of blood vessels delivering oxygen, and generates less force than fast-twitch muscle fibre but is able to resist fatigue.

SMART goal—Goal that is specific, measurable, attainable, realistic, and timely.

smokeless tobacco—Tobacco that is not smoked, such as chewing tobacco and snuff.

social–ecological model—A model that illustrates the interactions between living organisms and their environments.

social justice—Justice in terms of the distribution of wealth, opportunities, and privileges within a society.

social support—Support you get from family, friends, and members of your community that helps you succeed in life.

spa—Facility offering saunas, whirlpool baths, and other services such as massage and hair or skin care.

speed—Ability to perform a movement or cover a distance in a short time.

sport—Physical activity that is competitive (has winners and losers) and has well-established rules.

stage of exhaustion—Third stage of the general adaptation syndrome; occurs when the body is not able to resist a stressor well enough.

stage of resistance—Second stage of the general adaptation syndrome; occurs when the immune system starts to resist or fight the stressor.

state of being—Overall condition of a person.

static stretch—Stretch performed slowly as far as you can without pain, until you feel a sense of pulling or tension.

stimulant—A prescription drug most often used to treat attention-deficit/hyperactivity disorder [ADHD].

strength—Maximal amount of force your muscles can produce.

stress—Body's reaction to a demanding situation.

stressor—Something that causes or contributes to stress.

stroke—Condition in which the supply of oxygen to the brain is severely reduced or cut off.

sudden infant death syndrome (SIDS)—Sudden and unexpected death of an apparently healthy infant.

systolic blood pressure—Pressure in your arteries immediately after your heart beats.

tai chi—Ancient form of exercise that originated in China and whose basic movements have been shown to increase flexibility and reduce symptoms of arthritis in some people.

target ceiling—Your upper recommended limit of activity for optimally promoting fitness and achieving health and wellness.

team—A group of people working toward a common goal.

team building—A collective term used in many contexts, such as educational, business, and physical activity settings, in which teams must work cooperatively and collaboratively, within defined roles, to solve problems.

teamwork—Cooperative effort of all team members to strive for a common goal in the most effective way.

threshold of training—Minimum amount of overload you need in order to build physical fitness.

time—Length of a task; in the FITT formula (first "T"), it refers to the optimal length of an activity session designed to improve fitness and promote health and wellness.

Tolerable Upper Intake Level (UL)—Maximum amount of a vitamin or mineral that can be consumed without posing a health risk.

traditional family—A father and mother with children, sometimes referred to as a nuclear family.

trans-fatty acid—Product made from unsaturated fat that can be found in vegetable oil, for example, by means of a process that renders it solid at room temperature (such as solid margarine); also known as trans fat. It has been banned from food by the U.S. Food and Drug Administration.

transgender—Relating to the identity in which a person's gender is different from his or her biological sex (e.g., a person who has the sex organs of one sex but identifies with the other sex).

type—The specific kind of task; in the FITT formula (second "T"), it refers to the specific kind of physical activity that is performed.

uncontrollable risk factor—Risk factor that you cannot do anything to change.

underweight—Condition of having a weight less than the healthy range.

unsaturated fat—Fat that is liquid at room temperature; derived mostly from plants, such as sunflower, corn, soybean, olive, almond, and peanut.

vein—Vessel that carries blood filled with waste products from your muscle cells back to your heart.

vigorous aerobics—Aerobic activities intense enough to elevate your heart rate above your threshold of training and into your target zone for cardiorespiratory endurance.

vigorous recreation—Activity done during your free time that is fun and typically noncompetitive but intense enough to elevate your heart rate above your threshold of training and into your target zone for cardiorespiratory endurance.

vigorous sport—Sport activity that elevates your heart rate above your threshold of training and into your target zone for cardiorespiratory endurance.

walkability—A measure of how a community's or neighbourhood's physical spaces support walking.

web extension—Ending of a web address, such as .gov, .org, and .com.

weightlifting—Olympic sport involving free weights in which athletes try to lift a maximum load; includes two lifts, the snatch and the clean and jerk.

wellness—Positive component of health that involves having a good quality of life and a good sense of well-being as exhibited by a positive outlook.

windchill factor—Index used to determine when dangerously low temperatures and unsafe wind conditions exist.

win–win—A situation in which both parties involved benefit (i.e., you benefit and another person benefits).

withdrawal—Physical sickness that people with a physical dependence (addiction) develop when they cannot take the drug to which they are addicted.

yoga—Activity that originated in India and that in its traditional forms includes meditation, as well as the exercises and breathing techniques common to modern forms; involves poses called *asanas* that are similar to many flexibility exercises and can offer improved flexibility and other health benefits.

Index

Note: The italicized *f* and *t* following page numbers refer to figures and tables, respectively.